Treatment of Primary Glomerulonephritis

Treatment of Primary Glomerulonephritis

THIRD EDITION

Edited by

Claudio Ponticelli

Past Director of the Division of Nephrology
Istituto Scientifico Ospedale Maggiore Policlinico
Milan, Italy
and

Richard J. Glassock

Emeritus Professor
The David Geffen School of Medicine at the University of California
Los Angeles, California, USA

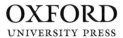
OXFORD
UNIVERSITY PRESS

OXFORD

UNIVERSITY PRESS

Great Clarendon Street, Oxford, OX2 6DP,
United Kingdom

Oxford University Press is a department of the University of Oxford.
It furthers the University's objective of excellence in research, scholarship,
and education by publishing worldwide. Oxford is a registered trade mark of
Oxford University Press in the UK and in certain other countries

© Oxford University Press 2019

The moral rights of the authors have been asserted

First Edition published in 1997
Second Edition published in 2009
Third Edition published in 2019

Impression: 2

Published in the United States of America by Oxford University Press
198 Madison Avenue, New York, NY 10016, United States of America

British Library Cataloguing in Publication Data

Data available

Library of Congress Cataloguing in Publication Data

Data available

ISBN 978–0–19–878408–1

Printed and bound by
CPI Group (UK) Ltd, Croydon, CR0 4YY

To my patients, my beloved wife Titti, and my children Alberto, Gisella, and Giorgio
—Claudio Ponticelli

To my wife Jo-Anne and my children, Ellen, Scott, Sharon and Mark and their children and grandchildren, for being a constant source of inspiration and joy.
—Richard J Glassock

Preface

In the last few years, many important advances have been made in the area of primary glomerulonephritis (PG): a new classification has been proposed for some diseases, such as focal glomerular sclerosis and membranoproliferative glomerulonephritis; the genome-wide associations have clarified the role of genetic abnormalities in IgA nephropathy, membranous nephropathy, thin basement nephropathy, etc.; the critical role of different podocyte proteins in regulating the glomerular filtration has been identified; the pathogenesis of membranous nephropathy, C3 nephropathy, and IgA nephropathy has been better elucidated; and a number of new therapeutic approaches have been proposed. In summary, since 2009 when the second edition of this book was delivered, a number of discoveries have changed the scenario of primary glomerular diseases.

When Oxford University Press asked us to prepare a third edition of *Treatment of Primary Glomerulonephritis*, both of us accepted the proposal with enthusiasm. With the help of old and new distinguished nephrologists, we personally reviewed and updated all the chapters. Although the book has been completely rewritten, we maintained the structure already used in the two previous editions. However, we have added a chapter to report the recent data on epidemiology and new classification of glomerulonephritis. We paid particular attention to the chapters focused respectively on symptomatic measures and on drugs currently used in immune-mediated glomerulonephritis. Each of the other chapters covers a single glomerulonephritis, with the exception of the last chapter, which deals with the less-common forms of primary glomerular diseases. For any disease, we report the definition, the pathology, the pathogenesis, the natural course, the prognostic factors, and the different treatments used. We then specify our suggestions and recommendations for handling the different aspects of glomerulonephritis, and we have added a subchapter reporting the results of kidney transplantation, including the risk of recurrence and the risk of *de novo* glomerulonephritis.

Although diabetic nephropathy and arterial hypertension are the most common causes of chronic kidney disease in Western countries, glomerulonephritis still represents the main prototype of renal disease. Assessing its clinical course and treatment remains a major issue for the clinician. The main goal of this book is to provide a synthetic but complete information guide on how a nephrologist may face the many problems presented by a patient with a PG, and when and how a treatment should be prescribed.

We thank our colleagues, who generously accepted to help us in the preparation of the book. We are confident that not only students and young specialists, but also some expert nephrologists may find the book of some utility in their daily practice.

Claudio Ponticelli
Richard J Glassock

Contents

List of abbreviations

ABAC1	ATP-binding cassette transporter A1	BSA	Bovine serum albumin
ACEi	Angiotensin-converting enzyme inhibitors	C3GN	C3 glomerulonephritis
		C3Nef	C3-nephritic factor
ACTH	Adrenocorticotropic hormone	CCBs	Calcium channel blockers
		CDC	Cell-mediated cytotoxicity
ADCC	Antibody-dependent cell-mediated cytotoxicity	CfH	Complement factor H
		CKD	Chronic kidney disease
AGEs	Advanced glycation end products	Cl	Chlorine
		CLCF-1	Cardiotrophin-like cytokine factor-1
aHUS	Atypical haemolytic-uraemia syndrome		
		CLL	Chronic lymphocytic leukaemia
AKI	Acute kidney injury		
Akt	Protein-kinase B	CMV	Cytomegalovirus
ALDH	Aldophosphamide-dehydrogenase	CNI	Calcineurin inhibitor
		COL4	Type-IV collagen
AMH	Anti-Mullerian hormone	CRP	C-reactive protein
ANCA	Anti-neutrophil cytoplasmic antibody	CsA	Cyclosporine A
		CVD	Cardiovascular disease
ANCA-SVV	ANCA-associated small vessel vasculitis	CYP3A	Cytochrome-P450 3A
		DAA	Direct-acting antiviral
ANGPTL4	Angiopoietin-like protein 4	DC	Dendritic cell
AP-1	Activator protein 1	DDD	Dense deposit disease
APC	Antigen presenting cell	DNAJB9	DNAJ Homolog Subfamily B Member 9
APIGN	Acute post-infectious glomerulonephritis		
		DNND	Diabetic nephropathy without diabetes
apoA	Apolipoprotein A		
apoB	Apolipoprotein B	DSG	15-Deoxyspergualin
apoE	Apolipoprotein E	DVT	Deep venous thrombosis
APOL1	Apoliprotein-L1	EGF	Epidermal growth factor
ARBs	Angiotensin receptor blockers	eGFR	Estimated glomerular filtration rate
ATG	Anti-thymocyte globulin		
AT-I	Angiotension I	EGPA	Eosinophilic granulomatosis with polyangiitis
AT-II	Angiotensin II		
AT-IV	Angiotensin IV	EMA	European Medicines Agency
AUC	Area under the curve	ENaC	Epithelial sodium channels
AZA	Azathioprine	ESRD	End-stage renal disease
BP	Blood pressure	FAS	Full age spectrum

FCGR	Fcγ receptor
FE IgG	Fractional excretion of IgG
FGGS	Focal and global glomerulosclerosis
FGN	Fibrillary glomerulonephritis
FKBP12	FK-binding protein 12
FLC	Free light chain
FSGS	Focal and segmental glomerulosclerosis
GAPHD	Glyceraldeide-3-phosphate-dehydrogenase
GBM	Glomerular basement membrane
GC	Glucocorticoid
GCR	Glucocorticoid receptor
GFR	Glomerular filtration rate
GI	Gastrointestinal
GN	Glomerulonephritis
GnRH	Gonadotropin releasing hormone
GPA	Granulomatosis with polyangiitis
GREs	Glucocorticoid response elements
GWAS	Genome-wide association studies
HACAs	human anti-chimeric antibodies
HBeAg	Hepatitis Be antigen
HBV	Hepatitis B virus
HDL	High-density lipoproteins
HIV	Human immunodeficiency virus
HMG-CoA	3-hydroxy-3methylglutaryl coenzyme A
HPLC	High-performance liquid chromatography
HSP	Heat shock protein
HSP	Henoch–Schönlein purpura/ IgA vasculitis
HUS	Haemolytic-uremic syndrome
ICGN	Immune complex-mediated GN
IDL	Intermediate-density lipoproteins

IF	Immunofluorescence
IgAN	Immunoglobulin A nephropathy
IgG4-RD	IgG4-related disease
IgM	Immunoglobulin M
IIF	Indirect immunofluorescence
IMPDH	Inosine monophosphate dehydrogenase
INR	International normalized ratio
IST	Immune-suppressive therapy
ITG	Immunotactoid glomerulopathy
IV	Intravenous
IVIg	Intravenous immunoglobulin
K	Potassium
KDIGO	Kidney Disease: Improving Global Outcomes
KLF	Kruppel-like factor 4
LAMP-2	Lysosomal membrane protein-2
LBW	Low birth weight
LDL	Low-density lipoproteins
LDL-A	LDL-apheresis
Lp(a)	Lipoprotein (a)
LPG	Lipoprotein glomerulopathy
LPS	Lipopolysaccharide
MAC	Membrane attack complex
MASP	MBL-associated serine protease
MBL	Mannose-binding lectin
MC	Mutation carrier
MCD	Minimal change disease
MCP-1	Macrophage chemotactic protein-1
MCR-1	Melanocortin receptor 1
MCR-2	Melanocortin receptor 2
MDR-1	Multidrug resistance gene-1
MESNA	Sodium 2-mercaptoethanesulphonate
MesPGN	Mesangial proliferative glomerulonephritis
MI	Myocardial infarction

MIF	Macrophage inflammatory factor	PAN	Puromycin aminonucleoside
miRNAs	MicroRNAs	PAP	Pulmonary alveolar proteinosis
MMF	Mycophenolate mofetil	PCP	Pneumocystis jiroveci pneumonia
MN	Membranous nephropathy		
MP	Methylprednisolone	PCR	Polymerase chain reaction
MPA	Microscopic polyangiitis	PECs	Parietal epithelial cells
MPA	Mycophenolic acid	P-gp	P-glycoprotein
MPAG	Acid glucuronide MPA	PI3-k	Phosphatydilinositol-3-kinase
MPGN	Membranoproliferative glomerulonephritis	PIGN	Post-infectious glomerulornephritis
MPO	Myeloperoxidase	PIIINP	Serum type-III procollagen peptide
MS	Mycophenolate sodium		
MSH	Melanocyte-stimulating hormone	PLA2R	Phospholipase A2 receptor
		PLA2R1	Phospholipase-A2 receptor 1
mTOR	Mammalian target of rapamycin	PLEX	Plasma exchange
		Plr	Plasmin receptor
mTORC1	mTOR complex 1/raptor complex	PML	Progressive multifocal leukoencephalopathy
mTORC2	mTOR complex 2/rictor complex	*PRTN3*	Proteinase 3 promoter gene
		PSGN	Post-streptococcal glomerulonephritis
MZB	Mizoribine		
Na	Sodium	QALYs	Quality-adjusted life years
NaCl	Sodium chloride	RAGEs	Advanced glycation end product receptors
NAPlr	Nephritis-associated plasmin receptor		
		RAS	Renin-angiotensin system
NEP	Neutral endopeptidase	RCTs	Randomized controlled trials
NF-AT	Nuclear factor of activated T cells	RTX	Rituximab
		RVT	Renal vein thrombosis
NFATc1	Nuclear factor of activated T-cells 1	SEGRAs	Selective GR agonists
		SLE	Systemic lupus erythematosus
NF-kB	Nuclear factor-kappa B	sMAC	Soluble membrane attack complex
NK	Natural killer		
NOAC	New oral anticoagulants	SMADs	Small intracellular signal transducer proteins
NOS	Not otherwise specified		
NS	Nephrotic syndrome	SNP	Single nucleotide polymorphisms
NSAIDs	Non-steroidal anti-inflammatory drugs		
		SPEB	Streptococcal pyrogenic exotoxin B
NSAP	Nephritis strain-associated protein	SPNSG	Southwest Pediatric Nephrology Study Group
O3FA	Omega-3 polyunsaturated fatty acids		
		STAT3	Signal transducer and activator of transcription 3 gene
PAI-1	Plasminogen activation inhibitor-1		

suPAR	Soluble urokinase-type plasminogen activator receptor
TAC	Tacrolimus
TBMN	Thin basement membrane nephropathy
TDM	Therapeutic drug monitoring
TES	Targeted exome sequencing
TG	Triglyceride
TGFβ	Transforming growth factor beta
TGFβ1	Transforming growth factor beta 1
TGNs	Thioguanine nucleotides
THSD7A	Thrombospondin type-1 domain-containing 7A
T-I	Tubulo-interstitial
TLRs	Toll-like receptors
TMP-SMX	Trimethoprim-sulfamethoxazole/ co-trimoxazole
TNF	Tumour necrosis factor

tPA	Tissue plasminogen activator
TPMT	Thiopurine methyltransferase
uACR	Albumin to creatinine ratio in urine
UGT	Uridine diphosphonate glucuronyl transferase
uPA	Urokinase type plasminogen activator
uPCR	Protein to creatinine ratio in urine
USFDA	US Food and Drug Administration
USRDS	US Renal Data System
VDBP	Vitamin D binding protein
VEGF	Vascular endothelial growth factor
VLDL	Very low-density lipoproteins
WBCs	White blood cells
WT1	Wilms tumour protein
YAP	Yes-associated protein
ZS9	Sodium zirconium cyclosilicate

Contributors

Giovanni Banfi
Formerly Nephrologist of
Department of Nephrology and
Urology, Istituto Scientifico,
Ospedale Maggiore di Milano,
Milan, Italy

Arthur H. Cohen
Formerly Professor of
Pathology, UCLA School
of Medicine, Los Angeles,
California, USA

Rosanna Coppo
Past Director of Nephrology
Dialysis and Transplantation
Unit, Regina Margherita
Children Hospital,
Turin, Italy

Fernando C. Fervenza
Director of the Nephrology
Collaborative Group, Mayo Clinic,
Rochester, Minnesota, USA

Richard J Glassock
Emeritus Professor, The David
Geffen School of Medicine at the
University of California, Los Angeles,
California, USA

Lee Hebert
Nephrologist, Wexner Medical
Centre, Ohio State University,
Ohio, USA

Kar Neng Lai
Emeritus Professor and Honorary
Clinical Professor, Department of
Medicine, University of Hong Kong,
Hong Kong

Gabriella Moroni
Nephrologist, Nephrology and
Dialysis Unit, Fondazione Ca'
Granda IRCCS Ospdale Maggiore
Policlinico, Milan, Italy

Patrick H. Nachman
Professor of Medicine, Division of
Renal Diseases and Hypertension,
University of Minnesota,
Minnesota, USA

Patrizia Passerini
Nephrologist, Nephrology and
Dialysis Unit, Fondazione Ca'
Granda IRCCS Ospdale Maggiore
Policlinico, Milan, Italy

Claudio Ponticelli
Past Director of the Division of
Nephrology, Istituto Scientifico
Ospedale Maggiore Policlinico,
Milan, Italy

Francesco Scolari
Associate Professor, Division of
Nephrology, Università di Brescia
and Ospedale di Montichiari,
Brescia, Italy

Chapter 1

A definition, modern classification, and global epidemiology of primary glomerulonephritis

Claudio Ponticelli and Richard J Glassock

Definition

The term *glomerulonephritis* (GN) nominally indicates an inflammation of glomeruli. Not all the glomerular diseases necessarily show an inflammatory component at histologic examination. Accordingly, some investigators feel correct to limit the term GN only to those glomerular diseases that show signs of inflammation (Sethi et al., 2016). On the other hand, primary GN diseases are caused by disorders of the adaptive immunity triggered by the activation of the innate immunity with consequent production of an inflammatory micro-environment. This may legitimate using the term GN to indicate all the diseases that mainly affect the glomeruli of both kidneys. Although the terms GN and glomerulopathy are interchangeable, GN is frequently used more from a traditional and historical perspective, rather than for accuracy.

Classification of glomerular diseases

Many different criteria exist for classifying the glomerular diseases, including those within the broad term of GN. Many classifications have been based on clinical features at presentation. At the beginning of the twentieth century, Friedrich Müller (1906) proposed the term *nephrosis* to define those kidney diseases characterized by degenerative lesions without any sign of inflammation. In 1914, Franz Volhard and Theodor Fahr introduced a novel classification of renal diseases based on differentiation between degenerative (nephroses), inflammatory (nephritides), and arteriosclerotic (scleroses) diseases. In 1947, Henry Christian of Boston first used the adjectival form of nephrosis—nephrotic syndrome (see Glassock et al., 2015). About ten years later, Berman and Schreiner (1958) and Derow (1958) proposed that the term *nephrotic syndrome* be used to indicate a condition characterized by marked proteinuria ≥3.5 g/24-hours associated with hypoalbuminaemia, and variable degrees of hyperlipidaemia and peripheral oedema. In contrast, the term *nephritic syndrome* was first used to indicate symptoms and signs that can be associated with inflammation of glomeruli, such as macroscopic or microscopic haematuria, often also associated with variable degree of proteinuria, hypertension and renal function deterioration (Wilson et al., 1947). Thus, according to the presence of either of these two syndromes a clinical classification of glomerular diseases can be based on nephrotic syndrome or nephritic syndrome. However, both syndromes may be concomitant (nephrosis-nephritis) in some instances and in other cases the initial symptoms and signs reliably predict the nature of the underlying glomerular damage.

Another classification of GN was based on the time of appearance and duration of the disease, i.e. acute, subacute or malignant, and chronic GN (Reubi, 1955). However, this classification was also affected by many biases and often led to misunderstanding between clinicians and pathologists (Mihatsch, 1979). Most current students of GN classification agree that the glomerular diseases should be differentiated into primary (the disease is caused by factors intrinsic to the kidney, and which are often unknown or idiopathic) and secondary (the glomerular disease is associated with systemic diseases such as diabetes mellitus or amyloidosis). Accordingly, a classification of glomerular diseases should take into account the possible aetiology and the diseases should be subdivided into primary or secondary forms. A clinical classification of GN can be also based on five major clinical syndromes: acute GN, rapidly progressive GN, chronic GN, the nephrotic syndrome, and asymptomatic urinary abnormalities (Glassock et al., 1991).

In 1946, Bell proposed the term *membranous* glomerulonephritis to describe a new category of glomerular disease. A few years later, kidney biopsy was introduced into clinical practice (Iverson and Brun, 1951; Kark and Muehrcke, 1954). This technique allowed to better elucidate the spectrum of morphologic types of glomerular lesions and their severity. In 1957, David Jones fully illustrated the special features of membranous nephropathy and demonstrated that they were not shared by other renal lesions. Pathologists also demonstrated that the so-called *lipoid nephrosis* in children was associated with minimal glomerular lesions at optical microscopy and by effacement of podocyte foot processes on electron microscopy, without significant deposits of immunoglobulins or complement on immunofluorescence (Joekes et al., 1958; Folli et al., 1958; Caulfield, 1964). In 1957, Arnold Rich reported that, in a number of children, some glomerular tufts in the juxtaglomerular region may show capsular adhesion and segmental sclerosis. These features were confirmed by other investigators, who proposed to adopt the term focal segmental glomerulosclerosis to define this pathological lesion (Kark et al., 1958; Heptinstall and Joekes, 1959; White et al., 1970; Habib and Gubler, 1973; Cameron et al., 1973). Habib and Kleiknecht (1971) pointed out that the glomerular lesions may be 'minimal', indicating that the glomeruli are normal or slightly modified, 'focal', indicating that, by light microscopy, a limited number of glomeruli are affected, and the remaining are normal, or 'diffuse', indicating generalized glomerular involvement, although not uniform in the degree or type.

With the exception of nephrotic syndrome in children, which is usually subdivided into steroid-sensitive and steroid resistant forms on the basis of clinical response to glucocorticoids, the most frequently used contemporary classification of glomerular diseases is a pathological one, mainly based on the results of optical microscopy, supplemented by immunofluorescence and electron microscopy. The current classification takes into consideration primary and secondary glomerular diseases. Among primary glomerular diseases, the clinical–pathological classification considers minimal change disease (MCD), focal and segmental glomerulosclerosis (FSGS), membranous nephropathy (MN), membranoproliferative GN (MPGN), infection-related GN, immunoglobulin A nephropathy (IgAN), and pauci-immune (renal limited) necrotizing and crescentic GN (KDIGO, 2012). However, recent advances in the knowledge of mechanisms responsible of GN impose the necessity to review and modify the current pathological classification. In some subtypes of primary GN in which the cause of GN has been identified the term *idiopathic is no longer relevant as a modifier*. For example, the term focal and segmental glomerulosclerosis refers to a phenotypic expression of different disorders that may have different pathogenesis, clinical outcome, and response to therapy. Primary FSGS is now considered as a podocytopathy characterized clinically by the presence of nephrotic syndrome in a patient with an FSGS lesion on light microscopy and widespread foot process effacement on electron microscopy. Thus, FSGS is a lesion, not a specific disease. Many genetic defects localized to the podocyte can be seen in children (Ranganathan, 2016) and adults (Gast et al., 2016) with FSGS. Exome capture has identified many new monogenic causes of familial FSGS. The presence of apoliprotein-L1 (APOL1) variants, related to the increased *APOL1* gene expression (Heymann et al., 2017), in patients of African descent confers seventeenfold higher odds for FSGS and twenty-nine-fold higher odds for HIV-associated nephropathy (Kopp et al., 2011), suggesting the existence of a particular form of APOL1-related FSGS. The cases of FSGS lesions characterized by the absence of nephrotic syndrome and the presence of segmental foot process effacement by electron microscopy are generally secondary to adaptive haemodynamic changes, infection, or exposure to drugs and should be considered as secondary forms (Sethi et al., 2015). The discovery that in most patients MN is caused by circulating antibodies directed against specific epitopes of some podocyte proteins identifies the disorder as an autoimmune disease and renders the term idiopathic obsolete (Beck et al., 2009; Glassock, 2012; Tomas et al., 2014; Fresquet et al., 2015; Kao et al., 2015). Six different pathologic variants of IgAN have been identified that can help to integrate prognostic significance independent of the clinical data (Working Group of the International IgA Nephropathy Network and the Renal Pathology Society, 2009). Until recently, MPGN has been classified as type I, type II, and type III based upon electron microscopy findings. Type I is characterized by immune deposits in the mesangium and subendothelial space. Type II (also called dense deposit disease, or DDD) is characterized by dense ribbon-like deposits along the basement membranes of the glomeruli and tubules. Type III is characterized by subepithelial deposits in addition to mesangial and subendothelial deposits. However, this classification cannot differentiate between immune complex-mediated and complement-mediated MPGN, an entity characterized by overactivation of the alternative pathway of complement (Servais et al., 2007). Thus, Sethi and Fervenza (2011 and 2012) proposed a new classification based on immunofluorescence results for immunoglobulin and complement deposition. Accordingly, it is now recognized that MPGN is a histological 'pattern of injury' in the same league as FSGS, and not a specific disease. This pattern may be caused either by immune-complexes or by dysregulation of the complement alternative pathway (e.g. C3 glomerulopathy), or, rarely, by chronic relapsing endothelial injury in thrombotic microangiopathy, without deposits of complement or immunoglobulins. Immunoglobulin-dominant MPGN, which is associated with autoimmune diseases, chronic infections, or monoclonal gammopathies with or without cryoglobulins, is now considered as a secondary GN. Instead, the cases in which the sole or dominant immunoreactant in the renal tissue is C3 are classified as primary GN and are defined as C3 glomerulopathy. The morphological phenotypic aspects of C3 glomerulopathy may be either those of DDD, characterized by dense osmiophilic deposits, or those of C3 glomerulonephritis, which shows isolated deposits and a histologic aspect of type I MPGN (Sethi and Fervenza, 2012; Pickering et al., 2013; Cook and Pickering, 2015). Many cases of crescentic GN have been discovered to be ANCA-positive vasculitis with predominant involvement of the kidney (Berden et al., 2010; Quintana et al., 2014). Finally, a number of less frequent primary GN are usually neglected in the different classifications used.

On the basis of the current knowledge, an aetiopathogenetic classification has been proposed by Mayo Clinic/Renal Pathology Society (Sethi et al., 2016). Five classes have been recognized:

1. Immune-complex GN

2. Pauci-immune GN

3. Anti-glomerular basement membrane GN

4. Monoclonal immunoglobulin GN

5. C3 Glomerulopathy

This classification is etymologically correct since it considers only GN characterized by increased glomerular hypercellularity caused by proliferation of indigenous cells and/or leukocyte infiltration. However, it does not include a number of proliferative GN, e.g. pure mesangial proliferative GN, IgM GN, C4 GN, and nonproliferative glomerular diseases, e.g. MCD, FSGS, MN, that may be considered as podocytopathies, but that are usually classified as GN (KDIGO, 2012). On the other hand, most glomerular diseases, including the so-called podocytopathies, are considered to be immune-related diseases (Couser and Johnson, 2014). It is now accepted by immunologists that the immune response is initiated by the activation of innate immunity with production of an inflammatory micro-environment. Thus, from a pathogenetic point of view, the immune-mediated glomerular diseases, including those without signs of inflammation at optic microscopy, might be classified as GN. Finally, the Mayo Clinic/Renal Pathology Society does not separate primary GN, in which the immune attack is limited to the kidney (Box 1.1), from secondary GN, in which the glomerular disease may be associated with systemic auto-immune diseases, infection, malignancy, or may be triggered by exposure to drugs or toxins. In this book we maintain the standard pathologic classification of primary GN, but the term C3 glomerulopathy and idiopathic MPGN will be used instead of MPGN.

Epidemiology of primary glomerular diseases

Little is known about the worldwide epidemiology of primary glomerular diseases. A large source of information comes from McGrogan and colleagues (2011), who conducted a systematic review of studies published between 1980 and 2007. The inclusion criteria were that the studies reported original work, that the study reported incidence of specific forms of glomerular disease with reference to a denominator population, that the estimates of population size and person-time contributed were accurate, and that efforts had been made to ascertain all incident cases. In most cases, primary GN was classified by renal

Box 1.1 List of primary glomerular diseases

- Minimal change disease
- Focal segmental glomerular sclerosis (excluding the histological pattern of FSGS secondary to well-defined causes)
- Membranous nephropathy
- Immunoglobulin A nephropathy
- C3 Glomerulopathy (DDD, C3 GN) and Idiopathic Immune Complex Membranoproliferative GN
- C4 Glomerulopathy (extremely rare)
- Infection-related and Renal-limited GN
- Renal Limited Vasculitis
- Collagenofibrotic glomerulopathy
- Thin basement membranes nephropathy
- Lipoprotein glomerulopathy
- 'Pure' mesangial proliferative GN
- IgM nephropathy
- C1q nephropathy
- Idiopathic nodular glomerulosclerosis (diabetic nephropathy without diabetes)

DDD = Dense Deposit Disease, GN = Glomerulonephritis

biopsy. From their large analysis McGrogan and colleagues (2011) found that the reported incidence rates of primary GN in adults varied between 0.2 and 2.5/100,000/year, depending on the specific disease considered. More recently, in children, the annual incidence of GN has been steady at five to ten cases per 100,000 population, with the peak incidence ranging between one and eight years of age (Grenbaum, 2012). In a retrospective cohort study using two large US administrative datasets, Wetmore and colleagues (2016) found a prevalence of primary GN of 306/100,000 persons.

Among the primary glomerular diseases, *minimal change disease* (MCD) accounts for over 75 per cent of cases of nephrotic syndrome in children. According to McGrogan and colleagues (2011), the incidence rates in children were between 0.23/100,000/year and 15.6/100,000/year, being between

0.23–2.8/100,000/year in Caucasian children, 2.4/100,000/year in Hispanic children, 3.4/100,000/year in Afro-Caribbean children, 7.2–11.6/100,000/ year in Arabian children, and 6.2–15.6/100,000/year in Asian children who resided in the UK. The exact prevalence is unknown, but it may be estimated at approximately ten to fifty cases per 100,000 children (Vivarelli et al., 2017). A systematic review on the epidemiology of histologically proven glomerular diseases in Africa between 1980 and 2014 reported that MCD was the most frequent primary GN accounting for 16.5 per cent (Okpechi et al., 2016). Another report showed that the incidence of idiopathic nephrotic syndrome in Japanese children is approximately three to four times higher than that in Caucasians (Kikunaga et al., 2017). This illustrates the great importance of geography, ancestry, and environment in determining the epidemiologic features of GN. In adults, MCD accounts for 10–15 per cent of all primary nephrotic syndrome cases undergoing renal biopsy (Waldman et al., 2007). In adolescents the incidence of MCD is similar to that observed in adults (Hogg et al., 1993).

The incidence of *FSGS* in prospective or retrospective studies, was between 0.2/100,000/year and 1.1/100,000/year (McGrogan et al., 2011). An Australian retrospective review reported higher rates of 2.5/100,000/year in males and 1.8/ 100,000/year in females (Briganti et al., 2001). In New York, the frequency of FSGS increased from 19.3 per cent (1986–1991) and 16.6 per cent (1992–1997) to 58.5 per cent in the period from 2002 (Dragovic et al., 2005). Recent reviews from different countries also reported that FSGS was the most common cause of nephrotic syndrome (Polito et al., 2009; Woo et al., 2010; Alwahaibi et al., 2013; Golay et al., 2013; Chavez-Valencia et al., 2014; Jegateesan et al., 2016; Murugapandian et al., 2016). A survey of renal biopsies performed in the US in adults with primary glomerulopathies found that FSGS was the most common lesion (38.9 per cent) across all race and ethnic groups. The lesion of FSGS was much more frequently seen in African-Americans and patients with FSGS had the highest rate of poverty (Sim et al., 2016). In the analysis from the NEPTUNE study, FSGS was the most frequent cause of nephrotic syndrome (Gipson et al., 2016). Even in children in the last 30 years the incidence of FSGS increased by three- to fivefold (Srivastava et al., 1999; Filler et al., 2003). It should be noted, however, that in an undefined number of cases, FSGS was secondary to other diseases or pathologic conditions.

The incidence of *membranous nephropathy* in children and adolescents ranged between 0.02/100,000/year to 0.09/100,000/year (McGrogan et al., 2011); in adults, MN develops between 50 and 60 years of age, with 2:1 male predominance (Couser, 2017). The estimated incidence of MN in adults is around 1.2/100,000/year (McGrogan et al., 2011; Couser, 2017). Surveys in different countries reported that MN was the most frequent cause of nephrotic syndrome among primary GN (Polenakovic et al., 2003; Zhou et al., 2011; Ozturk et al., 2014), particularly in elderly subjects (Moutzoris et al., 2009; Yokoyama et al., 2012; Jin et al., 2014; Rollino et al., 2014; Maixnerova et al., 2015), while in other series it was the second cause of nephrotic syndrome after FSGS (Chavez-Valencia et al., 2014; Gipson et al., 2016; Sim et al., 2016; Jegateesan et al., 2016; Murugapandian et al., 2016). It is generally assumed that MN is more frequent in males but McGrogan and colleagues (2011) determined that there was insufficient information to conclude reliably whether there is a difference in risk between males and females.

IgA nephropathy often presents with asymptomatic microscopic haematuria and mild or absent proteinuria. The different policies used for renal biopsy in patients with isolated microscopic haematuria may render difficult to estimate the real incidence of IgA nephropathy. At any rate, studies in children based on renal biopsy estimated an incidence ranging between 0.31 to 0.57/100,000/year (Sehic et al., 1997; Coppo et al., 1998), while a Japanese study based on screening reported an incidence of 4.5/100,000/year (Utsunomya et al., 2003). In McGrogan and colleagues (2011), most of the studies in adults were prospective, reporting rates from 0.2/100,000/year to 2.8/100,000/year; the retrospective studies reported a similar range of rates, from 0.4/100,000/year to 2.9/100,000/year. Taken together the available results, IgAN seems to be the most common histological feature in Europe, Asia, and the US (Gesualdo et al., 2004; Nair et al., 2006; Hanko et al., 2009; Riispere et al., 2012; Zaza et al., 2013; Xie et al., 2013; Sugiyama et al., 2013, Floege and Amann, 2016). IgAN is rare in subjects of African ancestry.

Until few years ago, the diagnosis of *membranoproliferative glomerulonephritis* was based on ultrastructural findings, namely interposition of the mesangium and a double contoured appearance of the glomerular basement membrane. As mentioned, today a histological appearance of MPGN associated with immunoglobulin deposits is generally secondary to infection or systemic diseases, while primary cases are generally associated with dysregulated activation of the alternative pathway of complement, hence the term *C3 glomerulopathy*. McGrogan and colleagues (2011) found that most cases defined as MPGN were actually secondary to acute post-infection glomerulonephritis or hepatitis B infection, making it difficult to evaluate the incidence of primary disease. According to the old classification, the general impression is that the incidence of this lesion among renal biopsies is decreasing in Western countries, while it seems to be increasing in the Danish and North-eastern Rumanian registries (Heaf et al., 1999; Volovat et al., 2013). However, the available data are deeply biased by the inclusion of cases associated with infection, cryoglobulinemia, or malignancy.

C3 glomerulopathy is often characterized by a membranoproliferative appearance at optical microscopy, with strong C3 deposition and without immunoglobulin deposits at immunofluorescence (Sethi and Fervenza, 2012). Within this histological pattern some cases are characterized by intramembranous DDD, which is more frequent and aggressive in younger subjects. The incidence of C3 glomerulopathy is quite low. A British study identified 80 cases, 21 with DDD and 59 with a MPGN pattern, with an incidence of around 0.1 per 100,000 population over the 17-year study duration in the Dublin and London areas (Medjeral-Thomas et al., 2014). In a smaller Indian study, C3 glomerulopathy accounted for 1 per cent of biopsy-proven primary GN, the most frequent histological pattern being that of MPGN (Mathur et al., 2015). Apart from C3 glomerulopathy, abnormal control of the complement alternative pathway can also result in atypical haemolytic uremic syndrome, as well as atypical postinfectious glomerulonephritis (Angioi et al., 2016).

The impact on renal survival of different subtypes of primary GN is discussed in the single chapters. A rough idea may be drawn by the data extracted from the US Renal Data System (USRDS) for adults, which considered six types of glomerular disease and vasculitis. Here we take into account only the four subtypes of primary glomerulonephritis reported in the USRDS study: FSGS, IgAN, MN, and MPGN. End stage renal disease (ESRD) attributed to diabetes and autosomal dominant polycystic kidney disease served as comparators. After a median follow-up of 2.5 years, the lowest crude mortality was seen in IgAN (3.7 deaths/100 person years). Compared to IgAN, adjusted mortality hazard ratio (HR) was higher in all other subtypes of glomerulonephritis (MN: HR 1.23; FSGS: HR 1.37; MPGN: HR 1.38) as well as in diabetes (HR 1.73), and in autosomal dominant polycystic kidney disease (HR 1.2; O'Shaughnessy et al., 2015).

Finally, it is important to recognize that in spite of the precautions taken by different investigators to prevent biases, the available epidemiological data suffer from a number of relevant discrepancies, the more relevant biases being:

i. the policy and indications for performance of kidney biopsy are quite variable, not only among countries, but also among practitioners and nephrologists in the same country;

ii. there are large differences in socio-economic and hygienic conditions among countries and among the regions of the same country; and

iii. there are differences in age, gender, and ethnicity in the available reports.

With these drawbacks in mind, it is reasonable to conclude that *IgAN* most likely represents the most frequent form of primary GN worldwide, except in equatorial Africa. Probably, its prevalence is even higher than generally estimated because many patients with isolated haematuria are not submitted to kidney biopsy. *Minimal change disease* is by far the most frequent cause of nephrotic syndrome in children and adolescents. However, its precise incidence and prevalence are difficult to evaluate, since most steroid-sensitive children do not receive kidney biopsy. *FSGS and membranous nephropathy* are the most frequent causes of nephrotic syndrome in adults, the former particularly in patients of African (West African) ancestry. However, it is possible that the relative impact of either of these two glomerular diseases may depend on the age and gender of patients. Indeed, it is likely that primary MN tends to be more frequent in the older adult. On the other hand, the higher the age of the patient, the less likely is his/her possibility of receiving a kidney biopsy, in spite of its documented usefulness in providing prognostic information and guiding therapeutic decisions (Bomback et al., 2012). Little information is available about the incidence of *C3 glomerulopathy*, since many diseases with the histological features of immunoglobulin deposits in the mesangium and basement membrane thickening have been wrongly classified among the label of MPGN. Finally, a number of rare primary glomerular diseases, e.g. collagenofibrotic glomerulopathy, thin basement membrane disease, IgM nephropathy, C1q nephropathy, etc., have never been considered in most of the available reports.

References

Alwahaibi NY, Alhabsi TA, Alrawahi SA. (2013). Pattern of glomerular diseases in Oman: A study based on light microscopy and immunofluorescence. Saudi J Kidney Dis Transpl. **24**: 387–91.

Angioi A, Fervenza FC, Sethi S, et al. (2016). Diagnosis of complement alternative pathway disorders. Kidney Int. **89**: 278–88.

Beck LH Jr, Bonegio RG, Lambeau G, et al. (2009). M-type phospholipase A2 receptor as target antigen in idiopathic membranous nephropathy. N Engl J Med. **361**: 11–21.

Bell, E.T. (1946). Glomerulonephritis. In *Renal Diseases*, pp. 141–253. Lea & Febiger, Philadelphia, PA.

Berden AE, Ferrario F, Hagen EC, et al. (2010). Histopathologic classification of ANCA-associated glomerulonephritis. J Am Soc Nephrol. **21**: 1628–36.

Berman LB, Schreiner GE. (1958). Clinical and histologic spectrum of the nephrotic syndrome. Am J Med. **24**: 249–67.

Bomback AS, Herlitz LC, Markowitz GS. (2012). Renal biopsy in the elderly and very elderly: Useful or not? Adv Chronic Kidney Dis. **19**: 61–7.

Briganti EM, Dowling J, Finlay M, et al. (2001). The incidence of biopsy-proven glomerulonephritis in Australia. Nephrol Dial Transplant. **16**: 1364–7.

Cameron JS, Ogg CS, Turner DR, et al. (1973). Focal glomerulosclerosis. Perspect Nephrol Hypertens. **1**: 249–61.

Caulfield JB. (1964). Application of the electron microscopy to renal diseases. N Engl J Med. **270**: 183–94.

Chávez Valencia V, Orizaga de La Cruz C, Guillermo Becerra Fuentes J, et al. (2014). Epidemiology of glomerular disease in adults: A database review. Gac Med Mex. **150** (Suppl 2): 186–93.

Cook HT, Pickering MC. (2015). Histopathology of MPGN and C3 glomerulopathy. Nat Rev Nephrol. **11**: 14–22.

Coppo R, Gianoglio B, Porcellini MG, et al. (1998). Frequency of renal diseases and clinical indications for renal biopsy in children (report of the Italian National Registry of Renal Biopsies in Children). Group of Renal Immunopathology of the Italian Society of Pediatric Nephrology and Group of Renal Immunopathology of the Italian Society of Nephrology. Nephrol Dial Transplant. **13**: 293–7.

Couser WG. (2017). Primary membranous nephropathy. Clin J Am Soc Nephrol. **12**: 983–97.

Couser WG, Johnson RJ. (2014). The etiology of glomerulonephritis: Roles of infection and autoimmunity. Kidney Int. **86**: 905–14.

Derow HA. (1958). The nephrotic syndrome. N Engl J Med. **258**: 77–82.

Dragovic D, Rosenstock JL, Wahl SJ, et al. (2005). Increasing incidence of focal segmental glomerulosclerosis and an examination of demographic patterns. Clin Nephrol. **63**: 1–7.

Filler G, Young E, Geier P, et al. (2003). Is there really an increase in non-minimal change nephrotic syndrome in children? Am J Kidney Dis. **42**: 1107–13.

Floege J, Amann K. (2016). Primary glomerulonephritides. The Lancet. **387**: 2036–48.

Folli G, Pollak VE, Reid RT, et al. (1958). Electron-microscopic studies of reversible glomerular lesions in the adult nephrotic syndrome. Ann Intern Med. **49**: 775–95.

Fresquet M, Jowitt TA, Gummadova J, et al. (2015). Identification of a major epitope recognized by PLA2R autoantibodies in primary membranous nephropathy. J Am Soc Nephrol. **2**: 302–13.

Gast C, Pengelly RJ, Lyon M, et al. (2016). Collagen (*COL4A*) mutations are the most frequent mutations in adult focal segmental glomerulosclerosis. Nephrol Dial Transplant. **31**: 961–70.

Gesualdo L, Di Palma AM, Morrone LF, et al. (2004). The Italian experience of the national registry of renal biopsies. Kidney Int. **66**: 890–4

Gipson DS, Troost JP, Lafayette RA, et al. (2016). Complete remission in the Nephrotic Syndrome Study Network. Clin J Am Soc Nephrol. **11**: 81–9.

Glassock RJ. (2012). The pathogenesis of membranous nephropathy: evolution and revolution. Curr Opin Nephrol Hypertens. **21**: 235–42.

Glassock RJ, Brenner BM. (1991). The major glomerulopathies. In JD Wilson, E Braunwald, KI Isselbacher, et al. (eds), *Harrison's Principles of Internal Medicine*, 12th edition, pp. 1170–80. MacGraw-Hill, Inc. New York.

Glassock RJ, Fervenza F, Hebert L, Cameron JS. (2015). Nephrotic syndrome redux. Nephrol Dial Transplant. **20**: 13–17.

Golay V, Trivedi M, Kurien AA, et al. (2013). Spectrum of nephrotic syndrome in adults: Clinicopathological study from a single center in India. Ren Fail. **35**: 487–91.

Greenbaum LA, Benndorf R, Smoyer WE. (2012). Childhood nephrotic syndrome-- current and future therapies. Nat Rev Nephrol. **8**: 445–58.

Habib R, Gubler MC. (1973). Focal sclerosing glomerulonephritis. Perspect Nephrol Hypertens. **1**: 263–78.

Habib R, Kleinknecht C. (1971). The primary nephrotic syndrome of childhood. Classification and clinicopathologic study of 406 cases. Pathol Annu. **6**: 417–74.

Hanko JB, Mullan RN, O'Rourke DM, et al. (2009). The changing pattern of adult primary glomerular disease. Nephrol Dial Transplant. **24**: 3050–4.

Heaf J, Løkkegaard H, Larsen S. (1999). The epidemiology and prognosis of glomerulonephritis in Denmark 1985–1997. Nephrol Dial Transplant. **14**: 1889–97.

Heptinstall RH, Joekes AM. (1959). Renal biopsy. Proc R Soc Med. **52**: 211–12.

Heymann J, Winkler CA, Hoek M, et al. (2017). Therapeutics for APOL1 nephropathies: Putting out the fire in the podocyte. Nephrol Dial Transplant. **32**: i65–70.

Hogg RJ, Silva FG, Berry PL, et al. (1993). Glomerular lesions in adolescents with gross hematuria or the nephrotic syndrome. Report of the Southwest Pediatric Nephrology Study Group. Pediatr Nephrol. **7**: 27–31.

Iverson P, Brun C. (1951). Aspiration biopsy of the kidney. Am J Med. **11**: 324–30.

Jegatheesan D, Nath K, Reyaldeen R, et al. (2016). Epidemiology of biopsy-proven glomerulonephritis in Queensland adults. Nephrology (Carlton). **21**: 28–34.

Jin B, Zeng C, Ge Y, et al. (2014). The spectrum of biopsy-proven kidney diseases in elderly Chinese patients. Nephrol Dial Transplant. **29**: 2251–9.

Joekes AM, Heptinstall RH, Porter KA. (1958). The nephrotic syndrome: A study of renal biopsies in 20 adult patients. Q J Med. **27**: 495–516.

Jones D. (1957). Nephrotic glomerulonephritis. Am J Pathol. **33**: 313–29.

Kao L, Lam V, Waldman M, et al. (2015). Identification of the immunodominant epitope region in phospholipase A2 receptor-mediating autoantibody binding in idiopathic membranous nephropathy. J Am Soc Nephrol. **26**: 291–301.

Kark RM, Muehrcke RC. (1954). Biopsy of kidney in prone position. The Lancet. **266**: 1047–9.

Kark RM, Pirani CL, Pollak VE, et al. (1958). The nephrotic syndrome in adults: A common disorder with many causes. Ann Intern Med. **49**: 751–4.

KDIGO. (2012). Clinical practice guideline for glomerulonephritis. Kidney Int. **2S** (2): 1–143.

Kikunaga K, Ishikura K, Terano C, et al. (2017). High incidence of idiopathic nephrotic syndrome in East Asian children: A nationwide survey in Japan (JP-SHINE study). Clin Exp Nephrol. **21**: 651–7.

Kopp JB, Nelson GW, Sampath K, et al. (2011). APOL1 genetic variants in focal segmental glomerulosclerosis and HIV-associated nephropathy. J Am Soc Nephrol. **22**: 2129–37.

Maixnerova D, Jancova E, Skibova J, et al. (2015). Nationwide biopsy survey of renal diseases in the Czech Republic during the years 1994-2011. J Nephrol. **28**: 39–49.

Mathur M, Sharma S, Prasad D, et al. (2015). Incidence and profile of C3 Glomerulopathy: A single center study. Indian J Nephrol. **25**: 8–11.

McGrogan A, Franssen CFM, de Vries CS. (2011). The incidence of primary glomerulonephritis worldwide: A systematic review of the literature. Nephrol Dial Trasplant. **26**: 414–43.

Medjeral-Thomas NR, O'Shaughnessy MM, O'Regan JA, et al. (2014). C3 glomerulopathy: Clinicopathologic features and predictors of outcome. Clin J Am Soc Nephrol. **9**: 46–53.

Mihatsch MJ. (1979). A modern classification of glomerulonephritis. A step forward for the pathologist. Path Res Pract. **164**: 35–48.

Moutzouris D-A, Herlitz L, Appel GB, et al. (2009). Renal biopsy in the very elderly. Clin J Am Soc Nephrol. **4**: 1073–82.

Müller F. (1906). Morbus brightii. Vehr Disch Pth Ges. **9**: 64.

Murugapandian S, Mansour I, Hudeeb M, et al. (2016). Epidemiology of glomerular disease in southern Arizona: Review of 10-year renal biopsy data. Medicine (Baltimore). **95**: e3633.

Nair R, Walker PD. (2006). Is IgA nephropathy the commonest primary glomerulopathy among young adults in the USA? Kidney Int. **69**: 1455–8.

Okpechi IG, Ameh OI, Bello AK, et al. (2016). Epidemiology of histologically proven glomerulonephritis in Africa: A systematic review and meta-analysis. PLoS One. **11**: e0152203.

O'Shaughnessy MM, Montez-Rath ME, Lafayette RA, et al. (2015). Patient characteristics and outcomes by GN subtype in ESRD. Clin J Am Soc Nephrol. **10**: 1170–8.

Ozturk S, Sumnu A, Seyahi N, et al. (2014). Demographic and clinical characteristics of primary glomerular diseases in Turkey. Int Urol Nephrol. **46**: 2347–55.

Pickering MC, D'Agati VD, Nester CM, et al. (2013). C3 glomerulopathy: Consensus report. Kidney Int. **84**: 1079–89.

Polenakovic MH, Grcevska L, Dzikova S. (2003). The incidence of biopsy-proven primary glomerulonephritis in the Republic of Macedonia-long-term follow-up. Nephrol Dial Transplant. **18** (Suppl 5): 26–7.

Polito MG, de Moura LA, Kirsztajn GM. (2009). An overview on frequency of renal biopsy diagnosis in Brazil: Clinical and pathological pattern based on 9617 native kidney biopsies. Nephrol Dial Transplant. **24**: 3050–4.

Quintana LF, Peréz NS, De Sousa E, et al. (2014). ANCA serotype and histopathological classification for the prediction of renal outcome in ANCA-associated glomerulonephritis. Nephrol Dial Transplant. **29**: 1764–9.

Ranganathan S. (2016). Pathology of podocytopathies causing nephrotic syndrome in children. Front Pediatr. **4**: 1–12.

Reubi F. (1955). Physiopathology and clinical manifestations of glomerulonephritis. J Urol Medicale Chir. **61**: 626–60.

Rich AR. (1957). A hitherto undescribed vulnerability of the juxtamedullary glomeruli in lipoid nephrosis. Johns Hopk Hosp Bull. **100**: 173–86.

Riispere Z, Ots-Rosenberg M. (2012). Occurrence of kidney diseases and patterns of glomerular disease based on a 10-year kidney biopsy material: A retrospective single-centre analysis in Estonia. Scand J Urol Nephrol. **46**: 389–94.

Rollino C, Ferro M, Beltrame G, et al. (2014). Renal biopsy in patients over 75: 131 cases. Clin Nephrol. **82**: 225–30.

Sehic AM, Gaber LW, Roy S III, et al. (1997). Increased recognition of IgA nephropathy in African-American children. Pediatr Nephrol. **11**: 435–7.

Servais A, Fremeaux-Bacchi V, Lequintrec M, et al. (2007). Primary glomerulonephritis with isolated C3 deposits: A new entity which shares common genetic risk factors with haemolytic uraemic syndrome. J Med Genet. **44**: 193–9.

Sethi S, Fervenza FC. (2011). Membranoproliferative glomerulonephritis: Pathogenetic heterogeneity and proposal for a new classification. Semin Nephrol. **31**: 341–8.

Sethi S, Fervenza FC. (2012). Membranoproliferative glomerulonephritis—a new look at an old entity. N Engl J Med. **366**: 1119–31.

Sethi S, Glassock RJ, Fervenza FC. (2015). Focal segmental glomerulosclerosis: towards a better understanding for the practicing nephrologist. Nephrol Dial Transplant. **30**: 375–84.

Sethi S, Haas M, Markowitz GS, et al. (2016). Mayo Clinic/Renal Pathology Society Consensus Report on Pathologic Classification, Diagnosis, and Reporting of GN. J Am Soc Nephrol. **27**: 1278–87.

Sim JJ, Batech M, Hever A, et al. (2016). Distribution of biopsy-proven presumed primary glomerulonephropathies in 2000-2011 among a racially and ethnically diverse US population. Am J Kidney Dis. **68**: 533–44.

Srivastava T, Simon SD, Alon US. (1999). High incidence of focal segmental glomerulosclerosis in nephrotic syndrome of childhood. Pediatr Nephrol. **13**: 13–18.

Sugiyama H, Yokoyama H, Sato H, et al. (2013). Japan Renal Biopsy Registry and Japan Kidney Disease Registry: Committee Report for 2009 and 2010. Clin Exp Nephrol. **17**: 155–73.

Tomas NM, Beck LH Jr, Meyer-Schwesinger C, et al. (2014). Thrombospondin type-1 domain-containing 7A in idiopathic membranous nephropathy. N Engl J Med. **371**: 2277–87.

Utsunomiya Y, Koda T, Kado T, et al. (2003). Incidence of pediatric IgA nephropathy. Pediatr Nephrol. **18**: 511–15.

Vivarelli M, Massella L, Ruggiero B, Emma F (2017). Minimal change disease. Clin J Am Soc Nephrol. **12**: 332–45.

Volhard FT. (1914). *Die Bright'sche Nierenkrankheit: Klinik, Pathologie und Atlas*. Springer. Berlin.

Volovăt C, Căruntu I, Costin C, et al. (2013). Changes in the histological spectrum of glomerular diseases in the past 16 years in the North-Eastern region of Romania. BMC Nephrol. **14**: 148.

Waldman M, Crew RJ, Valeri A, et al. (2007). Adult minimal-change disease: Clinical characteristics, treatment, and outcomes. Clin J Am Soc Nephrol. **2**: 445–53.

Wetmore JB, Guo H, Liu J, et al. (2016). The incidence, prevalence, and outcomes of glomerulonephritis derived from a large retrospective analysis. Kidney Int. **90**: 853–60.

White RH, Glasgow EF, Mills RJ. (1970). Clinicopathological study of nephrotic syndrome in childhood. Lancet. **1**: 1353–9.

Wilson HE, Saslaw S, Doan CA, et al. (1947). Reactions of monkeys to experimental mixed influenza and streptococcus infection. An analysis of the relative roles of humoral and cellular immunity, with the description of an intercurrent nephritic syndrome. J Exp Med. **85**: 199–215.

Woo KT, Chan CM, Mooi CY, et al. (2010). The changing pattern of primary glomerulonephritis in Singapore and other countries over the past 3 decades. ClinNephrol. **74**: 372–83.

Working Group of the International IgA Nephropathy Network and the Renal Pathology Society (2009). The Oxford classification of IgA nephropathy: Rationale, clinicopathological correlations, and classification. Kidney Int. **76**: 534–45.

Working Group of the International IgA Nephropathy Network and the Renal Pathology Society (2009). The Oxford classification of IgA nephropathy: pathology definitions, correlations, and reproducibility. Kidney Int. **76**: 546–56.

Xie J, Chen N. (2013). Primary glomerulonephritis in mainland China: An overview. Contrib Nephrol. **181**: 1–11.

Yokoyama H, Sugiyama H, Sato H, et al. (2012). Renal disease in the elderly and the very elderly Japanese: Analysis of the Japan Renal Biopsy Registry (J-RBR). Clin Exp Nephrol. **16**: 903–20.

Zaza G, Bernich P, Lupo A. (2013). Incidence of primary glomerulonephritis in a large North-Eastern Italian area: A 13-year renal biopsy study. Nephrol Dial Transplant. **28**: 367–72.

Zhou FD, Shen HY, Chen M, et al. (2011). The renal histopathological spectrum of patients with nephrotic syndrome: an analysis of 1523 patients in a single Chinese centre. Nephrol Dial Transplant. **26**: 3993–7.

Chapter 2

Symptomatic therapy

Richard J Glassock

Introduction and overview

Patients with glomerular diseases develop a wide variety of biochemical disturbances and pathophysiologic alterations leading to overt clinical manifestations (Glassock et al., 1995; Haraldsson et al., 2008; Ponticelli and Glassock, 2009; Floege and Feehally, 2015; Vaziri, 2016). These occur as a direct result of injury to the glomerular capillary wall and disturbances in normal glomerular function, including loss of filtration capacity and excessive transfer of erythrocytes and/or plasma proteins from blood to tubular lumina eventuating in haematuria and/or proteinuria. Proteinuria—which is believed to be the consequence of disturbed glomerular capillary wall permselectivity (Haraldsson et al., 2008)—when substantial, can lead to hypoproteinaemia (hypo-albuminaemia) and thereby to a reduction in plasma oncotic pressure and disordered Starling forces in the peripheral capillary network leading to increased interstitial fluid volume, sometimes at the expense of intravascular volume, if the transfers of fluid are rapid and severe. Secondary changes in the synthesis, turnover, and plasma concentration of various proteins and lipids develop and can lead to an imbalance of pro-thrombotic and anti-thrombotic factors promoting a *thrombophilic* state (Glassock, 2007). Primary disturbances in the renal handling of sodium chloride (NaCl) and water are often associated with oedema formation, expansion of intra-vascular volume, and/or hypertension (Schrier and Fassett, 1998). Finally, the rapid or slow loss of the glomerular filtration rate (GFR) due to damage of single nephrons (perhaps mediated in part by filtered proteins and their reabsorption) as well as by the 'drop out' of functioning nephrons from the overall population of nephrons in the two kidneys is responsible for ultimate progression to end-stage renal disease (ESRD) in many, but not all, of the primary glomerular disorders (Floege and Feehally, 2015).

Collectively these abnormalities give rise to 'syndromes' of glomerular disease. These 'syndromes' can be arbitrarily, but usefully, grouped into five general categories which may overlap to some degree; namely, the *acute nephritic syndrome, rapidly progressive glomerulonephritis, the nephrotic syndrome, 'symptomless' haematuria and/or proteinuria*, and *slowly progressive 'chronic' nephritis* (Glassock et al., 1995). The cardinal features of these syndromes and the diseases to which they are most closely associated are discussed in this monograph. This monograph will also deal largely with those glomerular diseases which *primarily* affect the kidneys and in which the extrarenal manifestations are the consequence of the impairment or disturbance of kidney function itself (the so-called *primary glomerular diseases*).

The clinical abnormalities resulting from these disturbances in renal pathophysiology require management in order to minimize or avoid disabling symptoms, often referred to as *symptomatic therapy*, and to distinguish the measures employed from those which are used in an attempt to ameliorate the specific underlying disease detailed in the chapters which follow, under the heading of *specific therapy*. Several aspects or targets of *symptomatic therapy* will be discussed here (see also Box 2.1), namely:

♦ Management of oedema arising from altered NaCl and fluid handling by the diseased kidney and the associated disturbances in the Starling forces operating within the peripheral capillaries.

♦ Treatment of hypertension developing because of extracellular and intravascular fluid volume expansion and vasoconstriction, possibly related incomplete suppression of the renin–angiotensin system, and other factors (such as reduced vasodilatory capacity [endothelial dysfunction] and/or reduced vascular compliance).

Box 2.1 Targets of symptomatic therapy of nephrotic syndrome

Oedema
Hypertension
Hyperlipidaemia (Hypercholesterolaemia and Hypertriglyceridaemia)
Hypercoagulable state (Thrombophilia)
Hypoproteinaemia/proteinuria
Progressive renal failure
Trace metal deficiencies
Endocrine disturbances
Fluid and electrolyte disorders
Infectious/immunodeficiency states

- Therapy of hyperlipidaemia (e.g. hypercholesterolaemia) and the tendency for accelerated atherogenesis.
- Management of the 'hypercoagulable' or 'thrombophilic' state accompanying hypoproteinaemic forms of glomerulonephritis (e.g. Nephrotic Syndrome).
- Non-disease-specific treatment of hypoproteinaemia and proteinuria, including protein-deficiency states.
- Non-disease-specific strategies designed to retard the progression of renal disease (loss of GFR) and prevention of the inexorable development of ESRD.
- Management of other disturbances, including trace metal deficiencies, endocrine perturbations, fluid and electrolyte disorders, immunodeficiency states, and enhanced risk of infection (usually bacterial in origin) occurring in the absence of the use of immunosuppressant agents for 'specific therapy'.

The extent to which each of these 'symptomatic' management principles can be successfully applied to specific glomerular diseases and to individual patients will vary depending upon the extent and magnitude of the underlying biochemical or pathophysiologic disturbances and their interactions with each other.

Oedema

Clinical features, pathogenesis, and pathophysiology

Oedema is common in glomerular disease, especially in those accompanied by marked proteinuria (nephrotic syndrome) (Glassock, 1997; Schrier and Fassett, 1998; Kim et al., 2007). The acute nephritic syndrome may also be associated with oedema, even when hypoproteinaemia is absent or mild, but it is usually less severe than that seen in nephrotic states. Oedema in glomerular disease usually first accumulates about the peri-orbital areas (where the interstitial pressure is low) and in dependent sites (ankle, feet, and pre-sacral areas). Pericardial effusions are very rare but pleural effusions and ascites may develop if the disease is severe and prolonged. Pulmonary oedema (increased lung interstitial water content) can occur, but seldom results in symptoms unless associated with disturbances in myocardial function (Marino et al., 2016).

In glomerular disease (acute nephritis and the nephrotic syndrome), the occurrence of oedema is usually related to hypoproteinaemia and/or augmented primary NaCl resorption at distal nephron (collecting duct) sites, conditioned by abnormalities of the Starling forces in the peripheral capillaries governing interstitial fluid formation and its re-uptake. Complicating congestive heart failure, advanced liver disease, pericardial effusions, or obstructions to venous/lymphatic disease may be a concomitant cause of oedema in some patients.

Except in oliguric patients or those with markedly impaired renal function, reduced NaCl excretion is not usually the consequence of reduced delivery to tubular reabsorptive sites because of impaired GFR per se.

The pathogenesis of oedema in glomerular disease in the absence of ESRD or severe acute renal failure is not fully understood (see Figure 2.1), but

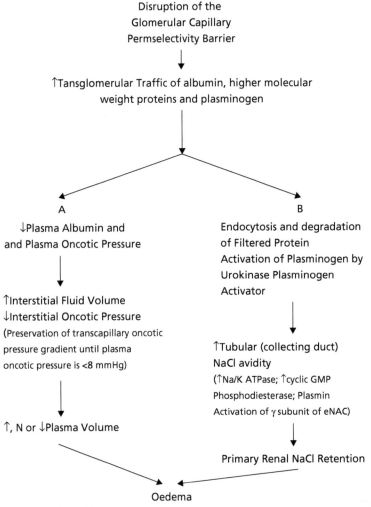

Figure 2.1 The pathophysiology of oedema formation in the Nephrotic Syndrome. Note that dependent on the interaction of A and B, the plasma volume may be reduced, normal, or increased. Due to intrinsic primary renal sodium retention, the plasma volume is commonly increased unless the plasma oncotic pressure is very low (<8 mmHg). See text for details.

considerable progress has been made in unravelling the complex processes underlying oedema formation in both the nephrotic syndrome and in acute nephritis (Lee and Humphreys, 1996; Deschenes et al., 2001; Donckerwolcke et al., 2003; Kim et al., 2006; de Seigneux et al., 2006; Doucet et al., 2007; Marino et al., 2016).

Two quite distinct pathophysiologic processes appear to be involved:

1. Disruption of the Starling equilibrium at the peripheral capillary level.

This particularly involves alterations in the factors governing the permeability of peripheral capillaries participating in the transfer of fluid from the vascular to the interstitial compartment (Joles and Koomans, 2001). In the nephrotic syndrome these abnormalities contribute to the redistribution of retained NaCl and water from the vascular to the interstitial compartments. If such transfers did not occur, the degree of primary NaCl retention seen in nephrotic syndrome would quickly lead to marked intravascular volume expansion and severe hypertension. Primary renal NaCl retention *without* an accompanying marked transfer of the retained fluid to the interstitial space appears to be involved in the development of volume-dependent hypertension observed in the acute nephritic syndrome

2. Marked primary renal NaCl retention occurring at distal (collecting duct) sites (Doucet et al., 2007; Marino et al., 2016).

This is the proximate cause of the retention of fluid in both nephritic and nephrotic states. Circulating hormones (e.g. aldosterone) play little role in the initiation of the salt-retaining state in these disorders.

While a decrease in plasma osmotic pressure (π) due to hypo-albuminaemia should result in a major displacement of intravascular fluid into the interstitial compartment, this generally does not occur unless the plasma π value falls well below 8 mmHg or 1 kPa (normal about 25 mmHg or 3.3 kPa) because of a corresponding fall in interstitial osmotic pressure, thus maintaining the transcapillary osmotic gradient (Joles and Koomans, 2001). However, a very *acute* decline in plasma π value, e.g. in rapidly developing nephrotic syndrome, may not be accompanied by a corresponding rapid decline in the interstitial π value; thus, a major displacement of fluid from the vascular compartment into the interstitial compartment may occur, leading to profound hypovolaemia. In more slowly developing conditions, oedema with expansion of the total extracellular volume occurs even when plasma π is only modestly reduced, and therefore other factors, in addition to the transcapillary osmotic gradient, must be involved in oedema formation (Joles and Koomans, 2001). In the nephrotic syndrome the peripheral capillaries increase the transfer of fluid from the intracapillary space to the interstitial space, where it traffics to the lymphatic system and ultimately to the thoracic duct, irrespective of the fundamental disease causing the abnormal glomerular permeability. Thus, the accumulation of retained fluid in the interstitial space (oedema) is the consequence of disturbed Starling forces in the peripheral capillary, but not usually due to the decrease in serum proteins (chiefly albumin) and thereby the plasma oncotic pressure (Joles and Koomans, 2001). This accounts for the variability in the severity of oedema in patients with the nephrotic syndrome, independent of the plasma albumin concentration and the π of the circulating fluids.

As a result, it is very clear that oedematous patients with hypoproteinaemia (hypo-albuminaemia) due to glomerular disease may have normal, expanded, or decreased intravascular volume (Joles and Koomans, 2001). The *underfilling* theory of renal NaCl retention in the nephrotic syndrome has been largely discarded, except in unusual circumstances. Those patients with clearly and unequivocally reduced intravascular volume constitute the minority of patients with nephrotic syndrome. Such patients typically have relatively *rapid* development of oedema and *minimal* glomerular structural abnormalities of glomeruli. Expansion of extracellular volume combined with normal or even increased intravascular volume in many patients with nephrotic syndrome points to an important contribution of primary renal processes in NaCl and fluid retention in the oedema of nephrotic syndrome (Doucet et al., 2007). On the other hand, the hypothesis that the great majority of subjects with the nephrotic syndrome have an *overfilled* vascular volume (due to primary renal NaCl retention) can also be criticized (Schrier and Fassett, 1998). These critiques have clinical implications as to how aggressively oedema is treated with diuretics. Subjects with '*underfilling*' of the intravascular volume in nephrotic syndrome may be very susceptible to decrements in arterial blood pressure (BP) or GFR with overly aggressive diuretic treatment of oedema.

Strong experimental evidence suggests that primary renal retention of NaCl is caused by intrarenal disturbances rather than by circulating hormonal factors or neural effects (Ichikawa et al., 1983; Doucet et al., 2007). Excess plasma renin activity or elevated circulating aldosterone levels, deficient atrial natriuretic factor production, or activation of the sympathetic nervous system do not fully account for the disturbances in NaCl handling by the kidney observed in nephrotic syndrome (Doucet et al., 2007). Furthermore, renal NaCl retention is related more to the onset and magnitude of proteinuria than the status of intravascular volume or the degree of hypo-albuminaemia. Indeed, NaCl retention appears before any reduction in serum protein concentration and a diuresis ensues in the absence of any significant change in serum protein concentration in nephrotic subjects. Infusions of hyperoncotic albumin, in the absence of diuretics, do not increase NaCl excretion, despite a rise in plasma oncotic pressure. Plasma renin activity, although sometimes modestly elevated, may show little clear relationship to intravascular volume; thus, it is possible that the renin–angiotensin system may be stimulated by intrarenal events rather than necessarily by a depletion of intravascular volume depletion.

The abnormal NaCl reabsorption within the nephron appears to be localized to the distal nephron and collecting ducts (Ichikawa et al., 1983). Post-receptor resistance to the action of atrial natriuretic factor due to enhanced activity of cyclic GMP phosphodiesterase may be involved (Lee and Humphries, 1996), but the dominant process appears to be an increased activity of Na^+/K^+ activated ATPase, perhaps abetted by alteration in the density of active epithelial sodium channels (ENaC) in the cortical collecting ducts (Deschenes et al., 2001; Kim et al., 2007; de Seigneux et al., 2006; Doucet et al., 2007). Increased abundance and apical targeting of the subunits of ENaC have been demonstrated in the cortical collecting ducts in experimental nephrotic syndrome (Doucet et al., 2007). ENaC activation is secondary to hyperaldosteronism (by recruitment of an intracellular pool of channels), but sodium retention and induction of Na^+-K^+ ATPase in the cortical collecting ducts are independent of hyperaldosteronism and increased ENaC may not be the rate limiting step in renal NaCl retention in experimental models of nephrotic syndrome (PAN nephrosis) (Lourdel et al., 2005). Primary renal NaCl retention can occur in the absence of aldosterone in experimental nephrotic syndrome (Doucet et al., 2007). Due to the *unilateral* retention of NaCl demonstrated in experimental models of nephrotic syndrome (Ichikawa et al., 1983), it is unlikely that any circulating factor is directly involved in primary renal NaCl retention observed in nephrotic states (Doucet et al., 2007).

A distinct linkage exists between abnormal glomerular permeability and increased exposure of tubules to, and subsequent reabsorption of, protein and primary renal NaCl retention. This indicates that enhanced glomerular permeability to protein may govern primary renal NaCl retention at the *individual* nephron level in nephrotic oedema. Functional changes in tubular cellular function consequent to expression of factors governing NaCl reabsorption in the collecting ducts (e.g. Na/K ATPase, ENaC) resulting from abnormally high concentrations of protein (including albumin) in tubular lumina appear to be involved, although this remains somewhat controversial (Zandi-Nejad et al., 2004; Yu et al., 2005; Doucet et al., 2007; see also 'Proteinuria and hypoalbuminaemia'). Specific filtered proteins (albumin, high-molecular weight proteins) may have differing effects on tubular reabsorptive phenomena. Intrinsic proteins may also have direct effects on NaCl reabsorption. For example, parvalbumin has been shown to have effects on the thiazide-sensitive

Na^+-Cl^- co-transporter and thus may be involved in both Na^+ and Ca^{++} handling in the distal convoluted tubule (Belge et al., 2007; Zacchia and Capasso, 2008).

In addition, compelling evidence has accumulated that plasminogen (a pro-serine protease) present in the tubular lumen in proteinuric states and cleaved by urokinase type plasminogen activator (uPA) to form plasmin can lead to activation of the epithelial sodium channel (ENaC) in collecting ducts by cleaving the γ subunit of ENac (Passero et al., 2010; Jacquillet et al., 2011; Staehr et al., 2015). These abnormalities can be a cause of volume expansion in nephrotic syndrome (Schork et al., 2016). Amiloride inhibits uPA and may therefore reduce the overactivity of ENaC in nephrotic syndrome (Staehr et al., 2015).

It is important to re-emphasize that the proteinuria-driven changes (luminal protein concentration) in cortical collecting tubule sodium avidity operates at the *individual nephron level*. Tubules which are not exposed to abnormal luminal protein concentration (i.e. tubules which are not affected in a focal glomerular disease process involving some but not all nephrons) are capable of excreting NaCl in a normal manner and these *normal* nephrons would be expected to excrete the NaCl retained by the *abnormal* nephrons in the mixed diseased/non-diseased nephron population. This phenomenon may explain why oedema is quite uncommon in subjects with very focal and segmental permselectivity defects (e.g. obesity-related glomerulopathy and other 'secondary' forms of focal segmental glomerulosclerosis). Tubular reabsorption of NaCl at more proximal sites (proximal tubule and ascending limb of the loop of Henle) is normal in nephrotic states, at least in the absence of acute hypovolaemia, diuretics, or an advanced decline in GFR. Reabsorption of NaCl at distal convoluted tubule sites where Na^+ and K^+ exchange occurs is also initially normal. Thus, potassium retention or potassium loss is generally not seen in nephrotic states in the absence of diuretics or aldosterone deficiency. However, potassium retention may be severe in acute nephritic syndrome, usually because of the attendant secondary hyporeninaemia, hypo-aldosteronism, and reduced capacity for K^+ excretion along with reduced GFR (Don and Schambelan, 1990).

Therapy

Mild oedema

If oedema is mild and well-tolerated, the best approach is to reduce dietary NaCl intake to levels below 3 g/day (42 mM Na^+ or about 0.5–0.6 mM/kg/day; Box 2.2). Bed rest should be avoided because of the tendency of these patients to develop thrombo-embolic complications (see 'Prophylaxis and therapy'). Support stockings and nocturnal leg elevation may be of value in some patients with mild oedema. Many patients will not require any more than these simple

Box 2.2 Management of oedema in nephrotic syndrome

Mild

Dietary NaCl restriction (to 3–4 g NaCl/day)
Support stockings
Hydrochlorothiazide 12.5–50 mg/day (if GFR >50 ml/min)
Furosemide 40–80 mg/day (if GFR <50 ml/min)

Moderate

Continue NaCl restriction, *add*
Furosemide 160–480 mg/day or bumetanide 1–2 mg/day *or* torsemide 40–160 mg/day
Mineralocorticoid receptor antagonists (spironolactone, eplerenone, finerenone). Spironolactone dosage is 25 mg two to four times daily; eplerenone dosage is 25–50 mg once daily; Finerenone dosage is 5–15 mg once daily. Use with caution if GFR <30 ml/min; monitor for hyperkalaemia.

Severe

Continue NaCl restriction, *add*
Oral or IV furosemide 160–480 mg/day (or bumetanide or torsemide) plus metolazone 2.5–10 mg/day.
Consider amiloride 5–10 mg/day.

Refractory

Continuous IV infusion of furosemide (20 mg/hour) or bumetanide (1 mg/hour) after a loading dose
or
Hyperoncotic salt-poor albumin (25–50 g) mixed with 120 mg of furosemide
or
Slow continuous venovenous ultrafiltration using a highly permeable (polysulfone) membrane.

measures. However, if they are unsuccessful, a diuretic may be added to the regimen. An oral thiazide-type diuretic (e.g. hydrochlorothiazide 12.5–50 mg/day or chlorthalidone 12.5–25 mg/day) is a reasonable first choice, providing the GFR is normal or near normal since the effectiveness of this class of agents is blunted when GFR is <30 mL/min (Ellison and Wilcox, 2008). If the serum creatinine is elevated (above 1.4 mg/dl; 120 μmol/l), thiazide-type diuretics are not likely to be very effective. Loop-acting diuretics (furosemide, ethacrynic acid, bumetanide, piretanide, or torsemide) are more effective choices when the GFR is reduced and when oedema is troublesome (Ellison and Wilcox, 2008). Because of the duration of action, furosemide should be given on a twice-daily regimen. Once-daily administration of loop-acting diuretics is not recommended. Because severe hypoproteinaemia may impair the rate of re-filling of the plasma volume, overly vigorous diuresis is to be avoided. Excessive diuresis may also activate the renin–angiotensin system and thereby promote thrombosis (see 'Hypercoagulability'). Oral furosemide 40–80 mg/day or oral bumetanide 1–2mg/day given in two or three divided doses, along with modest dietary NaCl (3g/day), should suffice in most instances of mild oedema.

Moderate oedema

More severe oedema may require more intensive regimens, such as high-dose oral furosemide (160–480 mg) given in two or three divided doses daily or by continuous intravenous infusion (see 'Severe or refractory oedema') (Glassock et al., 1997) (Box 2.2). Synergistic combinations of oral furosemide 160–320 mg daily or bumetanide 4–8 mg daily and the distally acting diuretic, metolazone 2.5–10 mg daily, are particularly effective, but may lead to pronounced kaliuresis requiring intensive potassium replacement. Very high doses of loop-acting diuretics, oral or intravenous, should be used with caution in patients with markedly impaired renal function because of the risks of transient or permanent deafness (Ellison and Wilcox, 2008). Mild diarrhoea may also be seen with very high doses of loop diuretics. The natriuretic effects of loop-acting diuretics are related to the urinary concentration of the diuretic (Brater, 1993). The relationship between diuretic excretion rate (in μg/min) and sodium excretion rate (in μEq/min) is described by a steep sigmoid curve. Different loop-acting diuretics differ only in potency, not in the shape of the curve (Brater, 1993). As mentioned earlier, because of the unique effects of amiloride on sodium handling in the distal nephron (Staehr et al., 2015), it may be uniquely suited to management of more severe oedema in nephrotic syndrome, especially when a kaliuresis has been promoted by thiazide-type agents. Adjunctive use of mineralocorticoid receptor antagonists (spironolactone, eplerenone, finerenone) may have value in promoting a natriuresis. They should be used with caution in subjects with GFR <30 ml/min, especially when renin-angiotensin system (RAS)-inhibition is used concomitantly. Serum potassium levels should be monitored (Lainscak et al., 2015). Gynaecomastia is also a troublesome side effect of spironolactone (Lainscak et al., 2015).

Potassium-sparing diuretics, e.g. spironolactone, eplerenone, triamterene, or amiloride, given alone are also of limited value but they may blunt the kaliuresis seen with thiazides or loop-acting diuretics and augment the resulting natriuresis when used in combination with other diuretics acting at different sites within the nephron. The special properties of amiloride on the ENaC (Staehr et al., 2015) might be a reason for use of this agent preferentially over other potassium-sparing diuretics. Used alone, the potassium-sparing diuretics are not usually very effective, but they can augment the effectiveness of both loop-acting diuretics and thiazide-type diuretics. These potassium-sparing diuretics should be used with great caution or not at all in patients with impaired GFR (<30 mL/min) or when hyperkalaemia is present. More rigorous dietary NaCl restriction (1 g/day) may also be required for short periods of time, but this will usually not be tolerated (or adhered to) over a period of longer than a few weeks.

Severe or refractory oedema

Anasarca is a relatively common severe oedematous state (anasarca) in which increasing doses of loop-acting diuretics combined with potassium-sparing diuretics (e.g. amiloride) and/or metolazone become increasingly less effective in inducing a natriuresis. This is so especially in patients with severe and massive proteinuria (>10 g/day), marked hypo-albuminaemia (<2.0 g/dl), and/ or impaired renal function (serum creatinine >2.0 mg/dl; see Glassock, 1997; Box 2.2).

At one time, the poor response to loop-acting diuretics (e.g. furosemide) was thought to be caused by binding of the drug to tubule fluid albumin, thereby preventing the action of the diuretic on the luminal side of the ascending limb of the loop of Henle to inhibit the $Na^+/K^+/2Cl^-$ reabsorptive pathway (Kirchner et al., 1993). This is no longer thought to be the case. An intravenous loading dose of furosemide or bumetanide followed by a slow intravenous infusion of the diuretic over 12–24 hours (20 mg/hour for furosemide and 1 mg/hour for bumetanide; Brater, 1993) may sometimes be effective when oral administration is not accompanied by a diuresis.

Excess compensatory 'upstream' distal-NaCl reabsorption (sites prior to the cortical collecting duct) may also be overcome by concomitant administration of a thiazide-type diuretic (Paton and Kane, 1977). Hyperoncotic (25 per cent) or iso-oncotic (5 per cent) human albumin infusions alone are seldom indicated to expand plasma volume, except when a rapid diuresis has resulted in clinical features of a plasma volume deficit, such as hypotension or a low central venous pressure. Such infusions should be used cautiously, if at all, in patients with impaired renal function and intrinsic cardiac disease because of the risk of precipitating congestive heart failure. Because of continued abnormal permselectivity, the infused albumin will be rapidly excreted in the urine (usually within 24–48 hours). Thus, the beneficial effects (if any) are short lived. The increased filtration of albumin can also result in further injury to the glomerular epithelial cells and or tubule. Indeed, some studies have suggested that use of intravenous albumin may inhibit the therapeutic responses to glucocorticoids in minimal change disease (MCD, Yoshimura et al., 1992). On the other hand, some investigators believe that intravenous albumin may be regarded as a useful vehicle for augmenting the delivery of loop-acting diuretics to tubular sites of action as mentioned previously. A natriuresis can be potentiated by the concomitant administration of a loop-acting diuretic and hyperoncotic albumin (furosemide mixed with 25 per cent human serum albumin) in equimolar concentrations (Brater, 1993; Kirchner, 1993), but the effect is usually limited and of short duration. In addition, some clinical investigators have challenged the usefulness of intravenous albumin in the treatment of nephrotic oedema, either alone or combined with diuretics, based on an exhaustive survey of the literature (Dorhout Mees, 1996). Loop-acting diuretics circulate bound to albumin and are delivered to their site of action in the ascending limb of the loop of Henle via the organic anion secretory pathway in the proximal tubule. When hypo-albuminaemia is present, both the volume of distribution and the extrarenal catabolism of loop diuretics are increased. Less drug is therefore delivered to secretory sites in the proximal tubule and the urinary excretion is diminished, leading to a blunted effect, even at high doses of the drug.

Intrinsic unresponsiveness of the renal tubule and impaired gastrointestinal (GI) absorption of furosemide have also been suggested as potential causes of diuretic refractoriness (Kirchner et al., 1992) but this does not appear to be of major importance, at least in the usual case of nephrotic syndrome. Non-steroidal anti-inflammatory drugs (NSAIDs), including aspirin, *antagonize* and angiotensin-converting enzyme inhibitors *potentiate* the action of loop-acting diuretics. Although hydrochlorothiazide and acetazolamide are poorly effective when used alone, they may be useful in resolving refractory oedema if given before furosemide (Fallahazadeh et al., 2017). Another possible treatment of refractory or massive oedema may consist in the administration of Tolvaptan, a selective oral vasopressin V2 receptor antagonist (Shimizu et al., 2014; Park et al., 2015). In exceptional patients who are truly refractory to all oral or parenterally based treatments (including high-dose loop-acting diuretics, metolazone, and/or amiloride), a course of slow, continuous ultrafiltration using a highly permeable (polysulfone) dialysis membrane and a venovenous circuit with systemic heparin anticoagulation can be used for temporary relief of anasarca (Fauchald et al., 1985). Because the oedema in the interstitial compartment can be partially mobilized when serum albumin concentration is increased by ultrafiltration, rapid rates of ultrafiltration (3–5 L/h) are usually well tolerated. The development of acute kidney injury in nephrotic patients, which is not uncommon in MCD (see also Chapter 4), may contribute to diuretic refractoriness. Such declines in GFR may be due to severe diffuse foot process effacement that interferes with hydraulic conductivity of the glomerular capillary wall (Drumond, 1994). It is often reversible with treated using steroids.

Hypertension

Clinical features, pathogenesis, and pathophysiology

Elevation of systolic and/or diastolic BP commonly occurs in patients with glomerular disease, especially when advanced reduction GFR is present (Wanner et al., 2016). The degree of hypertension is usually worse and its frequency more common in the acute nephritic syndrome and much less prominent in the nephrotic syndrome, unless a severe decrease in the GFR is present. Rapidly progressive glomerulonephritis appears to be an exception, as severe hypertension is decidedly uncommon in this syndrome. Severe hypertension (and volume overload) can lead to congestive heart failure and encephalopathy in patients with the acute nephritic syndrome, but this seldom occurs in those with the nephrotic syndrome or rapidly progressive glomerulonephritis, due to primary glomerular disease. Patients with hypertension due to primary glomerular disease tend not to have the normal decline in BP during sleep ('nondipper') when studied by 24-hour ambulatory BP monitoring (Tamura et al., 2008). The underlying pathophysiology of hypertension in primary glomerular disease remains a subject of intense investigation but several factors appear to be involved, namely:

- Primary renal NaCl retention leading to expansion of intravascular and extracellular fluid volumes (see 'Introduction and overview'); this is especially important in the acute nephritic syndrome.
- Intrarenal activation of the renin–angiotensin system despite relative vascular volume expansion; plasma renin activity and plasma aldosterone levels are markedly suppressed in the acute nephritic syndrome, but they may be inappropriately elevated in the presence of extracellular volume overload.

- ◆ Activation of the sympathetic nervous system, perhaps a consequence of the central actions of angiotensin II.
- ◆ The release, at the level of the vascular endothelial cell, of vasoconstrictor substances (e.g. thromboxane, endothelin) or deficiencies in the generation of vasorelaxant factors (e.g. nitric oxide, prostaglandins) may also participate.

A more pronounced effect on systolic pressure with widening of the pulse pressure suggests a prominent volume-mediated component and/or an effect of the disease on vascular compliance. Acute post-streptococcal glomerulonephritis is a classic example of volume-mediated hypertension in which the renin–angiotensin–aldosterone system is markedly suppressed (Don and Schambelan, 1990). Chronic forms of glomerulonephritis nearly always show an admixture of volume-mediated and vasoconstrictor pathophysiology. The concomitant presence of hypertension and nephrotic syndrome may alter the distribution of fluid between the intravascular and interstitial spaces and thus blunt the expected prohypertensive effect of fluid retention. In some exceptional patients with nephrotic syndrome, 'secondary' hyper-reninaemia and hyperaldosteronism are present without hypertension, indicative of a reduced plasma volume. These patients usually have minimal-change nephropathy and the rapid development of nephrotic syndrome (Meltzer et al., 1979).

Therapy

The management of hypertension accompanying glomerular disease is very important not only to reduce the risks of cardiovascular disease (stroke, myocardial infarction, peripheral vascular disease, congestive heart failure), but also potentially to blunt progressive renal insufficiency (see 'Reduction in GFR and progressive renal failure'). National guidelines are available concerning the best practices for management of hypertension (Verbeke et al., 2014; Agarwal, 2013). The management of hypertension in glomerular disease is based on two fundamental precepts:

1. Dietary NaCl restriction and/or diuretics in order to affect the volume-mediated influence on BP, and
2. To reduce the vasoconstrictor effect of an inappropriately activated renin–angiotensin or sympathetic nervous system.

Thiazide (hydrochlorothiazide, chlorthalidone, indapamide) or loop-acting diuretics may suffice in many patients (Roush and Sica, 2016) but it will often be ineffective if not accompanied by NaCl restriction, particularly when short-acting agents such as bumetanide or furosemide are used. When GFR is normal, the natriuretic effect of the furosemide lasts approximately six hours and thus, if this agent is administered on a once-daily basis, *in the absence of sodium restriction*, once the diuretic effect has dissipated, the sodium-avid kidney will reabsorb sodium to an extent that the 24-hour balance will be neutral. Diuretics with more prolonged action, e.g. thiazides or chlorthalidone, will not have this disadvantage. However, the natriuretic potency of these agents is considerably attenuated when the GFR is <30 mL/min.

If NaCl restriction and/or diuretics do not 'adequately' control BP (see later in this section for a discussion of what constitutes 'adequate' BP control), then additional antihypertensive agents can be added. For a variety of reasons, angiotensin-converting enzyme inhibitors (ACEi) or angiotensin II receptor blockers (ARB) appear to be the agents of choice. The use of drugs interfering with the action of the renin–angiotensin system is preferred as they:

- reduce protein excretion, presumably because of their intrarenal haemodynamic and other BP independent effects (Cravedi et al., 2007);

- have reno-protective properties *independent* of lowering BP and even their antiproteinuric effects, thus reducing the likelihood of future progression to ESRD (see 'Reduction in GFR and progressive renal failure') (Maschio et al., 1996; Ruggenenti et al., 2008);

- are well tolerated and are associated with minimal side effects (except cough and occasionally anaphylaxis with ACEi) and a good quality of life;

- are quite effective for lowering BP, particularly when combined with thiazide and/or loop diuretics and/or NaCl restriction (hyperkalaemia, allergic reactions—including angio-oedema—and agranulocytosis are relatively uncommon); and

  - favourably affect myocardial remodelling in hypertensive states and may protect from development or progression of congestive heart failure, especially when combined with neprilysin inhibition (Solomon et al., 2016).

A common troublesome side effect is a dry, non-productive cough associated with the use of ACEi but not usually with ARB, and is perhaps related to change in bradykinin activity. Cough is seen more commonly in individuals of Chinese or Japanese ancestry, but may also be seen in Caucasians. Combinations of ACEi and ARB may produce more side effects, including acute reductions of GFR and/or hyperkalaemia, particularly when used in patients with advanced renal failure or underlying cardiac disease (Cravedi et al., 2007). Theoretically, ACEi may also reduce thrombotic tendency because they lower plasminogen activation inhibitor-1 levels (see 'Hypercoagulability'; see also Kerins et al., 1995). Other antihypertensive agents such as β-adrenergic blockers (propranolol, atenolol), combined alpha/betablockers (labetalol), central or peripherally acting adrenergic inhibitors (clonidine), α-1 receptor blockers (doxazosin), dihydropyridine or non-dihydropyridine calcium channel blockers (CCBs), and direct-acting vasodilators (e.g. hydralazine, minoxidil, nitroprusside) may also be quite effective in lowering BP (Campese, 1995), but are not preferred as front-line agents in glomerular disease with proteinuria. Non-dihydropyridine CCBs (e.g. diltiazem, verapamil) may also reduce proteinuria, but to a lesser extent than ACEi (Gansevoort et al., 1995). Dihydropyridine CCBs have little effect on proteinuria or may actually increase protein excretion rates. Dihydropyridine CCBs should not be given in the absence of concomitant ACEi or ARB in patients with primary glomerular disease and proteinuria. Combinations of loop-acting diuretics, ACEi or ARB, and non-dihydropyridine calcium antagonists may be useful in difficult-to-manage cases. Refractory hypertension requires a multidrug approach, but control of volume expansion with diuretics and NaCl restriction is a critical component of therapy. Dihydropyridine CCBs (nifedipine, nisoldipine, amlodipine) are quite useful adjunctive antihypertensive agents but they tend not to be associated with a reduction in protein excretion and may aggravate oedema (Gansevoort et al., 1995). Furthermore, these latter agents do not appear to have renoprotective actions, independent of BP lowering. Small doses of aldosterone receptor antagonists (spironolactone, eplerenone, finerenone) may be very helpful for the control of BP in those subjects (mainly diabetics) who do not respond favourably to thiazides or loop-acting diuretics agents or ACEi/ARB, but caution about hyperkalaemia is warranted (Schjoedt et al., 2006). This class of agents also possess antiproteinuric effects, independent of BP control (Roush and Sica, 2016; Bakris et al., 2015). Hyperkalaemia can result from use of these agents, but serious hyperkalaemia is uncommon, especially with finerenone (Bakris et al., 2015). If troublesome hyperkalaemia develops with combined RAS-inhibition and aldosterone receptor antagonism, new well-tolerated and effective oral potassium-binding agents (patiromer or sodium zirconium cyclosilicate) can be of value (Sterns et al., 2016; Bushinsky et al., 2016; Rafique et al., 2015). Antihypertensive agents that can be administered on a once-a-day basis are preferred for chronic therapy. Administration of doses at bedtime may be helpful for subjects with 'non-dipping' or early morning surge in BP elevations (see also Table 2.1 for a description of recommendations for treatment of hypertension). When hyperkalaemia develops consequent to use of RAS inhibitors and/or aldosterone receptor antagonists it can be treated with oral administration of potassium-binding exchange resins (such as sodium polystyrene sulfonate [exchanging sodium for potassium] or patiromer [exchanging calcium for potassium]; Bushinsky et al., 2016; Sterns

Table 2.1 Therapy of hypertension in primary glomerular disease.

Goals:	Maintain systolic BP of 120–130 mmHg and diastolic BP of 70–80 mmHg. Do not allow diastolic BP to fall below 70 mmHg if symptomatic coronary artery disease is present.
Agents:	Angiotensin converting enzyme inhibitors (ACEi) or angiotensin receptor blockers (ARB) are preferred. Use NaCl restriction and/or diuretics (thiazides, loop acting, spironolactone, eplerenone, finerenone) to augment effectiveness. Combinations of ACEi and ARB may be used in selected circumstances, with careful attention to serum potassium and serum creatinine levels. Adjunctive therapy with calcium channel blockers (CCB) may be used for optimal BP control. Change in serum creatinine and potassium levels should be monitored at frequent intervals during the first month of initiating therapy. If serum creatinine levels rise >25 per cent from baseline, therapy may have to be interrupted.
Dosage:	For monotherapy with ACEi or ARB, the maximum tolerated dosage should be used, preferably to assure both daytime and night-time control of BP to desired goals. Ambulatory monitoring of 24-hour BP may be needed. For combination ACEi and ARB therapy the maximum recommended dosage of each agent should be used, with monitoring of serum potassium levels.

et al., 2016). Patiromer may be preferred as it is better tolerated and does not have the disadvantage of adding sodium to the extracellular fluid. Sodium polystyrene sulfonate combined with oral sorbitol (to prevent constipation) can be associated with serious side effects such as colonic ulceration and perforation. A new zirconium-based potassium binder (sodium zirconium cyclosilicate; ZS9) is approved by the USFDA and will very soon be added to the armamentarium for hyperkalaemia (Rafique et al., 2015).

The extent to which BP should be lowered for optimal or 'adequate' control remains a subject of ongoing investigation and controversy and depends on the specific disease (diabetes or non-diabetes related) being treated, the age of the patient, and the presence of comorbidity such as coronary artery disease, or a prior history of stroke (Agarwal, 2013; Verbeke et al., 2014). While specific details remain under intense discussion, for the time being a goal of 120–130 mm Hg for the systolic BP and 70–80 mmHg for the diastolic BP (mean arterial pressure of around 92 mmHg) appears prudent, a least for younger subjects with little comorbidity. In elderly subjects, a goal of 140/90mmHg may be more desirable, but this has been challenged by the reports of the SPRINT Trial of non-diabetic hypertension (SPRINT Research Group, 2015). However, the application of these findings to patients with non-diabetic chronic kidney disease (CKD), including those with primary glomerular disease, remains uncertain (Taler, 2016; Chrysant, 2016; Covic et al., 2015). Acute lowering of BP to levels <120/80 mmHg in subjects with encephalopathy (or carotid arterial stenoses) may be hazardous due to reduction in cerebral perfusion. Intravenous, short-acting antihypertensive agents (e.g. labetalol, enalaprilat, nitroprusside) may be useful for severe hypertension and associated acute left ventricular dysfunction with congestive heart failure. In more chronic states, it is not known whether lower levels of BP (<120 mmHg systolic or <70 mmHg diastolic) will be associated with any better protection from progressive renal failure; a low diastolic pressure (<70 mmHg) should be avoided in older patients with established coronary artery disease because of the risk of impairing coronary perfusion, which is *highly* dependent on diastolic pressure gradients (Messerli et al., 2006). Twenty-four-hour ambulatory BP recordings may be useful to detect 'non-dipping' status, which is associated with a greater degree of left-ventricular hypertrophy and a higher mortality rate from CVD (Hermida, 2007).

Hyperlipidaemia

Clinical features, pathogenesis, and pathophysiology

Elevation of plasma total cholesterol and triglycerides is commonly found to accompany glomerular disease, especially in those situations associated with heavy proteinuria and hypo-albuminaemia (nephrotic syndrome); see Box 2.3, Vaziri, 2016). The lowering of plasma albumin concentration and the increased protein excretion contribute separately to changes in lipoprotein metabolism in the nephrotic syndrome (Shearer et al., 2001; Vaziri, 2016). The underlying pathophysiology of hyperlipidaemia is only partially understood, but it appears to involve both enhanced synthesis and decreased metabolism of lipoproteins (Vaziri, 2016). The characteristic perturbation seen in nephrotic syndrome is an increase in low-density lipoproteins (LDL), very low-density lipoproteins (VLDL), and/or intermediate-density lipoproteins (IDL), but no change or a decrease in high-density lipoproteins (HDL). Apolipoprotein B and apolipoprotein CIII are increased, but apolipoprotein AI, AII, and CII are unchanged. The ratio of apolipoprotein CIII/CII is increased and contributes to a prevailing state of inhibition of lipoprotein lipase. HDL_3 is increased whereas HDL_2 is decreased. The combination of reduced HDL_2 and increased LDL/IDL increases greatly the *potential* risk for atherosclerotic cardiovascular disease, especially with the concomitant presence of smoking, obesity, diabetes, hyperuricemia, and hypertension. Circulating levels of lipoprotein

Box 2.3 Lipid dysregulation in nephrotic syndrome

Increased

Serum Very low-density lipoproteins
Serum Intermediate density lipoproteins
Serum Low density lipoproteins
Serum Apolipoprotein B
Serum Apolipoprotein CIII
Serum High-density lipoprotein-3
Serum Cholesterol ester transfer protein
Serum Lipoprotein (a)
Serum Total cholesterol
Serum Chylomicrons
Serum Triglycerides (when serum albumin <2 g/dl)
Serum Pro-protein convertase subtilisin kexin type 9 (PCSK9
Serum Free fatty acid (FFA) to albumin ratio
Serum Angiopoietin-like 4 protein (normally sialylated)
Upregulation of hepatic acyl-CoA cholesterol acyltransferase-2
Enhanced HMG-Co-reductase in liver

Unchanged

Serum Apolipoprotein AI
Serum Apolipoprotein AII
Serum Apolipoprotein CII
Decreased
Serum High density lipoprotein-2
Hepatic lipase
Serum Lipoprotein lipase activity
apoE and apoCII transfer to VLDL
glycosylphosphatidylinositol-anchor binding protein—1
VLDL receptor in muscle and adipose tissue
Downregulation of PDZ-containing kidney protein
Reduced reverse cholesterol transport

Data sourced from Vaziri ND. (2016) Disorders of lipid metabolism in nephrotic syndrome: mechanisms and consequences. Kidney Int. 90: 41–52.

(a) [Lp(a)] and fibrinogen are also increased in nephrotic syndrome and may have an additive effect on atherogenesis and on the predisposition to thrombotic events (Stenvinkel et al., 1993; Agrawal et al., 2018). The synthesis and cellular expression of LDL receptors is diminished in experimental nephrotic syndrome (Vaziri and Liang, 1996; Vaziri, 2016). A role for circulating levels of angiopoietin-like 4 protein in hypertriglyceridaemia (via inhibition of lipoprotein lipase) in nephrotic states has been advanced recently from studies in experimental forms of nephrotic syndrome (Mace and Chugh, 2014; Clement et al., 2015).

The net effects of the complex disturbance in lipid metabolism in nephrotic syndrome are many (Vaziri, 2016):

   i. decreased fatty acid delivery to fat and muscle;
  ii. impaired VLDL and chylomicron clearance leading to hypertriglyceridaemia;
 iii. increased cholesterol production by the liver and increased serum LDL-cholesterol; and
  iv. impaired reverse cholesterol transport.

It has also been suggested that proteinuria per se results in a disturbance of lipoprotein metabolism, perhaps because of the renal generation or urinary loss of a lipoprotein regulatory substance (Garber et al., 1984; Vaziri, 2016). It has long been known that elevated serum lipoproteins can occur even in glomerular proteinuria unaccompanied by nephrotic syndrome or hypo-albuminaemia.

These lipid abnormalities observed in nephrotic syndrome have important long-term consequences which deserve careful attention and appropriate management (Appel, 2001; Vaziri, 2016), but there is as yet little evidence-based data (e.g. randomized clinical trials) to guide rational management. Observational and controlled trials have proven atherogenesis to be accelerated in hypercholesterolaemic states (high LDL and low HDL cholesterol), and this leads to an increased risk for cardiovascular disease (CVD), including angina, myocardial infarction, strokes, and peripheral vascular disease. Concomitant hypertension, heavy smoking, obesity, diabetes (insulin resistance), physical in-activity, and/or a positive family history of coronary artery disease promote the risk of CVD in patients without renal disease. By inference, it is believed that the abnormal lipid patterns seen in glomerular disease also predispose to accelerated atherogenesis and atherosclerotic CVD complications. It is also postulated that abnormal plasma lipid concentrations contribute to progressive glomerular injury (see 'Reduction in GFR and progressive renal failure'; see also Vaziri, 2016) as a form of lipo-toxicity, which might provide an additional rationale for the use of hypolipidaemic agents (or metformin) to reduce progression of

CKD (Kim et al., 2015; Izquierdo-Lahuerta et al., 2016). However, the benefits and risks of statin therapy to slow progression of renal disease (independent of its benefits for dyslipidaemia) remains unproven and controversial (Strippoli et al., 2008; Tonelli, 2008). Further randomized trials will likely resolve this controversy. Statins may have lowering effects on established albuminuria, but whether this will translate into better outcomes is unknown (Douglas et al., 2006). Nevertheless, attempts to reduce the pro-atherogenic profile of lipid disturbances in patients with primary glomerular disease are worthwhile.

Therapy

Unfortunately, the management of hyperlipidaemia accompanying nephrotic syndrome is only fully successful in restoring the elevated levels to normal values when the underlying cause is remedied and long-term complete remissions of proteinuria are induced (see Table 2.2). Dietary therapy consisting of reduced cholesterol and saturated fat intake is generally ineffective and can make the HDL_2 reductions worse. Restriction of total fat intake has never been proven to alter the natural history of atherogenesis in subjects with the nephrotic syndrome. Even with strict dietary prescription and full compliance, LDL levels will usually fall a maximum of 15 to 20 per cent from baseline values. The long-term use of agents which interfere with the GI absorption of dietary cholesterol (such as ezetimibe [Zetia˚]) or exchange resins (e.g. cholestyramine, colestipol, psyllium colloids, oat bran, sevelamer) is incompletely evaluated in nephrotic syndrome, and they cannot be recommended at the present time.

Table 2.2 Hydroxy methyl glutaryl co-enzyme A reductase ('statin') therapy for hypercholesterolaemia in the nephrotic syndrome (adults).

◆ *Lovastatin:*	10–20 mg once daily in the evening (80 mg/day maximum dosage)
◆ *Simvastatin:*	20–40 mg once daily in the evening (80 mg/day maximum dosage)
◆ *Pravastatin:*	10–40 mg once daily (maximum dose 80 mg/day)
◆ *Fluvastatin:*	20–40 mg once daily (maximum dose 80 mg/day)
◆ *Atorvastatin:*	10–40 mg once daily (maximum dose 80 mg/day)
◆ *Rosuvastatin:*	5–20 mg once daily (maximum dose 40 mg/day)

A vegetarian–soy diet supplemented with amino acids may achieve the best results, but long-term compliance and overall efficacy of this dietary approach is not well known (D'Amico et al., 1992). Oral administration of bile-acid sequestering agents, e.g. cholestyramine, colestipol, psyllium colloid, are able to reduce modestly the total cholesterol but are relatively poorly tolerated and may aggravate underlying vitamin D deficiency. The impact of PCSK9 inhibitors on hypercholesterolaemia of nephrotic syndrome is not yet fully evaluated (Vaziri, 2016), but animal studies appear promising. These agents have a powerful effect to lower LDL cholesterol and in non-nephrotic subjects reduce the occurrence of major atherosclerotic events. Whether they are equally effective in hypercholesterolemia in nephrotic syndrome remains uncertain (Haas et al., 2016; Morris, 2016).

Fibric acid derivatives (gemfibrozil, fenofibrate) are more effective for hypertriglyceridaemia but are not very useful for the hypercholesterolaemia which accompanies nephrotic syndrome (Grundy, 1990). They may also be associated with muscle injury (Bridgman et al., 1972) and impaired renal function (Attridge et al., 2013). Nicotinic acid (niacin) will lower both LDL cholesterol and triglycerides (as well as phosphate levels) and also increase HDL cholesterol, but it is not well tolerated at the high dosage required, and such therapy has not been shown to reduce the development of CVD; it may even be harmful (Kalil et al., 2015). Probucol may be a useful agent since it lowers LDL cholesterol concentration by approximately 20 to 35 per cent and it may have other beneficial effects as an antioxidant (Neale et al., 1994). Unfortunately, it may also modestly reduce HDL_2 levels further. No controlled trials of probucol have been conducted in patients with glomerular disease.

Hydroxymethylglutaryl co-enzyme A reductase (HMG co-A reductase) inhibitors ('statins') are the current treatments of choice for hypercholesterolaemia of nephrotic syndrome (Appel, 2001; Vaziri, 2016). International guidelines also recommend statins for prevention of atherosclerotic CVD in patients with non-dialysis-dependent CKD (Wanner and Tonelli, 2014). All currently available preparations (lovastatin, simvastatin, pravastatin, fluvastatin, atorvastatin, rosuvastatin, etc.) will lower LDL and total cholesterol by approximately 25 to 45 per cent (atorvastatin and rosuvastatin are the most potent) despite continued proteinuria (see Box 2.4 for a listing of preparations and recommended dosage). These agents cause no changes or only a mild-modest elevation in HDL_2 and are generally well tolerated but rarely they may produce rhabdomyolysis and even acute renal failure, particularly at high dosage or combined with fibric acid derivatives (or possibly cyclosporin). High-dose rosuvastatin may be particularly apt to cause such events, and aggravate proteinuria (Vaziri, 2016). Asian patients might be more susceptible to these effects. Unfortunately,

Box 2.4 Therapy of lipid disturbances in nephrotic syndrome

Prudent diet, low in total cholesterol and saturated fat (relatively ineffective); vegetarian/soy diet

Stop smoking

Modest exercise

Avoid excessive alcohol

HMG co-reductase inhibitors (lovastatin, simvastatin, pravastatin, atorvastatin, rosuvastatin, fluvastatin, etc.)

Probucol (may lower HDL_2)

Bile acid sequestering agents (cholestyramine, colestipol, psyllium colloid)

PSCK9 inhibition (?)

---

statins have no or very limited effects on Lp(a) or fibrinogen levels (Wanner et al., 1994).

Although lowering serum cholesterol levels with a statin has the *potential* for significantly reducing the risk of coronary heart disease events in patients with and without pre-existing coronary heart disease in the absence of nephrotic syndrome or renal disease, their effects on prevention or regression of atherogenesis complicating human glomerular disease or on the progression of renal disease (loss of GFR) have not been unequivocally proven in a large prospectively designed randomized clinical trial in nephrotic subjects (Strippoli et al., 2008; Tonelli, 2008). Thus, treatment is largely 'on faith' that modest lowering of an atherogenic lipid (but not to normal ranges) will be accompanied by a lowered risk of subsequent cardiovascular events. (Scandinavian Simvastatin Survival Study, 1994; Tonelli et al., 2004). The SHARP Trial has clearly shown that treatment of diabetic and non-diabetic patients with CKD and proteinuria reduces the occurrence of atherosclerotic CVD events, but only in non-dialysis-dependent patients, but such treatment does not modify the progressive course of CKD (Baigent et al., 2011; Haynes et al., 2014).

The overall cost of this therapy is relatively high and the very long-term benefits (for survival) and the attendant risks uncertain, but most patients are so concerned about elevated total cholesterol and/or LDL levels that treatment can be justified as a means of reducing apprehension. Some evidence has been generated suggesting that statins given alone modestly reduce the level of proteinuria (Douglas et al., 2006), although at high doses in normal subjects they paradoxically increase albuminuria by interfering with tubular re-absorption of normally filtered protein by a direct action on tubules. Thus, for the present time at least, the indications for the use of statins in non-dialysis requiring CKD, even accompanied by the nephrotic syndrome, are the same as for their use in the general population (Clase, 2008; Wanner and Tonelli, 2014). Further evaluation in clinical trials (Vaziri, 2016) is necessary regarding the roles of PSCK9 inhibitors and acyl-coenzyme A:cholesterol acyl transferase inhibitors (Morris, 2016; Agrawal et al., 2018).

Regular moderate exercise, a prudent anti-atherogenic diet (low in total cholesterol, low in saturated and trans-fatty acids, low in fructose and sucrose, high in anti-oxidant content 'Mediterranean' style diet), complete avoidance of smoking, and rigorous control of BP (with ACEi and/or an ARB) and obesity may offer as much or more than drug management of serum cholesterol levels with respect to prevention of CVD and slowing the rate of progression of renal disease.

Hypercoagulability

Clinical features, pathogenesis, and pathophysiology

It has been known for many decades that patients with glomerular disease and marked (nephrotic range) proteinuria are at increased risk for venous and or arterial thrombotic or embolic events (thrombophilia), such as deep venous thrombosis (DVT), renal vein thrombosis, pulmonary embolism (PE), and arterial thrombi (Glassock, 2007; Mirrakhimiov et al., 2014; Christiansen et al., 2014, Kerlin et al., 2012; Barbano et al., 2013). This thrombophilic phenomenon has been attributed to an ill-defined hypercoagulable state in which an imbalance between naturally occurring pro-coagulant/prothrombotic factors and anticoagulant/antithrombotic factors promotes in situ thrombosis in deep veins or arteries (Glassock, 2007; see Box 2.5).

The biochemical nature of this thrombophilic state is probably multifactorial. The plasma concentration of fibrinogen is markedly increased in nephrotic syndrome. When this is combined with a low albumin level it leads to an almost universal increase in the erythrocyte sedimentation rate, irrespective of underlying inflammation. A mild thrombocytosis and increase in platelet adhesiveness and aggregability are also frequently present. Hypercholesterolaemia can lead to an increase in plasma viscosity. Urinary losses of proteins C, S, and antithrombin III may predispose to a low plasma concentration of these factors (Vaziri, 1983; Cameron, 1984), which tends to correlate with the severity of hypo-albuminemia (Huang et al., 2015). A genetically determined background of impaired resistance to activation of factor V (Leiden trait) may also

Box 2.5 Coagulation abnormalities in nephrotic syndrome

Increased (prothrombotic)

Fibrinogen
Platelets (and platelet adhesiveness)
Plasma viscosity (cholesterol, lipid)
Lipoprotein (a)
Plasminogen activator inhibitor
Decreased (antithrombotic)
Active protein C
Active protein S
Anti-thrombin III

predispose to thrombosis in the presence of these disturbances (Ridker et al., 1995; Sahin et al., 2013). Elevated Lp(a) levels may also contribute to impaired fibrinolysis (Kronenberg et al., 1996).

Evidence has accumulated linking local activation of the renin–angiotensin system with impaired endogenous fibrinolysis and a prothrombotic tendency. Angiotensin IV (AT-IV), a hexapeptide produced by the action of aminopeptidase on angiotensin II (AT-II), promotes endothelial cell synthesis of plasminogen activation inhibitor-1 (PAI-1) via interaction with an AT-IV specific receptor, not via the well-recognized AT-I and AT-II receptors (Kerins et al., 1995). Fibrinolysis may thus be inhibited leading to a prothrombotic state. It is possible that TGFβ (transforming growth factor β) is also involved in this interaction as angiotensin II is a strong promoter of TGFβ synthesis in tissue and TGFβ stimulates PAI-1 synthesis (Border and Noble, 1994). Angiotensin-converting enzyme inhibitors may reduce PAI-1 synthesis and because of concomitant elevated bradykinin levels, endothelial cell synthesis of tissue plasminogen activator (tPA) is enhanced (Kerins et al., 1995). The net effect of ACEi is to tilt the tPA/PAI-2 ratio in favour of a profibrinolytic rather than a prothrombotic state. ARBs would not be expected to have as favourable an effect on this ratio, and could even theoretically promote increased PAI-1 levels because of high AT-II (and thereby AT-IV) levels (Johnston, 1995). Similarly, diuretics that promote activation of the renin–angiotensin system and thereby the AT-II and AT-IV levels, could also promote a prothrombotic state by altering PAI-1 levels. High PAI-1 levels are known to be associated with increased risk of recurrent myocardial infarction in survivors of acute coronary thrombosis (Ridker et al., 1993).

Excess mortality from cardiovascular events in nephrotic syndrome (such as in membranous nephropathy (Lee et al., 2016; see also Chapter 6) could theoretically be explained, at least in part, by both hyperlipidaemia-related increased atherogenesis and a prothrombotic state induced by elevated PAI-1 evels driven by an activated renin–angiotensin system. Other concomitant processes such antiphospholipid auto-antibodies (usually seen in connection with systemic lupus erythematosus) and antiplasminogen auto-antibodies seen in systemic vasculitis (Anti-PR3 systemic vasculitis) may greatly affect the tendency to thrombosis in these diseases (Merkel et al., 2005; Bu et al., 2008). Anti-enolase auto-antibodies, strongly associated with membranous nephropathy and exerting an antifibrinolytic effect, could also be involved in the marked tendency of this disorder for thrombosis (Wakui et al., 1999).

Many of the disturbances associated with the thrombophilic state in nephrotic syndrome are correlated with the magnitude of depression of serum albumin levels or the ratio of proteinuria to serum albumin levels (Mahmoodi et al., 2008; Huang et al., 2015; Glassock, 2007; Lionaki et al., 2012). The concentration of albumin may therefore be used as 'surrogate' to approximate the magnitude of the hypercoagulable state and thereby the potential risk of thrombo-embolic events. Serum albumin concentrations <2.5–2.8 g/dl appear to be associated with an increased risk of thrombo-embolism. High levels of fibrinogen, low plasminogen activity, low antithrombin III, and high levels of PAI-1 may also predict the tendency for thrombosis (Glassock, 2007). A preceding thrombotic event (such as a DVT), recent abdominal, gynaecologic, or orthopaedic surgery, recent trauma, the presence of a lupus anticoagulant (antiphospholipid antibody), an antiplasminogen antibody, systemic vasculitis (Anti-PR3 systemic vasculitis), prolonged inactivity, obesity, and a family history of thrombophilia (such as might be present with a factor V Leiden trait), use of prothrombotic drugs (oral contraceptives), and use of central venous catheters are all predisposing factors for thrombotic events (Glassock, 2007; Kerlin et al., 2009; Mahmoodi et al., 2008; Mirrakhimov et al., 2014). The presence of *one or more* of these predisposing factors should influence the decision regarding use of measures to prevent thrombosis (oral anticoagulation with warfarin or use of heparin or enoxaparin) in individual patients (Glassock, 2007). The risk of thrombo-embolic events is highest in the first three months after development of nephrotic syndromes, but often continues for as long as the nephrotic state persists (Christiansen et al., 2014).

It also must be appreciated that the tendency for thrombosis is not uniform among the primary glomerular diseases leading to the nephrotic syndrome.

The disorders most prominently associated with thrombophilia are membranous nephropathy (MN), membrano-proliferative glomerulonephritis (MPGN), focal and segmental glomerulosclerosis (FSGS), and minimal change disease (Glassock, 2007; Mirrakhimov et al., 2014; Mahmoodi et al., 2008; Lionaki et al., 2012). The reasons underlying these disparities are incompletely understood. MN has been best studied (Glassock, 2007; Lionaki et al., 2012). DVT and/or renal vein thrombosis (RVT) may develop. The combined burden of both DVT and RVT in MN has been estimated to be about 45 per cent (Zhang et al., 2014). The development of RVT in MN is highly variable with reported prevalence ranging from 1.6 per cent to 60 per cent. The development of DVT is highly dependent on serum albumin concentration. A DVT prevalence of <3 per cent has been reported in those with a serum albumin >2.5 g/dl and 40 per cent in those with a serum albumin level of <2.5 g/dl (Bellomo and Atkins, 1993). A threshold value for serum albumin of <2.8 gm/dl was associated with the highest risk of venous thrombo-embolism in a study of MN (Lionaki et al., 2012). In many cases, the DVT or RVT are asymptomatic. Ventilation-perfusion lung abnormalities can be found in about 10 per cent of asymptomatic patients without any overt RVT or DVT, and in about 20 per cent of those with RVT alone accompanying the nephrotic syndrome. Higher values have been reported when pulmonary angiography is used for diagnosis. Thus, all patients with nephrotic syndrome should be considered at increased risk for thrombotic events, but those with MN, MPGN, MCD, and perhaps FSGS, appear to be at the highest risk, especially with the rapid development of severe nephrotic syndrome and profound hypo-albuminaemia. DVT is the most common, but spontaneous arterial thrombosis (pulmonary artery, axillary artery) may also occur when the nephrotic syndrome is very severe (Glassock, 2007). PE is the most feared and potentially lethal complication of thrombophilia in nephrotic syndrome. The diagnosis of venous thrombo-embolism rests on a high index of suspicion, physical examination, noninvasive testing for DVT, pulmonary ventilation-perfusion scans, CT scans (for RVT and PE) and often pulmonary angiography. Plasma D-dimer value may be greatly elevated, but nephrotic syndrome also increases D-dimer levels even in the absence of known DVT (Sexton et al., 2012). A normal plasma D-dimer value would make VTE unlikely. The Wells criteria for suspecting a PE may not be applicable to nephrotic syndrome, as emboli may originate from RVT. Serum albumin level is also not a variable in the Wells criteria. A spontaneous prolongation of the prothrombin time or severe thrombopaenia may be a sign of massive PE (Zhang et al., 2014).

Prophylaxis and therapy

Management of the thrombo-embolic complications of the thrombophilic state accompanying nephrotic syndrome in glomerular diseases may be divided into *prophylactic* and *therapeutic* strategies. As discussed, certain categories of renal diseases appear to be at higher risk for thrombo-embolic events, not entirely explained by the magnitude of proteinuria or hypo-albuminaemia. Such patients may be candidates for *prophylactic* anticoagulation with long-term oral warfarin or short-term anticoagulation with parenteral high molecular weight heparin or low molecular weight heparin derivatives, or even new oral anticoagulants (NOACs) to prevent thrombo-embolic phenomena (e.g. DVT, RVT, PE, arterial thrombosis). The NOACs (direct thrombin inhibitors or direct factor Xa inhibitors) have been sporadically used for treating thrombosis in NS rather than for prophylaxis in nephrotic subjects (Sexton et al., 2018). Decision analyses as well as systematic reviews have shown that an approach using oral warfarin theoretically will reduce the overall risk for serious thrombo-embolic events (e.g. PE) in excess of the induction of serious bleeding manifestations (Sarasin and Schifferli, 1994; Glassock, 2007) in subjects with nephrotic syndrome due to MN. A highly personalized approach employing decision analysis is preferred. However, no prospective randomized controlled studies have ever examined the overall efficacy and safety of a prophylactic approach to anticoagulation for patients with the nephrotic syndrome judged clinically to be at high risk for thrombo-embolic phenomenon, including those with MN. It is noteworthy that thrombo-embolism is rare in the 'placebo' arm of reports of controlled trials of therapy in MN (Glassock, 2007). It is unknown whether prophylactic oral warfarin anticoagulation is indicated in other glomerular diseases associated with hypo-albuminaemia. Short-term prophylactic, low-dose, subcutaneous heparin or enoxaparin may be indicated in patients with severe nephrotic syndrome who are massively oedematous and who are placed on bed rest or hospitalized for diuresis, trauma, surgery, or congestive heart failure (Medjeral-Thomas et al., 2014). Low molecular weight heparin should be used with caution in subjects with reduced renal function and only with appropriate dosage adjustment. Low-dose oral aspirin in nephrotic patients with higher levels of serum albumin could also theoretically be of benefit; however, this has not been proven in a randomized clinical trial (Medjeral-Thomas et al., 2014; Hofstra and Wetzels, 2016). A profound reduction in antithrombin III levels may be associated with resistance to the heparin anticoagulant effect. Patients with the Leiden trait (discussed earlier) may be at special risk and therefore may be candidates for a prophylactic approach (Glassock, 2007). A family history of venous thrombosis should always be sought and if positive, serious consideration should be given to prophylactic anticoagulation. The risk of anticoagulation cannot be overlooked, especially in the elderly and those with CNS or GI lesions (Glassock, 2007).

In summary, the decision to employ *prophylactic* anticoagulation in subjects with the nephrotic syndrome is dependent upon various factors, which include:

- The nature of the underlying disease (e.g. MN, MCD, FSGS);
- The severity of the nephrotic state (especially the level of serum albumin) and the rapidity of its onset (a high haemoglobin level may be a sign of plasma volume depletion which can promote thrombosis);
- The presence or absence of other predisposing factors (e.g. immobility, CHF, obesity, a family history of thrombophilia);
- A prior history of thrombosis; and
- The risks of anticoagulation (e.g. a central nervous system lesion, a prior history of GI bleeding, advanced age).

The final decision can only be made on a case-by-case basis (Glassock, 2007), aided by decision analysis algorithms (Lee et al., 2016).

Patients who have already experienced a thrombo-embolic event, such as DVT or PE, should be treated with long-term oral warfarin, after an initial course of intravenous standard high or low molecular weight heparin, unless some serous contraindication exists. Warfarin should never be administered alone, without initial heparin anticoagulation, because deficiency in active protein C and/or S may increase the risk of warfarin-induced skin necrosis. The warfarin should be continued for as long as the patients have marked hypo-albuminaemia (<2.8 gm/dl) and abundant proteinuria. The precise 'cut-off-point' for continuing or discontinuing warfarin is unknown, but it would be prudent to consider withdrawal of warfarin after *at least* six months of therapy if serum albumin is above 2.8–3.0 g/dl and urine protein is <3.5 g/day. The international normalized ratio (INR) for prothrombin time should be followed with the goal of maintaining the INR at about 1.8–2.0. Values over 3.0 are be associated with a marked increase in the risk of bleeding, particularly in the elderly. Values for INR between 2.0 and 2.9 are associated with a low risk of bleeding (about 5/100 patient years of treatment, but this risk may be higher in elderly subjects).

Initially, a search for an origination site of the thrombosis (DVT and/or RVT) in patients with an *overt* PE may not be very useful, since long-term anticoagulants will be used irrespective of the source of emboli. Patients with repeated episodes of PE despite anticoagulation should probably receive percutaneously placed inferior vena cava filters positioned above the renal veins.

The investigation of patients having *no* clinical, laboratory, or radiologic evidence of a thrombo-embolic event for the existence of a *covert* thrombosis, e.g. RVT or asymptomatic DVT, is probably not routinely warranted, especially if prophylactic warfarin is to be administered in any case, based on the individualized assessment of risks and benefits. Non-invasive screening studies, e.g. duplex Doppler ultrasonography, magnetic resonance imaging, are relatively sensitive and specific for RVT, but contrast CT venography is now the standard used for these comparisons (Rostoker et al., 1992; Zhang et al., 2014). Zhang and colleagues' (2014) study involving 512 nephrotic patients prospectively examined by CT angiography and CT renal venous angiography showed that 35 per cent had PE (28 per cent) and/or RVT (7 per cent). Most patients with PE were asymptomatic.

In most situations, a non-invasive test would be considered adequate and renal venous CT angiography is seldom required. At present, despite the demonstrated utility of these noninvasive studies, there is little reason to investigate asymptomatic patients for occult renal-vein or DVT since a *negative* noninvasive screening study at a particular point in time does not mean that a thrombosis cannot develop later. A *positive* non-invasive screening study, even in the absence of an *overt* PE, would likely be an indication for consideration of anticoagulation, but there are no studies to evaluate the safety or efficacy of such an approach to investigation and treatment in asymptomatic patients (Glassock, 2007).

Proteinuria and hypo-albuminaemia

Clinical features, pathogenesis, and pathophysiology

The mechanisms underlying proteinuria and hypo-albuminaemia in glomerular disease have been the subject of many recent reviews (Haraldsson et al., 2008; Cara-Fuentes et al., 2016). Proteinuria in glomerular disease is believed to be a consequence of a breakdown in the permselectivity barrier of the glomerular capillary wall (comprised of the endothelial cell, glomerular basement membrane, and the slit-pore diaphragm of the podocyte), although this time-honoured concept has been recently challenged by some experimental observations suggesting a role for impaired, proximal tubular reclamation of normally filtered proteins (Russo et al., 2007). Plasma proteins, principally albumin but including other plasma proteins as well, are allowed to pass through the glomerular capillary wall and into Bowman's space in variable amounts. The reabsorption of the filtered proteins is governed by the activity of cubulin and megalin in the brush border of the proximal tubular epithelial cell. The maximum tubular protein reabsorptive capacity is quickly exceeded resulting in overt proteinuria, which can range from barely above normal (200 mg/day) to massive (>20 g/day). Values >3.5 g/day in the adult signify nephrotic-range proteinuria (Glassock et al., 2015) and when accompanied by a serum albumin level below the lower limit of normal, the additional designation of nephrotic syndrome is appropriate (Glassock et al., 2015). The overall quantity of protein excreted above 3.5 g/day has little diagnostic significance per se, although 'massive' proteinuria (>20 g/day) is most commonly seen in amyloidosis, FSGS (collapsing variant), MN, and MCN. The excretion of higher molecular weight proteins in the urine (IgG, IgM-'non-selective' proteinuria) is thought to represent a more severe permselectivity defect and a greater degree of glomerular pathologic alterations (e.g. that seen in FSGS). The depression in serum albumin concentration and total-body albumin mass is the result of both increased renal catabolism and urinary excretion of albumin accompanied by an augmentation of hepatic albumin synthesis, which is insufficient to offset catabolic and excretory losses (Kaysen, 1993b). Alteration in the plasma and interstitial distribution of albumin may also contribute to altered plasma concentration. Hypo-albuminaemia is not the inevitable consequence of nephrotic-range proteinuria. Modest levels of nephrotic-range proteinuria (e.g. 4–6 g/day) can be well tolerated by well-nourished, robust individuals and serum albumin concentrations may remain normal presumably because of augmented hepatic synthesis (or alternatively, to slower rates of transfer of albumin into the interstitial space). Urinary protein excretion rates are also influenced by dietary protein intake, transglomerular hydraulic pressure gradients, serum protein concentrations, and GFR (Kaysen, 1993a). Increased dietary protein intake will augment urinary protein excretion and vice versa (Hutchinson et al., 1995). Lowered glomerular capillary pressure, as a result of ACEi- or ARB-induced efferent glomerular arteriolar dilatation, will lower urinary protein excretion (Gansevoort et al., 1995; Hutchinson et al., 1995; Hemmelder et al., 1996). Abnormal traffic of filtered protein along and through tubular epithelial cells can induce a phenotypic transformation in these cells, which then promotes local inflammation and fibrosis contributing to the progressive nature of renal disease (Abbate et al., 2006).

The degree of proteinuria seen in glomerular disease is generally classified according to quantity. Non-nephrotic or 'sub-nephrotic' proteinuria is generally defined as protein excretion between 0.5 and 3.5 g/day, while 'nephrotic' proteinuria is judged to be present when >3.5 g/day of protein are excreted in an adult (or 40 mg/h/m^2 in a child). Measurement of protein excretion based on 24-hour (timed) collections of urine has largely been replaced by random spot urine samples and assessment of protein (or albumin) to creatinine ratios (uPCR or uACR in mg/gm, mg/mg, or mg/mmol) due to the inaccuracies in timed urine collection. The values for the first morning specimen (obtained after overnight recumbency) will generally be less than that obtained during the day with normal upright activity—so one should always collect serial specimens at the same time of the day and under similar condition of hydration. However, even with meticulous care in specimen collection, the protein excretion rate in patients with glomerular disease can spontaneously vary over time, perhaps due to differences in physical activity, salt intake, or dietary protein intake. This sample-to-sample biologic variation is usually <20 per cent. A uPCR >3.0 mg/mg generally indicates a 'nephrotic range' proteinuria while values of <0.2 mg/mg would be regarded as normal. The accuracy of predicting 24-hour urine protein excretion for a uPCR (or uACR) value can be improved by multiplying the observed uPCR (or uACR) value be an estimated or measured urine creatinine excretion rate (Fotheringham et al., 2014; Abdelmalek et al., 2014). Measurement of uPCR on a presumed 24-hour collection or a 24-hour protein excretion is preferred for evaluation of nephrotic syndrome (Glassock, 2016).

It is vital to exclude 'tubular' proteinuria or 'overflow' proteinuria associated with primarily tubular disease or the presence of lower-molecular weight monoclonal proteins (light chains) respectively before concluding that the proteinuria is of glomerular origin. Tubular and glomerular proteinuria can co-exist. Elevated β_2 macroglobulin excretion relative to albumin excretion is a feature of tubular proteinuria. The 'quality' of the proteinuria, believed by some to have diagnostic, prognostic, or therapeutic significance, can be determined by measuring the rate of IgM, α, or β_2 microglobulin excretion, by assessing the fractional excretion of IgG (FE IgG), or by comparing the IgG to transferrin clearance in 'spot' urine samples (Bazzi et al., 2003; D'Amico and Bazzi, 2003; Deegens and Wetzels, 2007; Hofstra et al., 2008). The significance of these estimates of the 'selectivity' of proteinuria will be discussed further in the individual chapters that follow. It should also be stressed that the magnitude of proteinuria has different associations with the likelihood of progression of disease according to the individual diseases and is also influenced by gender (Cattran et al., 2008). The same amount on 24-hour proteinuria has much different associations with the rate of decline in GFR in MN nephropathy, FSGS, and IgA nephropathy. Nevertheless, the magnitude and persistence of proteinuria is an important determinant of the risk for progressive kidney disease and serves as a major target of treatment (Cravedi and Remuzzi, 2013). Both *time-averaged* and *time-varying* proteinuria may be useful metrics for evaluating the likelihood of progression and response to intervention, but the choice of an optimal metric may be, to some extent, disease-dependent (Barbour et al., 2015).

Therapy

It is obvious that the best approach to the management of proteinuria and hypo-albuminaemia in patients with glomerulonephropathies is to identify and correct the underlying disease. However, as pointed out in other chapters dealing with specific glomerular diseases (Chapters 5–11), this is not always possible. Exogenous infusion of hyperoncotic (salt-poor) human serum albumin will transiently increase the serum albumin concentration, but in the absence of any change in glomerular permselectivity, the infused albumin will be rapidly excreted in the urine, perhaps with adverse effects on glomerular and tubular structure and function.

Dietary measures that supplement oral protein intake are also often quite unsuccessful since urinary protein excretion almost invariably increases and total body albumin pools do not increase (Kaysen et al., 1998). Concomitant administration of ACEi and/or ARB will frequently reduce protein excretion rate by 30 to 60 per cent, depending upon the dose and prevailing NaCl intake (Gansevoort et al., 1995; Talal and Brenner, 2001; Pisoni et al., 2002; Cravedi and Remuzzi, 2013). These effects are probably mediated by intrarenal haemodynamic alterations independent of systemic arterial BP levels, but other specific effects of AT-II inhibition on glomerular permeability can also participate. In addition, a fall in systemic arterial BP appears to initiate the antiproteinuric effects of ACEi/ARB but the magnitude of the persistent antiproteinuric effect of ACEi/ARB are independent of the extent of BP reduction (Gansevoort et al., 1995). Modest protein restriction, combined with sufficient dosage of ACEi/ARB in the presence of restricted NaCl intake and/or diuretics, can not only reduce protein excretion rates, but can also increase the total body albumin pool and serum albumin concentration (Kaysen, 1993b). The addition of an inhibitor of the action of aldosterone (spironolactone, eplerenone, or finerenone), even in rather low doses not associated with a prominent risk of hyperkalaemia, can also lead to an additive antiproteinuric effect; it is not yet clear whether this effect is independent of the systemic arterial BP lowering effects of such agents. Active vitamin D analogues in addition to current regimens may also reduce proteinuria in CKD patients. In a systematic research of randomized controlled trials (RCTs) it has been observed a 16 per cent reduction of proteinuria in subjects given active vitamin D analogues compared to 6 per cent reduction in controls (de Borst et al., 2013). Such a treatment may also be useful to improve the blood levels of 25-OH vitamin D, which are usually reduced in patients with nephrotic syndrome (Aggarwal et al., 2016).

Combinations of ACEi and ARB given in maximum recommended dosages appear to have a greater antiproteinuric effect compared to monotherapy with individual agents also given in maximum recommended dosage (Kunz et al., 2008). However, this effect may be disease-dependent and is not seen in all primary glomerular diseases, and the risk of acute decline in GFR or hyperkalaemia may be augmented by such combination therapy. 'Supra-maximal' doses of some angiotensin-inhibiting agents may also have augmented antiproteinuric effects compared to 'conventional' doses, even though BP is not further reduced (Pisoni et al., 2001, 2002). The antiproteinuric response to ACEi and ARB, alone or in combination, varies among the categories of primary glomerular diseases (e.g. the antiproteinuric response to ACEi/ARB is poor in MN and in FSGS, but is very prominent in IgA N), and it is difficult to predict in individual patients what the response to this therapy will be in advance of a 'trial' of treatment, in adequate dosage. However, if urine protein excretion falls to 'sub-nephrotic' levels or below (partial remission) on such treatment and remains at or below this level, it is *likely* that the prognosis, in terms of progression to ESRD, is improved (Troyanov et al., 2004, 2005; Reich et al., 2007; Cravedi and Remuzzi, 2013).

The effects of ACEi/ARB on protein excretion rates may not be observed for several weeks and usually continue for several weeks once the drug is discontinued. The antiproteinuric effects of ACEi may also be related to polymorphisms in the ACE gene (Yoshida et al., 1995). Chronic administration of an ACEi may be associated with 'escape'—defined as a loss of the effect of ACEi on AT-II levels and aldosterone secretion rates (Werner et al., 2008). This phenomenon may have consequences for long-term use of agents in this class as monotherapy for proteinuria in glomerular disease.

NSAIDs, e.g. indomethacin, meclofenamate, ibuprofen, celecoxib, also exert a dose-dependent, antiproteinuric effect that is potentiated by NaCl depletion and which is independent of a change in GFR (Pisoni et al., 2001). The effects may be additive to the effects of ACEi in some circumstances, but are more rapid in onset and quickly dissipate when the drug is discontinued. NSAID will also interfere with the action of loop-acting diuretics and may, at times, cause acute renal failure due to an interstitial nephritis or acute tubular necrosis. The combination of ACEi and NSAIDs may also produce serious hyperkalaemia. For reasons of undesired side effects, NSAIDs are seldom used for their antiproteinuric effects.

Omega-3 polyunsaturated fatty acids (O3FA; e.g. eicosapentaenoic and docosahexaenoic acid) might have a modest and but inconsistent effect on proteinuria, but have only limited, and unconfirmed, renoprotective actions in certain diseases (Liu and Wang, 2012; Chou et al., 2012; see also Chapter 9 on IgA nephropathy).

In very unusual and fortunately rare circumstances, ablation of renal function by administration of nephrotoxic agents (such as high-dose indomethacin; 'medical nephrectomy') may become necessary if continued massive proteinuria results in severe life-threatening malnutrition (Glassock et al., 1995). Surgical bilateral nephrectomy or intentional arterial embolic infarction of the kidneys is seldom performed for massive proteinuria in current times.

GFR reduction and progressive renal failure

Clinical features, pathogenesis, and pathophysiology

Many glomerular diseases are associated with an acute or even progressive, albeit variable, degree of depression of GFR. In the acute nephritic syndrome, the loss of GFR may be quite abrupt and spontaneously reversible, even in the absence of specific therapy. In the syndrome of rapidly progressive nephritis, the loss of GFR may be abrupt or more insidious and, in the absence of specific therapy, the development of ESRD may be inexorable. In MCD, abrupt declines in GFR can also be observed (see Chapter 4). In the various causes of primary glomerular diseases, the decline of GFR is highly variable and depends on the persistence and magnitude of proteinuria and the level of control of BP (Cattran et al., 2008). Patients with 'symptomless' haematuria and/or proteinuria, by definition, have a normal GFR at the onset or presentation of disease, but in some instances, slow progression to ESRD may subsequently be observed.

The pace of development and progression of abnormal GFR varies widely among patients and between diseases and is determined by a multitude of factors (Jaber and Madias, 2005; Cattran et al., 2008). These include:

- the severity of the initial insult to glomerular architecture (proliferation, necrosis, obliteration of capillary network, obstruction or misdirection of the flow of the glomerular ultra-filtrate, and reduction of the trans-capillary hydraulic conductivity [Lp or Kf];
- the pathophysiologic response to injury (including maladaptive glomerular capillary hypertension/hypertrophy);
- the continued activity of the underlying disease process;
- concomitant systemic biochemical and circulatory abnormalities (such as hyperlipidaemia and hypertension);
- the noxious effect of proteinuria and/or haematuria on tubulointerstitial structure;
- the activity and dysregulation of the balance of mediator systems (such as complement, TGFβ, platelet-derived growth factor, and PAI-1);

- the loss of angiogenic factors contributing to capillary 'drop-out';
- the underlying genetic milieu and possibly gender; and
- nephron endowment at birth.

Each of these interact to determine the rate and manner of changes in individual nephron filtration rate as well as the extent and pace of nephron loss and thereby the concomitant decline in GFR and its potential for reversibility.

The level of renal function at the time of discovery of disease and during follow-up, the magnitude, quality, and duration of proteinuria, the severity of systemic and glomerular capillary hypertension and their control, and the extent of capillary loss, podocyte deficiency, tubular atrophy, and interstitial fibrosis stand out as major predictors of the long-term outcome of disease with respect to the eventual occurrence of ESRD.

Once a proportion of the functioning nephron mass is lost, a vicious cycle of events, unrelated to the initiating processes, is brought into play. Intraglomerular hypertension, residual nephron hyperfiltration glomerular hypertrophy, visceral epithelial cell (podocyte) injury, and tubulo-interstitial damage are principal components of these processes (Brenner et al., 1996; Taal and Brenner, 2001). Until we have a full and complete understanding of how the various pathophysiologic, cellular, and molecular events participate in progressive disease, our approach to ameliorating progression will remain relatively empiric, but as knowledge of these mechanisms improves so do the prospects for a rational and specific therapeutic approach to reduction, arrest, or even reversal of the progressive disease process (generically called reno-protection; Pisoni et al., 2001). Indeed, systematic clinical efforts to this end (renal remission clinics) are growing (Ruggenenti et al., 2008).

Increased filtration of protein and its eventual partial reabsorption by the proximal tubule is thought to play a major role in progression of renal injury (for a review, see Remuzzi and Bertani, 1998). Such events can lead to marked phenotypic changes in the tubule and the development of interstitial inflammation and fibrosis. The precise nature of proteins involved in stimulating this sequence of events and how injury to the glomerular filtration barrier produces their undesired effects is a subject of intense research interest (Remuzzi and Bertani, 1998; Kriz and LeHir, 2005; Zandi-Nejad et al., 2004). *Nevertheless, a reduction in urinary protein excretion (by whatever method) can slow the rate of progressive loss of GFR in many renal diseases* (Ruggenenti et al., 2008).

Assessment of GFR is the *sine qua non* for evaluating the degree of renal functional depression and its progression. Classically, serial measurements of serum creatinine concentrations have been used for this purpose. In recent years, formulae have been devised to use serum creatinine concentration to 'estimate' true GFR, since measurement of the 'true' value may not always be practical, e.g. estimated GFR (eGFR), corrected for body surface area (e.g. to standard body surface area of 1.73 m²; Stevens et al., 2006; Box 2.6; interested readers are referred to http://www.kidney.org/professionals/KDOQI/gfr_calculator. cfm for an online Internet-based calculation method). These formulas take into account variables of age, gender, and for some equations, race, and use a standardized method of determination of serum creatinine calibrated to a reference of isotope dilution mass spectrometry (Levey et al., 2007). These factors are added as 'surrogates' for the estimation of endogenous creatinine generation, a requirement for translation of serum creatinine levels into estimated clearance or GFR values. The CKD-EPI- creatinine equation is widely used, but other equations using Cystatin C as the biomarker of GFR may also have practical value (Inker et al., 2012; Levey and Inker, 2016). Many of the derived eGFR equations tends to have a negative bias (underestimate true GFR) at values above 60 mL/min/1.73m² and in the presence of marked obesity (Froissart et al., 2005; Issa et al., 2008).

Another formula, to estimate the creatinine clearance is the Cockcroft–Gault equation (which takes into account age and body weight and estimates creatinine clearance not adjusted for standard body surface, rather than GFR; Cockcroft and Gault, 1976). Creatinine clearance and eGFR equations using creatinine may be significantly altered (overestimate true GFR) in the presence of proteinuria and hypo-albuminaemia due to augmented tubular creatinine secretion (Branten et al., 2005). Current recommendations are to use the CKD-EPI creatinine or the CKD-EPI creatinine + cystatin C equation for estimating eGFR when monitoring patients with primary glomerular disease. The determination of whether the values obtained are normal or abnormal

---

Box 2.6 Estimation of the glomerular filtration rate (eGFR) by the modification of diet in renal disease (MDRD) abbreviated equation and the estimation of the endogenous creatinine clearance (C-G–Ccr) by the Cockcroft–Gault formula.

- MDRD eGFR (ml/min/1.73m² = 186.3 × (serum creatinine in mg/dl)$^{-1.154}$ × (age in years)$^{-0.203}$ × (1.212 if black) × (0.742 if female).
- C-G Ccr (ml/min) = (140–age in years) × (weight in kg)/72 × serum creatinine in mg/dl (× 0.85 if female).

should also take into account the expected decline in GFR with ageing and the fact that GFR is lower in females than in males, even after correcting for differences in body surface area (Wetzels et al., 2007). The variability of creatinine generation under the influence of drugs that modify muscle creatinine metabolism (e.g. corticosteroids) or tubular secretion of creatinine (e.g. trimethoprim) must be taken into account when interpreting serial values for eGFR using serum creatinine-based equations, which are based on a presumption of constancy of creatinine metabolism and renal handling. Cystatin C-based eGFR equations do not have this disadvantage, but they are affected by obesity, diabetes, inflammation, and perhaps by restriction of endothelial pore size (Cystatin C is a relatively large molecule—11,000 Daltons). A new formula, the full age spectrum (FAS) equation, may be particularly useful (Pottel et al., 2016).

Therapy

Obviously, eradication or control of the *underlying* disease process itself represents the best chance for improving GFR and preventing progression, providing it can be accomplished prior to the induction of irreversible or self-perpetuating injury. Falling short of this, consideration should be given to the employment of nonspecific strategies designed to ameliorate the pathophysiologic processes contributing to progressive renal damage, such as glomerular capillary (maladaptive) hypertension, proteinuria, glomerular and interstitial fibrosis, and capillary 'drop-out.' *Renoprotective agents* are a class of therapeutic compounds that affect these processes by slowing further nephron loss and delaying the development of ESRD, quite independent of control of the basic disease process itself (Pisoni et al., 2002; Ruilope, 2008). Control of systemic and/or intracapillary hypertension, reduction of plasma lipid concentrations, inhibition of thrombosis, retardation of fibrogenesis, promotion of angiogenesis to counteract capillary loss, and alteration of the regulation of cell cycle/cell growth could all be properly classed as potentially *renoprotective strategies*. ACEi and ARB both have renoprotective properties, independent of their BP-lowering effects, mentioned previously. Additional agents, including dihydropyridine calcium antagonists, do not have renoprotective actions, even though they reduce systemic arterial BP. Theoretically, HMG co-reductase inhibitors (statins) and NSAIDs may also be renoprotective, but RCTs are lacking, and the evidence for a beneficial renoprotective effect of these agents is weak or nonexistent (Tonelli, 2008). In patients with primary glomerular disease NSAIDs should be used with great caution and in the lowest effective dose due to their propensity to induce acute interstitial nephritis; they may also produce a fall in GFR because of haemodynamic effects.

Modest protein restriction (0.6–0.8 g/kg/day) combined with an ACEi/ARB *may* slow the rate of progression of renal disease in patients with heavy proteinuria and reduced GFR, i.e. 25–50 mL/min; see 'General management principles' (Klahr et al., 1994; Levey et al., 2006; Mandayam and Mitch, 2006; Menon et al., 2008), but protein malnutrition is a potential hazard of such an approach in patients with nephrotic syndrome. The benefit appears to be magnified by the concomitant use of ACEi/ARB.

As a class, renoprotective agents like ACEi/ARB should be considered in the management of *all* forms of glomerular disease accompanied by persisting moderate to severe proteinuria that have a demonstrated potential to progress to ESRD, providing contraindications to their use do not exist (e.g. hypersensitivity, hyperkalaemia, bilateral renal arterial stenosis). Patients with heavy and persistent proteinuria (>3.0 g/day), those with impaired GFR, and those whose renal biopsies demonstrate tubular atrophy and/or interstitial fibrosis should be considered as potential candidates for such treatment. Systemic arterial hypertension requires vigorous therapy, preferably with ACEi or ARB (see 'Hypertension'). The goal should be to reduce BP to the lowest level possible, usually 120–130/70–80 mmHg, around a mean arterial pressure of 90–92 mmHg, without impairing quality of life or inducing disabling symptoms. At times, three (or even four) drugs may be needed.

It must be recognized that the degree to which ACEi and/or ARB reduce proteinuria or delay the progression of declining GFR vary considerably between and among the individual diseases discussed in this volume. Thus, for example, a dosing regimen of an ACEi or ARB alone (or perhaps in combination) may be much more effective in IgA nephropathy than in MN. Unfortunately, very few large, long-term studies have been conducted in homogeneous groups of patients to provide information regarding the likely 'responsiveness' of the individual diseases to such therapy. In addition, the precise 'optimal' goals for proteinuria reduction have not been well defined for each entity (see Table 2.3; Cattran et al., 2008). In other words, reduction of proteinuria from 4 g/day to 2 g/day (a 50 per cent reduction) may have differing effects on the rate of subsequent progression of renal disease in each primary glomerular disease entity. It does appear that reduction of proteinuria is dose-dependent when an ACEi or an ARB is used, and that 'supra-maximal' doses (above those recommended by regulatory agencies and manufacturers) of these agents might have further beneficial effects on proteinuria without further lowering of BP (Pisoni, 2002; Weinberg et al., 2003). Combinations of an ACEi and an ARB are possibly more effective than either given alone in maximal recommended doses (e.g. in IgA nephropathy, less well understood in other lesions), but side effects (e.g. hyperkalaemia) need to be monitored more closely. It is vital to understand and

Table 2.3 The relationship of time averaged proteinuria (in g/d) to the progression of renal disease (in decline of eGFR in mL/min/year) in three primary glomerular diseases.

	Decline in eGFR (mL/min/year)					
	Time averaged proteinuria					
	<1 g/day	1–2 g/day	2–3 g/day	3–5 g/day	5–7 g/day	>7 g/day
IgA nephropathy:						
Males	<1	3.8	6.1	7.0	10.7	n/a
Females	<1	3.0	6.0	9.1	9.8	n/a
Focal segmental glomerulosclerosis:						
Males	2.1	2.5	3.1	4.0	10.9	18
Females	2.7	2.8	5.0	5.6	9.8	12
Membranous nephropathy:						
Males	1.3	1.5	1.6	1.4	4.0	12.0
Females	0.9	1.6	1.4	1.5	4.8	7.3

Data sourced from Cattran DC, Reich HN, Beanlands HJ, et al. (2008). The impact of sex in primary glomerulonephritis. Nephrol Dial Transplant. 23: 2247–53.

recognized the potential risks (hyperkalaemia and sudden declines in GFR). The addition of an aldosterone receptor antagonist in low dosage appears to have an additive effect on BP control and proteinuria reduction in patients who fail to achieve goal BP or proteinuria with ACEi and/or ARB; again caution must be exercised regarding the risk of hyperkalaemia in these combinations (Schjoedt et al., 2006; Chrysostomou et al., 2006; Epstein, 2006). When using ACEi and/or ARB for their antiproteinuric effects, careful attention is vital regarding the need for concomitant NaCl restriction, and the addition of diuretic appears to potentiate the antiproteinuric (and antihypertensive) action of these agents. Not uncommonly, the serum creatinine may rise (and the eGFR fall) following initiation of therapy with an ACEi and/or ARB. This is largely due to blunting of the intraglomerular maladaptive capillary hypertension and a reduction in the transcapillary hydraulic pressure gradients favouring filtration (due to efferent glomerular arteriolar dilatation). When the rise in serum creatinine is <25 per cent (e.g. a serum creatinine increases from 2.0 mg/dl to 2.3 mg/dl) one need not stop or modify therapy. However, progressive increase in serum creatinine above this threshold (e.g. serum creatinine increases from

2.0 mg/dl to 2.6 mg/dl), then the regimen should be interrupted. Such patients may have an underlying bilateral renal arterial stenosis or a unilateral stenosis in a solitary functioning kidney. ACEi and/or ARB can be used to retard progression even when the GFR is substantially reduced Hou et al., 2006); the risks of hyperkalaemia may require more intense monitoring, but adverse effects on eGFR may limit utility of ACEi/ARB therapy in advanced forms of CKD. A randomized trial to examine the effect of withdrawal of ACEi/ARB in advanced kidney diseases is in progress (Bhandari et al., 2016).

Fluid and electrolyte and acid-base disorders

Except for oedema, fluid and electrolyte disorders (hyponatraemia, hypernatraemia, hypokalaemia, hyperkalaemia, acidosis, or alkalosis) are uncommon in patients with primary glomerular diseases and well-preserved renal function and/or nephrotic syndrome or in the absence of treatment. Diuretics can be associated with hyponatraemia, hypokalaemia, or metabolic alkalosis. Inhibitors of the renin–angiotensin system and/or aldosterone receptor antagonists can be associated with hyperkalaemia. The anion gap is reduced when hypo-albuminaemia is severe in nephrotic syndrome, and the plasma bicarbonate may also be correspondingly elevated (Kraut and Madais, 2007).

General management principles

Patients with glomerular disease should be encouraged to consume a prudent diet, low in saturated fats, trans-fatty acids, cholesterol, and in NaCl content (6 g/day in the absence of oedema or 3 g/day in the presence of oedema). Caloric intake should be sufficient to maintain ideal body weight, around 35 kcal/kg. Caloric restriction is indicated in obese subjects with BMI >30 kg/m^2. Protein intake should be 0.8–1.0 g/kg/day plus any urinary protein losses if the GFR is >70 mL/min. Modest protein restriction to the level of 0.6–0.8 g/kg/day plus urinary losses could be used for patients with reduced GFR as long as malnutrition is not present. Protein should be of high biologic value and red meat should be discouraged. Fish, white meat, fruits, and coloured vegetables should be encouraged. A vegetarian/Mediterranean diet is best if the GFR is reduced. Increased protein intake (above 1.2 g/kg/day) is usually accompanied by increasing urinary protein excretion and, as mentioned, has little or no effect on albumin stores. Total fat should be limited to <30 per cent of total calories. Saturated fat should represent no more than 10 per cent of total calories. Cholesterol intake should be limited to 200 mg/day. Modest alcohol consumption (<60 mL of 30 to 40 per cent ethanol daily) is permitted. Supplementation of the diet with O3FA is permissible, but the benefits are uncertain.

Supplementation of the diet with antioxidant vitamins (e.g. vitamin C, ascorbic acid) is reasonable, but in the absence of malnutrition, supplementation with soluble vitamins B1, B2, B6, B12, or folate is not necessary; however, no harm would be done if such vitamins were given in doses equivalent to minimum daily requirements (especially to older patients). A normal intake of the fat-soluble vitamins E and K is suggested and supplementation is not needed. Oral vitamin D supplements (ergocalciferol, cholecalciferol) are useful in patients with heavy proteinuria, who are often deficient in 25-hydroxy vitamin D2 or D3 and may have a mild form of secondary hyperparathyroidism due to urinary losses of vitamin D combined with its receptor protein (Selewski et al., 2016; Agarwal et al., 2016). Oestrogen, androgen, and glucocorticoid-binding proteins are all excreted in the urine in excess in heavily proteinuric subjects (Harris and Ismail, 1994). Mild hypogonadism and altered glucocorticoid metabolism may ensue, but usually these abnormalities do not require active intervention. Copper, zinc, and iron are all excreted in the urine in patients with heavy proteinuria and deficiencies of these metals may occur (Harris and Ismail, 1994). Copper supplementation can be helpful for leg cramps. Zinc supplementation may be useful for dysgeusia, impotence, or poor wound healing. Iron supplementation is only indicated if iron deficiency is documented. Oral or intravenous (IV) iron preparations may not be efficacious if serum transferrin levels are very low due to excessive urinary losses not offset by enhanced hepatic transferrin synthesis (Prinsen et al., 2001). Oral calcium intake should be at least 1500 mg/day and supplementation of dietary calcium may be necessary. Phosphate intake need not be restricted unless GFR is <30 mL/min. Phosphate-binding compounds (calcium carbonate, calcium acetate, sevelamer hydrochloride or carbonate, lanthanum carbonate) can be prescribed if serum phosphorus is elevated, but the value and risks are uncertain. Aluminium-containing compounds should be avoided.

While less-frequently observed now than prior to the steroid-treatment era (circa 1960), infections remain a troublesome problem, particularly among children and in developing countries (Glassock et al., 1995). Not infrequently, spontaneous bacterial peritonitis may complicate severe oedema/ascites in children (Wang and Greenbaum, 2019). Encapsulated *Streptococcus* and *Hemophilus* species (e.g. *S. pneumoniae*) are frequently implicated, and in paediatric patients with severe oedema and ascites, a prophylactic approach with oral penicillin or IM benzathine penicillin (Bicillin˚) is indicated. Pneumococcal immunization programs may also reduce the incidence of this dreaded but now rare complication of nephrosis in children. The occurrence of fever, abdominal pain, and ascites is an indication for emergent paracentesis with culture and leukocyte counts. Cellulitis may become severe in profoundly oedematous patients and demands vigorous therapy with advanced generation cephalosporins and/or antistaphylococcal agents (e.g. nafcillin, methicillin, vancomycin, linezolid, daptomycin). Other localized and systemic infections, e.g. bacterial pneumonia, urinary tract infection, infectious diarrhoea, meningitis, can be treated in a standard fashion, taking into account the potential effects of hypo-albuminaemia and/or reduced GFR on pharmacokinetics and pharmacodynamics of individual agents. In patients who have or are receiving therapy with immunosuppressive agents, special care must be given to evaluation for opportunistic infections such as candidiasis, tuberculosis, toxoplasmosis, cryptococcosis, cytomegalovirus, herpesvirus, BK virus, or JC virus. Patients at high risk for human immunodeficiency viral (HIV) infection should always be studied with an appropriate serologic test for HIV antibody or by polymerase chain reaction (PCR) for virions.

IgG deficiency can arise, either from excessive urinary losses, extrarenal catabolism, or perhaps impaired synthesis (Giangiacomo et al., 1975). Sometimes this deficiency can be severe enough to impair the defence against bacterial infection (usually with encapsulated organisms). Exogenous polyvalent IV or intramuscular Ig replacement could be considered if bacterial infections are severe and recurrent. Vaccination with live, attenuated viruses is ordinarily well tolerated (but should be used with great caution in heavily immunosuppressed patients), although protective humoral immune responses may be impaired, particularly when renal failure is present (Garin et al., 1983). Some vaccines (e.g. Varicella) are well tolerated and highly effective even in the face of nephrotic syndrome (Furth et al., 2003) Although cell-mediated immunity may be impaired in patients with heavy proteinuria and/or mild renal insufficiency, there is no tendency for opportunistic infections unless severe renal failure is present or unless patients are receiving concomitant immunosuppressive therapy (Glassock et al., 1995).

To assess the benefits and harms of any prophylactic intervention for reducing the risk of infection in children and adults with nephrotic syndrome, the Cochrane Renal Group collected the RCTs and quasi-RCTs comparing any prophylactic interventions (pharmacological or non-pharmacological) for preventing any infection in children and adults with nephrotic syndrome. IVIG, thymosin, oral transfer factor, BCG vaccine, and Huangqi granules showed positive effects on the prevention of infection with no obvious serious adverse events in children with nephrotic syndrome. However, the methodological quality of all studies was poor, the sample sizes small, and all studies were from China; thus there is no strong evidence on the effectiveness of these interventions (Wu et al., 2012).

Regular aerobic or anaerobic exercise, and even engagement in competitive sport activities requiring short-time exposure to vigorous exercise, are not contraindicated. Indeed, such activity may promote fibrinolysis and prevent thrombotic events in those with the nephrotic syndrome. On the other hand, short-periods of bed rest may be advised for those with acute glomerulo-nephritis during periods of active NaCl retention and serious hypertension and oedema. Prolonged bed rest does not improve the chances for recovery from acute nephritis. Forced and extended periods of inactivity in overtly nephrotic subjects may have disastrous consequences by augmenting DVT or even PE. It is well appreciated that vigorous prolonged exercise (such as in marathon running) can result in an increase of proteinuria and/or haematuria. This effect is quite transient. While theoretically this can be harmful, no prospective studies have yet demonstrated that modest, regular exercise has any deleterious (or beneficial) effects on the progression of primary glomerular disease. Regular swimming may be the best advice, since it may be good for maintaining conditioning and does not apparently have any serious adverse effects.

Last, but not least, smoking should be avoided. Apart from the well- known risks for cancer and cardiovascular disease, smoking was reported to be a significant risk factor for future kidney failure in a large population-based sample (Hallan and Orth, 2011).

References

Abbate M, Zoja C, Remuzzi G. (2006). How does proteinuria cause progressive renal damage? J Am Soc Nephrol. 17: 2974–84.

Abdelmalek JA, Gansevoort RT, Lambers Heerspink HJ, Ix JH, Rifkin DE. (2014). Estimated albumin excretion rate versus urine albumin-creatinine ratio for the assessment of albuminuria: A diagnostic test study from the Prevention of Renal and Vascular Endstage Disease (PREVEND) Study. Am J Kidney Dis. 63: 415–21.

Agarwal R. (2013). Hypertension: KDIGO BP guidelines—more individualized, less prescriptive. Nat Rev Nephrol. 9: 131–3.

Aggarwal A, Yadav AK, Ramachandran R, et al. (2016). Bioavailable vitamin D levels are reduced and correlate with bone mineral density and markers of mineral metabolism in adults with nephrotic syndrome. Nephrology (Carlton). 21: 483–9.

Agrawal S, Zaritski J, Fornoni A, et al. (2018). Dyslipidaemia in nephrotic syndrome: mechanisms and treatment. Nat Rev Nephrol. 14: 57–70.

Appel G. (2001). Lipid abnormalities in renal disease. Kidney Int. 39: 169–83.

Attridge RL, Frei CR, Ryan L, Koeller J, Linn WD. (2013). Fenofibrate-associated nephrotoxicity: A review of current evidence. Am J Health Syst Pharm. 70: 1219–25.

Baigent C, Landray MJ, Reith C, et al. (2011). The effects of lowering LDL cholesterol with simvastatin plus ezetimibe in patients with chronic kidney disease (Study of Heart and Renal Protection): A randomised placebo-controlled trial. Lancet. 377: 2181–92.

Bakris GL, Agarwal R, Chan JC, et al. (2015). Effect of finerenone on albuminuria in patients with diabetic nephropathy: A randomized clinical trial. JAMA. **314**: 884–94.

Barbano B, Gigante A, Amoroso A, Cianci R. (2013). Thrombosis in nephrotic syndrome. Semin Thromb Hemost. **39**: 469–76.

Barbour SJ, Cattran DC, Espino-Hernandez G, Hladunewich MA, Reich HN. (2015). Identifying the ideal metric of proteinuria as a predictor of renal outcome in idiopathic glomerulonephritis. Kidney Int. **88**: 1392–401.

Bazzi C, Petrini C, Rizza V, et al. (2003). Fractional excretion of IgG predicts renal outcome and response to therapy in primary focal segmental Glomerulosclerosis: A pilot study. Am J Kidney Dis. **41**: 328–35.

Belge H, Gailly P, Schwaller B, et al. (2007). Renal expression of parvalbumin is critical for NaCl handling and response to diuretics. Proc Nat Acad Sci USA. **104**: 14849–54.

Bellomo R, Atkins RC. (1993). Membranous nephropathy and thromboembolism: Is prophylactic anticoagulation warranted? Nephron. **63**: 249–54.

Bhandari S, Ives N, Brettell EA, et al. (2016). Multicentre randomized controlled trial of angiotensin-converting enzyme inhibitor/angiotensin receptor blocker withdrawal in advanced renal disease: The STOP-ACEi trial. Nephrol Dial Transplant. **31**: 255–61.

Border W, Noble N. (1994). Transforming growth factor-β in tissue fibrosis. New Engl J Med. **331**: 1286–92.

de Borst MH, Hajhosseiny R, Tamez H, et al. (2013). Active vitamin D treatment for reduction of residual proteinuria: A systematic review. J Am Soc Nephrol. **24**: 1863–71.

Branten AJ, Vervoot G, Wetzels JF. (2005). Serum creatinine is a poor marker of GFR in nephrotic syndrome. Nephrol Dial Transplant. **20**: 707–11.

Brater DC. (1993). Diuretic resistance in patients with chronic renal insufficiency. In J Puschett, A Greenberg (eds), *Diuretics IV: Chemistry, Pharmacology and Clinical Application*, pp. 417–25. Elsevier, Amsterdam.

Brenner BM, Lawler EV, Mackenzie HS. (1996). The hyperfiltration theory: A paradigm shift in nephrology. Kidney Int. **49**: 1774–7.

Bridgman J, Rosen S, Thorp J. (1972). Complications during clofibrate therapy of nephrotic syndrome hyperlipoproteinaemia. Lancet. **ii**: 506–9.

Bu C, Li Z, Zhang C, Gao L, Cai G. (2008). IgG antibodies to plasminogen and their relationship to IgG anti-beta(2)-glycoprotein 1 antibodies and thrombosis. Clin Rheumatol. **27**: 171–8.

Bushinsky DA, Rossignol P, Spiegel DM, et al. (2016). Patiromer decreases serum potassium and phosphate levels in patients on hemodialysis. Am J Nephrol. **44**: 404–10.

Cameron JS. (1984). Coagulation thromboembolic complications in the nephrotic syndrome. Adv Nephrol. **13**: 75–97.

Campese V. (1995). Pathophysiology of essential hypertension. In S Massry and R Glassock (eds), *Textbook of Nephrology*, pp.1169–85. Lippincott, Williams and Wilkins, Philadelphia, PA.

Cara-Fuentes G, Clapp WL, Johnson RJ, Garin EH. (2016). Pathogenesis of proteinuria in idiopathic minimal change disease: Molecular mechanisms. Pediatr Nephrol. **31**: 2179–89.

Cattran DC, Reich HN, Beanlands HJ, et al. (2008). The impact of sex in primary glomerulonephritis. Nephrol Dial Transplant. **23**: 2247–53.

Chou HH, Chiou YY, Hung PH, Chiang PC, Wang ST. (2012). Omega-3 fatty acids ameliorate proteinuria but not renal function in IgA nephropathy: A meta-analysis of randomized controlled trials. Nephron Clin Pract. **121**: c30–5.

Christiansen CF, Schmidt M, Lamberg AL, et al. (2014). Kidney disease and risk of venous thromboembolism: A nationwide population-based case-control study. J Thromb Haemost. **12**: 1449–54.

Chrysant SG. (2016).The impact of SPRINT on the future treatment of hypertension: A mini review. Drugs Today (Barc). **52**: 193–8.

Chrysostomou A, Pedagogos E, MacGregor L, Becker GJ. (2006). Double-blind, placebo-controlled study on the effect of the aldosterone receptor antagonist spironolactone in patients who have persistent proteinuria and are on long-term angiotensin-converting enzyme inhibitor therapy, with or without an angiotensin II receptor blocker. Clin J Am Soc Nephrol. **1**: 256–62.

Clase CM. (2008). Statins for people with kidney disease. BMJ. **336**: 624–5.

Clement LC, Macé C, Del Nogal Avila M, et al. (2015). The proteinuria-hypertriglyceridemia connection as a basis for novel therapeutics for nephrotic syndrome. Transl Res. **165**: 499–504.

Cockcroft DW, Gault MH. (1976). Prediction of creatinine clearance from serum creatinine. Nephron. **16**: 31–41.

Covic A, Goldsmith D, Donciu MD, et al. (2015). From profusion to confusion: The saga of managing hypertension in chronic kidney disease! J Clin Hypertens (Greenwich). **17**: 421–7.

Cravedi P, Remuzzi G. (2013). Pathophysiology of proteinuria and its value as an outcome measure in chronic kidney disease. Br J Clin Pharmacol. **76**: 516–23.

Cravedi P, Ruggenenti P, Remuzzi G. (2007). Intensified inhibition of renin–angiotensin system: A way to improve renal protection? Curr Hypertens Rep. **9**: 430–6.

D'Amico C, Gentile M, Manna G, et al. (1992). Effect of vegetarian soy diet on hyperlipidaemia in nephrotic syndrome. Lancet. **339**: 1131–4.

D'Amico G, Bazzi C. (2003). Pathophysiology of proteinuria. Kidney Int. **63**: 809–25.

Deegens JK, Wetzels JF. (2007). Fractional excretion of high and low molecular weight proteins and outcome in primary focal and segmental Glomerulosclerosis. Clin Nephrol. **68**: 201–8.

Deschênes G, Gonin S, Zolty E, et al. (2001). Increased synthesis and avp unresponsiveness of Na,K-ATPase in collecting duct from nephrotic rats. J Am Soc Nephrol. **12**: 2241–52.

Don B, Schambelan M. (1990). Hyperkalemia in acute glomerulonephritis due to transient hypoproteinemic hypoaldosteronism. Kidney Int. **38**: 1159–63.

Donckerwolcke RA, France A, Raes A, Vande Walle J. (2003). Distal nephron sodium-potassium exchange in children with nephrotic syndrome. Clin Nephrol. **59**: 259–66.

Dorhout Mees EJ. (1996). Does it make sense to administer albumin to the patient with nephrotic oedema. Nephrol Dial Transplant. **11**: 1224–6.

Doucet A, Favre G, Deschenes G. (2007). Molecular mechanisms of edema formation in nephrotic syndrome: therapeutic implications. Pediatr Nephrol. **22**: 1983–90.

Douglas K, O'Malley PG, Jackson JL. (2006). Meta-analysis of the effect of statins on allbuminuria. Ann Intern Med. **145**: 117–24.

Drumond MC, Kristal B, Myers BD, et al. (1994). Structural basis for reduced glomerular filtration capacity in nephrotic humans. J Clin Invest. **94**: 1187–95.

Ellison DH, Wilcox C. (2008). Diuretics. In **B Brenner** (ed), *The Kidney*, 8th Edition, pp. 1646–78. Saunders Elsevier, Philadelphia, PA.

Epstein M. (2006). Aldosterone blockade: An emerging strategy for abrogating progressive renal disease. Am J Medicine. **119**: 912–19.

Fallahzadeh MA, Dormanesh B, Fallahzadeh MK, et al. (2017). Acetazolamide and hydrochlorothiazide followed by furosemide versus furosemide and hydrochlorothiazide followed by furosemide for the treatment of adults with nephrotic edema: A randomized trial. Am J Kidney Dis. **69**: 420–7.

Fauchald P, Noddeland H, Norseth J. (1985). An evaluation of ultrafiltration as treatment of diuretic resistant edema in nephrotic syndrome. Acta Med Scand. **17**: 127–31.

Floege J, Feehally J. (2015). Introduction to glomerular disease: Clinical presentations. In J Feehally, J Floege, R Johnson (eds), *Comprehensive Clinical Nephrology*, 5th edition, pp. 193–207. Mosby Elsevier, Edinburgh.

Fotheringham J, Campbell MJ, Fogarty DG, El Nahas M, Ellam T. (2014). Estimated albumin excretion rate versus urine albumin-creatinine ratio for the estimation of measured albumin excretion rate: Derivation and validation of an estimated albumin excretion rate equation. Am J Kidney Dis. **63**: 405–14.

Froissart M, Rossert J, Jacquot C, Paillard M, Houillier P (2005). Predictive performance of the modification of diet in renal disease and Cockcroft–Gault equations for estimating renal function. J Am Soc Nephrol. **16**: 763–73.

Furth SL, Arbus GS, Hogg R, et al. (2003). Varicella vaccination in children with nephrotic syndrome: A report of the Southwest Pediatric Nephrology Study Group. J Pediatr. **142**: 145–8.

Gansevoort R, Slinter W, Aemmelder M, et al. (1995). Antiproteinuric effect of blood pressure lowering agents: A meta-analysis of comparative trials. Nephrol Dial Transplant. **10**: 1963–74.

Garber D, Gottlieb B, Marsh J, et al. (1984). Catabolism of very low-density lipoproteins in experimental nephrosis. J Clin Invest. **79**: 1375–83.

Garin E, Sansville P, Richard G. (1983). Impaired primary antibody response and experimental nephrotic syndrome. Clin Exp Immunol. **52**: 595–603.

Giangiacomo J, Cleary T, Cole B, et al. (1975). Serum immunoglobulins in the nephrotic syndrome. New Engl J Med. **293**: 8–13.

Glassock RJ. (1997). Management of intractable edema in the nephrotic syndrome. Kidney Int. *58 (Suppl)*: s75–9.

Glassock RJ. (2007). Prophylactic anticoagulation in nephrotic syndrome: A clinical conundrum. J Am Soc Nephrol. **18**: 2221–5.

Glassock RJ. (2016). Evaluation of proteinuria redux. Kidney Int. **90**: 938–40.

Glassock RJ, Cohen A, Adler S. (1995). Primary glomerular disease. In **B Brenner** (ed), *The Kidney*, 6th Edition, pp. 1423–4. WB Saunders, Philadelphia, PA.

Glassock RJ, Fervenza FC, Hebert L, Cameron JS. (2015). Nephrotic syndrome redux. Nephrol Dial Transplant. **30**: 12–17.

Grundy SM. (1990). Management of hyperlipidemia of kidney disease. Kidney Int. **37**: 847–55.

Haas ME, Levenson AE, Sun X, et al. (2016). The role of proprotein convertase subtilisin/kexin type 9 in nephrotic syndrome-associated hypercholesterolemia. Circulation. **134:** 61–72.

Hallan SI, Orth SR. (2011). Smoking is a risk factor in the progression to kidney failure. Kidney Int. **80:** 516–23.

Haraldsson B, Nyström J, Deen WM. (2008). Properties of the glomerular barrier and mechanisms of proteinuria. Physiol Rev. **88:** 451–87.

Harris R, Ismail N. (1994). Extrarenal complications of the nephrotic syndrome. Am J Kidney Dis. **23:** 477–97.

Haynes R, Lewis D, Emberson J, et al. (2014). Effects of lowering LDL cholesterol on progression of kidney disease. J Am Soc Nephrol. **25:** 1825–33.

Hemmelder M, de Zeeuw D, Gansevoort R, et al. (1996). Blood pressure reduction initiates the antiproteinuric effect of ACE inhibitors. Kidney Int. **49:** 174–80.

Hermida RC. (2007). Ambulatory blood pressure monitoring and the prediction of cardiovascular events and effects of chronotherapy: Rationale and design of the MAPEC study. Chronobiol Int. **24:** 749–75.

Hofstra JM, Deegens JK, Willems HL, Wetzels JF. (2008). Beta-2-microglobulin is superior to N-acetyl-beta-glucosaminidase in predicting prognosis in idiopathic membranous nephropathy. Nephrol Dial Transplant. **23:** 2546–51.

Hofstra JM, Wetzels JF. (2016). Should aspirin be used for primary prevention of thrombotic events in patients with membranous nephropathy? Kidney Int. **89:** 981–3.

Hou FF, Zhang X, Zhang GH, et al. (2006). Efficacy and safety of benazepril for advanced chronic renal insufficiency. N Engl J Med. **354:** 131–40.

Huang MJ, Wei RB, Wang ZC, et al. (2015). Mechanisms of hypercoagulability in nephrotic syndrome associated with membranous nephropathy as assessed by thromboelastography. Thromb Res. **136:** 663–8.

Hutchinson F, Cui X, Webster, S. (1995). The antiproteinuric effects of angiotensin-converting enzyme is dependent on kinin. J Am Soc Nephrol. **6:** 1216–22.

Ichikawa, I, Rennke, H, Hoijer, J, et al. (1983). Role in intrarenal mechanisms in the impaired salt secretion of experimental nephrotic syndrome. J Clin Invest. **71:** 91–103.

Inker LA, Schmid CH, Tighiouart H, et al. (2012). Estimating glomerular filtration rate from serum creatinine and cystatin C. N Engl J Med. **367:** 20–9.

Issa N, Meyer KH, Arrigain S, et al. (2008). Evaluation of creatinine-based estimates of glomerular filtration rate in a large cohort of living kidney donors. Transplantation. **86:** 223–30.

Izquierdo-Lahuerta A, Martínez-García C, Medina-Gómez G. (2016) Lipotoxicity as a trigger factor of renal disease. J Nephrol. **29:** 603–10.

Jaber BL, Madias NE. (2005). Progression of chronic kidney disease: Can it be prevented or arrested? Am J Med. **118:** 1323–30.

Jacquillet G, Rubera I, Unwin RJ. (2011). Potential role of serine proteases in modulating renal sodium transport in vivo. Nephron Physiol. **119:** 22–9.

Johnston C. (1995). Angiotensin receptor antagonists: Focus on losartan. Lancet. **346:** 1403–7.

Joles JA, Koomans HA. (2001). Transcapillary fluid exchange in normal and pathologic states. In S Massry, R Glassock (eds), *Textbook of Nephrology*, 4th Edition, pp. 235–8. Lippincott, Williams and Wilkins, Philadelphia, PA.

Kalil RS, Wang JH, de Boer IH, et al. (2015). Effect of extended-release niacin on cardiovascular events and kidney function in chronic kidney disease: A post hoc analysis of the AIM-HIGH trial. Kidney Int. **87**: 1250–7.

Kaysen GA. (ed). (1993a). The nephrotic syndrome: Pathogenesis and consequences. Am J Med. **13**: 309–428.

Kaysen GA. (1993b). Plasma composition in the nephrotic syndrome. Am J Nephrol. **13**: 347–59.

Kaysen GA, Webster S, Al-Bander H, Jones H Jr, Hutchison FN. (1998). High-protein diets augment albuminuria in rats with Heymann nephritis by angiotensin II-dependent and -independent mechanisms. Miner Electrolyte Metab. **24**: 238–45.

Kerins D, Hao Q, Vaughan D. (1995). Angiotensin induction of PAI-1 expression is mediated by the hexapeptide angiotensin IV. J Clin Invest. **96**: 2515–20.

Kerlin BA, Ayoob R, Smoyer WE. (2012). Epidemiology and pathophysiology of nephrotic syndrome-associated thromboembolic disease. Clin J Am Soc Nephrol. **7**: 513–20.

Kerlin BA, Blatt NB, Fuh B, et al. (2009). Epidemiology and risk factors for thromboembolic complications of childhood nephrotic syndrome: a Midwest Pediatric Nephrology Consortium (MWPNC) study. J Pediatr. **155**: 105–10.

Kim DI, Park MJ, Heo YR, et al. (2015) Metformin ameliorates lipotoxicity-induced mesangial cell apoptosis partly via upregulation of glucagon like peptide-1 receptor (GLP-1R). Arch Biochem Biophys. **584**: 90–7.

Kim SW, de Seigneux S, Sassen MC, et al. (2006). Increased apical targeting of renal ENaC subunits and decreased expression of 11betaHSD2 in HgCl2-induced nephrotic syndrome in rats. Am J Physiol Renal Physiol. **290**: 674–87.

Kim SW, Frøkiaer J, Nielsen S. (2007). Pathogenesis of oedema in nephrotic syndrome: role of epithelial sodium channel. Nephrology (Carlton). **3**: s8–s10.

Kirchner K. (1993). Mechanisms of diuretic resistance in nephrotic syndrome. In J Puschett, A Greenberg (eds), *Diuretics. IV: Chemistry, Pharmacology and Clinical Applications*, pp. 435–44. Elsevier, Amsterdam.

Kirchner K, Voelker J, Brater D. (1992). Tubular resistance to frusemide contributes to the attenuated diuretic response in nephrotic rats. J Am Soc Nephrol. **2**: 1201–7.

Klahr S, Levey A, Beck G, et al. (1994). The effects of dietary protein restriction and blood pressure control on the progression of renal disease. New Engl J Med. **330**: 877–84.

Kraut JA, Madias NE. (2007) Serum anion gap: Its uses and limitations in clinical medicine. Clin J Am Soc Nephrol. **2**: 162–74.

Kriz W, LeHir M. (2005). Pathways to nephron loss from glomerular diseases-insights from animal models. Kidney Int. **67**: 404–19.

Kronenberg F, Utermann G, Dieplinger H. (1996). Lipoprotein (a) in renal disease. Am J Kidney Dis. **27**: 1–25.

Kunz R1, Friedrich C, Wolbers M, Mann JF. (2008). Meta-analysis: Effect of monotherapy and combination therapy with inhibitors of the renin–angiotensin system on proteinuria in renal disease. Ann Intern Med. **148**: 30–48.

Lainscak M, Pelliccia F, Rosano G, et al. (2015). Safety profile of mineralocorticoid receptor antagonists: Spironolactone and eplerenone. Int J Cardiol. **200**: 25–9.

Lee T, Derebail VK, Kshirsagar AV, et al. (2016). Patients with primary membranous nephropathy are at high risk of cardiovascular events. Kidney Int. **89**:1111–18.

Lee EY, Humphries MH (1996). Phosphodiesterase activity as a mediator of renal resistance to ANP in pathological salt retention. Am J Physiol. **271**: F3–F6.

Levey AS, Greene T, Sarnak MJ, et al. (2006). Effect of dietary protein restriction on the progression of kidney disease: Long-term follow-up of the Modification of Diet in Renal Disease (MDRD) study. Am J Kidney Dis. **48**: 879–88.

Levey AS, Coresh J, Greene T, et al. (2007). Expressing the Modification of Diet in Renal Disease Study equation for estimating glomerular filtration rate with standardized serum creatinine values. Clin Chem. **53**: 766–72.

Levey AS, Inker LA. (2016). GFR as the 'gold standard': Estimated, measured, and true. Am J Kidney Dis. **67**: 9–12.

Lionaki S, Derebail VK, Hogan SL, et al. (2012) Venous thromboembolism in patients with membranous nephropathy. Clin J Am Soc Nephrol. **7**: 43–51.

Liu LL, Wang LN. (2012). ω-3 fatty acids therapy for IgA nephropathy: A meta-analysis of randomized controlled trials. Clin Nephrol. **77**: 119–25.

Lourdel S, Loffing J, Favre G, et al. (2005). Hyperaldosteronemia and activation of the epithelial sodium channel are not required for sodium retention in puromycin-induced nephrosis. J Am Soc Nephrol. **16**: 3642–50.

Macé C, Chugh SS. (2014). Nephrotic syndrome: Components, connections, and angiopoietin-like 4-related therapeutics. J Am Soc Nephrol. **25**: 2393–8.

Mahmoodi BK, ten Kate MK, Waanders F, et al. (2008). High absolute risks and predictors of venous and arterial thromboembolic events in patients with nephrotic syndrome: Results from a large retrospective cohort study. Circulation. **117**: 224–30.

Mandayam S, Mitch WE. (2006). Dietary protein restriction benefits patients with chronic kidney disease. Nephrology (Carlton). **11**: 53–7.

Marino F, Martorano C, Tripepi R, et al. (2016). Subclinical pulmonary congestion is prevalent in nephrotic syndrome. Kidney Int. **89**: 421–8.

Maschio G, Alberti D, Janin G, et al. (1996). Effect of the angiotensin-converting-enzyme inhibitor benazepril on the progression of chronic renal insufficiency. The Angiotensin-Converting-Enzyme Inhibition in Progressive Renal Insufficiency Study Group. N Engl J Med. **334**: 939–45.

Medjeral-Thomas N, Ziaj S, Condon M, et al. (2014). Retrospective analysis of a novel regimen for the prevention of venous thromboembolism in nephrotic syndrome. Clin J Am Soc Nephrol. **9**: 478–83.

Meltzer JI, Keim HJ, Laragh JH, et al. (1979). Nephrotic syndrome: Vasoconstriction and hypervolemic types indicated by renin-sodium profiling. Ann Intern Med. **91**: 688–96.

Menon V, Wang X, Sarnak MJ, et al. (2008). Long-term outcomes in nondiabetic chronic kidney disease. Kidney Int. **73**: 1310–15.

Merkel PA, Lo GH, Holbrook JT, et al. (2005). Brief communication: High incidence of venous thrombotic events among patients with Wegener granulomatosis: the Wegener's Clinical Occurrence of Thrombosis (WeCLOT) Study. Ann Intern Med. **142**: 620–6.

Messerli FH, Mancia G, Conti CR, et al. (2006). Dogma disputed: Can aggressively lowering blood pressure in hypertensive patients with coronary artery disease be dangerous? Ann Intern Med. **144**: 884–93.

Mirrakhimov AE, Ali AM, Barbaryan A, et al. (2014). Primary nephrotic syndrome in adults as a risk factor for pulmonary embolism: An up-to-date review of the literature. Int J Nephrol. **2014**: 916760.

Morris AW. (2016). Nephrotic syndrome: PCSK9: A target for hypercholesterolaemia in nephrotic syndrome. Nat Rev Nephrol. **12**: 510.

Neale T, Ojha P, Exner M, et al. (1994). Proteinuria in passive Heymann nephritis is associated with lipid peroxidation and formation of adducts on type IV collagen. J Clin Invest. **94**: 1577–84.

Park ES, Huh YS, Kim GH. (2015). Is tolvaptan indicated for refractory oedema in nephrotic syndrome? Nephrology (Carlton). **20**: 103–6.

Passero CJ, Hughey RP, Kleyman TR. (2010). New role for plasmin in sodium homeostasis. Curr Opin Nephrol Hypertens. **19**: 13–19.

Paton R, Kane R. (1977). Long-term diuretic therapy with metolazone of renal failure and the nephrotic syndrome. J Clin Pharmacol. **17**: 243–51.

Pisoni R, Ruggenenti P, Remuzzi G. (2001). Renoprotective therapy in patients with non-diabetic nephropathies. Drugs. **61**: 733–45.

Pisoni R, Ruggenenti P, Sangalli F, et al. (2002). Effect of high-dose ramipril with or without indomethacin on glomerular selectivity. Kidney Int. **62**: 1010–19.

Pottel H, Hoste L, Dubourg L, et al. (2016). An estimated glomerular filtration rate equation for the full age spectrum. Nephrol Dial Transplant. **31**: 798–806.

Ponticelli C, Glassock RJ. (2009). *Treatment of Primary Glomerulonephritis*. 2nd Edition. Oxford University Press, Oxford.

Prinsen BH, de Sain-van der Velden MG, Kaysen GA, et al. (2001). Transferrin synthesis is increased in nephrotic patients insufficiently to replace urinary losses. J Am Soc Nephrol. **12**: 1017–25.

Rafique Z, Peacock WF, LoVecchio F, et al. (2015). Sodium zirconium cyclosilicate (ZS-9) for the treatment of hyperkalemia. Expert Opin Pharmacother. **16**: 1727–34.

Reich HN, Troyanov S, Scholey JW, et al. (2007). Remission of proteinuria improves prognosis in IgA nephropathy. J Am Soc Nephrol. **18**: 3177–83.

Remuzzi G, Bertani T. (1998). Pathophysiology of progressive nephropathies. N Engl J Med. **339**: 1448–556.

Ridker P, Hennekens C, Lindpainter K, et al. (1995). Mutations in the gene coding for coagulation factor V and the risk of myocardial infarction, stroke and venous thrombosis in apparently healthy men. New Engl J Med. **332**: 912–17.

Ridker P, Vaughan DE, Stampfer MJ, et al. (1993). Endogenous tissue-type plasminogen activator and risk of myocardial infarction. Lancet. **341**: 1165–8.

Rostoker G, Texier J, Jeandel B. (1992). Asymptomatic renal vein thrombosis in adult nephrotic patients: Ultrasonography and urinary fibrin–fibrinogen products: A prospective study. Eur J Med. **1**: 19–22.

Roush GC, Sica DA. (2016). Diuretics for hypertension: A review and update. Am J Hypertens. **29**: 1130–7.

Ruggenenti P, Perticucci E, Cravedi P, et al. (2008). Role of remission clinics in the longitudinal treatment of CKD. J Am Soc Nephrol. **19**: 1213–24.

Ruilope LM. (2008). Angiotensin receptor blockers: RAAS blockade and renoprotection. Curr Med Res Opin. **24**: 1285–93.

Russo LM, Sandoval RM, McKee M, et al. (2007). The normal kidney filters nephrotic levels of albumin retrieved by proximal tubule cells: Retrieval is disrupted in nephrotic states. Kidney Int. **71**: 504–13.

Sahin M, Ozkurt S, Degirmenci NA, et al. (2013). Assessment of genetic risk factors for thromboembolic complications in adults with idiopathic nephrotic syndrome. Clin Nephrol. **79**: 454–62.

Sarasin F, Schifferli J. (1994). Prophylactic oral anticoagulation in nephrotic patients with idiopathic membranous glomerulonephritis. Kidney Int. **45**: 578–85.

Scandinavian Simvastatin Survival Study. (1994). A randomized trial of cholesterol lowering in 4444 patients with coronary heart disease. Lancet. **344**: 1383–9.

Schjoedt KJ, Rossing K, Juhl TR, et al. (2006). Beneficial impact of spironolactone on nephrotic range albuminuria in diabetic nephropathy. Kidney Int. **70**: 536–42.

Schork A, Woern M, Kalbacher H, et al. (2016). Association of plasminuria with overhydration in patients with CKD. Clin J Am Soc Nephrol. **11**: 761–9.

Schrier R, Fassett RG. (1998). A critique of the overfill hypothesis of sodium and water retention in the nephrotic syndrome. Kidney Int. **53**: 1111–17.

de Seigneux S, Kim SW, Hemmingsen SC, et al. (2006). Increased expression but not targeting of ENaC in adrenalectomized rats wtih PAN-induced nephrotic syndrome. Am J Physiol Renal Physiol. **29**: F208–17.

Selewski DT, Chen A, Shatat IF, et al. (2016). Vitamin D in incident nephrotic syndrome: A Midwest Pediatric Nephrology Consortium Study. Pediatr Nephrol. **31**: 465–72.

Sexton DJ, Clarkson MR, Mazur MJ, et al. (2012). Serum D-dimer concentrations in nephrotic syndrome track with albuminuria, not estimated glomerular filtration rate. Am J Nephrol. **36**: 554–60.

Sexton DJ, de Freitas DG, Little MA, et al. (2018). Direct-acting oral anticoagulants as prophylaxis against thromboembolism in the nephrotic syndrome. Kidney Int Rep. **3**: 784–93.

Shearer GC, Stevenson FT, Atkinson DN, et al. (2001). Hypoalbuminemia and proteinuria contribute separately to reduced lipoprotein catabolism in the nephrotic syndrome. Kidney Int. **59**: 179–89.

Shimizu M, Ishikawa S, Yachi Y, et al. (2014). Tolvaptan therapy for massive edema in a patient with nephrotic syndrome. Pediatr Nephrol. **29**: 915–17.

Solomon SD, Claggett B, McMurray JJ, et al. (2016). Combined neprilysin and renin–angiotensin system inhibition in heart failure with reduced ejection fraction: A meta-analysis. Eur J Heart Fail. **18**: 1238–43.

SPRINT Research Group; Wright JT Jr, Williamson JD, et al. (2015). A randomized trial of intensive versus standard blood-pressure control. N Engl J Med. **373**: 2103–16.

Staehr M, Buhl KB, Andersen RF, et al. (2015). Aberrant glomerular filtration of urokinase-type plasminogen activator in nephrotic syndrome leads to amiloride-sensitive plasminogen activation in urine. Am J Physiol Renal Physiol. **309**: F235–41.

Stenvinkel P, Berglund L, Heimburger D. (1993). Lipoprotein (a) in nephrotic syndrome. Kidney Int. **44**: 1116–23.

Sterns RH, Grieff M, Bernstein PL. (2016). Treatment of hyperkalemia: Something old, something new. Kidney Int. **89**: 546–54.

Stevens LA, Coresh J, Greene T, et al. (2006). Assessing kidney function: Measured and estimated glomerular filtration rate. N Engl J Med. **354**: 2473–83.

Strippoli GF, Navaneethan SD, Johnson DW, et al. (2008). Effects of statins in patients with chronic kidney disease: Meta-analysis and meta-regression of randomised controlled trials. BMJ. **336**: 645–51.

Taal MW, Brenner BM. (2001). Evolving strategies for renoprotection: Non-diabetic renal disease. Curr Opin Nephrol Hypertens. **10**: 523–31.

Taler SJ. (2016). How Does SPRINT (Systolic Blood Pressure Intervention Trial) direct hypertension treatment targets for CKD? Am J Kidney Dis. **68**: 15–18.

Tamura K, Yamauchi J, Tsurumi-Ikeya Y, et al. (2008). Ambulatory blood pressure and heart rate in hypertensives with renal failure: Comparison between diabetic nephropathy and non-diabetic glomerulopathy. Clin Exp Hypertens. **30**: 33–43.

Tonelli M. (2008). Statins for slowing kidney disease progression: An as-yet unproven indication. Am J Kidney Dis. **52**: 391–4.

Troyanov S, Wall CA, Miller JA, et al. (2004). Idiopathic membranous nephropathy: Definition and relevance of a partial remission. Kidney Int. **66**: 1199–205.

Troyanov S, Wall CA, Miller JA, et al. (2005). Focal and segmental glomerulosclerosis: Definition and relevance of a partial remission. J Am Soc Nephrol. **16**: 1061–8.

Vaziri N. (1983). Nephrotic syndrome and coagulation and fibrinolytic abnormalities. Am J Nephrol. **3**: 1–6.

Vaziri ND. (2016). Disorders of lipid metabolism in nephrotic syndrome: Mechanisms and consequences. Kidney Int. **90**: 41–52.

Vaziri N, Liang KH. (1996). Down regulation of hepatic LDL-receptor expression in experimental nephrosis. Kidney Int. **50**: 887–93.

Verbeke F, Lindley E, Van Bortel L, et al. (2014). European Renal Best Practice (ERBP) position statement on the Kidney Disease: Improving Global Outcomes (KDIGO) clinical practice guideline for the management of blood pressure in non-dialysis-dependent chronic kidney disease: An endorsement with some caveats for real-life application. Nephrol Dial Transplant. **29**: 490–6.

Wakui H, Imai H, Komatsuda A, et al. (1999). Circulating antibodies against alpha-enolase in patients with primary membranous nephropathy (MN). Clin Exp Immunol. **118**: 445–50.

Wang CS, Greenbum LA. (2019). Nephrotic syndrome. Pediatr Clin North Am. **66**: 73–85.

Wanner C, Amann K, Shoji T. (2016). The heart and vascular system in dialysis. Lancet. **388**: 276–84.

Wanner C, Bohler J, Eckhardt H. (1994). Effects of simvastatin on lipoprotein (a) and lipoprotein composition in patients with nephrotic syndrome. Clin Nephrol. **41**: 138–43.

Wanner C, Tonelli M; Kidney Disease: Improving Global Outcomes Lipid Guideline Development Work Group Members. (2014). KDIGO Clinical Practice Guideline for

Lipid Management in CKD: Summary of recommendation statements and clinical approach to the patient. Kidney Int. **85**: 1303–9.

Weinberg MS, Kaperonis N, Bakris GL. (2003). How high should an ACE inhibitor or angiotensin receptor blocker be dosed in patients with diabetic nephropathy. Curr Hyperten Rep. **5**: 418–25.

Werner C, Baumhäkel M, Teo KK, et al. (2008). RAS blockade with ARB and ACE inhibitors: Current perspective on rationale and patient selection. Clin Res Cardiol. **97**: 418–31.

Wetzels JF, Kiemeney LA, Swinkels DW, et al. (2007). Age- and gender-specific reference values of estimated GFR in Caucasians: The Nijmegen Biomedical Study. Kidney Int. **72**: 632–7.

Wu HM, Tang JL, Cao L, et al. (2012). Interventions for preventing infection in nephrotic syndrome. Cochrane Database Syst Rev. (4): CD003964.

Yoshida H, Mitarai T, Kawamura T, et al. (1995). Role of deletion polymorphisms of the angiotensin converting enzyme gene in the progression and therapeutic responsiveness of IgA nephropathy. J Clin Invest. **96**: 2162–9.

Yoshimura H, Idenra T, Iwasaki S, et al. (1992). Aggravation of minimal change nephrotic syndrome by administration of serum albumin. Clin Nephrol. **37**: 109–14.

Yu Z, Schumacher M, Frey BM, et al. (2005). Regulation of epithelial sodium channel in puromycin aminonucleoside-induced unilateral experimental nephrotic syndrome in normal and analbuminemic Nagase rats. Nephron Physiol. **101**: 51–62.

Zacchia M, Capasso G. (2008). Parvalbumin: A key protein in early distal tubule NaCl reabsorption. Nephrol Dial Transplant. **23**: 1109–11.

Zandi-Nejad K, Eddy AA, Glassock RJ, et al. (2004). Why is proteinuria an ominous biomarker of progressive kidney disease? Kidney Int Suppl. **92**: S76–89.

Zhang LJ, Zhang Z, Li SJ, et al. (2014). Pulmonary embolism and renal vein thrombosis in patients with nephrotic syndrome: Prospective evaluation of prevalence and risk factors with CT. Radiology. **273**: 897–906.

Chapter 3

The pharmacology of old and new agents for specific therapy of primary glomerular diseases

Claudio Ponticelli and Richard J Glassock

Introduction and overview

A wide variety of pharmacologic agents having diverse mechanisms of action and potential adverse events are widely used in treatment of primary glomerular diseases. However, the indications for treating specific disease entities still represent a matter of controversy and discussion among nephrologists. Indeed, randomized controlled trials are relatively few in number and are often small, underpowered, and of short duration. Conversely, drugs such as glucocorticoids (GCs) and cytotoxic agents may exert beneficial effects in some glomerular diseases but may also be responsible of disquieting adverse events that can discourage their use in patients with indolent glomerulonephritis.

Recently, a number of biological agents have been developed to spare the use of potentially toxic agents while targeting the immune cells implicated in the pathogenesis of glomerular diseases. Thus far, however, many of them have failed to find a role in the clinical management of glomerular diseases. This chapter reports the main characteristics of the pharmacological classes of immunosuppressive agents that may be used in primary glomerular diseases.

Adrenocorticotropic hormone (ACTH)

The melanocyte-stimulating hormones (MSH) are a family of melanocortin polypeptides that include ACTH, α-MSH, β-MSH, and γ-MSH. Adrenocorticotropic hormone (ACTH) is secreted from the anterior pituitary in response to corticotrophin-releasing hormone by cleavage of a large precursor protein named pro-opiomelanocortin. ACTH stimulates the secretion of GCs, primarily cortisol, in the adrenal cortex and has little control over secretion of aldosterone.

In 1952, the US Food and Drug Administration (USFDA) authorized H.P. Acthar® gel (Mallinkrodt, St Louis) for use in diagnostic testing of adrenal function and for treatment of several disorders, including *idiopathic* nephrotic syndrome (NS) without 'uremia'. H.P. Acthar® gel is a porcine-derived, purified, sterile preparation of the natural form of ACTH in gelatine. This is a proprietary formulation, so the exact content is not precisely known. A synthetic peptide, tetracosactide, has also been created by isolating the first 24 amino acids from the 39-amino-acid ACTH. Sporadic reports suggest a potential therapeutic role both for natural and synthetic ACTH in idiopathic NS. In 2007 the USFDA authorized the use of synthetic ACTH only for diagnostic procedures or compassionate treatment.

Clinical pharmacology

ACTH contains 39 amino acids. The biologic (cortisol-stimulating effect) activity of ACTH resides in the N-terminal portion of the molecule and the 1-20 amino acid residue is the minimal sequence retaining full activity. Thus, the sequence of 24 amino acids in the tetracosactide formulation exerts the same activities of natural ACTH. The pharmacologic profile of synthetic ACTH is also similar to that of purified natural ACTH. A dose of 0.25 mg tetracosactide stimulates the adrenal cortex maximally and to the same extent as 25 units of natural ACTH. Following intravenous (IV) administration of tetracosactide 0.25 mg in patients with normal adrenocortical function, plasma cortisol concentrations begin to increase within five minutes and are approximately doubled within 15–30 minutes. After intramuscular administration of 0.25 mg in subjects with normal adrenocortical function, peak plasma cortisol concentrations are usually achieved within one hour and begin to decrease after two to four hours. The synthetic drug is rapidly removed from the plasma by many tissues, so the duration of action of tetracosactide is short. A long-acting synthetic 1-24-corticotropin has been developed. This depot formulation, which allows less-frequent administration, exhibits the same activity as natural ACTH with regard to all its biological activities.

Mechanisms of action

The main function of ACTH is to stimulate the production of cortisol from adrenal glands. Circulating ACTH selectively activates adrenal melanocortin receptor 2 (MCR-2), whereas the other melanocortin receptors can be activated by either ACTH or α, ß, γ, δ MSH (Dores et al., 2014). ACTH promotes a mild GC-mediated anti-inflammatory response but also exerts GC-independent anti-inflammatory actions. After binding to MCRs, ACTH can inhibit nuclear factor-kappa B (NF-κB) transcription and its translocation into the nucleus, where NF-κB triggers transcription of pro-inflammatory molecules (Arnason et al., 2013). ACTH and selective agonists for MCR-1 exert strong antiproteinuric effects in experimental models of membranous nephropathy by increasing the expression of MCR-1 in podocytes (Lindsgok et al., 2010). The activation of MCR-1 promotes an increase of catalase activity and reduces oxidative stress in podocytes. Moreover, MCR-1 agonists protect against podocyte apoptosis (Elvin et al., 2016). Furthermore, ACTH engenders down-modulating actions on immune system cells and the cytokines they synthesize. These anti-inflammatory and immunomodulating effects may account for the beneficial effects of ACTH in membranous nephropathy, idiopathic nephrotic syndrome, and other glomerular diseases.

Toxic effects

Hypercortisolism

A prolonged administration of ACTH (natural or synthetic) may result in symptoms and signs of hypercortisolism (exogenous Cushing syndrome, diabetes, hypertension, etc.), although the risk is lower than that observed with GCs themselves.

Pigmentation

Since ACTH has a chemical structure similar to that of MSH, its administration may cause freckling and a bronze coloration of the skin.

Allergic and anaphylactic reactions

Some patients may suffer from rash, itching, hives, or flushing. Exceptionally, patients may develop an anaphylactic reaction with difficult breathing, swelling of the face, lips, tongue, or other parts of the body. The risk is higher in patients with a history of allergy or asthma. We recommend that subjects under treatment with tetracosactide carry a vial of adrenaline in case of an anaphylactic reaction.

Clinical use in glomerular diseases

Intramuscular administration of natural ACTH was one of the earliest treatments used for managing acute glomerulonephritis and idiopathic NS, particularly minimal change disease (MCD) in children (infantile nephrosis in the older literature). In Europe a depot formulation of synthetic ACTH was approved decades ago for treating patients with NS, but this preparation is not approved for this use in the US. Both the synthetic (Ponticelli et al., 2006; Lindskog et al., 2010; Prasad et al., 2018) and natural ACTH (Bomback et al., 2012; Hogan et al., 2013; Gong et al., 2014; Madan et al., 2016) have been successfully used in some primary glomerular diseases with NS, especially membranous nephropathy (MN), and less frequently focal segmental glomerulosclerosis (FSGS) and MCD. No benefits on avoiding ESRD have yet been shown.

Glucocorticoids (GCs)

Two classes of steroids are synthesized from cholesterol and secreted by adrenal glands in response to ACTH: corticosteroids (21 carbons) and androgenic steroids (19 carbons). In turn, corticosteroids may be divided according to their metabolic activity into *glucocorticoids* (GCs), which interfere with intermediate metabolism, immunity, cellular survival, and repair, and inflammation and *mineralocorticoids*, which primarily regulate water and electrolyte (potassium and sodium) metabolism, but may also influence fibrosis generation.

Clinical pharmacology

The three natural GCs are cortisol (or hydrocortisone), cortisone, and corticosterone. They contain groups that are essential for anti-inflammatory activity, namely, a carbonyl group (CO) in position 17, a hydroxyl group (OH) in position 11, an oxygen (O) in position 3, and a double bound in position 4–5. Substitutions adjacent to critical sites increase anti-inflammatory activity and reduce mineralocorticoid activity.

Cortisol is produced in the zones fasciculata and reticularis of the adrenal cortex and represents about 90 per cent of corticosteroid output in humans. The circadian rhythm of cortisol is regulated by the central neural 'clock' located in the suprachiasmatic nucleus of the hypothalamus (Albrecht, 2012). In a normal subject, the secretion of cortisol is minimal at midnight, increases in the morning around 3 to 4 a.m., peaks around 8 a.m., then begins to decline. The release decreases through the afternoon and evening and reaches its lowest levels at midnight. The release of cortisol from the adrenal gland and ACTH from the anterior pituitary gland occurs in pulses with intervals of 40 minutes to eight hours. A variety of physical or psychological events can interrupt this circadian rhythm of secretion.

In blood, 90–93 per cent of cortisol is bound to plasma proteins. About 80 per cent is bound to transcortin, an α-2 globulin synthesized in the liver, another 10 per cent is bound to albumin, and a negligible amount is bound to other proteins. When the binding capacity of transcortin (about 25 mg/dl) is exceeded, binding to albumin increases. In normal conditions, only 10 per cent of cortisol circulates free in the blood; this fraction represents the active hormone. The hydrophobic GCs are filtered by the glomeruli, but almost 99 per cent are reabsorbed by the tubuli. To render them capable of renal elimination, GCs are first converted in the liver to inactive compounds through a series of reduction reactions and are then conjugated with glucuronide or sulfate. These water-soluble compounds are finally excreted by the kidney.

Synthetic GCs bind less efficiently to transcortin and therefore diffuse more rapidly into tissues where they converted, particularly in the liver, from inactive 11-ketoglucocorticoids to active 11-β-hydroxyl compounds by 11β-hydroxysteroid dehydrogenase enzymes, which are expressed in many tissues.

Cortisol is cleared from the plasma with a half-life of 70–120 minutes but its tissue half-life ranges between 8 and 12 hours. The half-lives of synthetic analogues are longer as their hepatic metabolism is lower. According to their duration of action, GCs may be divided into *short acting* (prednisone, prednisolone, methylprednisolone, and deflazacort, with a plasma half-life of 60–200 minutes and a tissue half-life between 12 and 36 hours); *intermediate acting* (paramethasone and triamcinolone, with a plasma half-life of about 300 minutes and a tissue half-life of about 48 hours); and *long acting* (dexamethasone and betamethasone, which suppress ACTH for more than 48 hours).

Mechanisms of action

GCs may exert genomic and non-genomic effects (see Table 3.1).

The *genomic* effects implicate the activation or repression of multiple genes. This action involves many steps and therefore takes effect with a time lag of about 4–24 hours. The genomic effects largely depend on the doses of synthetic GCs as well as density, availability, and affinity of GC receptors (GRs), i.e. DNA binding proteins that regulate transcription of specific genes and gene network. GCs are lipid-soluble molecules that can freely pass through the cell membrane after dissociation from carrier protein. In the cell, the GC actions are mediated by a specific nuclear receptor that regulates gene transcription. GR has two main isoforms: α and β. Isoform α is ubiquitously expressed and mediates the genomic actions of GCs, while isoform β is unable to bind GCs and may contribute to GC resistance through the formation of GRα/GRβ heterodimers. The GR is present in the cytoplasm in an inactive state as a multimeric complex with immunophilins and heat shock proteins (HSPs). GR are single polypeptides of 90–95 kDa with three functional domains: the ligand-binding domain (domain A), which interacts with the specific steroid; the DNA-binding domain (domain B), which recognizes specific sequences of the DNA called hormone-responsive elements; and an immunogenic domain (domain C) in the amino terminal region. When GR binds its ligand, immunophilins and HSP dissociate and the receptor becomes active. An important role in this step is played by the co-ordinated action of HSP 70 and 90. While HSP 70 inactivates GR through partial unfolding, HSP 90 reverses this inactivation as it acts in the later stages

Table 3.1 Genomic and nongenomic effects of glucocorticoids.

Genomic effects	Non-genomic effects
Transactivation	Class 1
Mechanisms	*Mechanisms*
Transcription factors bind to promoter regions that increase gene expression	Interactions with cell membranes (at high doses of steroid).
Effects	*Effects*
Anti-inflammatory activity	Immunosuppression
Immunosuppressive activity	Class 2
Adverse events	*Mechanisms*
Hypertension	Interaction with membrane-bound GRs
Infection	*Effects*
Diabetes mellitus	Rapid T-cell immunosuppressive action
Obesity, metabolic syndrome	Class 3
Neuropsychiatric disorders	*Mechanisms*
Osteomuscular complications	Activation of phospholipase 2
Ocular complications	*Effects*
Growth retardation	Production of vasodilating prostaglandins
Transrepression	and inflammatory leukotrienes
Mechanisms	Class 4
Inhibition of transcription factors NF-κB and AP-1	*Mechanisms*
	Inhibition of norepinephrine reuptake
Effects	*Effects*
Anti-inflammatory activity	Vasoconstriction
Immunosuppressive activity	

of folding by binding to partially folded intermediates (Kirschke et al., 2014). Upon dissociation and activation, the GR undergoes a conformational change that triggers its translocation to the nucleus. Here, GRs bind to specific GC response elements (GREs) in the promoter region of the target genes, resulting in the regulation of a number of genes that control many aspects of cell physiology, including the transcription of anti-inflammatory genes. This process of gene transcription is called *transactivation* (Kadmiel and Cidlowski, 2013). On the other hand, activated GRs can bind to DNA in the same site where other transcription factors would bind. The inhibited activity of key transcription factors, like NF-κB and activator protein 1 (AP-1), can repress the activity of many important pro-inflammatory genes. This process of impaired transcription is called *transrepression* (Granner et al., 2015). Thus, GC action is predominantly mediated through the GRs (Figure 3.1). Sensitivity to GCs varies among individuals. Low mRNA expression of GRs (Zahran et al., 2013) and multidrug resistance-1 gene polymorphisms (Dhandapani et al., 2015) may cause steroid resistance. The high number of GR isoforms highlighting the

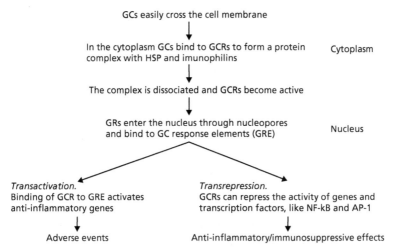

Figure 3.1 Genomic effects of glucocorticoids (GCs).
After entering the cytoplasm, GCs bind to their receptors (GCRs) which are complexed with heat-shock proteins (HSPs) and immunophilins. The binding of GCs with GCRs dissociates HSP and immunophilins. After dissociation GCRs become active, undergo a conformational change, and enter the nucleus where they bind to elements (GRE) that can activate anti-inflammatory genes or repress transcription factors that activate inflammatory genes.

dynamic nature of hormone signalling may also explain the different sensitivity to GCs (Ramamoorthy and Cidlowski, 2016).

Non-genomic effects are also dose-dependent. They are characterized by rapid onset (seconds to minutes) and short duration of action (60–90 minutes). These effects may depend on interactions of GCs with a non-classical membrane-bound GR and can occur in cells that do not have nucleus (Mitre-Aguilar et al., 2015). Alternatively, the binding of GC to the nuclear GR may transduce a rapid steroid response at the membrane, or may regulate a critical component of the signalling cascade of a distinct membrane GR (Nahar et al., 2016). GCs may also exert direct effects on podocyte function and survival (see 'Clinical use in glomerular diseases').

Anti-inflammatory and immunosuppressive effects

GCs are very effective anti-inflammatory agents and can also interfere with the immune response, cellular immunity being more susceptible than humoral immunity. These and other actions that involve most cells of the body occur simultaneously and are mainly mediated by the inhibition of the pro-inflammatory transcription factors NF-κB and AP-1. NF-κB is a rapid-acting transcription factor that regulates genes responsible for both the innate and adaptive immune response, by controlling transcription of DNA, cytokine production, and cell survival. AP-1 regulates gene expression in response to a variety of stimuli, including cytokines, growth factors, stress, and bacterial and viral infections.

Effects on inflammation

Inflammation is critical for an organism to respond to and remove pathogens and danger signals. The inflammatory response is characterized by a number of events involving innate immunity, the local vascular system, and various cells and cytokines within the injured tissue. Any type of injury can alarm toll-like receptors (TLR). The activation of these sentinels triggers an intracellular signalling cascade that culminates in the activation of the AP-1, NF-κB, and other pro-inflammatory transcription factors that induce vasodilation, increased vascular permeability, extravasation of plasma proteins, and leukocyte accumulation in the affected tissue.

GCs can induce inhibitory or stimulatory effects on inflammation. GRs play a critical role that may be considered as cellular rheostats to ensure the proper response. GCs, acting through GRs, can stimulate the pro-inflammatory transcription factors AP-1, NF-κB, and STAT3. On the other hand, GCs can promote the resolution of inflammation, by stimulating the secretion of proresolving molecules, inducing neutrophil and T-cell apoptosis, promoting a wound-healing and anti-inflammatory phenotype in macrophages (Fan et al., 2014), and promoting the removal of apoptotic cells. The ability of GRs to accomplish these pleiotropic actions depends on several factors, including post-translational modifications, extracellular environment, ligand availability and duration of signalling, cell type-specific cofactors and binding partners, and chromatin accessibility (Busillo and Cidlowski, 2013).

When given intravenously, methylprednisolone can be incorporated into cell membranes, leading to changes in the physicochemical properties of the membrane; can reduce the generation of superoxide anion radicals; can inhibit the production of the platelet-activating factor, a lipid mediator of glomerular inflammation; can modify the chemical composition of the glomerular basement membrane (GBM), with consequent reduced proteinuria; and can inhibit complement-induced granulocyte aggregation without producing long-lasting abnormalities of polymorphonuclear functions. IV methylprednisolone shows a rapid peak and a serum half-life of three hours.

Effects on the immune response

GCs have pleiotropic effects on the immune system. However, a clear picture of the cellular and molecular basis of GC action has remained elusive (Cain and

Cidlowski, 2017). GCs can modulate the expression of cytokines and cell adhesion molecules, the traffic, maturation, and differentiation of immune system cells, the expression of substances involved in molecular adhesion, and cell migration. As a consequence, GCs may inhibit both innate and acquired immunologic functions. T-cells are particularly sensitive to the inhibitory effects of GCs. In children with nephrotic syndrome even a short-term administration of high-dose prednisone may induce a significant reduction of circulating CD4+ and CD8+ T-cells (Baris et al., 2016). Such an effect can be due to an enhanced programmed cell death during T-cell activation (Xing et al., 2015). By inhibiting IL-1 and TNFα, GCs can also interfere with macrophage functions that are associated with antigen presentation to T-cells (Coutnho and Chapman, 2011). Moreover, by influencing dendritic cell maturation and function and promoting the development of regulatory IL-10-producing T-cells, GCs may favour the development of tolerance to specific antigens (Podestà et al., 2015). At elevated doses GCs also induces lymphocyte apoptosis (including B-cells) and can prevent in vitro differentiation of B-cell into plasma cells (Haneda et al., 2014). Large concentrations of steroid are also likely to interfere with Fcγ receptor signalling, including the inhibitory FcγRIIb, which acts as a key negative modulator of B-cell function and controls bone marrow plasma cell apoptosis (Xiang et al., 2007). When given intravenously at very high doses, GCs can inhibit IL-6 and TNFα receptors (Matsui et al., 2015) and can induce a rapid, dramatic, and transient increase in circulating regulatory T-cells (Mathian et al., 2015).

Toxic effects

GCs can elicit a variety of adverse events, which are usually dose- and time-dependent. Many adverse events can be attributed to the ability of the GRs to transactivate genes producing metabolic effects. By contrast, the anti-inflammatory effects of GCs are due to transrepression of pro-inflammatory genes (Newton et al., 2010).

Diabetes mellitus

GCs at physiological levels are essential for many homeostatic processes, including glycaemic controls; however, an endogenous or exogenous GC excess can cause hyperglycaemia and insulin resistance through the activity of protein mediators at molecular and tissue-specific level (Patel et al., 2014). The risk of diabetes is increased. Usually diabetes develops after some weeks or months of oral GC therapy. However, immediately after the administration of IV high-dose methylprednisolone severe hyperglycaemia can occur. It usually reverses spontaneously but, in a few patients, this hyperglycaemia heralds the development of an often-persisting severe diabetes requiring the chronic administration of insulin or hypoglycaemic agents.

Hyperlipidaemia

Being a member of the nuclear receptor superfamily of transcription factors, the GR translocates into the cell nucleus upon GC binding, where it serves as a transcriptional regulator of distinct GC-responsive target genes that can be associated with lipid regulatory pathways and can thereby control both physiological and pathophysiological systemic lipid homeostasis (de Guia and Herzig, 2015). GCs may enhance the activity of acetyl coenzyme A carboxylase and free fatty acid synthetase, may increase hepatic synthesis of VLDL, may downregulate LDL receptor activity of 3-hydroxy-3methylglutaryl coenzyme A (HMG-CoA) reductase, and may inhibit lipoprotein lipase. These effects can result in *increased* levels of VLDL, total cholesterol, and triglycerides and *decreased* levels of HDL depending on the doses and duration of treatment. Through increases in caloric and dietary fat intake, along with increased hydrolysis of circulating triglycerides by lipoprotein lipase activity, GCs increase the amount of fatty acids in circulation. These combined effects may be pro-atherogenic.

Obesity and metabolic syndrome

Body weight gain is common in patients given GCs and some patients may develop a true obesity. GCs regulate appetite and adiposity. Recent evidence shows that GCs possess the ability to increase hepatic endocannabinoid signalling, which is known to regulate appetite, energy balance, and metabolic processes through both central and peripheral pathways (Bowles et al., 2015). Moreover, GCs promote pre-adipocyte conversion to mature adipocytes, causing hyperplasia of the adipose tissue. GCs also have acute anti-lipolytic effect on adipocytes, whereas their genomic actions facilitate increased lipolysis (Peckett et al., 2011). GCs could also induce visceral adiposity through by expressing Dexras1, a small G protein which is expressed by GCs. Dexras1 can link GC signalling to the insulin-like growth factor-1 signalling pathway in adipogenesis (Kim et al., 2016).

Steroid-induced obesity can aggravate other risk factors triggered by GCs and eventually lead to a true metabolic syndrome, including insulin-resistance, visceral obesity, hypertension, dyslipidaemia, and an increased risk of cardiovascular diseases. These effects are mainly related to increased intracellular GC reactivation catalysed by the enzyme 11β-hydroxysteroid dehydrogenase type-1 in obese adipose tissue (Morton, 2010). A low-calorie diet should be prescribed to patients for whom a prolonged administration of GCs is foreseen.

Hypercoagulability

Some suggestions have been made that GCs increase the risk for deep venous thrombosis. The mechanisms involved in the thromboembolic complications are endothelial dysfunction, hypercoagulability, and stasis (Cohelo et al., 2014). Obesity can also contribute to hypercoagulability (Samad and Ruf, 2013).

Hypertension

Arterial hypertension may occur in 20 per cent of normotensive subjects treated with high doses of synthetic GCs. The mechanisms for GC-induced hypertension are incompletely understood, but are probably multifactorial. GCs decrease the production of endothelial nitric oxide (Williamson et al., 2015), while enhancing the effects of vasoconstrictors (Peppa et al., 2011). There is also evidence that vascular endothelial GR can have a critical role in generating and maintaining GC-mediated hypertension (Goodwin et al., 2011). On the other hand, GCs can increase the extra-cellular volume by activating the NaCl cotransporter (Ivy et al., 2016). Thus, GCs may be responsible both of increased peripheral resistance and increased circulatory volume and cardiac output.

Cardiovascular disease

GCs increase the risk of cardiovascular disease through multiple pathways. GCs can cause adverse systemic effects including arterial hypertension, obesity, hyperglycaemia, and metabolic syndrome. Furthermore, GCs have direct effects on the heart and blood vessels, mediated by both GC and mineralocorticoid receptors and modified by local metabolism of GCs by the 11β-hydroxysteroid dehydrogenase enzymes. These effects influence vascular function, atherogenesis, and vascular remodelling following intravascular injury or ischemia (Walker, 2007). Finally, GC-inducible kinase 1 regulates NF-κB and plays a pivotal role in the progression of intimal narrowing following arterial injury and in vascular inflammation during atherogenesis (Zhong et al., 2014; Borst et al., 2015).

Dermatologic effects

The most typical aesthetic complication is represented by *Cushingoid appearance*, with facial and neck fullness, 'buffalo hump', increased supraclavicular and suprasternal fat, and truncal obesity. These features are usually dose-dependent and are caused by abnormal adipose tissue redistribution. These effects may be reversible after interruption of steroids.

Acne is extremely frequent. Its severity is usually dose-related. Facial erythrosis and rosacea can also occur. Acne occurs early on the cheeks, forehead, chin, and chest. Rarely, the lesions may progress to nodulocystic transformation (*acne conglobata*). A complication seen almost constantly in patients given prolonged

GC administration is the so-called *Bateman's purpura*. It consists of irregular purpuric areas that develop spontaneously or after minor trauma, mainly on the extensor surfaces of the hands, forearms, and legs, often with spontaneous star-shaped pseudo-scars. *Striae rubrae* are wide and violaceous stripes, mainly located over the abdomen, thighs, and buttocks. They are usually irreversible, although they tend to become pale after interruption of GCs. Some patients have increased *hair growth* mainly on the face and back. Of importance, the skin of patients under prolonged GC treatment can become thin, *atrophic*, and *friable*. Topical retinoic acid at concentrations ranging from 0.01 to 0.05 per cent may improve this complication. Some patients, however, complain of ir-ritation. Ammonium lactate 6–12 per cent creams are usually better tolerated.

Peptic ulcer

A meta-analysis of double-blind randomized trials showed a similar risk of peptic ulcer in patients in the placebo group—9 of 3267, or 0.3 per cent—and in patients in the steroid group—13 of 3335, or 0.4 per cent (Conn and Poynard, 1994). In physiologic conditions GCs may be even gastroprotective by maintaining local defensive factors and inhibiting pathogenic elements (Filareterova, 2011).

Adrenal insufficiency

Synthetic GCs suppress the release of both ACTH and cortisol. A recent meta-analysis concluded that adrenal insufficiency after discontinuation of GC occurs frequently and there is no administration form, dosing, treatment dur-ation, or underlying disease for which adrenal insufficiency can be excluded with certainty (Broersen et al., 2015). However, some measures may reduce suppression of the hypothalamic–pituitary–adrenal axis. *Steroids should be ad-ministered in a single morning administration not later than between 7 and 9 a.m.* Some synthetic GCs (such as prednisone) induce less profound adrenal suppression than others (e.g. betamethasone). Whenever possible, the admin-istration of a *dose every other day* may reduce the inhibitory effect of synthetic GCs. After long-term steroid administration, the dosage of GCs should be gradually reduced and discontinued only after reaching minimal doses (i.e. prednisone 2.5 mg every other day). In case of serious infection, operation, or injury, patients should receive supplementary steroid administration. The degree of the hypothalamic–pituitary–adrenal axis suppression cannot be re-liably estimated from the dose of GC, the duration of therapy, or the basal plasma concentration. The corticotrophin-releasing hormone test and the insulin–hypoglycaemia test are considered to be more reliable tests to assess the pituitary–adrenal response.

Infection

The risk of infection increases as the dose of GC increases, but risk may vary according to the age, the clinical conditions of the patient, the concomitant administration of other drugs interfering with the immune response, and the type of underlying disease. Indeed, glucocorticoids can promote neutrophil survival, by inhibiting their apoptosis. However, this effect may be undesired since it accentuates neutrophilic inflammation (Saffar et al., 2011). Any kind of infection—bacterial, viral, fungal, parasitic—can occur. Attention should be given to the possibility of a pre-existing infection before starting GC therapy. Reactivation of tuberculosis can occur but may be masked by the steroid-induced inhibition of tuberculin reaction. Isoniazid may be needed to prevent dissemination or reactivation of latent tuberculosis.

Neuropsychiatric complications

Glucocorticoids exert profound and complex actions on the central nervous system, many of which are mediated by the GRs that are recruited to Klf 9 upstream regions in a hormone-dependent manner (Bonett et al., 2009; Bagamasbad et al., 2012). *Psychiatric reactions* may occur in up to one-third of patients. Patients with psychological difficulties experience more frequent and severe reactions. Decreasing the doses of steroids may improve the symptoms. Lithium carbonate is effective, while tricyclic antidepressants may worsen the steroid-induced depression. *Sleeplessness* is frequent. It may be reduced by administering short-acting GCs in a single morning administration. *Pseudotumour cerebri*, characterized by intracranial hypertension and papilloedema, may occur in children when GC doses are rapidly decreased. Pseudotumour cerebri can be managed with lumbar taps or increased doses of GCs.

Muscular complications

Steroid-induced *myopathy* is a frequent but often underestimated adverse effect of steroid treatment. GCs have a direct catabolic effect on muscle, decreasing protein synthesis and increasing the rate of protein catabolism leading to muscle atrophy. Creatinine production can be markedly decreased giving to overestimation of true GFR by creatinine-based eGFR formulas. Clinical presentation of myopathy may differentiate two features: the less frequent acute myopathy, essentially observed in patients treated with high dosages, and the more frequent insidious, painless, chronic myopathy, characterized by a progressive symmetrical proximal deficit, especially of the lower extremities. The first complaint is an inability to climb stairs. Muscle enzymes are normal. The treatment is based on reduction or discontinuation of the steroid. Fluorinated GCs, e.g.

dexamethasone, should be replaced with nonfluorinated GCs, e.g. prednisone (Pereira and Freire de Carvalho, 2011). In a murine model, intermittent, rather than daily, GC regimen promoted sarcolemmal repair and muscle recovery from injury while limiting atrophic remodelling (Quattrocelli et al., 2017).

Spontaneous *tendon rupture* is a rare complication which occurs mainly with prolonged therapy. This should be taken into account for patients engaged in active sports, e.g. tennis, basketball. Muscle cramps are common during tapering after high-dose regimens.

Bone complications

GCs may cause an imbalance in bone remodelling through different mechanisms. GCs decrease the net intestinal calcium absorption, increase urinary calcium excretion, inhibit the secretion of growth hormone, and decrease the production and/or the bioactivity of some skeletal growth factors, e.g. insulin-like growth factor 1 and transforming growth factor beta 1 (TGFβ1). However, the main deleterious effect of GCs is a direct inhibition of bone formation, as they inhibit osteoblast differentiation, induce apoptosis in mature osteoblasts, and favour the production of reactive oxygen species and autophagy that play a key role in increasing osteoclast formation and bone resorption (Frenkel et al., 2015; Shi et al., 2015). The final result is a decreased bone mineral density, but persistent and severe inhibition of bone formation leads to further bone loss and progressively increased fracture risk. While trabecular bone is particularly vulnerable, cortical bone is relatively spared even in the long-term therapy. Calcium, vitamin D, weight-bearing exercise, and osteoporosis-prevention treatment can be used to prevent and/or treat osteoporosis (Hant and Bolster, 2016). Bisphosphonates, which are potent inhibitors of bone resorption, are considered the most effective and first-line agents for increasing bone mineral density and decreasing the risk of fracture. Human parathyroid hormone has also emerged as a promising agent for the treatment of severe osteoporosis when used alone or in combination with a bisphosphonate. There is also clinical evidence that twice yearly subcutaneous administrations of denusomab, a fully human monoclonal antibody to the receptor activator of NF-κB ligand, can obtain significant reductions in vertebral, nonvertebral, and hip fractures in postmenopausal women with osteoporosis (Cummings et al., 2009).

Aseptic necrosis of femoral head and more rarely knees or shoulders usually occurs after long-term therapy but may also develop in the first weeks of treatment. Unilateral hip or knee pain is the most common initial symptom. The pathogenetic mechanisms of steroid-related aseptic necrosis are still unclear, but it is likely that GCs can contribute by increasing apoptosis of osteoblasts and osteocytes (Ding et al., 2015).

Ocular complications

Bilateral posterior subcapsular *cataract* is a common complication. It is usually dose- and time-related but can occur even after short-term steroid therapy. *Increased intraocular* pressure, caused by decreased aqueous outflow, is a dose-related complication that can reverse after prompt cessation of therapy. Patients with diabetes myopia or a familial history of glaucoma have an increased risk.

Growth retardation

Chronic administration of GCs can impair statural growth in children and pre-pubertal adolescents. This adverse event is partly related to the doses of GCs. In a study on children with steroid-dependent nephrotic syndrome, there was no negative impact on growth seen at doses of prednisolone of less than 0.75 mg/kg/day (Simmonds et al., 2010). The effect on growth is due to an abnormal spontaneous secretion as well as to a reduced response to the stimulation of growth hormone. GCs also interfere with growth hormone receptors and reduce the local production of insulin-like growth factor. Since the major growth spurts occur in infancy before the age of two years and at puberty, steroid therapy may cause severe loss of height at these times. Recombinant human growth hormone may be effective and safe for paediatric patients with growth retardation. However, self-injection by children can be problematic. Injection pens or needle-free devices enable easy self-injection by children, minimize medication reconstitution and storage requirements, and reduce injection pain.

Pregnancy

GCs may predispose the pregnant woman to hypertension and pre-eclampsia when used at high doses. These agents easily traverse the placenta, but 90 per cent of the maternal dose is metabolized within the placenta by 11-beta- hydroxysteroid dehydrogenase-2, which converts cortisol, prednisone, and methylprednisolone into inactive products, while dexamethasone and betamethasone are less well metabolized. Since only inert products of prednisone or analogues cross the placenta the foetus is protected from adverse effects. However, a small reduction of size at birth and adrenal suppression may occur when GCs are used at high doses. There has been concern about a possible increase of oral-facial clefts in newborns to mothers receiving GCs. However, this risk is approximately 1.3 to 3.3 for every 1,000 pregnancies exposed during the critical period versus a birth population prevalence of 1 per 1,000, suggesting that the risk associated with prenatal exposure to GCs is minimal (Chambers et al., 2006). Prednisolone has been assigned to pregnancy category C by the USFDA (Table 3.2).

Table 3.2 Classification of foetal risk according to the US Food and Drug Administration criteria.

A	No foetal risk in controlled studies.
B	No risk to human foetus. Possible animal risk or no risks in animal studies, but human studies lacking.
C	Human risk cannot be ruled out. Animal studies may or may not show risk.
D	Evidence of risk to human foetus.
X	Contra-indicated in pregnancy.

Measures to reduce toxicity of glucocorticoids (GCs)

While waiting for new classes of GCs or other GR agonists with reduced toxicity, some measures can be adopted to minimize the toxicity of GCs without diminishing efficacy (Ponticelli and Locatelli, 2018).

Single morning-dose therapy

Endogenous cortisol has peak values at about 8 a.m. and a nadir at about noon. As a consequence, a synthetic short-acting agent given in a single morning dose will produce only a slight adrenal suppression, while the same dose given at midnight will bring about a nearly complete suppression of the adrenal secretion for at least 24 hours. Furthermore, while 10 mg of prednisone given at 8 a.m. does not cause adrenal suppression, four administrations of 2.5 mg each given to the same subjects at evenly spaced intervals may produce a considerable adrenal suppression. Therefore, for long-term therapy, there is a preference for a short-acting agent and the entire amount should be given (if possible) in a single dose between 7 and 9 a.m. or even earlier (the peak levels are reached two to three hours after oral administration), so allowing normal hypothalamic stimulation.

Alternate-day therapy

Even more innocuous is alternate-day therapy based on the administration of a short-acting agent in a single double dose between 6 and 8 a.m. every 48 hours. This regimen minimizes the interference with the pituitary-adrenal axis and reduces the side-effects of a divided-dose regimen. It can also be used to help restoration of the pituitary–adrenal axis following prolonged daily administration. Alternate-day therapy is particularly indicated for maintenance therapy when the activity of a renal disease has been quenched by previous treatment. A sudden switching from daily to alternate-day therapy can be complicated by fever, arthralgias, and asthenia on the 'off' day. In the case of previous prolonged daily steroid therapy, it is advisable to switch to alternate-day administration by modifying the doses gradually.

Hygienic measures

Patients receiving continuous steroid treatment should follow a hypocaloric diet to prevent obesity, diabetes, and hyperlipidaemia. Salt intake should be limited to prevent hypertension and oedema. Physical activity is highly recommended in order to prevent myopathy, osteopenia, and obesity. It is mandatory to stop smoking, which can aggravate many of side effects of GCs.

Hypo-adrenalism

Many of the signs and symptoms of hypo-adrenalism are non-specific and can be mistaken for symptoms of intercurrent illness or the underlying condition being treated with GC therapy (weakness, hypotension, hypoglycaemia, myalgia, arthralgias). Levels of serum cortisol <85 nmol/l indicate a severe hypo-adrenalism. Symptomatic adrenal suppression should be treated with daily physiologic replacement doses of GC plus 'stress doses' during physiological stress, e.g. intercurrent illness, injury, or surgery.

Methylprednisolone (MP) pulse therapy

First used in kidney transplantation for managing acute rejection, high-dose (500 mg–1000 mg per dose) 'pulses' of IV methylprednisolone (MP) are the standard initial treatment in patients with rapidly progressive renal disease. Although no formal studies have compared conventional oral high-dose and pulse steroid therapy in rapidly progressive pauci-immune glomerulonephritis or other primary glomerular diseases, the clinical impression is that MP pulses can obtain more profound anti-inflammatory effects, faster recovery from symptoms, and lower toxicity in comparison with high-dose oral steroids. Their effects are probably mediated by non-genomic actions within the cells.

MP pulse administration is generally safe, but, exceptionally, severe complications—including seizures, sudden death, and anaphylaxis—have been reported, particularly when the steroid was injected rapidly and/or was given through a central venous line. These complications occurred generally in severely ill patients and the relationship with methylprednisolone has not always been established. Some patients may suffer from complex ventricular arrhythmias; others complain of flushing, tremor, nausea, and altered taste. These symptoms, which may be exacerbated by the use of high-dose furosemide, spontaneously disappear within a few hours. Steroid pulses can produce severe hyperglycaemia and a transient hypercoagulable state through the activation of the tissue factor, FVII. IV MP pulses may also induce a transient reduction of glomerular filtration rate (GFR). Renal dysfunction is more likely to occur in patients with renal insufficiency or severe nephrotic syndrome, suggesting that sodium and water retention may be responsible for interstitial oedema. Renal dysfunction spontaneously reverses within few days. To minimize the possible side-effects of IV high-dose MP, some precautions should be taken:

i. Serum potassium should be checked before infusion;

ii. Patients with cardiac problems should be monitored with electrocardiogram during infusion;

iii. Patients with severe hypo-albuminaemia should receive prophylactic injection of low molecular weight heparin for three days before, during, and after infusion to prevent thromboembolism;

iv. MP should be infused in a peripheral vein over 30–60 minutes;

v. Outpatients should stay in the surgery for at least two hours after infusion; and

vi. In case of hyperglycaemia, further administrations should be delayed until glycaemia returns to normal values.

Locally acting glucocorticoids

The enteric formulation of budesonide targeted to ileocecal region reduced significantly proteinuria and serum creatinine in 16 patients with IgA nephropathy (Smerud et al., 2011). In a large randomized clinical trial, targeted-release budesonide 16 mg/day added to optimized renin-angiotensin-system blockade significantly reduced proteinuria in patients with IgA nephropathy (Fellstrom et al., 2017).

Selective GR agonists

Selective GR agonists (SEGRAs) might optimize genomic GC effects by modulating NF-κB and AP-1 in order to induce transrepression with little or no transactivating activity. In preclinical studies, the novel SEGRAs, mapracorat and Compound A, potently inhibited the production of a variety of inflammatory mediators including cytokines and prostaglandin E2, with limited side effects. On the other hand, systemic pharmacologic inhibition of GR using mifepristone reduced proteinuria, preserved renal function and podocyte numbers, deactivated parietal epithelial cells, and inhibited formation of proliferative lesions in a mice model of crescentic GN. These effects were similar to those obtained by high–dose GC treatment (Kuppe et al., 2017).

Clinical use in glomerular diseases

In clinical practice, oral or IV GCs have been used with variable success in all the types of primary glomerular diseases (see specific chapters in this volume). One of the main problems with the use of GCs is represented by their low therapeutic index. Prednisone, prednisolone, and methylprednisolone are the short-acting GCs most frequently used in clinical practice. These agents have a similar anti-inflammatory activity, but methylprednisolone has a considerably higher antilymphocyte potency than prednisolone. When given at high doses intravenously, methylprednisolone may also exert nongenomic effects that allow a more rapid and intense anti-inflammatory and immunosuppressive activity.

Of note, GCs may directly protect podocytes from injury, independently of their systemic effects. GRs are expressed in the podocyte and experimental studies show that GCs can have a direct effect on the podocyte via rearrangement of actin cytoskeleton, inhibiting apoptosis, and regulating protein trafficking of critical slit diaphragm proteins (Ransom et al., 2005; Guess et al., 2010). The phosphorylation of nephrin is important for maintaining normal podocyte function. In human cultured podocytes treated with dexamethasone for 24 hours the phosphorylation of podocytes significantly increased, suggesting that in human glomerulonephritis GC may exert its function by regulating the phosphorylation of nephrin (Ohashi et al., 2011; Agrawal et al., 2011). MicroRNAs (miRNAs) are essential for podocyte homeostasis. Downregulation of miRNAs induced in experimental animals by puromycin aminonucleoside (PAN), lipopolysaccaride (LPS), or TGF-β can cause podocyte cytoskeletal damage and apoptosis. GC treatment maintains miRNA-30 expression in cultured podocytes treated with TGF-β, LPS, or PAN and in the podocytes of PAN-treated rats. These data suggest that the renoprotective activity of GCs in some podocytopathies may be related to their effects on microRNA-30 family (Wu et al., 2014). GCs can also increase podocyte regeneration by augmenting the number of podocyte progenitors (Zhang et al., 2013). Finally, dexamethasone can regulate the response of glomerular podocytes to vasoactive factors in cultured murine podocytes (Lewko et al., 2015) and can increase the podocyte expression of Krüppel-like factor 15, a transcription factor that regulates podocyte differentiation and protect podocyte against injury (Mallipattu et al., 2017). In vitro, GCs decrease cellular crescent formation and inhibit proliferation and migration of parietal epithelial cells (Kuppe et al., 2017).

Calcineurin inhibitors (CNI)

Cyclosporine

Cyclosporine A (CsA) is an undecapeptide of molecular weight 1203 kDa, derived from the Norwegian fungus *Tolypocladium inflatum*. The amino acids in positions 1, 2, 3, and 11 form a hydrophilic active immunosuppressive site. CsA crystallizes from acetone to give white prismatic needles that dissolve easily in most organic solvents, but only poorly in water. The drug is available as oral solution, capsules, and IV infusion. It is stabilized with olive oil vehicles for oral administration and with castor oil (Cremophor) for IV infusion. The relative bio-equivalence of oral to IV doses is 1:3. A micro-emulsion formulation of CsA (Sandimmun Neoral®) is now preferred to the old formulation, having better bio-availability and more predictable pharmacokinetics. It is a preconcentrate that, upon contact with aqueous gastrointestinal fluids, immediately forms a micro-emulsion, making CsA available for absorption. CsA is usually administered twice daily. After the patency for CsA expired a number of generic formulations have been made available.

Clinical pharmacokinetics

After oral administration, CsA is absorbed from the upper small intestine into the vascular compartment via a bile-dependent process. In blood, almost 60 per cent of CsA is bound to erythrocytes, 33 per cent is distributed in the plasma, mainly bound to high-density and low-density lipoproteins, while only a small fraction circulates free. CsA is extensively metabolized in the liver and intestine by cytochrome-P450 3A (CYP3A), predominantly CYP3A4 and CYP3A5 isoenzymes and by the efflux P-glycoprotein (P-gp), a protein product of the *ABCB1* gene (De Jonge et al., 2012). P-gp has a major role in limiting distribution of CsA to tissues such as the brain, placenta, lymphocytes, and kidney. Inactivating polymorphisms and inhibition of P-gp have the potential to significantly increase CNI exposure in these tissues with possible implications for toxicity and efficacy. Many single-nucleotide polymorphisms in *CYP3A4*, *CYP3A5*, and *ABCB1* genes have been identified to account for the variability in the pharmacokinetics of CsA (Staatz et al., 2010). The metabolites are primarily excreted in the bile and to a small extent (about 6 per cent) in the urine. CsA is extensively distributed to the tissues. Liver accounts for most of the body stores, but CsA can also be found in ectodermic tissues (skin, gingiva, central nervous system) and mesodermic tissues.

There are differences between the old formulation of CsA and the micro-emulsion Neoral. With the old formulation the gastrointestinal absorption is slow, incomplete, and variable. The average bio-availability widely ranges between 5 and 89 per cent, with a mean of 30 per cent. Peak concentrations in blood also vary considerably between one and eight hours, with a mean of 3.8 hours. With the micro-emulsion the absorption is more rapid (time to maximum concentration 1.5 vs. 2.1 hours) and complete with almost one-third higher area under the curve (AUC). With the old formulation of CsA the AUC is about 60 per cent higher when the drug is given with food than without food. The blood levels increase even more after introduction of olive oil, corn oil, or grapefruit. Instead, eating does not influence absorption when Neoral is used.

A number of variables can influence the bio-availability and the pharmaco-kinetics of CsA:

i. Diversion of bile flow from intestine impairs the absorption of the lipophilic CsA.

ii. Patients with diarrhoea or with short-bowel syndrome show poor absorption and lower than expected blood levels.

iii. The clearance of CsA is accelerated in children and slowed in elderly patients (Shi et al., 2015).

iv. Hypercholesterolaemia can reduce blood levels of CsA.

v. Variations in the gene's polymorphism may be associated with variations on the bio-availability and the pharmacokinetics of CsA. Among them, CYP3A5*3 allele seems to be particularly important for tacrolimus and CYP3A4*22 allele for CsA. Its determination may improve CsA dosing (Lunde et al., 2014).

vi. CsA trough levels increase during bacterial and fungal infections and return to pre-infection levels once the infection was resolved (Hegazy et al., 2015).

vii. Co-administration of drugs or grapefruit that interact at the gut level with the cytochrome P-450 system or P-gp may affect CsA metabolism and interfere with blood levels (Vanhove et al., 2016; see Table 3.3).

Mechanisms of action

Cyclosporine suppresses the immune system and acts selectively on T-cells by slowing down their growth. CsA exerts its actions through the inhibition of a calcium-dependent phosphatase, called calcineurin, a calcium and calmodulin dependent serine/threonine protein phosphatase. After entering the blood circulation, the lipophilic CsA easily diffuses through the cell membrane. Within cells, CsA binds to a specific protein receptor, called cyclophilin, a 17 kDa ubiquitous isomerase that catalyses a rate-determining isomerization in protein folding in vitro. Cyclophilin mediates the cis–trans- isomerization of proline

Table 3.3 Drugs and conditions that can alter the blood levels and area under the curve of calcineurin inhibitors by interfering with cytochrome P-450 metabolites and/or P-glycoprotein.

Conditions and drugs that can increase CNI blood levels	Conditions and drugs that can decrease CNI blood levels
Elderly	Childhood
Infection	Afro-American individuals
Grapefruit	Bile diversion
Cytochrome P 450 genetic variants	Diarrhoea
Fluconazole	Phenobarbital
Itraconazole	Phenytoin
Ketoconazole	Carbamazepine
Clarithromycin	Nafcillin
Erythromycin	Rifampin
Diltiazem	Rifabutin
Verapamil	Dexamethasone (?)
Nicardipine	
Carvedilol	

imino bonds and so allows the slow refolding phase in which proteins fold to their native three-dimensional structure, which is necessary for their function as enzyme or structural protein. The complex CsA-cyclophilin binds to and inhibits calcineurin, a protein phosphatase which has a key role in T-cell activation. Calcineurin removes phosphates from a family of transcription factors, called nuclear factors of activated T-cells (NF-AT). Dephosphorylation allows cytosolic factors (NF-ATc) to enter the nucleus, where they dimerize with another protein induced by a signal from T-cell receptors (NF-ATn) to form a heterodimeric active nuclear factor. This binds to and activates the gene for IL-2, ultimately resulting in IL-2 secretion. As its dephosphorylation is inhibited by CsA, NF-AT cannot enter the nucleus and cannot encode and synthesize IL-2 and other cytokines produced by T-helper-1 cells. As a consequence of the inhibited production of IL-2, the proliferation and differentiation of cytotoxic and other effector T-cells are both inhibited (Kapturczak et al., 2004). Moreover, as the secretion of IL-2 by Th1 cells activates B cells to secrete antibodies, the production of humoral antibodies is also reduced. CsA also blocks the activation of June-N terminal kinases and p38 signalling pathways triggered by antigen recognition, making the drug a highly specific inhibitor of T-cell activation. Other important mechanisms of action are represented by the increased expression of TGF-ß1 and inhibited synthesis of IFγ, colony-stimulating factor, and macrophage-activating factor, which provide signals activating macrophages and monocytes and play an important role in inflammatory processes. All these effects are rapid in onset, dose-dependent, and often quickly reversible after stopping treatment (Barbarino et al., 2013).

Apart from its systemic immunosuppressive activity, CsA could exert protective effect on podocytes by different mechanisms. CsA blocks the calcineurin-mediated dephosphorylation of synaptopodin, an actin-associated protein that modulates actin-based shape and motility of renal podocyte foot processes (Faul et al., 2008). By stabilizing synaptopodin, CsA can also prevent intrapodocyte TRPC6 channel localization and activity, which contributes to podocyte dysfunction and proteinuria (Yu et al., 2016). The inhibited access to the nucleus of NF-AT prevents its binding to the gene promoter encoding uPAR, which activates β3 integrin pathway (Zhang et al., 2012). The impaired cholesterol extrusion from fatty podocyte in NS is mediated by NF-AT activation, which is inhibited by CsA (Pedigo et al., 2016). Finally, murine podocytes express the IL-2R which upregulates pro-apoptotic molecules and induces podocyte injury. CsA can inhibit activation of IL-2R by blocking the synthesis of IL-2 (Zea et al., 2016).

Toxic effects

The therapeutic index (the ratio between toxic and effective dose) of CsA is low, about 2–3 (Ericson et al., 2017). Thus, patients on long-term therapy are particularly susceptible to severe side effects. Therapeutic drug monitoring (TDM) is often used in clinical practice to improve efficacy and reduce adverse events of CsA. However, the role of TDM is limited. Local exposure to CsA is probably more important than systemic exposure in triggering side effects (Naesens et al., 2009). The use of low-dose CsA and careful monitoring of serum creatinine and clinical conditions of the patient are strongly recommended whenever long-term treatment with CsA is prescribed.

Nephrotoxicity

Nephrotoxicity is the major side effect of CsA (Table 3.4). Nephrotoxicity is usually dose-dependent but it is also related to different intra- and interindividual bio-availability and sensitivity and various additional risk factors. It is possible to separate CsA-nephrotoxicity into acute and chronic.

Acute nephrotoxicity is caused by the increased renal vascular resistances. It is characterized by reduced GFR and by an even more profound decrease of renal blood flow with a consequent increased filtration fraction. This nephrotoxicity

Table 3.4 Main side effects of calcineurin inhibitors and factors that can increase their renal toxicity.

Adverse event	Cyclosporine	Tacrolimus	Factors increasing renal toxicity
Nephrotoxicity	+++	+++	Renal insufficiency
Hypertension	+++	+	Hypertension
Neurotoxicity	++	+++	Elderly age
Diabetes	++	+++	NSAIDs
Hyperlipidaemia	++	+	Amphotericin-Azoles
Gum hyperplasia	+++	-	Cidofovir
GI toxicity	+	++	Aminoglycosides
Hypertrichosis	+++	-	Dehydration-Diuretics

is functional and reversible but it may also induce histologic lesions, predominantly in the proximal tubular cells, including giant mitochondria, isometric vacuolization, and microcalcifications caused by calcification of Tamm–Horsfall protein casts. Clinically, acute CsA nephrotoxicity is characterized by increase in serum creatinine and uric acid, weight gain, hypertension, decrease of urine volume, together with low urinary sodium and chloride. The presence of these clinicopathologic features should lead the clinician to modify the doses of CsA and/or to stop the use of concomitant nephrotoxic therapies to prevent the development of chronic lesions.

Chronic nephrotoxicity is a result of long-term administration of CsA, which may induce chronic renal injuries such as arteriolar lesions, interstitial fibrosis, tubular atrophy, and glomerular sclerosis; all can be progressive and lead to irreversible end-stage renal disease (ESRD). Although no histologic finding is specific for CsA toxicity, muscular arteriolar hyaline deposits predominate in CsA-treated patients (Snanoudj et al., 2011). The vascular lesions mainly affect afferent arterioles, while interlobular and arcuate arteries are usually spared. CsA-related arteriolopathy may be characterized by nodular protein deposits that permeate the arteriolar wall and/or by a mucinoid thickening of the intima that results in narrowing of the lumen. Severe vascular lesions, interstitial fibrosis, and tubular atrophy are irreversible and usually lead to progressive renal failure. A common lesion seen in kidneys that develop progressive CsA nephrotoxicity is segmental or diffuse glomerular sclerosis. Clinically, CsA-associated chronic nephropathy is characterized by progressive deterioration of renal function and arterial hypertension.

Different mechanisms can collaborate in inducing CsA-related chronic nephrotoxicity. An important role in initiating these structural lesions is played by micro-RNA that can induce tubular epithelial cell epithelial-mesenchymal transition (Yuan et al., 2015). The activation of the vasoconstriction systems can cause endothelial dysfunction, increase smooth vascular reactivity, and induce episodic hypoxia in nephron segments (Fahling et al., 2017). An important role is played by oxidative stress. CsA induces endoplasmic reticulum stress and increases mitochondrial reactive oxygen species production: this modifies the redox balance and causes lipid peroxidation and induces nephrotoxicity. Moreover, CsA may activate a variety of signalling pathways that increase growth factors, e.g. TGF-β1 and angiotensin II, inhibit P-glycoprotein, and induce apoptosis in renal tubular epithelial cells (Wu et al., 2018).

Arterial hypertension

CsA significantly increases blood pressure compared to placebo in a dose-related fashion. The drug increases sympathetic nervous activity, activates the renin–angiotensin system, and increases the production of renal thromboxane A_2 and the renal synthesis of endothelin while reducing the expression of vasodilating prostaglandins and nitric oxide. Moreover, CsA can significantly increase the reactivity of vascular smooth muscle cells in Wistar rats by increasing the calcium influx in the cytoplasms (Grzésk et al., 2016). The resulting vasoconstrictive effect on afferent preglomerular arterioles decreases GFR and natriuresis leading to salt and water retention. This latter effect is potentiated by the epithelial action of CsA that can directly activate the thiazide-sensitive Na-Cl cotransporter of the distal convoluted tubule, whereas its effect on Na-K-2Cl cotransporter is more complex and requires concomitant stimulation by arginine vasopressin (Blankenstein et al., 2017). Therefore, post-transplant hypertension can be considered as a sodium-dependent hypertension associated with an increase of peripheral vascular resistances. Although the plasma renin levels are often normal, they should be considered inappropriately elevated in front of volume expansion, and may concur in causing hypertension. Elevated blood pressure may increase the risk of stroke, myocardial infarction (MI), heart failure, and other adverse cardiovascular events (Robert et al., 2010).

Managing hypertension in CsA-treated patients is not easy. Thiazide diuretics may be indicated but they can increase serum levels of creatinine and uric acid. Calcium channel blockers (CCBs) are probably the most effective drugs for treating CsA-induced hypertension. However, in association with CsA, CCBs may cause gum hypertrophy. Moreover, non-dihydropyridinic calcium channel blockers (e.g. diltiazem, verapamil) may substantially increase the blood levels of CsA. Renin-angiotensin system (RAS) inhibitors are not particularly effective in CsA-mediated hypertension, since the serum levels of renin and angiotensin are usually low. Moreover, RAS inhibitors may increase serum creatinine, and it may be difficult for clinicians to recognize whether a mild increase in serum creatinine should be referred to the effects of RAS inhibitors or CsA. Finally, a randomized trial in kidney transplant recipients treated with calcineurin inhibitors reported that ramipril compared with placebo did not lead to a significant reduction in doubling of serum creatinine, end-stage renal disease, or death in kidney transplant recipients with proteinuria (Knoll et al., 2016).

Dermatologic complications

The skin is one of the principal sites of accumulation of CsA. The drug, which is highly lipophilic, may partly be eliminated through the sebaceous glands. This may explain the frequent pilosebaceous lesions observed in CsA-treated patients. A frequent complication of CsA is represented by *hypertrichosis,* which is more frequent and severe in children. Hypertrichosis is characterized by thick and pigmented hair appearing over the trunk, back, shoulder, arms, neck, forehead, helices, and malar areas. Hypertrichosis is particularly disturbing not only in children but also in black-haired women. A possible mechanism for CsA-induced hypertrichosis is the increased activity of alpha-reductase, an enzyme that transforms androgens into dihydrotestosterone in peripheral tissues. The alpha-reductase inhibitor finasteride and the antiandrogenic cyproterone acetate may improve hypertrichosis. This and other aesthetic changes caused by CsA may improve after drug withdrawal.

Gingival hyperplasia

Gum hypertrophy occurs in about one-third of patients treated with CsA. It is characterized by hyperplasia of epithelial and connective tissue components. These effects are probably caused by the anti-apoptotic activity of CsA in human gingival fibroblast (Rao et al., 2017). This complication generally occurs after three or more months of treatment and can be worsened by the concomitant administration of calcium channel blockers or phenytoin. Gingival overgrowth is at least partially preventable with careful oral hygiene. Initially, a hyperplasia of the anterior interdental papillae occurs which subsequently spreads to the whole gum also involving the inner side. A five-day treatment with azithromycin, a macrolide antimicrobial agent, may improve gingival overgrowth and the subjective symptoms. The most severe cases require gingivectomy.

Gastrointestinal and hepatic complications

About 10 per cent of patients complain of anorexia, nausea, and/or vomiting. These side-effects are rarely severe.

CsA alters calcium fluxes across hepatocyte cell membranes in vitro, elevates serum bile acids, and decreases bile flow. As a consequence, a slight increase in the bilirubin level unaccompanied by abnormalities in transaminases is common. An increased incidence of cholelithiasis and choledocholithiasis may also occur.

Neurologic complications
Tremor, burning paraesthesias, headache, flushing, depression, confusion, and somnolence have been reported in about 20 per cent of renal transplant recipients treated with CsA. These complications respond slowly to dose reduction. A few cases of convulsions have also been reported, more often in transplanted children. Seizures may be favoured by an increased water content in the brain because of hypertension, by hypomagnesaemia, or by concomitant therapy with IV methylprednisolone, all of which would enhance the distribution of CsA into the nervous system (Ponticelli and Campise, 2005).

A reversible *posterior leukoencephalopathy* can develop even at levels of CsA within the normal range, being that occipital white matter particularly vulnerable to the adverse effects of CsA. Children are more susceptible to this cerebral complication (Hacihamdioğlu et al., 2014). The clinical symptoms include headache, vomiting, confusion seizures, cortical blindness, and other optic abnormalities. Neuro-imaging studies typically show low density white matter lesions suggestive of oedema in the posterior areas of cerebral hemispheres, but abnormalities may also involve other cerebral areas, the brain stem, or the cerebellum.

Other rare complications are *hearing loss, tinnitus, or otalgia*. These symptoms are often reversible with the reduction or withdrawal of the offending drug.

Glucose intolerance
CsA can induce glucose intolerance by a number of mechanisms, including both insulin resistance and insulin secretion (Chakkera et al., 2017). Older or obese patients, carriers of hepatitis C virus, and individuals with a familial history of diabetes are at increased risk of developing diabetes. In patients with open diabetes thiazolidinediones do not display any pharmacological interaction with CsA, but their safety and efficacy need to be confirmed in large-scale randomized trials. Sulfonylureas should be used with caution regarding the suspected interaction of some of them with CsA. If needed, insulin regimens may be adopted.

Hyperlipidaemia
CsA-induced hyperlipidaemia represents a significant clinical issue. CsA may increase LDL and VLDL cholesterol levels, VLDL triglyceride levels, as well as apolipoprotein B and lipoprotein (a), while reducing HDL concentration.

CsA can interfere with lipolysis by inhibiting calcineurin, which can activate lipolysis (Suk et al., 2013). Furthermore, CsA can increase genes and/or proteins involved in hepatic lipogenesis (Fuhrmann et al., 2014) and may inhibit 26-hydroxylase, an enzyme involved in the formation of bile acids from cholesterol, so decreasing the transport of cholesterol to the intestines. On the other hand, hyperlipidaemia may diminish the expression and the functional activity of P-glycoprotein, leading to increased CsA exposure (Brocks et al., 2014).

HMG-CoA reductase inhibitors (statins) are the drugs of choice for treating hypercholesterolaemia. As both CsA and statins are metabolized by the P450 cytochrome enzymatic system, there are bilateral pharmacokinetics interactions that can increase the AUC of statins. To prevent any possible side-effects, when giving statins to CsA-treated patients the doses of statins should not exceed 10–20 mg/day for simvastatin, atorvastatin, and pravastatin, 20–40 mg/day for fluvastatin. Ezetimibe can be used as a second-line lipid-lowering medication if statin therapy is not tolerated or cholesterol targets are not reached by statins alone.

Hyperuricaemia

Hyperuricaemia is a frequent complication of CsA treatment. The specific mechanism for CsA-induced hyperuricaemia is unknown, but it probably involves alterations in tubular transport of uric acid. In a number of cases plasma urate levels considerably increase and may lead to the development of severe acute gouty arthritis and chronic tophaceous gout. Hyperuricaemia can be aggravated by concomitant diuretic therapy, which increases urate reabsorption. Patients respond well to allopurinol or febuxostat. However, these drugs cannot be used in patients taking azathioprine, since allopurinol blocks xanthine oxidase leading to an unpredictable accumulation of 6-mercaptopurine. Whether hyperuricaemia is an independent risk factor for chronic renal dysfunction or only a marker of reduced GFR is still disputed.

Electrolyte abnormalities

The most noticeable change in electrolyte handling is the decreased reabsorption of magnesium, with consequent hypomagnesaemia. Deficiency in magnesium may cause hyperexcitability, muscular symptoms, fatigue, apathy, confusion, and tachycardia.

There is a decreased secretion of potassium and hydrogen ions by the distal tubules, leading to mild hyperkalaemia and acidosis.

Musculoskeletal pain

Isolated musculoskeletal pain may develop during therapy with CsA. The pain mainly involves the joints, but tendons may also be affected. Rare cases of tendon rupture may occur. An increased risk of myopathy and exceptional cases of rhabdomyolysis have been reported in patients given CsA and statins.

Neoplasia

CsA can lead to an increased risk of cancer, which is dose- and time-dependent. This effect is mainly related to its immunosuppressive effect that interferes with the immune surveillance. However, CsA can also promote cancer progression both by a direct cellular effect related to an increased production of TGF-β (Suthantiran et al., 2009) and by promoting tumour angiogenesis through increasing production of mitochondrial reactive oxygen species (Zhou and Rhyeom, 2014).

Pregnancy

CsA may increase the risk of hypertension and pre-eclampsia in pregnant women. Women with solid-organ transplants receiving CsA are at risk for premature birth, low birth weight, caesarean delivery, and hypertensive disorders of pregnancy. The USFDA classifies CsA as category C, meaning that human risk cannot be ruled out (Table 3.2), However, the drug does not appear to be teratogenic (Durst and Rampersad, 2015; Ponticelli and Moroni, 2015; Gotestam Skorpen et al., 2016). Also, lactation is safe (Constantinescu et al., 2014). Nonetheless, long-term effects in humans prenatally exposed to this drug require further evaluation.

Clinical use in glomerular diseases

CsA has been mainly used in patients with GN and nephrotic syndrome. In patients with MCD, FSGS, or MN, CsA should be considered as a second or third treatment option in case of failure, poor tolerance, or contraindications to the standard primary treatment. Instead, poor results have been reported in IgA nephritis or C3 glomerulopathy. We recommend selecting patients before administering CsA. Patients with severe hypertension and eGFR ≤30 ml/min are not good candidates for CsA. Serum creatinine and blood pressure should be monitored every seven to ten days in the early period and at least every month after four weeks. If serum creatinine increases >30–50 per cent over the baseline, the doses should be reduced; if the increase is ≥75–100 per cent over the baseline CsA should be stopped and started again only when serum creatinine returns to the baseline levels. CsA should be given at the smallest effective dose for at least six months. If proteinuria is not reduced by 50 per cent by the end of this time frame, an alternate therapy should be considered, although in some cases the response may occur later. Treatment targets should include complete or partial remission of proteinuria, maintenance of stable GFR (not more than 30 per cent of pre-treatment level), avoiding hypertension. Measuring blood levels is not strictly necessary but some random checks may be useful to verify the adequacy of doses. We suggest keeping trough blood levels between 150–250 ng/ml in the first three to four months and progressively reducing the dosage by keeping trough blood levels <100–150 ng/ml. If complete remission occurs, CsA should be tapered off over three to four months. For partial remission, CsA should be given at the lowest doses able to prevent nephrotic proteinuria for an additional one to two years and perhaps maintained at a non-toxic level indefinitely if renal function is stable and/or the patient has previously failed other forms of treatment. Alternatively, CsA could be tapered slowly over two to three years and increased as required following any relapses. If there is no response to CsA or if a response occurs with adverse effects, an alternative therapy should be considered. In order to minimize the risk of renal toxicity some guidelines should be respected. Unfortunately, most patients who attain complete disappearance of proteinuria with CsA show early relapse of proteinuria after CsA is stopped or even reduced, possibly due to dissipation of local effects on podocytes. However, the rate of relapses may be reduced if CsA is given in low dosage for a prolonged period and then tapered off gradually, even though this may expose to the nephrotoxic effects of the agent.

Tacrolimus (TAC)

Tacrolimus (also known as FK-506) is a macrolide immunosuppressant derived from the fungus *Streptomyces tsukubaensis*. It has a molecular mass of 822 kDa and is poorly soluble in water while it is very soluble in ethanol, methanol, propylene glycol, and polyethylene glycol. The drug inhibits cellular immune responses and humoral immune responses to a less extent. TAC is available for IV and oral administration.

There are three main formulations of tacrolimus. The immediate release formulation of tacrolimus (Prograf®) is given in a twice-daily administration. A once-daily formulation of tacrolimus (Astagraf XL™, Astellas Pharm US, Inc., Northbrook, IL) has been approved for use by European authorities in 2007 and by the USFDA in 2013. Astagraf XL™ or Advagraf® is modified to be released slowly by adding ethylcellulose, hypromellose, and lactose monohydrate in order to modify water penetration and form a protective polymer coating around the drug. A revision of studies of conversion from twice-daily to once-daily extended-release TAC in renal transplant recipients showed that mean serum creatinine levels remained stable during two years of observation. TAC trough levels were significantly reduced at one to two weeks, at one month, six months, 12 months, and at 24 months after conversion. Regarding the safety profile, no significant changes were noted in blood glucose, potassium, and magnesium. Approximately 35 per cent of recipients preferred the extended-release formula tacrolimus to twice-daily tacrolimus (Tran et al., 2014). A novel once-daily extended-release TAC (Envarsus®) is also available (Rostaing et al., 2016). All the three formulations proved to be effective in preventing acute rejection in kidney transplant recipients (Jouve et al., 2017).

Metabolism

After oral administration TAC is rapidly, but incompletely, absorbed in the gastrointestinal tract. Peak plasma concentrations are usually reached within one hour, but sometimes up to four hours. The oral bio-availability is poor with wide ranges of 6–56 per cent, with a mean of 25 per cent. Its half-life is also variable with ranges of 3.5–40.5 hours, with a mean value of 11.3 hours. TAC is highly distributed into red blood cells. Plasma protein binding approaches 99 per cent with the majority of the drug binding to α1-acid glycoprotein and albumin. TAC is almost completely metabolized by the cytochrome P450 CYP3A4 isoenzymes in the liver. Even a single polymorphism of these isoenzymes may alter TAC pharmacokinetics. As an example, patients expressing CYP3A5 have a dose requirement that is around 50 per cent higher than non-expressers (De Jonge et al., 2011; Tang et al., 2016). Of note, the POR*28 variant allele is associated with increased in vivo CYP3A5 activity for TAC in CYP3A5 expressers (Elens et al., 2014). Intestinal mucosa also concurs to metabolize the parent drug by P450 CYP3A4 isoenzymes and the efflux protein P-gp. Most metabolites do not show immunosuppressive properties. While tacrolimus and its metabolites are primarily eliminated by biliary tract and excreted in faeces, less than 2 per cent of the drug is eliminated unchanged in the urine.

With the extended release formulation, the trough levels were 40 per cent lower than that of regular release TAC at six weeks after administration. The total daily dose requirement also tended to be at least 10 per cent higher with extended release TAC as compared to the regular release TAC (Ho et al., 2013). Some groups used a 1:1.25 dose conversion ratio between regular TAC and extended release TAC to avoid underimmune suppression post conversion, but this did not prevent the need for subsequent dose modifications.

TAC and its extended release formulation have a large inter- and intra-individual variability. African-Americans and Hispanics have a poorer bio-availability than Caucasians. Children may have a higher clearance of TAC than adults (Kim et al., 2005), while the clearance is reduced in elderly subjects and in patients with liver dysfunction (Shi et al., 2015). Since polymorphism of genes encoding P450 isoenzymes is associated with low initial TAC exposure and increased dose requirements, CYP3A5 genotyping might be useful to improve initial dosing of TAC (Lunde et al., 2014; Ito et al., 2017; Sanghavi et al., 2017). A number of drugs may interact with TAC and CsA by affecting bio-availability.

TAC disposition is more susceptible to these interactions compared with CsA because CsA is itself a moderately strong CYP3A4 inhibitor and strong P-gp inhibitor (Vanhove et al., 2016), blunting the effect of additional inhibitors (Table 3.3). In view of its low therapeutic index, the doses of the drug should be adjusted in most patients. Whole blood drug monitoring can help in optimizing treatment.

Mechanisms of action

TAC shares a number of immunosuppressive properties with CsA. Through the inhibition of calcineurin, both the drugs strongly inhibit the induction of the synthesis of IL-2 and other cytokines and this is the key to their immunosuppressive action. As CsA, TAC is a lipophilic prodrug. It easily enters the cell wall and binds to its cytoplasmic receptor, called FK-binding protein 12 (FKBP12), which is structurally different from cyclophilin. The drug-receptor complex undergoes an allosteric conformational change which allows it to bind to calcineurin. This binding inhibits the activity of calcineurin, which, as discussed, is a complex of phosphatases particularly important for the entry into the nucleus of cytosolic factors (NF-AT), which can promote transcription of cytokine genes. Thus, both cyclophilin and FKBP12 represent part of a signal transduction pathway used during T-cell activation, which is important for the activation of select cytokine genes. FK-binding protein and cyclophilin are related and one may be transformed into the other by the enzyme rotamase. TAC interacts with its binding protein with greater affinity than CsA binds to cyclophilin. CsA and TAC can cause different effects on TGF-ß1, which is an important immune modulator but also a strong profibrotic factor. Neither CsA nor TAC can induce TGF-ß1 biosynthesis (Minguillon et al., 2005). However, the ligand to FKBP12, an important inhibitor of TGF-ß1 receptor (Chiasson et al., 2012), may result in an increased activity of TGF- ß1. TAC, like CsA, may also have direct (and reversible) effects on podocytes to suppress proteinuria (see 'Mechanisms of action' of CsA).

Toxic effects

Patients treated with TAC may suffer from the same potential adverse events that may occur with CsA. Some differences can be found in the prevalence and intensity of clinical side effects. Most of side effects are dose- and duration-dependent.

Nephrotoxicity

The mechanisms responsible of nephrotoxicity are probably similar for CsA and TAC (Table 3.4). However, patients with TAC nephrotoxicity exhibit increased expression of profibrogenic genes compared to CsA nephrotoxicity (Khanna et al., 2002). This may be explained by the binding of TAC to FKBP12. As a consequence, there is a reduced inhibition of TGF-ß1 receptor, allowing aberrant TGF-β receptor signalling that can eventually result in arteriolar hyalinosis and interstitial kidney fibrosis (Chiasson et al., 2012; Kern et al., 2014). At any rate, the prevalence of nephrotoxicity is similar with TAC and CsA. In particular, morphologic changes associated with toxic drug effects in the kidney are indistinguishable from one another, i.e. tubular lesions, arteriolopathy, microangiopathic changes in glomeruli and vessels. A meta-analysis of studies comparing TAC with CsA in renal transplant recipients concluded that treating 100 patients with TAC instead of CsA for the first post-transplant year avoided 12 patients having acute rejection and two losing graft, but caused insulin-dependent diabetes in five patients (Webster et al., 2005).

Hypertension

The clinical impression is that arterial hypertension is less pronounced with TAC than with CsA, probably because of the lower interference of TAC with the reactivity of the vascular smooth muscular cells (Grzesk et al., 2016).

Diabetes mellitus

One of the most frequent and severe complications of TAC is the onset of a dose-dependent *de novo* diabetes mellitus (Penfornis and Kury-Paulin, 2006). It seems to be caused both by a decrease in insulin secretion (Ozbay et al., 2011) and by an increase in insulin resistance (Li et al., 2015). There is agreement that TAC is more diabetogenic than CsA. Zucker rats treated with TAC showed reduced beta-cell proliferation and *Ins2* gene expression in comparison with CsA (Rodriguez-Rodriguez et al., 2013). HCV infection, impaired fasting glucose, a family history of diabetes, male gender, and elevated body mass index can increase the risk of diabetes. TAC should probably not be used in obese or pre-diabetic subjects.

Gastrointestinal symptoms

Gastrointestinal troubles, particularly diarrhoea, are relatively frequent with TAC and can be worsened by the concomitant use of mycophenolate salts (Savvidaki et al., 2014).

Neurological complications

These complications are more frequent and more severe with TAC in comparison with CsA. Tremors, paraesthesias, insomnia are common. Convulsions, aphasia, paralysis, disabling pain syndrome, and leukoencephalopathy can also occur (Ponticelli and Campise, 2005). Hearing loss is more frequent with TAC than with CsA. Cases of posterior reversible encephalopathy have been reported (Song et al., 2016).

Hyperlipidaemia

Serum total cholesterol, triglyceride, Apo A1, Apo B, and LDL levels may be increased in patients treated with high doses of TAC. However, these levels are usually lower than those seen in CsA-treated patients. Beneficial effect on lipid levels has been reported in renal transplant recipients after conversion from CsA to TAC.

Electrolyte disturbances

About one-third of patients show an increase of potassium in the blood. Hypomagnesaemia is also frequent.

Malignancy

The risk of malignancy is similar to that of CsA. However, the incidence of lymphoproliferative disorders in the first year after kidney transplantation has been reported to be higher with TAC than CsA (Akar Özkan et al., 2014).

Pregnancy

TAC may favour the development of diabetes or hypertension in pregnant women. The FDA classifies TAC as category C, meaning that human risk cannot be ruled out, because the human studies are lacking and the experimental studies are either positive for risk or lacking. However, in newborns from transplant recipients the risk of major malformations was low—similar to that of CsA (Durst and Rampersad, 2015; Piccoli et al., 2017). The patterns of defects were so variable that it is difficult to attribute malformations to TAC. No lingering effects due to breastfeeding have been found in infants who were breastfed while their mothers were taking TAC (Constantinescu et al., 2014).

Clinical use in glomerular diseases

There are no formal indications for TAC in the treatment of primary glomerular diseases (for more information, see specific chapters in this volume). However, promising results with TAC alone or in combination with other immunosuppressive drugs have been reported in different glomerular diseases resistant to previous treatments. As for CsA, most patients suffered from relapse of nephrotic syndrome when TAC was interrupted. At present, TAC may be considered to have the same role and the same limits than CsA in treating glomerular diseases. TAC is more expensive and may cause diabetes and neurologic symptoms more frequently than CsA. However, TAC can be effective even at low doses, causes less frequent hypertension and hyperlipidaemia in comparison with CsA, and does not cause aesthetic changes. Recommendations with the use of TAC in glomerulonephritis are similar to those given for CsA. The initial doses may range between 0.1 and 0.2 mg/kg/day, with gradual reduction, and treatment should be interrupted if no change in proteinuria is seen after six months of therapy. Checking blood levels is not strictly needed in adults (although some sporadic checks may be useful to control the bio-availability and the adherence to prescription). In children it is recommended to check the trough blood levels, at least in the first period, being that the bio-availability and the pharmacokinetics of TAC are variable and unpredictable. The trough blood levels should be maintained between 5–10 ng/ml in the initial period and between 4–6 ng/ml for maintenance.

Nucleotide synthesis inhibitors

Azathioprine

Azathioprine is an N-methylnitroimidazole thiopurine which was developed in the early 1950s. It is a prodrug, being a modification of 6-mercaptopurine, which in turn is an analogue of the purine base hypoxanthine. Azathioprine has been mainly used in clinical transplantation, vasculitis, and in auto-immune diseases. The possible indications for azathioprine in primary glomerular diseases are still a matter of controversy. The drug is available for oral use, in the form of tablets, and as a sodium salt for IV injection (rarely used).

Thiopurine metabolism

Azathioprine is a mercaptopurine prodrug, with poor bio-availability, large interindividual variability, and a less pronounced intraindividual variability. After oral administration, about 40–44 per cent of azathioprine is absorbed and rapidly transformed into 6-mercaptopurine by hepatic and erythrocytic glutathione. The peak plasma concentration of 6-mercaptopurine ranges between one and two hours after oral administration. The mean half-life of 6-mercaptopurine is about 74 minutes, but there is wide day-to-day variability.

Mercaptopurine is rapidly biotransformed into mercaptopurine nucleotides (thioinosine monophosphate, thioguanine and 6-thioguanine nucleotides). The thioguanine nucleotides (TGN) are the mono-, di-, and triphosphates of thioguanosine. They incorporate into DNA and inhibit *de novo* purine synthesis by the methylmercaptopurine nucleotides. TGN are eliminated slowly. The main pathway of degradation is direct oxidation catalysed by the enzyme xanthine oxidase. However, TGN should first be catalysed to methylated derivatives by the enzyme methionine S-methyltransferase, with subsequent oxidation. The degradation process leads to formation of 6-thiouric acid, a final product devoid of immunosuppressive effects, and which is eventually eliminated by the kidney (Figure 3.2). There are differences in S-methylation. 'Low' methylators are more susceptible to myelosuppression (Dewitt et al., 2011), while 'fast' methylators may have a poor response to azathioprine. However,

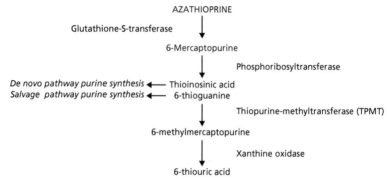

Figure 3.2 About 40–44 per cent of AZA is absorbed and transformed into 6-mercaptopurine (that contains thioinosinic acid and thioguanine). Phosphoribosyltransferase releases thioguanine nucleotides from 6-mercaptopurine. Thioinosinic acid inhibits the *de novo* pathway of purine synthesis and 6-thioguanine inhibits the salvage pathway. Thioguanine nucleotides are broken slowly by thiopurine methyltransferase (TPMT) and oxidated to inactive thiouric acid by xanthine oxidase.

difference in S-methylation does not predict other adverse effects, nor does it explain most cases of thiopurine resistance. Other genetic polymorphisms, such as single nucleotide polymorphism in NUDT15 and in the class II HLA locus have been shown to predict thiopurine-related leukopenia and pancreatitis (Roberts and Barclay, 2015).

Mechanisms of action

The pharmacological activity of azathioprine rests on the formation of the active intracellular nucleotides thioinosinic acid and 6-thioguanine. Thioinosinic acid inhibits enzymes that mediate the first step of *de novo* pathways of purine synthesis from smaller molecular weight precursors, while 6-thioguanine interferes with the salvage pathway by inhibiting enzymes required for the interconversion of purine bases. By depleting cellular purine stores, these nucleotides inhibit the synthesis of DNA, RNA, and various proteins and coenzymes, so halting the proliferation of lymphocytes, which require purines during their proliferative phase. The immunosuppressive effects of azathioprine are more potent on T- than on B-cells. The drug may also block antigen recognition by alkylating thiol groups on T-cell surface membranes.

Toxic effects

The occurrence of adverse effects is a major drawback in the use of azathioprine. Iatrogenic effects are usually dose-dependent but may also be caused by a genetic defect of thiopurine methyltransferase (TPMT), which mediates

S-methylation of 6-mercaptopurine. 'Slow' methylators are particularly suscep-tible to myelotoxicity from the drug. It has been suggested that subjects who are prescribed azathioprine should have the TPMT activity measured beforehand so as to avoid unexpected toxicity myelosuppression with 'normal' dosage. The activity of TPMT is regulated by a common genetic polymorphism. One in 300 individuals lack enzyme activity and 11 per cent are heterozygous for a variant low activity allele and have an intermediate activity. Very low TPMT activity is associated with grossly abnormal thiopurine drug metabolism, excess pro-duction of cytotoxic metabolites and profound life-threatening myelotoxicity, in patients taking thiopurine drugs (Lennard, 2014). Rapid clinical assays of the enzyme are now available (Burchard et al., 2014). However, the presence of the normal TPMT activity genotypes cannot preclude the development of side effects (Liu et al., 2015). Thus, regular monitoring of the white blood cell is re-commended during azathioprine treatment.

Bone marrow inhibition

Thioguanine is incorporated into human bone marrow cells. Leukopenia is the most common manifestation of bone marrow toxicity, thrombocytopenia and megaloblastic anaemia may also occur. As only inactive metabolites are excreted by the kidney, renal insufficiency does not lead to accumulation of me-tabolites with immunosuppressive effects. However, due to the increased sensi-tivity of uraemic bone marrow to thioguanine, a reduction of azathioprine dose is advisable in patients with renal failure.

Concomitant administration of azathioprine and drugs which block xanthine oxidase, engenders the hazard of severe bone marrow suppression because these dugs inhibit the oxidation of 6-mercaptopurine to inactive metabolites. *Whenever allopurinol or febuxostat is introduced, azathioprine should be reduced to at least one-third of the previous dosage and blood cell count should be checked at least every week for the first four weeks.*

Liver toxicity

Liver toxicity is a rare, but potentially severe, complication of azathioprine. Rare cases of *hypersensitivity* and liver toxicity have been reported. *Hepatotoxicity* is relatively uncommon. Clinically it is characterized by a reversible increase in serum transaminases and bilirubin. At liver biopsy, hepatocellular and cana-licular cholestasis with mild portal and periportal inflammation may be seen (Siramolpiwat and Sakonlaya, 2017). *Veno-occlusive hepatic disease* is a rare but severe complication characterized histologically by a fibrous obliteration of terminal hepatic venules. This condition causes mild liver enzymatic increases and eventually leads to portal hypertension and death. Early discontinuation of azathioprine may improve the outcome. Another exceptional complication is *nodular regenerative hyperplasia* of the liver, which may occur in patients given high doses of thioguanines and/or in those with elevated liver enzymes (Musumba, 2013). This complication, characterized by a diffuse nodular involvement of the liver and by absence of fibrosis, may lead to intrahepatic portal hypertension and/or chronic anicteric cholestasis. Exceptionally idiosyncratic reactions with acute leukopenia, fever, rash, and hepatitis may develop a few days after the first administration of azathioprine.

Pancreatitis
Azathioprine has been linked to subsequent acute pancreatitis in case reports and small case series. In a large retrospective series, the incidence rate for acute pancreatitis among all users of azathioprine was one per 659 treatment year (Floyd et al., 2003).

Gastric intolerance
About 10 per cent of patients may complain of gastric discomfort, which only exceptionally leads to drug discontinuation.

Dermatological complications
Rare cases of febrile neutrophilic dermatitis have been reported. The complete resolution after azathioprine withdrawal speaks in favour of azathioprine hypersensitivity syndrome (Aleissa et al., 2017). Thinning of the hair and scalp hair loss, changes of colour or texture of the hair, and actinic keratoses may occur in azathioprine-treated patients, particularly after extensive sunlight exposure.

Neoplasia
Azathioprine is considered as an oncogenic drug as it is incorporated into the DNA of the genome. Experience with azathioprine in organ transplantation suggested that patients might have an excess risk of tumours, including lymphoma and skin tumours. The risk of malignancy mainly depends on the duration and cumulative dosage of azathioprine treatment as well as on the association with other drugs or infections that may impair the immunological surveillance, with the cumulative risk of tumours increasing over time (Weaver, 2012).

The oncogenic risk of azathioprine in auto-immune diseases is difficult to assess. A systematic review aimed to determine the trade-off between the benefits and risks of azathioprine in multiple sclerosis hypothesized that a long-term risk of cancer from azathioprine may be related to a treatment duration above ten years and cumulative doses above 600 g (Casetta et al., 2007). There is little information about the risk of malignancy in primary glomerulonephritis but sporadic cases of cancer in azathioprine-treated patients have been reported. The problem is complicated by the fact that, in some cases, glomerulonephritis is secondary to cancer.

Infections

The interference of azathioprine with cellular immunity may theoretically account for a high rate of infections, particularly in leukopenic patients. Usually, however, azathioprine is well tolerated and its use does not account for an increased risk of infections, except for patients with bone marrow suppression.

Interstitial nephritis

Rare cases of interstitial nephritis after the administration of azathioprine have been reported.

Pregnancy

Only inactive metabolites pass into the foetal circulation. The USFDA classified azathioprine as a drug at potential risk of teratogenic effects (Class C) on the basis of animal studies. However, clinical studies did not show an excess of malformations in women exposed to azathioprine during pregnancy (Ponticelli and Moroni, 2015). The long-term consequences of in-utero exposure to azathioprine are unknown.

Clinical use in glomerular diseases

Azathioprine has been used in several types of primary glomerulonephritis. The results have not been very impressive and after initial enthusiasm, azathioprine has almost been abandoned. However, it is still used for maintenance treatment in patients with renal vasculitis or lupus nephritis.

The drug is administered at doses ranging between 1.5 and 3 mg/kg/day. During treatment, circulating leukocytes should be checked regularly, every seven to ten days initially and at longer intervals when leukocytes maintain stable levels with a fixed dose of azathioprine. We suggest not attempting to induce leukopenia deliberately, since there is no evidence that leukopenia improves the response to azathioprine, while it certainly does increase the risk of infections. As mentioned, should the use of allopurinol or febuxostat be necessary, the dose of azathioprine must be reduced to one third. Liver transaminases should be checked regularly in the case of prolonged therapy with azathioprine. Today genetic tests are available that can identify the five main genes of thiopurine methyltransferase. This may include low methylators and high methylators.

Mycophenolate salts

Two mycophenolate salts are commercially available: mycophenolate mofetil (MMF) and an enteric coated formulation of mycophenolate sodium (MS). Both of them are prodrugs that release the active mycophenolic acid (MPA). MPA is a reversible and non-competitive inhibitor of the inosine monophosphate dehydrogenase (IMPDH) enzyme by which guanine is synthesized from inosine. As a consequence, the *de novo* pathway of purine synthesis is inhibited. Unlike azathioprine, MPA is not incorporated into DNA and has no pro-oncogenic effects. Since activated lymphocytes rely more than other cells on *de novo* pathway, T- and B-cells are preferentially affected by MPA, which causes an accumulation of lymphocytes at the G1-S phase of the cell cycle. MMF and MS are available for oral use in the form of tablets. A tablet of the enteric coated formulation of 360 mg is equivalent to a tablet of 500 mg of MMF.

MPA metabolism

(Figure 3.3)

After oral administration, mycophenolate salts are rapidly reabsorbed and hydrolysed by esterases to the active moiety MPA. There is a peak in plasma concentration of MPA between 0.5 and 1.0 hour after oral administration of MMF. Differently from MMF, the enteric coated formulation does not release MPA under acidic conditions (pH <5), i.e. in the stomach, but is highly soluble in neutral pH conditions, i.e. in the intestine. Therefore, MPA reaches a peak concentration in plasma later with MS, between 1.5 and 2.75 hours.

In the blood, MPA is bound to albumin >98 per cent. MPA is metabolized in the liver by uridine diphosphonate glucuronyl transferase (UGT) to acid

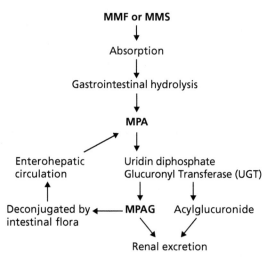

Figure 3.3 After oral administration, MMF is rapidly absorbed and hydrolysed to MPA in the stomach while MMS is hydrolysed later in the intestine. MPA is glucoronated by hepatic UGT to inactive MPAG and in minimal part to active acylglucoronide. MPAG is deconjugated by intestinal flora to active MPA, thus originating a second peak of MPA in the serum. MPAG and acylglucoronide are eventually eliminated by the kidney.

glucuronide MPA (MPAG). MPAG is secreted in the bile and is deconjugated by gut flora into MPA, which is reabsorbed in the blood producing a second peak approximately six to eight hours after drug administration. The majority of MPA dose administered is eliminated in the urine primarily as MPAG (>60 per cent) and approximately 3 per cent as unchanged MPA. MPAG may accumulate in renal failure but it does not cause toxic effects, since it does not have pharmacologic activity. The mean elimination half-lives of MPA and MPAG are 8–16 hours, and 13–17 hours, respectively. MPA exposure is increased in patients with renal dysfunction taking macrolides owing to enhanced MPAG enterohepatic circulation (Colom et al., 2014). Genetic variants within genes involved in MPA metabolism (*UGT1A9, UGT1A8, UGT2B7*), cellular transportation (*SLCOB1, SLCO1B3, ABCC2*), and targets (IMPDH) have been reported to affect MPA pharmacokinetics and/or response (Staatz and Tett, 2014).

Mechanisms of action

MPA is an uncompetitive and reversible inhibitor of inosine monophosphate dehydrogenase and induces a striking conformational change in IMPDH protein in intact cells, resulting in the formation of annular aggregates of protein with concomitant inhibition of IMPDH activity. As a result, MPA produces a marked reduction of guanosine triphosphate necessary for DNA synthesis and inhibits the *de novo* pathway of guanosine nucleotide synthesis. T- and B-lymphocytes are more dependent on this pathway than other cell types are. Moreover, MPA is a fivefold more potent inhibitor of the type II isoform of IMPDH, which is expressed in activated lymphocytes, than of the type I isoform of IMPDH, which is expressed in most cell types. MPA has therefore a more potent cytostatic effect on lymphocytes than on other cell types. This is the principal mechanism by which MPA exerts immunosuppressive effects. Three other mechanisms may also contribute to the immunosuppressive efficacy of MPA:

i. MPA can induce apoptosis of activated T-lymphocytes.

ii. by depleting guanosine nucleotides, MPA suppresses glycosylation and the expression of some adhesion molecules, thereby decreasing the recruitment of lymphocytes and monocytes into sites of inflammation.

iii. by depleting guanosine nucleotides, MPA also depletes tetrahydrobiopterin, a co-factor for the inducible form of nitric oxide synthase (Allison and Eugui, 2000).

MPA is not a nucleotide and therefore does not require incorporation into DNA, as does azathioprine. Because T- and B-lymphocytes are critically dependent for their proliferation on *de novo* synthesis of purines, whereas other cell types can utilize salvage pathways, MPA has potent cytostatic effect on both

T- and B-cells. Experimental studies have also found that MMF can attenuate the progression of renal fibrosis by inhibiting TGF-β1- and TNF-α-induced fibronectin synthesis (Yung et al., 2015).

Toxic effects

Most of the following adverse effects are dose dependent.

Bone marrow toxicity

The risk of leukopenia is increased in patients with high circulating levels of free MPA, which may occur in case of hypo-albuminaemia. Interaction between MPA and valacyclovir may also lead to neutropenia. Thrombocytopenia is uncommon and usually attributable to the underlying disease or to a complicating infection, often viral in nature, or to a thrombo-embolic event. Rare cases of agranulocytosis have been reported (Matsui et al., 2010).

Gastrointestinal toxicity

Nausea, vomiting, and, in particular, diarrhoea are relatively frequent in patients treated with mycophenolate salts. The gastric adverse effects are irritative in nature and are often reversible. However, in a number of patients they may require a dose change or even the discontinuation of the drug. As gastric symptoms are related to the peak blood concentration, it is advisable to subdivide the daily dose of MMF in two or even three amounts for administration. MS has a later and lower peak concentration in the blood and might mitigate the incidence and the impact of gastrointestinal disturbances in comparison with MMF (Manger et al., 2015).

Lung toxicity

In rare cases, MMF may cause dry cough and dyspnoea. In most patients, symptoms develop within the third month and may raise problems of differential diagnosis with pneumonitis. Exceptionally, MMF may lead to pulmonary fibrosis and acute respiratory failure. The clinical symptoms completely reverse after MMF discontinuation.

Acute inflammatory syndrome

A paradoxical pro-inflammatory reaction of polymorphonuclear cells, characterized by fever, arthralgias, oligoarthritis, and increased levels of reactive C protein may exceptionally occur (Maes et al., 2002). The syndrome is completely reversible with the discontinuation of the drug.

Neoplasia

Although MPA may theoretically favour an increased risk of tumour through an impairment in the immune surveillance, it has been shown to have an antiproliferative activity against leukaemia and lymphoma and anti-tumour and anti-angiogenetic effects against solid cancer. The antineoplastic activity of MPA is probably related to its inhibition of IMPDH, which is up-regulated in many tumours. Furthermore, MPA may downregulate a number of genes and proteins with promigratory functions and upregulate genes with antimigratory functions (Dun et al., 2013).

Infections

Like all other immunosuppressive agents, mycophenolate may render the patients more susceptible to infections. In organ transplant recipients given mycophenolate, the risk of cytomegalovirus (CMV) infection is increased. The risk is dose dependent and is highly influenced by the concomitant use of GCs or other immunosuppressive agents. Patients at high risk of CMV infection should avoid mycophenolate. An increased risk of polyoma BK virus interstitial nephritis has been reported in patients given the association tacrolimus with mycophenolate.

Progressive multifocal leukoencephalopathy (PML)

Cases of PML have been reported in renal transplant recipients or lupus patients treated with MMF. The USFDA has warned against the possible risk of PML in patients treated with mycophenolate.

Pregnancy

Use of mycophenolate during pregnancy is associated with an increased risk of first trimester pregnancy loss and increased risk of congenital malformation, especially external ear and other facial abnormalities, including cleft lip and palate, and anomalies of the distal limbs, heart, oesophagus, and kidney. FDA classifies these drugs as Category D, i.e. with positive evidence of human foetal risk. Women being considered for treatment with mycophenolate should always have a negative pregnancy test and should employ at least two methods of contraception during its use. If pregnancy occurs, the drug should be stopped. Azathioprine can be substituted for mycophenolate under these circumstances. Instead, paternal exposure to MPA did not increase the risk of adverse birth outcomes in children fathered by male kidney transplanted patients. These data support the continuation of paternal MPA treatment before, during, and after conception (Midtvedt et al., 2017).

Clinical use in glomerular diseases

Both MMF and MS are being largely used in lupus nephritis and renal vasculitis. However, the indications, the dosage, the duration of treatment, and the possible benefits and risks in primary glomerular diseases are still unclear. Good short-term results have been reported in steroid-dependent MCD. In FSGS and MN controlled and uncontrolled studies reported the possible effectiveness of MMF in reducing proteinuria, but complete remission was rare and relapses were very common. In IgA nephropathy (IgAN), a meta-analysis of eight randomized trials found that MMF had no significant effects in reducing proteinuria or protecting renal function. compared with other therapies (Chen et al., 2014). Although mycophenolate salts may yet find a niche in the management of proteinuric renal diseases, well-designed randomized trials are needed to better evaluate their proper evidence-based role in patients with primary glomerulonephritis.

The large variability in metabolism and pharmacokinetics of MPA is a major issue with the use of mycophenolate. It should be reminded that mycophenolate salts are metabolized to the inactive mycophenolic acid glucuronide by uridine diphosphate glucuronosyltransferases, which have several promoter polymorphisms that affect their activity and can thus increase or decrease exposure to MPA. Moreover, some drugs can reduce the absorption of MMF (including amoxicillin, rifampin, fluoroquinolones, and proton pump inhibitors), while other drugs may increase the risk of leukopenia (such as acyclovir, ganciclovir, valacyclovir, valganciclovir). Some investigators feel that to obtain an adequate therapeutic drug monitoring, the AUC of MPA should be established for any single patient (Saint Marcoux et al., 2011; Abd Rahman et al., 2014; Sobiak et al., 2015). On the other hand, many studies indicate relatively good correlation between trough concentration and the AUC in patients treated with mycophenolate. In clinical practice, the therapeutic drug monitoring of MPA is often based on the C0 measured approximately 12 hours post-dose (Streicher et al., 2014). The threshold of 3 mg/L can potentially be recommended as a target trough value in patients with glomerular disease (Łuszczyńska and Pawiński, 2015).

Mizoribine (MZB)

Mizoribine, also called bredinin, is an imidazole nucleoside which demonstrated immunosuppressive activity in various animal models, in renal transplant recipients, and in Japanese patients with idiopathic nephrotic syndrome, IgA nephritis, or lupus nephritis. It is administered orally in form of tablets. It is approved for use in Asia, but not in the US or in Europe.

Clinical pharmacology

Pharmacokinetic studies of MZB showed that the peak serum level appeared two to four hours after oral administration of 50–200 mg, with a linear relationship between the dose and the peak serum MZB level. The elimination rate from serum depends on kidney function, and the elimination rate constant is well correlated with the endogenous creatinine clearance. No circadian rhythm is apparent. The absorption rate of MZB from the gastrointestinal tract may be affected by gastrointestinal diseases. Dosage adjustment based on the renal function is suggested.

Mechanisms of action

MZB exerts activity through selective inhibition of monophosphate synthetase and guanosine monophosphate synthetase, resulting in the complete inhibition of guanine nucleotide synthesis without incorporation into nucleotides. Thus, MZB blocks the *de novo* synthesis of the purine guanosine. It arrests DNA synthesis in the S phase of cellular division. The proliferation of T- and B-cells is especially sensitive to inhibition by MZB. On the other hand, most non-immune cells are resistant to the drug because they can meet their requirements for guanosine by using enzymes in the salvage pathway. MZB has immunosuppressive effects comparable to those of azathioprine. MZB can also attenuate the expression of monocyte chemoattractant protein-1 in human mesangial cells and may exert a suppressive effect on activated macrophages and intrinsic renal cells. Moreover, MZB might also prevent podocyte injury through correction of the intracellular energy balance and nephrin biogenesis in cultured podocyte and rat models (Tanaka et al., 2015).

Toxicity

MZB exerts less toxicity on bone marrow and liver than azathioprine as it does not cause damages to normal cells and normal nucleic acid. The principal adverse reactions associated with the use of MZB were leukopenia (0.8–6.6 per cent), abnormal hepatic function (1.1–4.1 per cent), rash, increased levels of uric acid (0.4–2.5 per cent), and gastrointestinal troubles (0.4–1.5 per cent); the incidence depends on the type of disease and dosage of the drug (Kawasaki, 2009). These side effects may be prevented by keeping the serum levels below 0.5 μg/ml.

Clinical use in glomerular diseases

The mechanisms of action and the indications of MZB are similar to those of mycophenolic acid. Most reports on this drug come from Japan, where MZB is produced. MZB has been mostly used in idiopathic nephrotic syndrome, in lupus nephritis, and in kidney transplantation. The drug has also been successfully administered in patients with FSGS, MN, and IgAN in observational studies without serious adverse effects. However, it is unclear which is the best regimen. Usually, MZB was administered at a dose of 100–200 mg/day either given in a single dose or three times in a day. Due to its large bio-availability, it has been suggested to tailor the dosage of MFB on the basis of its blood concentration at three hours after administration (Fuke et al., 2012). In severe lupus nephritis MZB has also been used intermittently at high dosage (10 mg/kg) to obtain higher peak serum levels and higher efficacy. To better assess the role of MZB in primary glomerular diseases, well-designed, prospective, randomized trials are needed. It is not approved for use by the USFDA or the European Medicines Agency (EMA).

Leflunomide

Leflunomide is an isoxazole derivative—a prodrug that releases the active compound A771726. Leflunomide has proved to be effective and well tolerated in patients with rheumatoid arthritis (RA) and is currently approved for this use by the USFDA and EMA. Leflunomide produces neither myelotoxicity nor nephrotoxicity and does not require dose adjustment in case of renal insufficiency. It is available in form of tablets. The initial dosage in patients with RA is 100 mg/24 hours for three days followed by a dose of 10–20 mg/day.

Clinical pharmacology

After absorption leflunomide is converted to its active metabolite A771726, a malononitrilamide, in the gut wall, in plasma, and in the liver. Peak plasma concentrations of A771726 are reached 6–12 hours after leflunomide administration and appear to be linear across the dosage range of 5–25 mg/day. The drug undergoes enterohepatic circulation and biliary recycling may contribute to its long elimination half-life (15–18 days). Plasma levels of A771726 remain above 0.02 mg/L (the level above which teratogenic effects could still occur) for up to two years after stopping leflunomide. The active metabolite is extensively protein bound (>99 per cent) and is cleared by biliary and renal excretion.

Mechanisms of action

The active metabolite A771726 binds to mitochondrial enzyme dihydro-orotate dehydrogenase, which is involved in the synthesis of pyrimidines. This leads to a reduction in uridine triphosphate levels and pyrimidine synthesis by lymphocytes. The action of the enzyme tyrosine kinase is also reduced. These effects result in changes in DNA and RNA synthesis and T- and B-cell proliferation in addition to suppression of immunoglobulin production and interference with cell adhesion. Indeed, leflunomide inhibits the T-cell receptor signal and CD28 signal. Moreover, leflunomide inhibits the T–B cell interaction and T-independent antibody formation. Leflunomide may also exert anti-viral effects against polyoma BK virus and herpes virus 1, while its efficacy against cytomegalovirus infection is controversial.

Toxic effects

Gastrointestinal effects
Diarrhoea, nausea, and dyspepsia may occur in 10–20 per cent of patients when leflunomide is administered at a dose of 20 mg/day.

Bone marrow toxicity
Transient cases of thrombocytopenia, leukopenia, and eosinophilia may occur.

Infections
The risk of infections in patients with RA given leflunomide at a dose of 20 mg/day is similar to that observed with standard methotrexate therapy.

Hepatotoxicity
Increase in liver enzymes may occur in 2–4 per cent of patients treated with leflunomide.

Hypertension
Up to 10 per cent of patients may develop hypertension, perhaps caused by an increased sympathetic drive.

Pregnancy

Animal studies indicate that the exposure to leflunomide during pregnancy has teratogenic and foetotoxic effects. The drug should not be used in women who are pregnant or who are contemplating pregnancy. Since leflunomide metabolites are detectable in plasma for a long period, pregnancy should be postponed at least two years after discontinuation of leflunomide.

Clinical use in glomerular diseases

Apart from its use in RA, leflunomide has been used in Chinese patients with IgAN (Cheng et al., 2015; Liu et al., 2016; Min et al., 2017) and primary MN (Yang et al., 2013). It is also used in renal transplant recipients to mitigate the effects of polyoma BK virus infection. It is not approved for use in glomerular disease by the USFDA or by the EMA.

Alkylating agents

Alkylating agents are so called because they have in common the capacity to contribute alkyl groups to biologically vital macromolecules such as DNA. These drugs have been used in primary glomerular diseases with variable results. No alkylating agent is approved for use in glomerular disease in the US or in Europe. The two alkylating agents most frequently used in clinical nephrology are cyclophosphamide and chlorambucil.

Cyclophosphamide

Cyclophosphamide is an oxazaphosphorine with two chloroethyl groups on the exocyclic nitrogen atom. The drug is supplied as tablets and as a powder for IV injection.

Clinical pharmacology

Cyclophosphamide is a prodrug that is activated primarily in the liver. The hepatic cytochrome P-450 monooxygenase enzymes convert cyclophosphamide to the active metabolite, 4-hydroxycyclophosphamide (4-OH CYC) which exists in equilibrium with its tautomer aldophosphamide. Aldophosphamide is oxidized by aldehyde dehydrogenase (ALDH) to inactive metabolites such as carboxycyclophosphamide. A small proportion of aldophosphamide is transported by the circulatory system to the target cells, where it is cleaved to phosphoramide mustard and acrolein. The cytotoxic effects of cyclophosphamide are mainly related to the total amount of phosphoramide mustard (Figure 3.4). In other words, the biological activity of the drug is more affected by detoxification and by elimination than by changes in the rate of generation of the activated metabolites. Some individuals, termed 'low' carboxylators, excrete minimal amounts of metabolites with consequent accumulation of aldophosphamide and increased toxicity and efficacy.

There is a large interpatient variability in the pharmacokinetics and metabolism of cyclophosphamide. This may be influenced by polymorphism of genes, such as *CYP2B6* and *CYP2C19* (Veal et al., 2016). The protein binding capacity

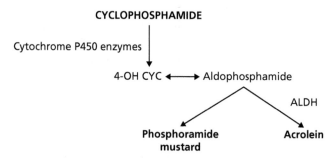

Figure 3.4 Metabolism of cyclophosphamide.
After oral administration the drug is rapidly absorbed and transformed by enzymes of the P450 cytochrome to 4-hydroxycyclophosphamide (4-OHCYC), which is in equilibrium with its tautomer aldophosphamide. The enzyme aldophosphamide-dehydrogenase (ALDH) splits aldophosphamide into acrolein and phosphoramide mustard, which exerts cytotoxic effects by alkylating various nucleophilic moieties. CYP2B6*9 and ABCB1 C3435T genetic polymorphism and hypo-albuminaemia may interfere with the disposition of cyclophosphamide and 4-OHCYC.

of cyclophosphamide is low at between 13 to 20 per cent. Maximal concentrations in plasma are usually achieved one hour after oral administration, and the drug is nearly completely cleared from plasma by 24 hours after its administration. The half-life of cyclophosphamide ranges between five and eight hours in adults and between three and six hours in children. Phosphoramide mustard, carboxycyclophosphamide, and acrolein are the principal metabolites found in urine.

Mechanisms of action

Phosphoramide mustard forms irreversible covalent linkages by alkylating various nucleophilic moieties such as phosphate, amino, sulfhydryl, hydroxyl, carboxyl, and imidazole groups, so preventing DNA replication and leading to cell apoptosis. By these mechanisms, cyclophosphamide impairs cell growth, mitotic activity, differentiation, and function. The drug exerts a marked action against cells in the dividing phase and may also alkylate quiescent cells, but in non-proliferating cells the process of alkylation is not a lethal event since the DNA repair systems correct lesions in the DNA prior to the next cellular division.

Both T and B lymphocytes are sensitive to the effects of cyclophosphamide. The drug is particularly effective at reducing antibody production by mature B-cells (plasmablasts and plasma cells). However, some subsets of T-cells may have different sensitivity to the drug, related to the differential ALDH expression. Total circulating CD19 positive B-cell counts fall slowly with cyclophosphamide therapy. Phosphoramide mustard is only formed in cells that have low levels of ALDH. Since regulatory T-cells increase expression of ALDH, they become cyclophosphamide resistant (Kanakry et al., 2015).

Toxic effects

Bladder toxicity

The excretion in the urine of acrolein, an inactive metabolite of aldophosphamide, can exert toxic effects on the bladder epithelium. As a consequence, a sterile haemorrhagic cystitis characterized by gross or microscopic haematuria (typically isomorphic/normomorphic) and voiding symptoms (dysuria, frequency, urgency) can develop. More rarely, prolonged treatments with cyclophosphamide may be complicated by bladder fibrosis and bladder cancer (transitional cell carcinoma). In a Scandinavian study on patients with cANCA-associated vasculitis, the risk of bladder cancer was 3.6 times greater for patients who received >36 g of cyclophosphamide than for those given fewer than 36 g or no cyclophosphamide at all (Faurschou et al., 2008). In a retrospective study of 1,018 patients treated with cyclophosphamide, less than 2 per cent developed haemorrhagic cystitis (median time ten months) and 0.19 per cent developed bladder cancer (median time eight years) over 4,224 patient-years (Ylmaz et al., 2015).

Usually, cumulative doses of cyclophosphamide is the main risk-factor for urotoxicity but there is a large individual variability. To prevent bladder toxicity, frequent voiding, generous fluid intake, or diuretic therapy in the case of nephrotic syndrome, are recommended. For these reasons it is more convenient to give the drug in the morning. Some drugs can bind acrolein and reduce urotoxicity. The most used agent is sodium 2-mercaptoethanesulphonate (MESNA), which binds acrolein and prevents its direct contact with the uroepithelium. MESNA can be given orally or intravenously. However, a number of patients may develop haemorrhagic cystitis despite treatment with MESNA (Ylmaz et al., 2015). A possible explanation may rest on the observation that cyclophosphamide causes two waves of apoptosis, one peaking at two hours and a second at 48 hours. The first wave is independent of acrolein and results from the cleavage of caspase 3/7 from caspase-1 (Hughes et al., 2013). The anti-oxidant acetylcysteine, resveratrol, hyperbaric oxygen therapy, and bladder instillation of hyaluronic acid or formalin are alternative therapies. All cyclophosphamide-treated patients who receive long-term treatment should have urinary cytologic evaluation, even after cyclophosphamide treatment has been stopped. In the case of macroscopic haematuria, a cystoscopic evaluation is mandatory.

Bone marrow toxicity
The haematopoietic system is particularly susceptible to the toxic effects of cyclophosphamide. Leukocytes are the most vulnerable cells, while significant thrombocytopenia is less common. Agranulocytosis is more frequent in patients with serum cholinesterase activity lower than 200 U/L. With IV administration, the nadir for leukocytes is generally reached 8–14 days later, with recovery after 18–25 days. While some clinicians think that the immunosuppressive effect is related to the degree of leukopenia, we do not seek to produce leukopenia in patients with renal diseases. On the contrary, we recommend to reduce the dose if the white blood cell count decreases below 5,000/μL, and we stop the drug if leukocytes fall below 3,000/μL in order to reduce the risk of infection.

Both cyclophosphamide and its metabolites are cleared from the kidney; moreover, renal insufficiency seems to reduce the resistance of the bone marrow to cytotoxic agents. Thus, in patients with eGFR values <40 ml/min it is more prudent to halve the standard doses of cyclophosphamide and to reduce it to one-third or less for those on dialysis treatment. Since the bone marrow of elderly patients is particularly susceptible to the toxic effects of alkylating agents, it is advisable to halve the standard doses in patients over 65 years. Either granulocyte colony-stimulating factor or granulocyte-macrophage colony-stimulating factor can obtain a rapid leukocyte mobilization in cases of agranulocytosis following an intensive treatment with cyclophosphamide.

Infection
The most serious complications from cyclophosphamide-induced myelo-suppression are life-threatening opportunistic infections or sepsis. The risk of severe infection is increased in patients with neutropenia.

Hyponatraemia
High doses of cyclophosphamide can cause a syndrome of inappropriate se-cretion of antidiuretic hormone with water retention and hyponatraemia. This complication may occur without changes in vasopressin. Experiments in the rat kidney showed that cyclophosphamide may activate vasopressin-2 receptors and induce upregulation of aquaporin-2 in the absence of vasopressin stimu-lation, suggesting the possibility of drug-induced nephrogenic syndrome of inappropriate antidiuresis (Kim et al., 2015). Hyponatraemia usually develops at doses higher than 50 mg/kg, which are not used in clinical nephrology. However, a case of severe hyponatraemia has been reported in a man with acute glomerulonephritis after IV infusion of 500 mg of cyclophosphamide (Esposito et al., 2017).

Gonadal toxicity
In males, cyclophosphamide can induce aplasia of the germinal epithelium of the testis, with consequent oligospermia or even permanent azoospermia. This complication is dose-, time-, and age-dependent. Although it is not easy to find out the threshold dosage, it is generally accepted that azoospermia in children does not develop for cumulative doses lower than 19 grams/m² (Meistrich, 2009). In a study of meta-analysis in children with idiopathic nephrotic syn-drome, no safe threshold for a cumulative amount of cyclophosphamide was found in males, but there was a marked increase in the risk of oligo- or azoo-spermia with higher cumulative doses. The authors recommended not ex-ceeding a maximum cumulative dosage of 250 mg/kg, i.e. 2 mg/kg/day for 18 weeks or 3 mg/kg/day for 80 days (Latta et al., 2001). The simultaneous use of high-dose GCs may increase the gonadal toxicity of cyclophosphamide. In the study by Arnaud and colleagues (2017), GC-treated male systemic lupus erythematosus (SLE) patients had higher levels of luteinizing hormone and more frequent bioactive testosterone deficiency than their matched controls. In some cases, recovery from azoospermia can be observed three or more years after drug discontinuation. Since the testicular toxicity of cyclophosphamide is

caused by oxidative stress, it has been suggested to use anti-oxidant agents, such as vitamin E or melatonin, to protect the male reproductive system (Ghobadi et al., 2017). In men who wish to retain fertility and who require long-term and/or high-dose cyclophosphamide therapy semen cryopreservation is recommended before starting the drug.

In females, amenorrhea and ovarian failure may develop when prolonged treatments are used, particularly in women over the age of 30 years. In a multivariate analysis the most important risk factors for menstrual abnormalities were duration of treatment and cumulative dose of cyclophosphamide (Apphenzeller et al., 2008). In a retrospective study, the serum titres of anti-Mullerian hormone (AMH), a marker for ovarian dysfunction, were comparable in lupus women never treated with cyclophosphamide and in those given a cumulative dose of 3 g of cyclophosphamide administered intravenously, while the serum levels of AMH were significantly lower in women who received >6 g of cyclophosphamide (Tamirou et al., 2017). The use of gonadotropin releasing hormone (GnRH) agonist leuprolide acetate proved capable of reducing the risk of ovarian failure in women treated with chemotherapy for cancer is advisable (Song et al., 2013; Hasky et al., 2015).

Dermatologic effects

Alopecia is a well-known, dose-related side-effect of cyclophosphamide. Studies in mice suggested that alopecia may be the result of premature and aberrant catagen mediated by the epidermal growth factor receptor signals (Bicksel et al., 2013). Hair growth will usually return after stopping the drug, but the newly grown hair may be curly and 'kinky'. Mucosal ulcerations, transverse riding of the nails, and increased skin pigmentation can also develop.

Gastrointestinal effects

Nausea and vomiting are common, particularly after IV high-dose administration. These symptoms usually occur 6–10 hours after infusion. A chronic, fastidious nausea may also occur in some patients with oral administration. Concomitant administration of antimotility and anti-emetic drugs, such as metoclopramide, can reduce this side effect.

Liver toxicity

Cyclophosphamide can induce an increase in serum transaminases and, rarely, jaundice and hepatitis. These disorders are usually reversible after the discontinuation of the drug. Hepatotoxicity is more likely to occur in patients with low serum cholinesterase levels. As cyclophosphamide induces a reduction of cholinesterase activity, the drug should be discontinued if cholinesterase activity is lower than 200 U/L. The use of the anti-oxidant vitamin E could exert protective effect in experimental animals (Cuce et al., 2015).

Cardiac toxicity

High-dose cyclophosphamide can, rarely, lead to cardiac necrosis, myocarditis, and/or pericarditis. Acrolein seems to be heavily implicated in the onset of cardiotoxicity (Nishikawa et al., 2015). Cardiac involvement may be checked by measurement of brain natriuretic peptide and endothelin levels, which rise before cardiomyocyte necrosis. These parameters are much more sensitive indicators of myocardial injury than functional tests, such as echocardiography, whereas diastolic functional parameters are more sensitive predictors of early cyclophosphamide-induced cardiotoxicity. However, with the oral doses used in renal patients, cardiac complications are extremely rare.

Lung toxicity

When given at high doses and for prolonged periods, cyclophosphamide can induce lung fibrosis. This side-effect is unusual with the dosages used in clinical nephrology, but exceptional cases of fulminant interstitial pneumonitis may develop two to six weeks after the initiation of cyclophosphamide. These cases, clinically characterized by rapidly progressive dyspnoea and a non-productive cough, are thought to be hypersensitivity reactions, as shown by the presence of aggregates of histiocytes at lung biopsy. In a few patients a course with GCs resulted in recovery from this life-threatening complication (Ochoa et al., 2012).

Neoplasia

Cyclophosphamide is a carcinogenic drug. The oncogenic risk is mainly dependent on intensity and length of treatment. The use of other immunosuppressive agents and/or exposure to radiation may enhance the risk of cancer. The most frequent malignancies associated with cyclophosphamide are lymphomas, leukaemia, skin cancer, and bladder cancer. A meta-analysis of studies in patients with ANCA-associated vasculitis treated with cyclophosphamide reported an increased risk of late-occurring malignancies, particularly nonmelanoma skin cancer, leukaemia, and bladder cancer, with standardized incidence rates of 5.18, 4.89, and 3.84 respectively (Shang et al., 2015). The pathogenesis of haematologic malignancies is probably related to chromosomal abnormalities caused by the prolonged use of cyclophosphamide; the risk of haematologic malignancy seems to be higher in patients who developed agranulocytosis. Bladder cancer is probably due to the chronic mucosal inflammation and irritation caused by acrolein, although it is not possible to rule out a direct oncogenic effect of cyclophosphamide or other metabolites on the urothelium.

Most of the available data come from patients with systemic diseases. We lack information for patients with primary glomerular diseases. Anecdotal cases of leukaemia and solid tumours in cyclophosphamide-treated patients have been reported, but there is not a systematic study on this problem. Theoretically, it is possible that the peculiar immune status of auto-immune glomerular diseases makes patients more susceptible to haematologic malignancies and that cytotoxic therapy may further increase this risk. Recent data suggest that auto-immune stimulation critically interferes with the rapid cell division, somatic hypermutation, class switch recombination, and immunological selection of maturing B-cells in the germinal centre and causes damage contributing to transformation (Hemminki, 2016). At any rate, it would be prudent not to use cyclophosphamide for more than 6–12 months, not exceeding a cumulative dose of 360 mg/kg.

Pregnancy

Miscarriages and preterm deliveries have been reported in mothers taking cyclophosphamide. Teratogenicity of cyclophosphamide is well demonstrated in animals. Cases of malformation have been described in newborns of mother who received cyclophosphamide. Cyclophosphamide is contra-indicated in pregnancy (USFDA Class D). All women contemplating its use *must* have a negative pregnancy test *before* commencing on the drug and at least two methods of contraception should be used by sexually active women in the reproductive age group during the administration of the agent.

Clinical use in glomerular diseases

Cyclophosphamide has been successfully used in MCD, in MN, in lupus nephritis, and in ANCA-associated vasculitis, while it is ineffective in steroid-resistant FSGS and of highly uncertain value in IgAN. The drug may be administered orally or by IV infusion. Studies in dogs reported no difference in drug exposure to 4-OHCP after IV or oral administered cyclophosphamide (Warry et al., 2011). Compared to the oral route, intermittent IV use needs long infusion times and risk of extravasation. Some studies in lupus nephritis have shown that high-dose IV pulses of cyclophosphamide given intermittently may show lower risk of infections, haemorrhagic cystitis, or neoplasia in comparison with standard daily doses of oral cyclophosphamide. However, these data have been challenged by a comprehensive review of the literature, which did not find hard evidence to support the superiority of long-term IV cyclophosphamide in terms of complications (Wetzels, 2004). There is little experience with intermittent IV pulses of cyclophosphamide in primary glomerular diseases. Small controlled trials in patients with FSGS and MN did not report favourable results. Whatever the route of administration, it should be pointed out that genetic polymorphisms of CYP2B6*9 and ABCB1 C3435T may decrease the cyclophosphamide bio-activation. Moreover, alterations in serum proteins, urine protein excretion, and kidney function, all common to glomerulonephritis, may alter cyclophosphamide metabolites disposition. Cyclophosphamide is only 20 per cent bound in plasma so variability in pharmacokinetics secondary to serum albumin is not relevant. However, cyclophosphamide metabolites are moderately bound to plasma proteins (50 and 67 per cent) and the pharmacokinetic disposition of total metabolite concentrations may be influenced by alterations in serum albumin. In patients with lupus nephritis, reductions in serum albumin and increases in urinary protein excretion resulted in reduced exposure to the 4-hydroxycyclophosphamide metabolite (Joy et al., 2012).

In summary, cyclophosphamide may be effective in different glomerular diseases. However, because of its potential toxicity, cyclophosphamide should be used only in selected cases by experienced clinicians. The cumulative doses should be as low as possible in order to prevent disquieting toxicity. Repeated courses should be avoided whenever possible as the toxicity is cumulative. Several precautions should be taken to minimize the potential side-effects. To reduce the risk of agranulocytosis the dose should be halved if white blood cells (WBCs) are <5,000/μL and stopped if WBCs <3,000/μL until WBCs raise >5,000/μL. Although cyclophosphamide pharmacokinetics is not altered by the worsening of renal function (de Miranda Silva et al., 2009), in patients with renal failure and in elderly subjects the oral doses should be decreased to 0.05–1 mg/kg, being that bone marrow in these patients is particularly vulnerable to the toxic effect of alkylating agents (Ponticelli et al., 2018). To prevent bladder toxicity, frequent voiding and forced diuresis are recommended. If high doses of IV cyclophosphamide are given, patients should receive IV MESNA. Patients with haematuria should receive a cystoscopy. To reduce the oncogenic risk, cumulative doses >36 g with cyclophosphamide or >3 g with chlorambucil should not be used. The risk of haematological neoplasia is increased in patients who developed agranulocytosis. To prevent gonadal toxicity, the cumulative dose of cyclophosphamide should be ≤250 mg/kg. Sperm collection is advisable if long-term treatment is scheduled. In females the risk of ovarian failure is more frequent in women over 30 years of age. Suppression of ovulation with leuprolide may protect from ovarian failure.

Chlorambucil

Chlorambucil is an *N, N*-bis (2-chloroethyl)-amino-phenyl-butyric acid. The drug has been widely used in the therapy of chronic lymphocytic leukaemia, polycythaemia vera, Waldenstrom's macroglobulinaemia, and as an adjuvant therapy for various types of cancer. In primary glomerular diseases chlorambucil has been mostly used in MCD and in MN. The drug is supplied in tablets that should be kept at 4°C.

Clinical pharmacology

Chlorambucil is passively absorbed in the upper gastrointestinal tract. The absorption is adequate and reliable with peak levels occurring 15–30 minutes after oral administration. The oral bio-availability is close to 100 per cent and is not influenced by food. After absorption, chlorambucil rapidly disappears from plasma, with a half-life of one hour, but has a delayed onset of action. The drug is beta-oxidized in the liver to phenylacetic acid mustard, which seems to have cytotoxic properties similar to those of its parent compound. The uptake into cells is unaffected by metabolic inhibitions and does not take place against a concentration gradient. Chlorambucil and its metabolites may be fixed in several tissues, including adipose tissue, from which they are removed very slowly. This might account for some delayed effects of chlorambucil. There are large inter- and intra-individual variations in the pharmacokinetics of chlorambucil, which are even more pronounced for the cytotoxic metabolite phenylacetic acid mustard. When incorporated in a long-circulating nano-emulsion, chlorambucil shows an improved pharmacokinetic profile and better therapeutic efficacy (Ganta et al., 2010). At any rate, both this metabolite and its parent compound are almost completely metabolized, as shown by their extremely low urinary excretion of less than 1 per cent.

Mechanisms of action

The pharmacological and cytotoxic actions of chlorambucil are similar to those of cyclophosphamide.

Toxic effects

Although most side-effects of chlorambucil are similar to those of cyclophosphamide, chlorambucil is neither a vesicant nor does it produce urothelial damage and bladder toxicity. In haematologic malignancies chlorambucil is better tolerated than purine nucleoside analogues (Lepretre et al., 2015).

Bone marrow toxicity

The myelosuppressive effects of chlorambucil are clearly dose-dependent. As for other immunosuppressive agents along with chlorambucil, we do not seek leukopenia, but rather we halve the dose if the leukocyte count decreases below 5,000/µL and we stop the drug if leukocytes fall below 3,000/µL. Chlorambucil is reintroduced at half of the previous dosage only when leukocytes are above 5,000/µL. The bone marrow of elderly and uraemic patients is particularly vulnerable. In these instances, the administration of chlorambucil should be very careful (starting dose ≤0.1 mg/kg) with frequent monitoring of blood cells. It must be pointed out that leukopenia can develop late, sometimes after chlorambucil treatment has already been stopped. This is probably due to the tissue accumulation of the drug, with slow release.

Ocular complications

Diplopia, papillary oedema, and keratitis are possible, although rare, side-effects.

Neurological complications

Hallucination, seizures, and electroencephalographic changes have been reported in children treated with chlorambucil. In a meta-analysis, seizures were reported in 3.6 per cent of children with idiopathic nephrotic syndrome treated with chlorambucil (Latta et al., 2001).

Gonadal toxicity

Gonadal toxicity of chlorambucil is well established. In males, chlorambucil can induce azoospermia which may or may not be reversible, largely depending on the cumulative dosage. It is difficult to fix a threshold cumulative dose because of different individual sensitivities. It is not known whether the post-pubertal testis is more or less resistant than the pre-pubertal testis to chlorambucil. At any rate, in male children it is unsafe to exceed a cumulative dose of chlorambucil of more than 1.4 g/m^2 (Meistrich, 2009). In young males, it is advisable to collect the sperm in a semen bank before beginning chlorambucil therapy. During treatment, the monitoring of plasma follicular stimulating hormone, which increases in cases of testicular germinal epithelium damage, may be useful for deciding when to discontinue the drug. The recovery of sperm production depends on the survival of the spermatogonial stem cells and their ability to differentiate. There is little information about the risk of ovarian failure in women treated with chlorambucil. To be on the safe side, it is better to use the drug at a dose ≤0.1 mg/kg/day for no longer than two to three months.

Gastrointestinal effects

In some patients, anorexia, nausea, and vomiting may occur, leading to treatment being stopped in 1–2 per cent of cases. Rarely, a mild and reversible increase of liver transaminases can occur.

Malignancy

Chlorambucil has been recognized by the International Agency for Research on Cancer as a potential human carcinogen, with bone marrow specificity. Chlorambucil has highly reactive electrophilic centres that react with DNA to form mutagenic adducts and cross-linking. This effect is dose-dependent and cumulative. A marked increase of acute leukaemia has been noted in patients given long-term chlorambucil. This risk is particularly high for patients with polycythaemia vera, breast cancer, or ovarian cancer. However, patients with primary neoplasia (polycythaemia is considered to be a pre-leukaemic condition) are particularly exposed to the hazard of a second cancer. Most patients who developed malignancy had been given chlorambucil for many months or years.

In rheumatic patients, no cases of leukaemia were seen in patients who received less than 1 g of chlorambucil and in whom the duration of treatment was less than six months. We have little information about the leukaemogenic effect of chlorambucil in renal patients. Cases of acute myeloid leukaemia have been reported in patients with ANCA-associated vasculitis who received high cumulative doses of chlorambucil, often in association with other cytotoxic agents over treatment periods up to 43 months.

The relative risk for the other types of cancer seems not to be increased by treatment with chlorambucil, at least in rheumatic patients. As for other immunosuppressive agents, there is a lack of solid data about the oncogenicity of chlorambucil in renal diseases. In the meta-analysis of Latta and colleagues (2001), out of 1,504 children who received cytotoxic therapy for idiopathic nephrotic syndrome, 14 cases of malignancy occurred (0.9 per cent) in patients treated with high doses of either cyclophosphamide or chlorambucil. In adults with primary MN who received chlorambucil for three months, the risk of cancer was similar to that reported in general population (Ponticelli et al., 1998). Since the oncogenic effect depends on the dose and the duration of treatment, it is prudent not to prolong cumulative therapy for more than three months and not to re-expose to the drug those patients who developed agranulocytosis or chromosomal abnormalities.

Pregnancy

Chlorambucil can induce gene mutations which are dose-dependent and cumulative. The drug is contraindicated in pregnancy (USFDA Class D).

Clinical use in glomerular diseases

The indications to chlorambucil in primary glomerular diseases may be similar to those of cyclophosphamide. Chlorambucil proved to be able to prolong remission in steroid-dependent patients with MCD and FSGS. In association with GCs, chlorambucil could obtain remission and protect renal function in patients with MN. However, nephrologists prefer the use of cyclophosphamide as they are more familiar with this drug, which is also easier to use than chlorambucil. In some instances, the characteristics of each agent may influence the choice. For example, epileptic patients should not be given cyclophosphamide, as barbiturates and other anti-epileptic drugs stimulate the microsomal liver enzymes that activate cyclophosphamide and can therefore cause unexpected toxicity. On the other hand, chlorambucil may also cause seizures in 3–4 per cent of children, but very rarely in adults.

Mammalian target of rapamycin (mTOR) inhibitors

Sirolimus (rapamycin), and its derivate everolimus, inhibit mTORC1, a master regulator of cell growth and metabolism. These drugs are very similar for mechanisms of action and potential toxicity, but differ in pharmacokinetics.

Clinical pharmacology

The mTOR is a serin-threonin kinase that nucleates at least two distinct multi-protein complexes: mTOR complex 1 (mTORC1) or raptor complex, and mTOR complex 2 (mTORC2) or rictor complex. The mTORC1, which comprises five different proteins, positively regulates cell growth and proliferation by promoting many anabolic processes, including biosynthesis of proteins, lipids, and organelles, and by limiting catabolic processes, e.g. autophagy. The mTORC2, composed by six different proteins, regulates the actin cytoskeleton dynamics as well as ion transport and growth via SGK1 phosphorylation.

Sirolimus is macrolide lactone naturally produced by *Streptomyces hygroscopicus* containing a diketoamide moiety similar to that present in tacrolimus. The compound is insoluble in water. The drug has a long half-life, about 62 hours, and a high concentration in the brain. Its derivate *everolimus* has a similar chemical structure but a covalently bound 2-hydroxyethyl group was introduced at position 40 to improve bio-availability and reduce the half-life to about 26 hours. The compounds are absorbed rapidly with a peak concentration one to two hours after an oral dose. The steady state is achieved after four days with everolimus and after eight days with sirolimus. The mTOR inhibitors are actively and reversibly taken up by erythrocytes. The oral bio-availability of both drugs is minimal and is affected by food with a reduction of 60 per cent with high-fat meals in comparison to fasting state. Both sirolimus and everolimus are metabolized by the hepatic P450 (CYP) enzymes. The metabolites do not exert immunosuppressive activity. The clearance ranges around 8–9 L/h, but is reduced in patients with hepatic impairment. There is a strong interaction with other drugs metabolized by hepatic cytochrome enzymes, e.g. calcineurin inhibitors.

Mechanisms of action

After oral administration, mTOR inhibitors enter the cells and bind to a specific cytoplasmic receptor, the FK-binding protein 12, the same receptor of TAC. However, differently from TAC, the complex drug-receptor does not inhibit the enzymatic activity of calcineurin but blocks the serine-threonine kinase mTORC1. This kinase is the downstream effector of phosphatydilinositol-3-kinase (PI3-k), which, together with a protein-kinase B (Akt), governs several signal pathways by phosphorylating a cascade of other kinases that provide the signals for cell proliferation. A number of different stimuli—including IL-2, IL-15, oncogenic proteins, insulin, nutrients, vascular endothelial growth factor (VEGF), and some viruses, such as CMV—may activate PI3-k, which provides the signal for cell proliferation through the phosphorylation of different kinases, including p70-S6 (S6K1) and 4E-BP1. The inhibited activity of mTORC-1 interferes with the signals leading to T-cell proliferation. Apart from the immunosuppressive activity, these agents show protective effects on the endothelium by inhibiting the VEGF that stimulates the endothelial cell proliferation and angiogenesis through the family of kinases governed by PI3-k. Of importance, mTOR antagonists can exert anti-tumour activity in cancers caused either by overactivity of PI3-k, or by overexpression of mTOR caused by deficiency of PTEN, the physiological inhibitor of PI3-k.

Both sirolimus and everolimus have important immunosuppressive properties and may synergize with CNIs. While CsA and TAC interfere with the synthesis of IL-2 and other cytokines, mTOR antagonists inhibit the response to IL-2 and IL-15. CNIs interfere with the cell cycle between G0 and G1, while mTOR antagonists inhibit the cell cycle between G1 and S. There are also pharmacological interactions between CsA and mTOR inhibitors. CsA increases the AUC of mTOR inhibitors, but not vice versa. The interference between TAC and mTOR inhibitors is still poorly investigated but TAC does not seem to increase the exposure to mTOR inhibitors (Ponticelli, 2014).

Toxicity

The side effects of mTOR antagonists are mainly related to their antiproliferative activities.

Hyperlipidaemia

Increase in blood lipids is the most frequent side effect of mTOR-inhibitors. It is characterized by increased serum levels of total cholesterol, LDL-cholesterol, triglycerides, and Apo C-III. These abnormalities are probably the result of complex interferences of mTOR inhibitors on the insulin signalling pathway that may increase adipose tissue lipase activity and/or decrease lipoprotein lipase activity, reduce the catabolism of VLDL apoB100-containing lipoproteins, and/or impair the bile salt synthesis with consequent hypercholesterolaemia. It has also been demonstrated that the TORC1 pathway is involved in neutral lipid homeostasis in yeast (Madeira et al., 2015). Accordingly, the inhibition of mTORC1 might originate a derangement in lipid metabolism, which may be aggravated by co-administration of drugs like CsA and GCs. Statins should be part of drug regimen in patients with hypercholesterolaemia. These drugs may reduce LDL lipoproteins with a small increase in HDL lipoproteins and a slight decrease of triglycerides.

Bone marrow toxicity

Thrombocytopenia and anaemia may occur in patients treated with mTOR inhibitors, their frequency and severity depending on the dosage. Also, mTOR inhibitors may cause growth inhibition of erythroid precursor cells and diminished globin synthesis, contributing to microcytic anaemia (Diekman et al., 2012).

Proteinuria

In experimental animals, mTOR inhibitors can exert antiproliferative and apoptotic effects on epithelial tubular cells that may be so severe to lead to tubular collapse, vacuolization, and nephrocalcinosis. In clinical studies, the development of proteinuria in patients given mTOR inhibitors is frequently associated with increased urinary excretion of markers of tubular toxicity. Accordingly, proteinuria may be attributed to an impaired tubular reabsorption of albumin and small proteins (Franz et al., 2010). However, mTOR inhibitors might also exert a direct effect on the glomerular filtration barrier. In cultures of human podocytes, sirolimus significantly reduced the expression of nephrin and other slit diaphragm proteins essential for podocyte integrity, such as podocin, C2AP, and actin. As a consequence, podocyte adhesion to GBM and motility are reduced with possible passage of proteins in the extraglomerular space (Stallone et al., 2011). The concomitant use of ACE inhibitors may reduce the incidence of proteinuria caused by mTOR inhibitors (Mandelbrot et al., 2015). On the other hand, in mice podocytes intoxicated with puromycin aminonucleoside, rapamycin can inhibit the mTOR/P70S6K/4EBP1 signalling pathway and activate podocyte autophagy, consequently reducing podocyte apoptosis (Jin et al., 2018).

Haemolytic-uraemic syndrome (HUS)

Cases of *de novo* HUS caused by thrombotic microangiopathy have been reported in transplant patients given mTOR inhibitors in the context of contemporaneous or contiguous administration of CNI. It may be hypothesized that, by downregulating VEGF, mTOR inhibitor may induce anti-angiogenic activity with late repair of endothelial lesions caused by CNI, rejection, or virus infection. The withdrawal of the offending drug may obtain resolution of the disease, if the diagnosis is made early.

Wound healing

Retarded wound healing after surgery and increased risk of lymphocele have been noted in organ transplant recipients treated with mTOR inhibitors, probably as a consequence of their antiproliferative activity. The high dosage of these drugs and the association with GCs facilitate these complications.

Interstitial pneumonia

Interstitial pneumonia more frequently occurs in patients treated with high doses of mTOR inhibitors for cancer. However, cases of pulmonary alveolar proteinosis (PAP) have also been reported in kidney transplant recipients. PAP is a progressive lung disease characterized by the accumulation of surfactant-like material in the lungs leading to decreased pulmonary function with shortness of breath and cough as common symptoms (Kadikoy et al., 2010). The respiratory symptoms usually have insidious onset, but in severe cases can ultimately result in severe respiratory failure. Drug discontinuation or reduction may lead to resolution within three weeks in most cases. The pathophysiology is unknown but the response to drug discontinuation and/or GCs may suggest that pneumonitis might be related to a hypersensitivity reaction.

Mouth ulcers

Painful oral ulcers have been reported in 10–24 per cent of patients treated with mTOR inhibitors. Ulcers are more frequent when high doses of mTOR inhibitors are used or when sirolimus or everolimus are combined with mycophenolate. Lowering the dosage of the drug and treatment with clobetasol propionate may reduce pain and shorten healing times.

Joint pain

Joint pain may occur in up to 25 per cent of patients given high doses of mTOR inhibitors. Pain may be disabling, but usually may resolve with dose reduction or drug withdrawal in more severe cases. It is possible that pain is caused by changes of circulation in the bone, perhaps induced by a reflex sympathetic dystrophy syndrome.

Oedema

Eyelid and/or leg oedemas may occur. These oedemas are dose dependent, are usually mild to moderate, and may reverse with low-dose furosemide. Oedemas are probably related to the impaired endothelial barrier function caused by protein kinase C-α activation and disruption of the p120-vascular endothelial cadherin interaction (Habib et al., 2013).

Neoplasia

Sirolimus and everolimus are believed to possess anti-neoplastic properties. Both drugs and the derivate tesirolimus are currently used in different types of cancer in which the PI3K/mTOR kinase pathway is enhanced.

Pregnancy

The mTOR inhibitors increase the mortality of foetus in experimental animals. However, no teratogenic effects have been seen either in rats or rabbits. There is insufficient information about pregnant women treated with these drugs. Anecdotal cases of healthy newborns from mothers receiving mTOR inhibitors have been reported. The USFDA classifies these drugs as Category C (teratogenic risk cannot be ruled out because of lack of information).

Clinical use in glomerular diseases

Since mTORC1 activation triggers the unfolded protein response in podocytes and leads to nephrotic syndrome (Ito et al., 2011), both everolimus and sirolimus have been used in experimental models of glomerular diseases. Everolimus could prevent the formation of FSGS during chronic anti-Thy1 nephritis (Wittman et al., 2008). Sirolimus prevented podocyte injury in passive Heymann nephritis and in an in vitro model of puromycin amino nucleotide-cultured podocytes (Wu et al., 2014). Sirolimus also slowed progression of IgAN in rats (Tian et al., 2014), but worsened glomerular pathology in other models.

The few attempts of treating human primary glomerular diseases with mTOR inhibitors generally proved to be unsuccessful or even impaired kidney function or aggravated proteinuria. However, good results have been obtained with a combination of low-dose sirolimus, ACE inhibitors, and statins in patients with IgA nephropathy (Cruzado et al., 2011). Contrasting results have been reported in FSGS. In some anecdotal reports, the use of rapamycin resulted in induced FSGS and severe proteinuria (Dogan et al., 2011), while in anecdotal steroid-resistant cases it obtained reversal of proteinuria (Tsagalis et al., 2009).

Intravenous immunoglobulins (IVIg)

IVIg are purified IgG extracted from the plasma of thousands of blood donors. IVIg are mainly used in primary immune deficiencies and infections. However, IVIg are also used in auto-immune diseases since they may also exert immunomodulatory and anti-inflammatory effects. The commercially available products include certain characteristics:

    i. IVIg should be prepared out of at least 1,000 different human donors;

    ii. All four IgG subgroups, i.e. 1–4, should be present;

    iii. The IgG should maintain biological activity and a lifetime of at least 21 days;

    iv. The product cannot contain samples which are HIV-, hepatitis B-, or hepatitis C-positive;

    v. The product must be screened and treated in a manner that destroys viruses.

IVIg are administered by infusion. Dosage of IVIg is dependent on indication. In renal diseases IVIg are usually given at a dose of 400 mg/kg of body weight every three to four weeks.

Mechanisms of action

The precise mechanism by which IVIg suppress harmful inflammation has not been definitively established but it is believed that they can exert multiple functions:

    i. IVIg may bind to natural antibodies, cytokines, or superantigens and pathogens;

    ii. they may provide a "sink" that could divert proinflammatory complement fragments;

    iii. they may prevent the lytic effects of the terminal complement complex C5b-9 (the membrane attack) by scavenging complement components and diverting membrane attack from cellular targets;

    iv. they may immunoregulate the anti-idiotype antibodies by neutralizing the activity-inhibition of the binding to the respective autoantigen;

    v. they may modulate cytokines by triggering the production of IL-1 receptor antagonists;

    vi. they may interact with the membrane molecules of antigen-presenting-cells, T-cells, and B-cells, and may inhibit the differentiation and maturation of dendritic cells (Gilardin et al., 2015); or

    vii. they may bind to Fc receptors so triggering anti-inflammatory pathways (Tedla et al., 2015).

Toxic effects

Influenza-like syndrome

The most common adverse effects occur soon after infusions and can include fever, headache, flushing, chills, myalgia, wheezing, tachycardia, lower back pain, nausea, and hypotension. If this happens during an infusion, the infusion should be slowed or stopped. If symptoms are anticipated, a patient can be premedicated with antihistamines and IV hydrocortisone.

Allergic reaction

Serious anaphylactoid reactions occur soon after the administration of IVIg to patients with IgA deficiency. These reactions are caused by the production of anti-IgA antibodies. This occurs in one out of 500–1000 patients. Anaphylaxis associated with sensitization to IgA in patients with IgA deficiency can be prevented by using IgA-depleted immune globulin. The presence of IgG anti-IgA antibodies is not always associated with severe adverse reactions to IVIg.

Acute kidney injury (AKI)

An uncommon, but life-threatening and potentially irreversible, adverse event is AKI. This complication occurred with a sucrose-stabilized formulation, and products containing sucrose as a stabilizer have an elevated osmolality and are mainly associated with AKI through the mechanism of osmotic nephrosis. No case of AKI has been reported with the D-sorbitol–stabilized formulation. The issue of nephrotoxicity should be fully considered when prescribing IVIg to a renal patient. Apart from unmodifiable risk factors, e.g. pre-existing renal disease and old age, another important risk factor for such toxicity is represented by volume depletion. A correct level of hydration is mandatory before or during the infusion of IVIg.

Thrombosis

Case reports and observational studies indicate that IVIg may cause thrombo-embolic events, leading the USFDA to require a boxed warning in 2013. These complications are more frequent when products with high osmolality are used and in patients with underlying risk factors such as hypertension, hypercholesterolaemia, atrial fibrillation, history of vascular disease and stroke, and deep venous thrombosis. However, the mechanism leading to thrombosis remains hypothetical, and the consensus that IVIg infusion causes an increased risk of thromboembolic events may be unwarranted, as supporting evidence does not exist (Basta, 2014).

Haemolysis

Haemolysis can be seen when high titre anti-A or anti-B isohaemagglutinins are present in the IVIg preparation.

Pregnancy

IVIg have been largely used in pregnancy. The tolerance is usually good. No adverse impact on the foetus has been reported.

Clinical use in glomerular diseases

There are anecdotal encouraging reports on the efficacy of prolonged IVIg in MNs resistant to conventional therapy. However, the exact success rate, optimal dosage, and clinical indications remain undetermined. IVIg have also been used in the setting of kidney transplant for desensitization of antibodies to achieve a negative cross-match and permit transplant or for treating an antibody-mediated rejection. Treatment with IVIg is expensive and is not devoid of side effects. Patients for whom a treatment with IVIg is prescribed should be closely monitored and receive adequate hydration to correct volume depletion, which, together with renal disease, represents a risk factor for nephrotoxicity.

Monoclonal antibodies

Rituximab (RTX)

Rituximab is a chimeric human/murine monoclonal antibody with a high affinity for the CD20 antigen, a membrane protein expressed on B-cells. Its role in B-cell development includes regulation of activation for cell cycling and B-cell differentiation. The main indication of RTX is follicular non-Hodgkin's B-cell lymphoma, but it has been also used off-label in organ transplantation and in a number of auto-immune diseases, including SLE, and some forms of primary glomerular diseases. RTX is available in vials. The usual dosage is 375 mg/m^2 or 500–1000 mg to be repeated at different intervals according to the clinical response and the count of B-cells (as assessed by the loss of CD-19, a B-cell specific marker). Some auto-immune protocols involve giving 1000 mg at two intervals two weeks apart. Either course virtually assures nearly complete elimination of circulating CD19+ and CD20+ B-cells, but has no effect on mature plasma cells, which lack the CD20 antigen. Because of the risk of allergic reactions and massive lymphocyte destruction the first dose should be infused slowly, with antihistamines and hydrocortisone, under surveillance of a doctor or a specialized nurse.

Clinical pharmacology

Following IV administration, RTX distributes in both the intravascular and extravascular compartments. Serum levels and the half-life of RTX are extremely variable. However, the elimination half-life of rituximab tends to increase from a mean of 76.3 ± 31.1 hours after the first infusion to 205.8 ± 95.0 hours after the fourth and final infusion. A more rapid disappearance may be seen in patients with nephrotic syndrome (Counsilman et al., 2015). A close correlation of the excretion of RTX to the excretion of IgG molecules has been found suggesting selectivity of proteinuria as the determining factor of RTX excretion (Stahl et al., 2017). In these patients, the serum half-life of RTX can be extremely short, which may explain the poor results of RTX in some patients with massive proteinuria.

Mechanisms of action

RTX induces a very rapid elimination of circulating B-cells (measured in hours) that may be maintained for weeks or months. RTX targets CD20 on B lymphocytes. A large body of evidence shows that RTX depletes CD20+ B-cells through three main mechanisms of action: antibody-dependent cell-mediated cytotoxicity (ADCC), cell-mediated cytotoxicity (CDC), and apoptosis leading to cell death (Figure 3.5). In the ADCC-mediated mechanism, the Fc of antibody bound to the target cell binds to the Fcγ receptor on macrophages and natural killer cells and induces phagocytosis of the target cell to which the antibody is bound (Amoroso, 2011; Maloney et al., 2002). However, the role of ADCC still needs to be better elucidated. Preclinical studies suggest that single nucleotide polymorphisms in the Fcγ receptor (FCGR) genes may influence the response to RTX. However, in follicular lymphoma, the FCGR3A and FCGR2A single nucleotide polymorphisms did not confer differential responsiveness to RTX (Kenkre et al., 2016). CDC is probably the main mechanism of RTX killing in vivo. The classical pathway of complement is activated by the binding

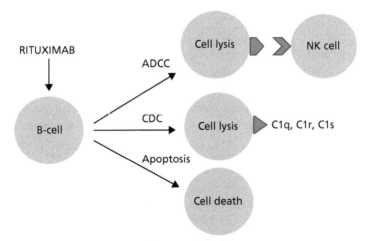

Figure 3.5 The main mechanisms of action of RTX.
In antibody-dependent cell-mediated cytotoxicity (ADCC), the Fc of RTX bound to the target cell binds to the Fcγ receptor of natural killer (NK) cell triggering NK activation and death of target cell. In cell-mediated cytotoxicity (CDC), RTX activates the classical pathway of complement with eventual production of membrane attack complex and lysis of the target cell. The third mechanism rests on direct signalling of apoptosis.

of the Fc portion of IgG to C1q, which triggers a proteolytic cascade that eventually leads to the activation of the membrane attack complex (Abulayha et al., 2014). However, the degree to which CMC contributes to the clinical response to therapy is still unclear (Weiner, 2010). The third mechanism through which RTX may induce cell death is apoptosis. RTX may overcome the anti-apoptotic proteins BCL-2 and BCL_{xl}.

On the other hand, the fact that the maximal clinical response is obtained after several weeks or months suggests that other phenomena may be involved. RTX may cause direct cellular effects by inducing lipid raft modifications of B-cell membranes, and by exerting killing effects through various intracellular signalling pathways, including activation or deregulation of kinase (PI3k and mTOR) and caspase. These actions may deplete memory cells, abolish the antigen presentation by B-cells, and increase the number and function of regulatory T-cells (Bezombes et al., 2011; Abulayha et al., 2014).

Apart from its effects on B lymphocytes, RTX can also bind sphingomyelin phosphodiesterase acid-like 3b protein and regulate acid sphingomyelinase activity, therefore protecting from injury podocytes and foot processes and reducing proteinuria by a direct action on podocytes (Fornoni et al., 2011).

Toxicity

Cytokine release syndrome

The first dose of RTX can cause a massive lysis of B-cells with release of cytokines, and can be associated with fever, chills, rigor, orthostatic hypotension, irregular heart rhythms, and bronchospasm. This reaction correlates with the number of circulating CD20 cells and is more frequent in patients with tumour while it is milder in patients with auto-immune disease. In patients with pre-existing cardiac morbidity, arrythmias, angina, and acute respiratory distress syndrome have been reported. Infusion should be interrupted in case of severe bronchospasm. Premedication with GCs or antihistamine agents can reduce the intensity of symptoms.

Infection

RTX abates CD20 lymphocytes and decreases the serum levels of immunoglobulin M (IgM). In the long-term, some patients may show IgG levels <500 mg/dl (Fujnaga et al., 2016). Severe infections may occur in heavily immunosuppressed patients (Nixon et al., 2017) and in patients with renal insufficiency (Fabrizi et al., 2015). Although most observations are limited by the retrospective nature of the studies, the off-label use of rituximab in patients with GN is justified. However, this agent should be used with caution in patients who are receiving strong immunosuppression. The majority of infections are caused by bacterial or opportunistic viral agents and generally develop 30 days to 11 months after the end of therapy. Serious infectious events include sepsis and hepatitis B virus (HBV) re-activation with related fulminant hepatitis (Yilmaz, 2016). RTX should be avoided in the presence of active significant infections and in carriers of hepatitis infection (HBs antigen positive or anti-HBc antibody positive). A few cases of fatal PML, probably caused by reactivation of JC virus, have also been reported (Carson et al., 2009; Felli et al., 2014). These patients were also receiving other immunomodulating drugs and were severely immunosuppressed. In lymphoma patients treated with RTX, pneumocystis jiroveci pneumonia (PCP) is frequently reported.

Bronchiolitis obliterans and interstitial lung disease
In clinical studies and post-marketing surveillance, there have been a limited number of reports of bronchiolitis obliterans presenting up to six months post-RTX infusion. Interstitial lung disease is a rare, but potentially fatal, complication of RTX therapy. A systematic review of the literature reported 120 cases. The mean time of onset from the last RTX infusion until symptom development or relevant abnormal radiological change was 30 days (range 0–158 days). Abnormal radiological findings were similar in all patients with diffuse bilateral lung infiltrates. Hypoxaemia was seen in all cases and pulmonary function tests were uniformly abnormal with a characteristic diffusion capacity deficit and restrictive ventilatory pattern. The disease was fatal in 18 cases (Hadjinicolaou et al., 2012). Prompt and aggressive treatment with GCs may lead to resolution of the disease. Patients who worsen despite GCs have a poor outcome. The safety of resumption or continued administration of RTX in patients with pneumonitis or bronchiolitis obliterans is unknown.

Major cardiac events
Cardiovascular complications have been reported during or a short time after RTX infusion. Exceptionally, MI may occur 24 hours later (Mehrpooya et al., 2015).

Haematologic events
Severe decreases in red and platelets may occur with RTX. Prolonged leucopenia is frequent. Agranulocytosis may develop in about 10 per cent of children with nephrotic syndrome. It usually resolves in a few days (Kamei et al., 2015).

Immunogenicity
The incidence of antibody positivity in an assay is highly dependent on the sensitivity and specificity of the assay and may be influenced by several factors, including sample handling, concomitant medications, and underlying disease. For these reasons, the incidence of human anti-chimeric antibodies (HACAs) to RTX may be misleading. In clinical studies of patients with low-grade or

follicular non-Hodgkin's lymphoma receiving RTX as a single therapy, HACAs were detected in 1.1 per cent patients.

Malignancy

There are few data about the risk of malignancy in patients treated with RTX. In patients with RA the risk of malignancy was higher in patients treated with RTX than in those receiving infliximab (Aaltonen et al., 2015).

Hypersensitivity reactions

As a chimeric protein, RTX may be associated with serum sickness-like reactions and rarely by anaphylaxis.

Pregnancy

According to the USFDA, a teratogen risk cannot be excluded for RTX (Category C). However, despite counselling to avoid pregnancy, women may inadvertently become pregnant during or after RTX treatment. Chakravarty and colleagues (2011) used the global drug safety database of RTX and identified 231 pregnancies associated with maternal RTX exposure. Of 153 pregnancies with known outcomes, 90 resulted in live births. Twenty-two infants were born prematurely, with one neonatal death at six weeks. Eleven neonates had haematologic abnormalities; none had corresponding infections. Four neonatal infections were reported. Two congenital malformations were identified: clubfoot in one twin, and cardiac malformation in a singleton birth. One maternal death from pre-existing auto-immune thrombocytopaenia occurred. A reversible B-cell deficiency has been noted in infants born of mothers who received RTX during pregnancy. According to current guidelines, women should avoid pregnancy for about 12 months after RTX exposure. The administration of RTX to a pregnant woman should be discouraged unless the benefits outweigh the potential risk for the foetus.

Clinical use in glomerular diseases

Although the mechanisms of action of RTX are still poorly defined, non-controlled studies and a few randomized trials have reported good results in frequently relapsing MCD, steroid-sensitive FSGS, MN, pauci-immune GN, and ANCA-associated vasculitis. Anecdotal reports also pointed out the possibility of inducing remission (usually partial) in cases of FSGS recurring after transplantation. However, the optimal schedule, the interactions with other immunosuppressives, and predictive factors for response or resistance to RTX remain unanswered questions. Despite being well tolerated (Bonanni et al., 2018), the possibility that the perturbation of the immune system caused by RTX might induce long-term side effects (including infection and multifocal leukoencephalopathy) has not been ruled out. Randomized clinical trials in patients with different types of glomerular disease are under way and hopefully will allow better definition of the actual role of RTX in treating these diseases. Prophylaxis of PCP with trimethoprim-sulfamethoxazole is suggested.

Ofatumumab

Ofatumumab is a humanized anti-CD20 monoclonal antibody approved by the USFDA and EMA for the treatment of multidrug-resistant chronic lymphocytic leukaemia (CLL), with efficacy against RTX-resistant B-cell cancers.

Mechanisms of action

Ofatumumab induces killing of B-cells via activation of complement-dependent cytotoxicity and antibody-dependent cell-mediated cytotoxicity in vitro. Compared with RTX, which is a chimeric anti-CD20 antibody, ofatumumab has stronger complement-dependent cytotoxicity, as well as a slower off-rate and more stable CD20 binding. It also binds a different epitope of CD20 than RTX (Laurenti et al., 2016).

Toxicity

Adverse events are usually limited to grade 1 and 2 infusion-related reactions, which tend to decrease throughout the treatment. Infections are frequent but usually not severe. In CLL patients treated with Ofatumumab the risk of pneumonia ranged around 5 per cent, neutropenia developed in 16 per cent of patients, and anaemia in 8 per cent (Byrd et al., 2014).

Clinical use in glomerular diseases

At a dose of 300 mg/1.73 m^2 of body surface area for the first week, followed by 2000 mg/1.73 m^2 weekly for five infusions, ofatumumab obtained remission in a few patients with steroid- and RTX-resistant nephrotic syndrome (Basu et al., 2014; Vivarelli et al., 2017). Ofatumumab is a feasible alternative in patients intolerant to RTX (Fujinaga and Sakuraya, 2018).

Eculizumab

Eculizumab is a humanized monoclonal antibody that inhibits the terminal portion of complement cascade (C5). It is approved for the treatment of paroxysmal nocturnal haemoglobinuria and atypical HUS. It may also find a role in the treatment of other complement-mediated renal diseases, including C3 glomerulopathy, antibody-mediated rejection, anti-phospholipid syndrome, etc. Unfortunately, the indications of eculizumab are limited by its astronomic cost. Eculizumab is given intravenously over 25–45 minutes. Each vial of 30 ml contains 300 mg of eculizumab.

Clinical pharmacology

Eculizumab is a fully humanized monoclonal antibody directed against the complement protein C5. The monoclonal antibody has a molecular weight of 148 kDa. Its mean elimination half-life is 11.3 ± 3.4 days. The onset of steady state is predicted to be approximately 49–56 days. There is significant interpatient variability in eculizumab clearance, ranging from 16 to 237 mL/hr/70 kg in the induction phase (Jodele et al., 2016). The disappearance rate of eculizumab may be increased in the presence of nephrotic syndrome, due to urinary losses of the infused antibody. No dose adjustment is required for patients with renal insufficiency. However, plasma exchange can halve eculizumab concentrations following a one-hour intervention and the elimination half-life of eculizumab can be reduced to 1.3 hours. Supplemental dosing is recommended when eculizumab is administered to patients receiving plasma infusion or exchange.

Mechanisms of action

By binding to C5 with high-affinity eculizumab inhibits its cleavage to C5a and C5b and prevents the generation of the anaphylatoxin C5a and the inflammatory terminal complement complex C5b-9 (also called membrane-attack complex), which exerts haemolytic activity. Eculizumab preserves the early components of complement activation that are essential for opsonization of micro-organisms and clearance of immune complexes.

Toxic effects

Meningococcal meningitis

Eculizumab blocks the terminal complement pathway required for serum bactericidal activity. Because treated patients are at more than a thousandfold increased risk of meningococcal disease, vaccination is recommended. Patients should be vaccinated or revaccinated with a meningococcal vaccine at least two weeks prior to receiving the first dose of eculizumab. However, vaccination may not be sufficient to prevent meningococcal infection. This is probably due to the inhibition of C5a, an upregulator of phagocytosis (Konar and Granoff, 2017). Patients should be monitored closely for early signs of meningococcal infections and evaluated immediately if infection is suspected, and treated with antibiotics if necessary.

Infusion reactions

Administration of eculizumab may result in infusion reactions or immunogenicity that could cause allergic or hypersensitivity reactions. Headache, nasopharyngitis, back pain, cough, and nausea may occur in the period following injection.

Other systemic infections

Eculizumab should be administered with caution to patients with active systemic infections. Patients may have increased susceptibility to infections, especially with *Streptococcus pneumoniae* and *Haemophilus influenzae* (Wiseman, 2016).

Pregnancy

In animals, eculizumab crosses the placenta and may cause increased rates of development abnormalities. Rare cases of retinal dysplasia have been reported in newborns from mothers treated with eculizumab. Some reports outline an increased mortality in males. Theoretically, eculizumab may also cause terminal complement inhibition in the foetal circulation. However, in a study on two newborns from a mother treated with eculizumab during pregnancy, the antibody neither accumulated in foetal plasma nor impaired the complement function in the newborns (Hallstensen et al., 2015). According to the manufacturer, the drug should be administered to pregnant women only if benefits may justify the potentially increased risk for the foetus. Women of childbearing potential must use effective contraception during treatment and up to five months after treatment. It is unknown whether eculizumab is excreted into human breastmilk. However, because of the potential for serious adverse reactions in nursing infants, breastfeeding should be discontinued during treatment and up to five months after treatment.

Clinical use in glomerular diseases

Eculizumab has been largely used in patients with dense deposit disease and C3 glomerulonephritis. Eculizumab proved to be an effective treatment for patients with crescentic, rapidly progressive C3 glomerulopathy. Its benefit in patients with non-rapidly progressing forms is limited (Le Quintrec et al., 2018).

The mechanism of action of eculizumab renders this monoclonal antibody potentially attractive for treating many complement-mediated renal diseases. The main limitation to its use is represented by its excessive cost.

Alemtuzumab

Alemtuzumab (Campath 1H) is an unconjugated, fully humanized, monoclonal antibody directed against the cell surface antigen CD52 on lymphocytes and monocytes. The drug was withdrawn from the markets in the US and Europe in 2012 to prepare for a higher-priced relaunch of Lemtrada aimed at multiple sclerosis.

Anti-TNFα antibodies (infliximab and adalimumab)

These monoclonal antibodies are directed against TNF-α, but not TNFβ. Both drugs are approved by regulatory authorities for treatment of RA, ankylosing spondylitis, plaque psoriasis, and psoriatic arthritis. Adalimumab is administered by subcutaneous injection while infliximab is injected intravenously.

Clinical pharmacology

The pharmacokinetics of infliximab and adalimumab are similar to those of other monoclonal antibodies, notably with an elimination half-life of approximately two to three weeks.

Infliximab is an antibody with high affinity to both membrane-bound and soluble TNFα. It has a bio-availability of 100 per cent, being administered intravenously. Its half-life is 9.5 hours. Infliximab is metabolized by the reticulo-endothelial system. Both body weight and sex were found to influence infliximab pharmacokinetics, and its clearance increased thrice in the presence of antibodies against infliximab.

Adalimumab is a complete human antibody against TNFα. It has a volume of distribution of 4.7–6.0 L and an average bio-availability of 65 per cent. Its pharmacokinetics were linear over the dose range of 0.5 to 10.0 mg/kg following a single dose. The mean terminal half-life is approximately two weeks, with a range of 10–20 days across studies. No gender-related pharmacokinetic differences were observed after correction for a patient's body weight.

No pharmacokinetic data are available for these drugs in patients with hepatic or renal impairment or nephrotic syndrome.

Mechanisms of action

The TNF family is a group of naturally occurring cytokines that are involved in normal inflammatory and immune responses. The best-known member of this family is TNFα. Little is known about TNF-β, which is inhibited by IL-10. TNF can bind two receptors: TNFR1 and TNFR2. This binding causes a conformational change to occur in the receptor, leading to the dissociation of the inhibitory protein SODD from the intracellular death domain. This dissociation enables the adaptor protein TRADD to serve as a platform for subsequent protein binding. Following TRADD binding, three pathways can be initiated:

i. activation of NF-κB, which is involved in inflammation and anti-apoptotic factors;

ii. activation of JNK (Jun N-terminal kinase), which is involved in cell differentiation and has apoptotic activity; or

iii. recruitment of caspase-8, which causes cell apoptosis.

Therefore, different and even contrasting effects may be induced by TNF.

Infliximab and *adalimumab* are in the subclass of 'anti-TNFα antibodies' (in the form of naturally occurring antibodies) and are capable of neutralizing all forms (extracellular, transmembrane, and receptor-bound) of TNFα. These monoclonal antibodies have high specificity for TNFα and do not neutralize TNFβ, a related but less-inflammatory cytokine that utilizes the same receptors as TNFα. They neutralize the biological activity of TNFα by binding with high affinity to the soluble (free-floating in the blood) and transmembrane (located on the outer membranes of T-cells and similar immune cells) forms of TNFα and inhibit or prevent the effective binding of TNFα with its receptors. The anti-TNFα antibodies have the capability of lysing cells involved in the inflammatory process. No differences in rates of drug response or remission were observed between the two anti-TNFα monoclonal antibodies.

Toxic effects

Infections
The risk of infection of anti-TNFα agents is difficult to evaluate as most patients receiving these drugs are also treated with GCs or immunosuppressive agents. However, the rate of serious infections such as tuberculosis, sepsis, and fungal infections appears to be increased in anti-TNFα-treated subjects compared to the expected rate (Singh et al., 2011). Some of these infections can be severe and life threatening. Individuals with active infections should not be treated with anti-TNFα antibodies.

Neurologic toxicity
Optic neuritis, polyneuropathy, and Guillain Barré syndrome may seldom occur.

Malignancies
Because of the role of TNF in host defence, it was hypothesized that its inhibition might lead to an increased risk of malignancies. However, it is difficult to assess the oncogenic risk of anti-TNF agents, as patients given these agents have also been treated with other immunosuppressive drugs, often given at high doses and for prolonged periods of time. Moreover, patients with RA have a higher rate of cancers than the general population. At any rate, the National Register for Biologic Treatment in Finland reported a lower incidence of cancer in patients with RA treated with infliximab in comparison to conventional disease-modifying antirheumatic drug (Aaltonen et al., 2015).

Immunogenicity
Antibodies to the TNFα receptor portion or other protein components of the drug product may be detected in sera of adult patients treated with anti-TNFα agents. The prevalence of anti-infliximab antibodies in patients with RA varies

from 12 per cent to 44 per cent and seems to be inversely proportional to the level of seric infliximab and therapeutic response. The prevalence of anti-adalimumab antibodies ranges from 1 per cent to 87 per cent (Aikawa et al., 2012).

Induction of auto-immune disease

A number of auto-immune diseases, including non-cutaneous leukocytoclastic vasculitis, lupus, interstitial lung diseases, auto-immune hepatitis, and nephrotic syndrome have been reported in patients treated with anti-TNF drugs (Ramos-Casals et al., 2007).

Pregnancy

The few available data about pregnancy mainly come from case reports or retrospective studies. From the small numbers available, there was no excess of birth defects reported with infliximab. However, exposed newborns were more likely to be born prematurely and to be lower in body weight than other newborns from mothers with RA (Chambers et al., 2006). The FDA includes anti-TNFα agents in Category B (no documented increased risk for structural defects).

Clinical use in glomerular diseases

Anti-TNFα antibodies have been used successfully in some cases of renal vasculitis and lupus nephritis, but trials with infliximab in these diseases failed. Experimental studies and clinical observations support a role for TNFα in the pathogenesis of acute and chronic renal disease. It has been shown that TNF receptors are significant prognostic biomarkers for MN (Lee et al., 2014) and elevated concentrations of circulating TNFRs at baseline are early biomarkers for subsequent renal progression in patients with IgAN (Oh et al., 2015). Anecdotal cases of remission of MN (Santoro et al., 2012) or crescentic glomerulonephritis (Zaenker et al., 2004) after treatment with anti-TNFα therapy have been reported. Instead, no benefit was observed in patients with FSGS treated with adalimumab (Trachtman et al., 2015). Caution should be used before considering anti-TNFα agents for treatment of primary glomerular diseases. Given their dual functions in inflammation and immune regulation, TNF may mediate both pro-inflammatory as well as immunosuppressive effects, particularly in kidney diseases. As mentioned, blockade of TNFα may lead to the development of auto-antibodies, SLE, or vasculitis in patients affected by other auto-immune diseases. These data raise concerns about using TNF-blocking therapies in renal disease as the kidney may be especially vulnerable to the manifestation of auto-immune processes. On the other hand, there are sporadic reports emphasizing good results with the use of anti-TNFα agents in lupus nephritis and vasculitis, i.e. the same diseases that may be triggered by their administration.

Fusion proteins

Etanercept

Etanercept is a soluble fusion protein produced by recombinant DNA that binds specifically to TNF and acts as a TNF inhibitor.

Clinical pharmacology

After a single subcutaneous injection of 25 mg of etanercept, the mean half-life is 102 ± 30 hours and the time to maximal concentration is 69 ± 34 hours. After six months of twice weekly administration of 25 mg there is a two- to sevenfold increase in peak serum concentrations and approximately fourfold increase in the AUC. Pharmacokinetic parameters are not different between men and women and do not vary with age in adult patients.

Mechanisms of action

Etanercept binds specifically to tumour necrosis factor (TNF) and blocks its interaction with cell surface TNF receptors. Etanercept is a dimeric soluble form of the p75 TNF receptor that can bind to two TNF molecules. It inhibits the activity of TNF in vitro.

Toxic effects

The risk of adverse events, immunogenicity, and auto-immune disorders is similar for etanercept, infliximab, and adalimumab.

Injection site reactions

About 14 per cent to 37 per cent of patients may complain of mild to moderate reactions (erythema and/or itching, pain, or swelling) at the site of injection of etanercept. Injection site reactions generally occur in the first month and subsequently decrease in frequency. The mean duration of injection site reactions is three to five days. Systemic side effects are headache, rash, nausea, and stomach upset.

Neurotoxic effects

Exceptional cases of demyelinating disease have been reported in patients treated with etanercept.

Infections

As for anti-TNF antibodies, it is difficult to estimate the risk for infection in etanercept-treated patients. However, in hospitalized patients with RA, etanercept and infliximab had significantly higher hazard ratios of hospitalized infection compared to abatacept (Yun et al., 2015).

Malignancy

No difference in the incidence of lymphoma was seen between etanercept and other biologic agents in patients with RA (Singh et al., 2011).

Clinical use in glomerular diseases

The pros and cons for the use of etanercept are the same already exposed for anti-TNFα antibodies. In a child with recurrent post-transplant FSGS resistant to plasmapheresis, twice weekly etanercept injections followed by infliximab-sustained partial remission (Bitzan et al., 2012). No beneficial effects were reported in patients with ANCA-associated vasculitis. Instead, cases of *de novo* MN, IgAN, or necrotizing glomerulonephritis developed in patients treated with etanercept (Piga et al., 2014).

CTLA-4 fused proteins (abatacept and belatacept)

Abatacept is a fusion protein composed of the Fc region of the immunoglobulin IgG1 fused to the extracellular domain of CTLA-4 a receptor of Ig superfamily with a structure analogue to CD28. The drug inhibits the activation of T-cells by blocking the interaction between the costimulatory molecules CD80 and CD86 on the antigen presenting cell (APC) and the CD28 on the surface of T-cells. The drug is approved for clinical use in patients with RA. It may be administered by IV infusion or subcutaneous injection. Belatacept is another protein similar to abatacept. However, belatacept differs by two amino acids, allowing for greater binding affinity for CD80–CD86 adhesion molecules in comparison with abatacept. Belatacept is used in organ transplantation where it can help avoid the use of calcineurin inhibitors in kidney transplantation.

Clinical pharmacology

The pharmacokinetics of abatacept is comparable in patients with RA and in normal volunteers. The terminal half-life is about 16.7 hours after a single infusion and about 13.1 hours after multiple infusions. After multiple IV infusions, the pharmacokinetics of abatacept showed proportional increases of peak and AUC over the dose range of 2 mg/kg to 10 mg/kg. At 10 mg/kg, serum concentration appeared to reach a steady-state by day 60 with a mean trough concentration of 24 mcg/ml (1 to 66 mcg/ml). No systemic accumulation of abatacept occurred upon continued repeated treatment with 10 mg/kg at monthly intervals. Age and gender do not affect clearance, but increasing body weight is associated with higher clearance of abatacept. Renal and liver function do not affect the abatacept clearance.

Following multiple doses of 5 or 10 mg/kg, belatacept demonstrates linear pharmacokinetics with low variability, and concentration-dependent pharmacodynamics. The median belatacept elimination half-life is eight to nine days. Belatacept exhibits concentration-dependent binding to CD86 receptors. The clearance of belatacept is not affected by renal or liver function or dialysis.

Mechanisms of action

Naïve T-cells require two signals to be activated. The first signal is provided by the contact between the alloantigen presented by antigen-presenting cells and the specific receptor located on the surface of T-cells. However, this is an anergic/apoptotic signal. A second signal (costimulation) is needed to rescue T-cells from apoptosis and to activate them. This signal is given by the contact between proteins located on the APCs, such as B7-1 and B7-2 (also called CD80 and CD86) and CD28 located on the surface of T- cells. B7 molecules have a great affinity for CTLA-4. Thus, the administration of abatacept or belatacept can prevent the second signal and the activation of T-cells.

It has been reported that B7-1 molecules can be expressed also on podocytes of patients with several different types of glomerular disease, including FSGS and diabetic nephropathy (Yu et al., 2013). However, other studies have not confirmed the increased B7-1 expression in glomeruli in FSGS (Benigni et al., 2014).

Toxic effects

Infusion-related reactions
Nausea, flushing, urticaria, cough, pruritus, rash, and wheezing may occur in <1 per cent of patients. Rarely, cardiopulmonary symptoms, e.g. hypotension, increased blood pressure, dyspnoea, may also develop.

Anaphylactic reactions
Anaphylaxis or anaphylactoid reactions can occur after the first infusion and can be life threatening. If an anaphylactic or other serious allergic reaction occurs, administration of abatacept should be stopped immediately with appropriate therapy instituted, and its use should be permanently discontinued.

Infections
Life-threatening infections, including sepsis and pneumonia, have been reported. Infections are more frequent and severe in patients on concomitant immunosuppressive therapy.

Malignancy
Treatment with CTLA-4 fusion proteins can increase the risk for lymphoma is approximately 3.5 times higher than expected in an age- and gender-matched general population. The risk is particularly elevated in patients without

anti-Epstein-Barr virus antibodies. Other malignancies, included lung, skin, breast, and uterine cancers, have been reported.

Clinical use in glomerular diseases

Normally, podocytes do not express B7-1. However, certain glomerulopathies may be associated with the presence of B7-1 on the surface of podocytes. The abnormal expression of this costimulatory protein reduces the ability of podocytes to attach to the surrounding GBM and favours proteinuria. Mechanistically, B7-1 promotes podocyte migration through inactivation of the $\beta1$ integrin. In vitro studies demonstrated that abatacept can bind to B7-1 on podocytes, stabilize β_1-integrin activation, and inhibit podocyte migration and proteinuria. A report of five patients suggested that abatacept could be used in corticoresistant relapse of FSGS after kidney transplantation, inducing partial or even complete remission of proteinuria (Yu et al., 2013). Thus, abatacept might be indicated in glomerulopathies associated with an increase on the surface of podocytes of B7-1 (Trimarchi, 2015). However, in some studies, proteinuria remained unchanged after abatacept therapy in patients with primary or recurrent FSGS after transplantation despite the presence of mild B7-1 glomerular expression (Garin et al., 2015). Belatacept is mainly indicated in patients with organ transplantation, since it may avoid the use and side effects of calcineurin inhibitors. It might theoretically find an indication in patients with glomerular diseases characterized by high expression of B7-1 (CD80) on podocytes. Promising results have been reported in anecdotal cases of MCD with elevated urinary B7-1 (Garin et al., 2015).

Proteasome inhibitors

Bortezomib

Bortezomib is an N-protected dipeptide that binds the catalytic site of the 26S proteasome with high affinity and specificity. Bortezomib is approved for treating patients with multiple myeloma and has been used also in patients with mantle lymphoma. The drug is available in vials of 1 mg that are administered intravenously usually twice a week with ten days of interval. New proteasome inhibitors, including carfilzomib and ixazomib, that can be taken by mouth have been recently approved by the USFDA and the EMA for treating multiple myeloma. Due to its mechanism of action, bortezomib has also been employed as a rescue treatment of antibody-mediated rejection or glomerular diseases associated with monoclonal gammopathy.

Clinical pharmacology

After IV injection, peak plasma levels maintained only for about five minutes, after which the levels rapidly drop as the drug distributes to tissues. Both IV and subcutaneous routes provide equal drug exposures and generally comparable therapeutic efficacy. Elimination half-life is approximately 9–15 hours and the drug is cleared primarily by hepatic metabolism, while its renal excretion is neglectable.

Mechanisms of action

There are multiple mechanisms to ensure that nascent polypeptides are properly folded and mature proteins maintain their functional conformation. When proteins misfold, either because of normal or pathological stimuli or mutations, they must be refolded correctly or recycled. In the absence of these corrective processes, they may become toxic to the cell. A central role in the regulation of proteins is played by a multisystem enzyme complex called proteasome. Before a protein is degraded, it is first conjugated with a polyubiquitin chain. Multiple ubiquitination cycles resulting in a polyubiquitin chain are required for targeting a protein to the proteasome for degradation. The proteasome regulatory cap binds the polyubiquitin chain, denatures the protein, and feeds the protein into the proteasome's proteolytic core. The multisubunit 26S proteasome recognizes, unfolds, and degrades polyubiquitinated substrates into small peptides (Amm et al., 2014). Therefore, the proteasome regulates protein expression and function by degradation of ubiquitylated proteins, and also cleanses the cell of abnormal or misfolded proteins. This function can also maintain the immortal phenotype of myeloma cells.

While multiple mechanisms are likely to be involved, proteasome inhibition may prevent degradation of pro-apoptotic factors, permitting activation of programmed cell death. Moreover, bortezomib can cause a rapid and dramatic change in the levels of intracellular peptides that are produced by the proteasome. These effects are particularly vigorous in neoplastic cells.

Toxic effects

Systemic toxicity

Asthenia, fever, headache, and gastrointestinal symptoms can develop in 40–65 per cent of patients.

Haematologic side effects

Anaemia, neutropenia, and thrombocytopenia are relatively frequent, being largely dependent on the dosage.

Neurological side effects

About one-third of patients complain of dizziness, paraesthesia, or insomnia. A manageable peripheral neuropathy is frequent and probably underestimated. In a series, this complication developed in 70 per cent of patients with multiple myeloma (Zaroulis et al., 2014). Rigours are less frequent.

Infection

Viral and bacterial infection may occur in about 10 per cent of patients, with the lung and urinary tract being the most common locations. A case of acute interstitial nephritis has been reported in a patient treated with bortezomib, although renal function improved after GC therapy and discontinuation of bortezomib (Cheungpasitporn et al., 2015).

Muscle toxicity

Experimental studies demonstrate that in primary human myoblasts, bortezomib at low concentrations leads to excessive storage of lipid droplets together with structural mitochondrial abnormalities. This may result in a reversible myopathy characterized by a proximal muscle weakness involving lower limbs (Guglielmi et al., 2017).

Pregnancy

Bortezomib has caused embryo-foetal lethality in animal studies at doses lower than the clinical dose. There are no controlled data in human pregnancy. Pregnancy is contra-indicated and effective contraception is recommended for women of childbearing potential. The excretion of bortezomib in breastmilk is unknown. Lactation is not recommended.

Clinical use in glomerular diseases

Good results with bortezomib have been reported in murine models of lupus-like nephritis. In clinical nephrology, bortezomib has been successfully used in cases of monoclonal gammopathies associated with proliferative glomerulonephritis. In a patient with MN a single administration of bortezomib resulted in an almost complete remission (Hartono et al., 2014). The drug has also been used as a rescue treatment in antibody-mediated rejection of kidney transplantation. Theoretically, bortezomib or other proteasome inhibitors may find possible applications in lupus, IgAN, idiopathic nephrotic syndrome, and renal fibrosis (Coppo, 2014).

Miscellaneous immunomodulating drugs

Levamisole

Levamisole is a synthetic imidazothiazole derivative that has been used for many years as an anthelmintic drug. After exhibiting immunomodulatory properties levamisole has been used as a steroid-sparing agent in patients with MCD and frequent relapses of the nephrotic syndrome. The drug is available in some countries in form of tablets. Levamisole was banned by the USFDA in 1998, probably because it was used as a cutting agent in cocaine to enhance its euphoric properties among users.

Clinical pharmacology

Levamisole is a levo-isomer of tetramisole. After administration by mouth it is rapidly and completely absorbed with a plasma peak after two to four hours. The drug is metabolized by the liver. The opening of the thiazolic ring produces the metabolite DL-2-oxy-3 (2-mercaptoethyl)-5 phenylimidazoline, which has immunomodulating effects. The drug is mainly excreted by the kidney and by the gastrointestinal tract. The plasma half-life is about four hours. Only 5 per cent of the drug is excreted unmodified in the urine. The pharmacokinetic parameters are similar in children and adults, although the elimination rate was slightly higher in children (Kreeftmeijer-Vegter et al., 2015).

Mechanisms of action

Levamisole enhances the specific immune response and restores immunity in immune-deficient hosts. The drug stimulates the differentiation of T-cells, restores their function, and increases the activity of macrophages when the immune system is depressed, thus amplifying the immune response. It also increases the motility of neutrophils. The exact mechanism of action in renal disease is still poorly defined. It has been hypothesized that the sulphur contained in levamisole may release a factor that would interfere with T-cell function in a way similar to thymic hormone. Moreover, the imidazole group increases the cellular content of GMP. The consequent increased intracellular ratio GMP/AMP stimulates the immunological response and enhances the production of cellular clones. Experimental studies showed that levamisole can also protect against podocyte injury in a puromycin aminonucleoside-treated cell model, probably by increasing the expression of GRs and activating GR signalling (Jiang et al., 2015).

Toxic effects

Adverse reactions are usually mild and consist of fatigue, arthralgias, and fever often associated with nausea, diarrhoea, and metallic taste. Significant neutropenia may occur in about 10 per cent of nephrotic patients. Rarely, the drug may be responsible for tremors, agitation, seizures, and confusion.

Cutaneous complications

Cutaneous vasculitis and other skin complications are a cause of discontinuation of the drug. Allergic reactions can also result in difficult breathing, constriction of the throat, and swelling of the lips, tongue, or face.

Vasculitis

Levamisole is frequently used to adulterate cocaine. Such an association can frequently cause systemic vasculitis (Sirvent et al., 2016) or necrotizing glomerulonephritis with MN (Carrara et al., 2016).

Pregnancy

Levamisole has not been studied for use by pregnant women. It is unknown whether levamisole may be dangerous for the foetus. Although it is unlikely that the drug produces teratogenic effects, it has been classified in Category C (insufficient information) by the USFDA. It is better to avoid the use of levamisole during pregnancy.

Clinical use in glomerular diseases

Levamisole has been used in children with MCD on the assumption that the drug might restore abnormal T-cell function. It is also possible that levamisole can increase the resistance of podocytes to injury. The drug is mainly used in children with frequent relapses of idiopathic nephrotic syndrome to increase the time to relapse (Gruppen et al., 2018). At doses of 60 mg/m^2 once daily until urine is protein-free for six days, followed by a dose of 60 mg/m^2 every other day with progressive reduction every week for 16 weeks, the drug is well tolerated. Non-controlled studies emphasized the effectiveness of levamisole but the results of randomized trials are less optimistic. At present the drug is not commercially available in many Western countries.

Deoxyspergualin

15-Deoxyspergualin (DSG) is a synthetic analogue of spergualin, a natural product of the bacterium *Bacillus laterosporus*. DGS has been initially developed as an anti-cancer drug, but strong immunosuppressive properties were later discovered in several animal models of transplantation and of auto-immune disease. DGS has been successfully used in patients with recurrent kidney transplant rejections. DGS comes in the form of white powder and is easily dissolved in water. The drug is supplied for IV or subcutaneous injection. The European Commission has assigned to DGS the status of *orphan drug* treatment of ANCA-associated vasculitis.

Clinical pharmacology

DGS is a 1-amino-19-guanidino-11-hydroxy-4, 9, 12-triazanona-decane-10, 1–3-dione with a molecular weight of 497. A small fraction of DSG is excreted unmetabolized in the urine. The amount of DSG in the urine correlates strongly to renal function. Pharmacokinetics are otherwise not affected by the degree of renal function. Therefore, the drug can safely be given to patients with impaired renal function.

Mechanisms of action

DGS binds to the immunophilin Hsc 70, a nuclear translocator of NF-κB involved in the refolding and allosteric changes of proteins, but the mechanism of action is not well understood. DGS can inhibit several immunologic functions, such as the development of plaque-forming cells, but, in particular, it inhibits lysosomal enzyme release and superoxide production by monocytes. It has, therefore, been suggested that DGS may be immunosuppressive via a predominantly antimonocyte-macrophage effect. The drug may also inhibit lymphocyte proliferation in response to mitogenic and allogenic stimuli and antibody production by B cells.

Toxic effects

Leukopenia

Neutropenia is frequent but it is usually transient and reversible. In contrast to neutrophil counts, lymphocyte and monocyte counts are less affected by DSG. However, a slight decrease in absolute lymphocyte counts of ~20 per cent below the normal range may be observed.

Infections

Infections, mostly of the upper respiratory tract, may occur. They usually resolve quickly with the use of antibiotics without further consequences. Opportunistic infections are rare but may develop in patients taking concomitantly other immunosuppressive drugs.

Gastrointestinal troubles

Some patients complain of gastric discomfort and flushing.

Pregnancy

There is no information about the use of DGS in pregnant women.

Clinical use in glomerular disease

Anecdotal reports showed the efficacy of DGS in lupus nephritis, proliferative glomerulonephritis, and crescentic glomerulonephritis. A phase I/II study in patients with active lupus nephritis showed a significant reduction in proteinuria for those patients who completed a course of nine cycles with DGS (Lorenz et al., 2011).

Imatinib

Imatinib mesylate is a protein-tyrosine kinase inhibitor approved for treatment of chronic myeloid leukaemia, gastrointestinal stromal tumours, and some brain tumours. The drug may also exert favourable effects in some rheumatic diseases. It is available in form of rigid capsules that should be taken in a single daily administration during a meal with a glass of water.

Clinical pharmacology

Imatinib is well absorbed after oral administration with a peak in plasma concentration achieved within two to four hours post-dose. Mean absolute bioavailability is 98 per cent. Following oral administration in healthy volunteers, the elimination half-lives of imatinib and its major active metabolite, the N-demethyl derivative, are approximately 18 and 40 hours, respectively. At clinically relevant concentrations of imatinib, binding to plasma proteins in in vitro experiments is approximately 95 per cent, mostly to albumin and a1-acid glycoprotein.

CYP3A4 is the major enzyme responsible for metabolism of imatinib. Other cytochrome P450 enzymes play a minor role in its metabolism. The main circulating active metabolite in humans is the N-demethylated piperazine derivative, which shows in vitro potency similar to the parent imatinib. The plasma protein binding of N-demethylated metabolite CGP74588 is similar to that of the parent compound. Approximately 81 per cent of the dose is eliminated mostly as metabolites within seven days in faeces (68 per cent) and urine (13 per cent). Unchanged imatinib accounts for 25 per cent of the dose.

Mechanisms of action

Imatinib is a 2-phenylaminopyrimidine derivative that functions as a specific inhibitor of a number of tyrosine kinase enzymes. It occupies the TK active site, leading to a decrease in activity. In particular, imatinib inhibits the bcr-abl tyrosine kinase, the constitutive abnormal tyrosine kinase created by the Philadelphia chromosome abnormality in chronic myeloid leukaemia. Imatinib inhibits proliferation and induces apoptosis in bcr-abl positive cell lines as well as fresh leukaemic cells from Philadelphia chromosome positive chronic myeloid leukaemia. Imatinib inhibits colony formation in assays using ex vivo peripheral blood and bone marrow samples.

On the immune system, imatinib has antiproliferative activity and immunomodulatory effects in lymphocytes, macrophages, mast cells, and dendritic cells, with abrogating multiple signal transduction pathways involved in pathogenesis of auto-immune diseases, e.g. inhibiting IFN-γ, TNF-α, IL-1β, and IL-17 pro-inflammatory cytokines (Azizi and Mirschafey, 2013).

Toxic effects

Most patients complain of adverse events during treatment with imatinib, such as nausea, vomiting, muscle cramps and bone pain. However, serious side effects are not frequent.

Hepatotoxicity

Cases of acute hepatitis with five to more than 20 times the upper normal levels of transaminases or four times the upper normal values of bilirubin have been reported in 0.4–3.5 per cent of patients. Data about liver histology varies between reports from focal periportal necrosis with mixed lymphocyte, neutrophil, and plasmocyte infiltration to massive hepatic necrosis or cytolytic acute hepatitis. The time between beginning treatment and development of liver toxicity varies from 11 days to 49 weeks. Hepatotoxicity is usually resolved with imatinib dose reduction or interruption. However, permanent imatinib discontinuation for hepatic toxicity may be required in 0.5 per cent of patients. Exceptionally, deaths from hepatic failure have been reported (Ridruejo et al., 2007).

Oedema

Most patients present peri-orbital and leg oedema. Sometimes fluid retention may be severe, with pleural and/or pericardial effusion.

Gastrointestinal side effects

Nausea, vomiting, and diarrhoea may occur in 40–70 per cent of patients.

Pain

Muscle cramps, skeletal, or abdominal pain are common but mild. They may be managed with medication without reducing the prescribed dosage.

Cardiac complications

Severe congestive cardiac failure is an uncommon but well-recognized side effect of imatinib. Mice treated with large doses of imatinib show toxic damage to their myocardium. Early concerns regarding imatinib-related cardiotoxicity have not been confirmed in large prospective randomized trials, with reports indicating a low incidence of approximately 0.2–0.4 per cent (Ben Ami and Demetri, 2016).

Bone marrow toxicity

Anaemia and cytopenia have been rarely described. A very few case reports of bone marrow aplasia following imatinib therapy have been reported so far.

Pregnancy

Imatinib has been found to be teratogenic in rats and is not recommended for use during pregnancy. There is a paucity of data regarding patients on imatinib mesylate becoming pregnant and completing pregnancy. Among 28 pregnancies in women who received imatinib, 19 (67.9 per cent) were uneventful while the remaining pregnancies ended in adverse events (Iqbal et al., 2014).

Clinical use in primary glomerulonephritis

Experimental studies showed that imatinib can suppress cryoglobulinaemia and secondary membranoproliferative glomerulonephritis (Iyoda et al., 2009; Wallace et al., 2012), may slow the progression of anti-glomerular basement membrane nephritis (Iyoda et al., 2013), and may attenuate the effects of chronic anti-thy1 glomerulosclerosis towards tubulointerstitial fibrosis and renal insufficiency (Wang-Rosenke et al., 2013). These data may render imatinib of potential interest for treating some primary proliferative glomerulonephritis (such as IgAN), but the serious side effects of therapy remain a significant concern.

References

Aaltonen KJ, Joensuu JT, Virkki L, et al. (2015). Rates of serious infections and malignancies among patients with rheumatoid arthritis receiving either tumor necrosis factor inhibitor or rituximab therapy. J Rheumatol. 42: 372–8.

Abd Rahman AN, Tett SE, Staatz CE. (2014). How accurate and precise are limited sampling strategies in estimating exposure to mycophenolic acid in people with autoimmune disease? Clin Pharmacokinet. 53: 227–45.

Abulayha A, Bredan A, El Enshasy H, et al. (2014). Rituximab: Modes of action, remaining dispute and future perspective. Future Oncol. 10: 2481–92.

Agrawal S, Guess AJ, Benndorf R, et al. (2011). Comparison of direct action of thiazolidinediones and glucocorticoids on renal podocytes: protection from injury and molecular effects. Mol Pharmacol. 80: 389–99.

Aikawa NE, Pereira RM, Lage L, et al. (2012). Anti-TNF therapy for polymyalgia rheumatica: Report of 99 cases and review of the literature. Clin Rheumatol. 31: 575–9.

Akar Özkan E, Özdemir BH, Deniz EE, et al. (2014). Post-transplant lymphoproliferative disorder after liver and kidney transplant. Exp Clin Transplant. 12 (Suppl 1): 142–8.

Albrecht U. (2012). Timing to perfection: The biology of central and peripheral circadian clocks. Neuron. 74: 246–60.

Aleissa M, Nicol P, Godeau M, et al. (2017). Azathioprine hypersensitivity syndrome: Two cases of febrile neutrophilic dermatosis induced by azathioprine. Case Rep Dermatol. 9: 6–11.

Allison AC, Eugui EM. (2000). Mycophenolate mofetil and its mechanisms of action. Immunopharmacology. 47: 85–118.

Amm I, Sommer T, Wolf DH. (2014). Protein quality control and elimination of protein waste: The role of the ubiquitin-proteasome system. Biochim Biophys Acta. **1843**: 182–96.

Amoroso A, Hafsi S, Militello L, et al. (2011). Understanding rituximab function and resistance: Implications for tailored therapy. Front Biosci (Landmark Ed). **16**: 770–82.

Appenzeller S, Blatyta PF, Costallat LT. (2008). Ovarian failure in SLE patients using pulse cyclophosphamide: Comparison of different regimes. Rheumatol Int. **28**: 567–71.

Arnason BG, Berkovich R, Catania A, et al. (2013). Mechanisms of action of adrenocorticotropic hormone and other melanocortins relevant to the clinical management of patients with multiple sclerosis. Mult Scler. **19**: 130–6.

Arnaud L, Nordin A, Lundholm H, et al. (2017). Effect of corticosteroids and cyclophosphamide on sex hormone profiles in male patients with systemic lupus erythematosus or systemic sclerosis. Arthritis Rheumatol. **69**: 1272–9.

Azizi G, Mirshafiey A. (2013). Imatinib mesylate: An innovation in treatment of autoimmune diseases. Recent Pat Inflamm Allergy Drug Discov. **7**: 259–67.

Bagamasbad P, Ziera T, Borden SA, et al. (2012). Molecular basis for glucocorticoid induction of the Kruppel-like factor 9 gene in hippocampal neurons. Endocrinology. **153**: 5334–45.

Barbarino JM, Staatz CE, Venkataramanan R, et al. (2013). PharmGKB summary: Cyclosporine and tacrolimus pathways. Pharmacogenet Genomics. **23**: 563–85.

Baris HE, Baris S, Karakoc-Aydiner E, et al. (2016). The effect of systemic corticosteroids on the innate and adaptive immune system in children with steroid responsive nephrotic syndrome. Eur J Pediatr. **175**: 685–93.

Basta M. (2014). Intravenous immunoglobulin-related thromboembolic events—an accusation that proves the opposite. Clin Exp Immunol. **178**: 153–5.

Basu B. (2014). Ofatumumab for rituximab-resistant nephrotic syndrome. N Engl J Med. **370**: 1268–70.

Ben Ami E, Demetri GD. (2016). A safety evaluation of imatinib mesylate in the treatment of gastrointestinal stromal tumor. Expert Opin Drug Saf. **15**: 571–8.

Benigni A, Gagliardini E, Remuzzi G. (2014). Abatacept in B7 1 positive proteinuria kidney disease. N Engl J Med. **370**: 1261–3.

Bezombes C, Fournié JJ, Laurent G. (2011). Direct effect of rituximab in B-cell-derived lymphoid neoplasias: Mechanism, regulation, and perspectives. Mol Cancer Res. **9**: 1435–42.

Bichsel KJ, Gogia N, Malouff T, et al. (2013). Role for the epidermal growth factor receptor in chemotherapy-induced alopecia. PLoS One. **8**: e69368.

Bitzan M, Babayeva S, Vasudevan A, et al. (2012). TNFα pathway blockade ameliorates toxic effects of FSGS plasma on podocyte cytoskeleton and β3 integrin activation. Pediatr Nephrol. **27**: 2217–26.

Blankenstein KI, Borschewski A, Labes R, et al. (2017). Calcineurin inhibitor cyclosporine A activates renal Na-K-Cl cotransporters via local and systemic mechanisms. Am J Physiol Renal Physiol. **312**: F489–F501.

Bomback AS, Canetta PA, Beck LH Jr, et al. (2012). Treatment of resistant glomerular diseases with adrenocorticotropic hormone gel: A prospective trial. Am J Nephrol. **36**: 58–67.

Bonanni A, Calatroni M, D'Alessandro M, et al. (2018). Adverse events linked with the use of chimeric and humanized anti-CD20 antibodies in children with idiopathic nephrotic syndrome. Br J Clin Pharmacol. **84**: 1238–49.

Bonett RM, Hu F, Bagamasbad P, et al. (2009). Stressor and glucocorticoid-dependent induction of the immediate early gene kruppel-like factor 9: Implications for neural development and plasticity. Endocrinology. **150**: 1757–65.

Borst O, Schaub M, Walker B, et al. (2015). Pivotal role of serum- and glucocorticoid-inducible kinase 1 in vascular inflammation and atherogenesis. Arterioscler Thromb Vasc Biol. **35**: 547–57.

Bowles NP, Karatsoreos IN, Li X, et al. (2015). A peripheral endocannabinoid mechanism contributes to glucocorticoid-mediated metabolic syndrome. Proc Natl Acad Sci USA. **112**: 285–90.

Brocks DR, Chaudhary HR, Ben-Eltriki M, et al. (2014). Effects of serum lipoproteins on cyclosporine. A cellular uptake and renal toxicity in vitro. Can J Physiol Pharmacol. **92**: 140–8.

Broersen LH, Pereira AM, Jørgensen JO, et al. (2015). Adrenal insufficiency in corticosteroids use: Systematic review and meta-analysis. J Clin Endocrinol Metab. **100**: 2171–80.

Burchard PR, Abou Tayoun AN, Lefferts JA, et al. (2014). Development of a rapid clinical TPMT genotyping assay. Clin Biochem. **47**: 126–9.

Busillo JM, Cidowski JA. (2013). The five Rs of glucocorticoid action during inflammation: Ready, reinforce, repress, resolve, and restore. Trends Endocrinol Metab. **24**: 109–19.

Byrd JC, Brown JR, O'Brien S, et al. (2014). Ibrutinib versus ofatumumab in previously treated chronic lymphoid leukemia. N Engl J Med. **371**: 213–23.

Cain DW, Cidlowski JA. (2017). Immune regulation by glucocorticoids. Nat Rev Immunol. **17**: 233–47.

Carrara C, Emili S, Lin M, et al. (2016). Necrotizing and crescentic glomerulonephritis with membranous nephropathy in a patient exposed to levamisole-adulterated cocaine. Clin Kidney J. **9**: 234–8.

Carson KR, Focosi D, Major EO, et al. (2009). Monoclonal antibody-associated progressive multifocal leucoencephalopathy in patients treated with rituximab, natalizumab, and efalizumab: A review from the Research on Adverse Drug Events and Reports (RADAR) Project. Lancet Oncol. **10**: 816–24.

Casetta I, Iuliano G, Filippini G. (2007). Azathioprine for multiple sclerosis. Cochrane Database Syst Rev. **4**: CD003982.

Cattran DC, Alexopoulos E, Heering P, et al. (2007). Cyclosporin in idiopathic glomerular disease associated with the nephrotic syndrome: Workshop recommendations. Kidney Int. **72**: 1429–47.

Chakkera HA, Kudva Y, Kaplan B, et al. (2017). Calcineurin inhibitors: Pharmacologic mechanisms impacting both insulin resistance and insulin secretion leading to glucose dysregulation and diabetes mellitus. Clin Pharmacol Ther. **101**: 114–20.

Chakravarty EF Murray ER, Kelman A, et al. (2011). Pregnancy outcomes after maternal exposure to rituximab. Blood. **117**: 1499–506.

Chambers CD, Tutunku ZM, Johnson D, et al. (2006). Human pregnancy safety for agents used to treat rheumatoid arthritis: Adequacy of available information and strategies for developing post-marketing data. Arthritis Res Ther. **8**: 215–25.

Chen Y, Li Y, Yang S, et al. (2014). Efficacy and safety of mycophenolate mofetil treatment in IgA nephropathy: A systematic review. BMC Nephrol. **15**: 193.

Cheng G, Liu D, Margetts P, et al. (2015). Valsartan combined with clopidogrel and/ or leflunomide for the treatment of progressive immunoglobulin A nephropathy. Nephrology (Carlton). **20**: 77–84.

Cheungpasitporn W, Leung N, Rajkumar SV. (2015). Bortezomib-induced acute interstitial nephritis. Nephrol Dial Transplant. **30**: 1225–9.

Chiasson VL, Jones KA, Kopriva SE, et al. (2012). Endothelial cell transforming growth factor-β receptor activation causes tacrolimus-induced renal arteriolar hyalinosis. Kidney Int. **82**: 857–66.

Coelho MC, Dos Santos CV, Vieira Neto L, et al. (2014). Adverse effects of glucocorticoids: Coagulopathy. Eur J Endocrinol. **173**: M11–21.

Colom H, Lloberas N, Andreu F, et al. (2014). Pharmacokinetic modeling of enterohepatic circulation of mycophenolic acid in renal transplant recipients. Kidney Int. **85**: 1434–43.

Conn HO, Poynard T. (1994). Corticosteroids and peptic ulcer: Meta-analysis of adverse events during steroid therapy. J Intern Med. **236**: 619–32.

Constantinescu S, Pai A, Coscia LA, et al. (2014). Breast-feeding after transplantation. Best Pract Res Clin Obstet Gynaecol. **28**: 1163–73.

Coppo R. (2014). Proteasome inhibitors in progressive renal diseases. Nephrol Dial Transplant. **29** (Suppl 1): i25–i30.

Counsilman CE, Jol-van der Zijde CM, Stevens J, et al. (2015). Pharmacokinetics of rituximab in a pediatric patient with therapy-resistant nephrotic syndrome. Pediatr Nephrol. **30**: 1367–70.

Coutinho AE, Chapman KE. (2011). The anti-inflammatory and immunosuppressive effects of glucocorticoids, recent developments and mechanistic insights. Mol Cell Endocrinol. **335**: 2–13.

Cruzado JM, Poveda R, Ibernón M, et al. (2011). Low-dose sirolimus combined with angiotensin-converting enzyme inhibitor and statin stabilizes renal function and reduces glomerular proliferation in poor prognosis IgA nephropathy. Nephrol Dial Transplant. **26**: 3596–602.

Cuce G, Çetinkaya S, Koc T, et al. (2015). Chemoprotective effect of vitamin E in cyclophosphamide-induced hepatotoxicity in rats. Chem Biol Interact. **232**: 7–11.

Cummings SR, San Martin J, McClung MR, et al. (2009). Denosumab for prevention of fractures in postmenopausal women with osteoporosis. N Engl J Med. **361**: 756–65.

Dhandapani MC, Venkatesan V, Rengaswamy NB, et al. (2015). Association of ACE and MDR1 gene polymorphisms with steroid resistance in children with idiopathic nephrotic syndrome. Genet Test Mol Biomarkers. **19**: 454–6.

De Guia RM, Herzig S. (2015). How do glucocorticoids regulate lipid metabolism? Adv Exp Med Biol. **872**: 127–44.

De Jonge H, de Loor H, Verbeke K, et al. (2012). In vivo CYP3A4 activity, CYP3A5 genotype, and hematocrit predict tacrolimus dose requirements and clearance in renal transplant patients. Clin Pharmacol Ther. **92**: 366–75.

De Jonge H, Metalidis C, Naesens M, et al. (2011). The P450 oxidoreductase *28 SNP is associated with low initial tacrolimus exposure and increased dose requirements in CYP3A5-expressing renal recipients. Pharmacogenomics. **12**: 1281–91.

de Miranda Silva C, Fernandes BJ, Donadi EA, et al. (2009). Influence of glomerular filtration rate on the pharmacokinetics of cyclophosphamide enantiomers in patients with lupus nephritis. J Clin Pharmacol. **49**: 965–72.

Dewit O, Moreels T, Baert F, et al. (2011). Limitations of extensive TPMT genotyping in the management of azathioprine-induced myelosuppression in IBD patients. Clin Biochem. **44**: 1062–6.

Dogan E, Ghanta M, Tanriover B. (2011). Collapsing glomerulopathy in a renal transplant recipient: Potential molecular mechanisms. Ann Transplant. **16**: 113–16.

Dores RM, Londraville RL, Prokop J, et al. (2014). Molecular evolution of GPCRs: Melanocortin/melanocortin receptors. J Mol Endocrinol. **52**: T29–T42.

Diekmann F, Rovira J, Diaz-Ricart M, et al. (2012). mTOR inhibition and erythropoiesis: Microcytosis or anaemia? Nephrol Dial Transplant. **27**: 537–41.

Ding H, Wang T, Xu D, et al. (2015). Dexamethasone-induced apoptosis of osteocytic and osteoblastic cells is mediated by TAK1 activation. Biochem Biophys Res Commun. **460**: 157–63.

Dun B, Sharma A, Teng Y, et al. (2013). Mycophenolic acid inhibits migration and invasion of gastric cancer cells via multiple molecular pathways. PLoS One. **8**: e81702.

Durst JK, Rampersad RM. (2015). Pregnancy in women with solid-organ transplants: A review. Obstet Gynecol Surv. **70**: 408–18.

Elens L, Hesselink DA, Bouamar R, et al. (2014). Impact of POR*28 on the pharmacokinetics of tacrolimus and cyclosporine A in renal transplant patients. Ther Drug Monit. **36**: 71–9.

Elvin J, Buvall L, Lindskog Jonsson A, et al. (2016). Melanocortin 1 receptor agonist protects podocytes through catalase and RhoA activation. Am J Physiol Renal Physiol. **310**: F846–56.

Ericson JE, Zimmerman KO, Gonzalez D, et al. (2017). A systematic literature review approach to estimate the therapeutic index of selected immunosuppressant drugs after renal transplantation. Ther Drug Monit. **39**: 13–20.

Esposito P, Domenech MV, Serpieri N, et al. (2017). Severe cyclophosphamide-related hyponatremia in a patient with acute glomerulonephritis. World J Nephrol. **6**: 217–20.

Fabrizi F, Cresseri D, Fogazzi GB, et al. (2015). Rituximab therapy for primary glomerulonephritis: Report on two cases. World J Clin Cases. **3**: 736–42.

Fähling M, Mathia S, Scheidl J, et al. (2017). Cyclosporin a induces renal episodic hypoxia. Acta Physiol (Oxf). **219**: 625–39.

Fan H, Kao W, Yang YH, et al. (2014). Macrophage migration inhibitory factor inhibits the antiinflammatory effects of glucocorticoids via glucocorticoid-induced leucine zipper. Arthritis Rheumatol. **66**: 2059–70.

Faul C, Donnelly M, Merscher-Gomez S, et al. (2008). The actin cytoskeleton of kidney podocytes is a direct target of the antiproteinuric effect of cyclosporine. Nat Med. **14**: 931–8.

Faurschou M, Sorensen IJ, Mellemkjaer L, et al. (2008). Malignancies in Wegener's granulomatosis: Incidence and relation to cyclophosphamide therapy in a cohort of 293 patients. J Rheumatol. **35**: 100–5.

Felli V, Di Sibio A, Anselmi M, et al. (2014). Progressive multifocal leukoencephalopathy following treatment with rituximab in an HIV-negative patient with non-Hodgkin lymphoma: A case report and literature review. Neuroradiol J. **27**: 657–64.

Fellström BC, Barratt J, Cook H, et al. (2017). Targeted-release versus placebo in patients with IgA nephropathy (NEFIGAN): A double-blind, randomised, placebo-controlled phase 2b trial. Lancet. **389**: 2117–27.

Filaretova L. (2011). Glucocorticoids are gastroprotective under physiologic conditions. Ther Adv Chronic Dis. **2**: 333–42.

Floyd A, Pedersen L, Nielsen GL, et al. (2003). Risk of acute pancreatitis in users of azathioprine: A population-based case-control study. Am J Gastroenterol. **98**: 1305–8.

Fornoni A, Sageshima J, Wei C, et al. (2011). Rituximab targets podocytes in recurrent focal segmental glomerulosclerosis. Sci Transl Med. **3**(85): 85ra46.

Franz S, Regeniter A, Hopfer H, et al. (2010). Tubular toxicity in sirolimus- and cyclosporine-based transplant immunosuppression strategies: An ancillary study from a randomized controlled trial. Am J Kidney Dis. **55**: 33–43.

Frenkel B, White W, Tuckermann J. (2015). Glucocorticoid-induced osteoporosis. Adv Exp Med Biol. **872**: 179–215.

Fuhrmann A, Lopes P, Sereno J, et al. (2014). Molecular mechanisms underlying the effects of cyclosporin A and sirolimus on glucose and lipid metabolism in liver, skeletal muscle and adipose tissue in an in vivo rat model. Biochem Pharmacol. **88**: 216–28.

Fujinaga S, Ozawa K, Sakuraya K, et al. (2016). Late-onset adverse events after a single dose of rituximab in children with complicated steroid-dependent nephrotic syndrome. Clin Nephrol. **85**: 340–5.

Fujinaga S, Sakuraya K. (2018). Single infusion of low-dose ofatumumab in a child with complicated nephrotic syndrome with anti-rituximab antibodies. Pediatr Nephrol. **33**: 527–8.

Fuke T, Abe Y, Hibino S, et al. (2012). Mizoribine requires individual dosing due to variation of bioavailability Pediatr Int. **54**: 885–91.

Ganta S, Sharma P, Paxton JW, et al. (2010). Pharmacokinetics and pharmacodynamics of chlorambucil delivered in long-circulating nanoemulsion. J Drug Target. **18**: 125–33.

Garin EH, Reiser J, Cara-Fuentes G, et al. (2015). Case series: CTLA4-IgG1 therapy in minimal change disease and focal segmental glomerulosclerosis. Pediatr Nephrol. **30**: 469–77.

Ghobadi E, Moloudizargari M, Asghari MH, et al. (2017). The mechanisms of cyclophosphamide-induced testicular toxicity and the protective agents. Expert Opin Drug Metab Toxicol. **13**: 525–36.

Gilardin L, Bayry J, Kaveri SV. (2015). Intravenous immunoglobulin as clinical immune-modulating therapy. CMAJ. **187**: 257–64.

Gong R. (2014). Leveraging melanocortin pathways to treat glomerular diseases. Adv Chronic Kidney Dis. **21**: 134–51.

Goodwin JE, Zhang J, Gonzalez D, et al. (2011). Knockout of the vascular endothelial glucocorticoid receptor abrogates dexamethasone-induced hypertension. J Hypertens. **29**: 1347–56.

Gotestam Skorpen C, Hoeltzenbein M, Tincani A. (2016). The EULAR points to consider for use of antirheumatic drugs before pregnancy, and during pregnancy and lactation. Ann Rheum Dis. **75**: 795–810.

Granner DK, Wang JC, Yamamoto KR. (2015). Regulatory actions of glucocorticoid hormones: From organisms to mechanisms. Adv Exp Med Biol. **872**: 3–31.

Grześk E, Malinowski B, Wiciński M, et al. (2016). Cyclosporine-A, but not tacrolimus significantly increases reactivity of vascular smooth muscle cells. Pharmacol Rep. **68**: 201–5.

Gruppen MP, Bouts AH, Jansen-Van der Weide MC, et al. (2018). A randomized clinical trial indicates that levamisole increases the time to relapse in children with ssteroid-sensitive idiopathic nephrotic syndrome. Kidney Int. **93**: 510–18.

Guess A, Agrawal S, Wei CC, et al. (2010). Dose- and time-dependent glucocorticoid receptor signaling in podocytes. Am J Physiol Renal Physiol. **299**: F845–53.

Guglielmi V, Nowis D, Tinelli M, et al. (2017). Bortezomib-induced muscle toxicity in multiple myeloma. J Neuropathol Exp Neurol. **76**: 620–30.

Habib A, Karmali V, Polavarapu R, et al. (2013). Sirolimus-FKBP12.6 impairs endothelial barrier function through protein kinase C-α activation and disruption of the p120-vascular endothelial cadherin interaction. Arterioscler Thromb Vasc Biol. **33**: 2425–31.

Hacihamdioğlu DÖ, Gökhan A, Cihan M, et al. (2014). Cyclosporin A-induced posterior reversible encephalopathy syndrome in an adolescent with steroid-resistant nephrotic syndrome. Int Urol Nephrol. **46**: 2055–6.

Hadjinicolaou AV, Nisar MK, Parfrey H, et al. (2012). Non-infectious pulmonary toxicity of rituximab: A systematic review. Rheumatology (Oxford). **51**: 653–62.

Hallstensen RF, Bergseth G. Foss S, et al. (2015). Eculizumab treatment during pregnancy does not affect the complement system activity of the newborn. Immunobiology. **220**: 452–9.

Haneda M, Owaki M, Kuzuya T, et al. (2014). Comparative analysis of drug action on B-cell proliferation and differentiation for mycophenolic acid, everolimus, and prednisolone. Transplantation. **97**: 405–12.

Hant FN, Bolster MB. (2016). Drugs that may harm bone: Mitigating the risk. Cleve Clin J Med. **83**: 281–8.

Hartono C, Chung M, Kuo SF, et al. (2014). Bortezomib therapy for nephrotic syndrome due to idiopathic membranous nephropathy. J Nephrol. **27**: 103–6.

Hasky N, Uri-Belapolsky S, Goldberg K, et al. (2015). Gonadotrophin-releasing hormone agonists for fertility preservation: Unraveling the enigma? Hum Reprod. **30**: 1089–101.

Hegazy SK, Adam AG, Hamdy NA, et al. (2015). Effect of active infection on cytochrome P450-mediated metabolism of cyclosporine in renal transplant patients. Transpl Infect Dis. **17**: 350–60.

Hemminki K, Liu X, Ji J, et al. (2016).Origin of B-cell neoplasms in autoimmune disease. PLoS One. **11**: e0158360.

Ho ET, Wong G, Craig JC, et al. (2013). Once-daily extended-release versus twice-daily standard-release tacrolimus in kidney transplant recipients: A systematic review. Transplantation. **9**: 1120–8.

Hughes FM Jr, Corn AG, Nimmich AR, et al. (2013). Cyclophosphamide induces an early wave of acrolein-independent apoptosis in the urothelium. Adv Biosci Biotechnol. **4**. DOI: 10.4236/abb.2013.48A2002

Iqbal J, Ali Z, Khan AU, et al. (2014). Pregnancy outcomes in patients with chronic myeloid leukemia treated with imatinib mesylate: Short report from a developing country. Leuk Lymphoma. **55**: 2109–13.

Ito N, Nishibori Y, Ito Y, et al. (2011). mTORC1 activation triggers the unfolded protein response in podocytes and leads to nephrotic syndrome. Lab Invest. **91**: 1584–95.

Ito A, Okada Y, Hashita T, et al. (2017). Sex differences in the blood concentration of tacrolimus in systemic lupus erythematosus and rheumatoid arthritis patients with CYP3A5*3/*3. Biochem Genet. **55**: 268–77.

Ivy JR, Oosthuyzen W, Peltz TS, et al. (2016). Glucocorticoids induce nondipping blood pressure by activating the thiazide-sensitive cotransporter. Hypertension. **67**: 1029–37.

Iyoda M, Hudkins KL, Becker-Herman S, et al. (2009). Imatinib suppresses cryoglobulinemia and secondary membranoproliferative glomerulonephritis. J Am Soc Nephrol. **20**: 68–77.

Iyoda M, Shibata T, Wada Y, et al. (2013). Long- and short-term treatment with imatinib attenuates the development of chronic kidney disease in experimental anti-glomerular basement membrane nephritis. Nephrol Dial Transplant. **28**: 576–84.

Jiang L, Dasgupta I, Hurcombe JA, et al. (2015). Levamisole in steroid-sensitive nephrotic syndrome: usefulness in adult patients and laboratory insights into mechanisms of action via direct action on the kidney podocyte. Clin Sci (Lond). **128**: 883–93.

Jin J, Hu K, Ye M, et al. (2018). Rapamycin reduces podocyte apoptosis and is involved in autophagy and mTOR/ P70S6K/4EBP1 signaling. Cell Physiol Biochem. **48**: 765–72.

Jodele S, Fukuda T, Mizuno K, et al. (2016). Variable eculizumab clearance requires pharmacodynamic monitoring to optimize therapy for thrombotic microangiopathy after hematopoietic stem cell transplantation. Biol Blood Marrow Transplant. **22**: 307–15.

Jouve T, Rostaing L, Malvezzi P. (2017). New formulations of tacrolimus and prevention of acute and chronic rejections in adult kidney-transplant recipients. Expert Opin Drug Saf. **16**: 845–55.

Joy MS, La M, Wang J, et al. (2012). Cyclophosphamide and 4-hydroxycyclophosphamide pharmacokinetics in patients with glomerulonephritis secondary to lupus and small vessel vasculitis. Br J Clin Pharmacol. **74**: 445–55.

Kadikoy H, Paolini M, Achkar K, et al. (2010). Pulmonary alveolar proteinosis in a kidney transplant: A rare complication of sirolimus. Nephrol Dial Transplant. **25**: 2795–8.

Kadmiel M, Cidlowski JA. (2013). Glucocorticoid receptor signaling in health and disease. Trends Pharmacol Sci. **34**: 518–30.

Kamei K, Takahashi M, Fuyama M, et al. (2015). Rituximab-associated agranulocytosis in children with refractory idiopathic nephrotic syndrome: Case series and review of literature. Nephrol Dial Transplant. **30**: 91–6.

Kanakry CG, Ganguly S, Luznik L. (2015). Situational aldehyde dehydrogenase expression by regulatory T-cells may explain the contextual duality of cyclophosphamide as both a pro-inflammatory and tolerogenic agent. Oncoimmunology. **20**: e974393.

Kapturczak MH, Meier-Kriesche HU, Kaplan B. (2004). Calcineurin inhibitor antagonists. Transplant Proc. **36**(2 Suppl): 25S–32S.

Kawasaki Y. (2009). Mizoribine: A new approach in the treatment of renal diseases. Clin Dev Immunol. 2009: 681482.

Kenkre VP, Hong F, Cerhan JR, et al. (2016). Fcγ Receptor 3A and 2A Polymorphisms do not predict response to rituximab in follicular lymphoma. Clin Cancer Res. **22**: 821–6.

Kern G, Mair SM, Noppert SJ. (2014). Tacrolimus increases Nox4 expression in human renal fibroblasts and induces fibrosis-related genes by aberrant TGF-beta receptor signalling. PloS One. **9**: e96377.

Khanna A, Plummer M, Bromberek C, et al. (2002). Expression of TGF-beta and fibrogenic genes in transplant recipients with tacrolimus and cyclosporine nephrotoxicity. Kidney Int. **62**: 2257–63.

Kim JS, Aviles DH, Silverstein DM, et al. (2005). Effect of age, ethnicity, and glucocorticoid use on tacrolimus pharmacokinetics in pediatric renal transplant patients. Pediatr Transplant. **9**: 162–9.

Kim HJ, Cha JY, Seok JW, et al. (2016). Dexras1 links glucocorticoids to insulin-like growth factor-1 signaling in adipogenesis. Sci Rep. **27**: 28648.

Kim S, Choi HJ, Jo CH, et al. (2015). Cyclophosphamide-induced vasopressin-independent activation of aquaporin-2 in the rat kidney. Am J Physiol Renal Physiol. **309**: F474–83.

Kirschke E, Goswami D, Southworth D, et al. (2014). Glucocorticoid receptor function regulated by coordinated action of the Hsp90 and Hsp70 chaperone cycles. Cell. **157**: 1685–97.

Knoll GA, Fergusson D, Chassé M, et al. (2016). Ramipril versus placebo in kidney transplant patients with proteinuria: A multicentre, double-blind, randomised controlled trial. Lancet Diabetes Endocrinol. **4**: 318–26.

Konar M, Granoff DM. (2017). Eculizumab treatment and impaired opsonophagocytic killing of meningococci by whole blood from immunized adults. Blood. **130**: 891–9.

Kreeftmeijer-Vegter AR, Dorlo TP, Gruppen MP, et al. (2015). Population pharmacokinetics of levamisole in children with steroid-sensitive nephrotic syndrome. Br J Clin Pharmacol. **80**: 242–52.

Kuppe C, van Roeyen C, Leuchtle K, et al. (2017). Investigations of glucocorticoid action in GN. J Am Soc Nephrol. **28**: 1408–20.

Latta K, von Schnakenburg C, Ehrich JH. (2001). A meta-analysis of cytotoxic treatment for frequently relapsing nephrotic syndrome in children. Ped Nephrol. **16**: 271–82.

Laurenti L, Innocenti I, Autore F, et al. (2016). New developments in the management of chronic lymphocytic leukemia: Role of ofatumumab. Onco Targets Ther. **9**: 421–9.

Lee SM, Yang S, Cha RH, et al. (2014). Circulating TNF receptors are significant prognostic biomarkers for idiopathic membranous nephropathy. PLoS One. **9**: e104354.

Lennard L. (2014). Implementation of TPMT testing. Br J Clin Pharmacol. **77**: 704–14.

Lepretre S, Dartigeas C, Feugier P, et al. (2015). Systematic review of the recent evidence for the efficacy and safety of chlorambucil in the treatment of B-cell malignancies. Leuk Lymphoma. **8**: 1–14.

Le Quintrec M, Lapeyraque AM, Lionet A. (2018). Patterns of clinical response to eculizumab in patient with C3 glomerulopathy. Am J Kidney Dis. **72**: 84–92.

Lewko B, Waszkiewicz A, Maryn A, et al. (2015). Dexamethasone-dependent modulation of cyclic GMP synthesis in podocytes. Mol Cell Biochem. **409**: 243–53.

Li Z, Sun F, Zhang Y, et al. (2015). Tacrolimus induces insulin resistance and increases the glucose absorption in the jejunum: A potential mechanism of the diabetogenic effects. PLoS One. **10**: e0143405.

Lindskog A, Ebefors K, Johansson ME, et al. (2010). Melanocortin 1 receptor agonists reduce proteinuria. J Am Soc Nephrol. **21**: 1290–8.

Liu Y, Xiao J, Shi X, et al. (2016). Immunosuppressive agents versus steroids in the treatment of IgA nephropathy-induced proteinuria: A meta-analysis. Exp Ther Med. **11**: 49–56.

Liu YP, Xu HQ, Li M, et al. (2015). Association between thiopurine s-methyltransferase polymorphisms and azathioprine-induced adverse drug reactions in patients with autoimmune diseases: A meta-analysis. PLoS One. **10**: e0144234.

Lorenz HM, Schmitt WH, Tesar V, et al. (2011). Treatment of active lupus nephritis with the novel immunosuppressant 15-deoxyspergualin: An open-label dose escalation study. Arthritis Res Ther. **13**: R36.

Lunde I, Bremer S, Midtvedt K, et al. (2014). The influence of CYP3A, PPARA, and POR genetic variants on the pharmacokinetics of tacrolimus and cyclosporine in renal transplant recipients. Eur J Clin Pharmacol. **70**: 685–93.

Łuszczyńska P, Pawiński T. (2015). Therapeutic drug monitoring of mycophenolic acid in lupus nephritis: A review of current literature. Ther Drug Monit. **37**: 711–17.

Madan A, Mijovic-Das S, Stankovic A, et al. (2016). Acthar gel in the treatment of nephrotic syndrome: A multicenter retrospective case series. BMC Nephrol. **17**: 37.

Madeira JB, Masuda CA, Maya-Monteiro CM, et al. (2015). TORC1 inhibition induces lipid droplet replenishment in yeast. Mol Cell Biol. **35**: 737–46.

Maes B, Oellerich M, Ceuppens JL, et al. (2002). A new acute inflammatory syndrome related to the introduction of mycophenolate mofetil in patients with Wegener's granulomatosis. Nephrol Dial Transplant. **17**: 923–6.

Mallipattu, SK, Guo Y, Revelo MP, et al. (2017). Krüppel–like factor 15 mediates glucocorticoid-induced restoration of podocyte differentiation markers J Am Soc Nephrol. **28**: 166–84.

Maloney DG, Smith B, Rose A. (2002). Rituximab: Mechanism of action and resistance. Sem Oncol. **29**(Suppl 2): 2–9.

Mandelbrot DA, Alberú J, Barama A, et al. (2015). Effect of ramipril on urinary protein excretion in maintenance renal transplant patients converted to sirolimus. Am J Transplant. **15**: 3174–84.

Manger B, Hiepe F, Schneider M, et al. (2015). Impact of switching from mycophenolate mofetil to enteric-coated mycophenolate sodium on gastrointestinal side effects in patients with autoimmune disease: A Phase III, open-label, single-arm, multicenter study. Clin Exp Gastroenterol. **8**: 205–13.

Mathian A, Jouenne R, Chader D, et al. (2015). Regulatory T-cell responses to high-dose methylprednisolone in active systemic lupus erythematosus. PLoS One. **10**: e0143689.

Matsui M, Okuma Y, Yamanaka J, et al. (2015). Kawasaki disease refractory to standard treatments that responds to a combination of pulsed methylprednisolone and plasma exchange: Cytokine profiling and literature review. Cytokine. **74**: 339–42.

Matsui K, Shibagaki Y, Sasaki H, et al. (2010). Mycophenolate mofetil-induced agranulocytosis in a renal transplant recipient. Clin Exp Nephrol. **14**: 637–40.

Meistrich ML. (2009). Male gonadal toxicity. Pediatr Blood Cancer. **53**: 261–6.

Mehrpooya M, Vaseghi G, Eshraghi A, et al. (2015). Delayed myocardial infarction associated with rituximab infusion: A case report and literature review. Am J Ther. **23**: 283–7.

Midtvedt K, Bergan S, Reisæter AV, et al. (2017). Exposure to mycophenolate and fatherhood. Transplantation. **101**: e214–17.

Min L, Wang Q, Cao L, et al. (2017). Comparison of combined leflunomide and low-dose corticosteroid therapy with full-dose corticosteroid monotherapy for progressive IgA nephropathy. Oncotarget. **8**: 48375–84.

Minguillón J, Morancho B, Kim SJ, et al. (2005). Concentrations of cyclosporin A and FK506 that inhibit IL-2 induction in human T-cells do not affect TGF-beta1 biosynthesis, whereas higher doses of cyclosporin A trigger apoptosis and release of preformed TGF-beta1. J Leukoc Biol. **77**: 748–58.

Mitre-Aguilar IB, Cabrera-Quintero AJ, Zentella-Dehes A. (2015). Genomic and non-genomic effects of glucocorticoids: Implications for breast cancer. Int J Clin Exp Pathol. **8**: 1–10.

Morton NM. (2010). Obesity and corticosteroids: 11β-Hydroxysteroid type 1 as a cause and therapeutic target in metabolic disease. Mol Cell Endocrinol. **316**: 154–64.

Musumba CO. (2013). Review article: The association between nodular regenerative hyperplasia, inflammatory bowel disease and thiopurine therapy. Aliment Pharmacol Ther. **38**: 1025–37.

Nahar J, Ramamoorthy S, Cidlowski JA. (2016). Corticosteroids: Mechanisms of action in health and disease. Rheum Dis Clin North Am. **42**: 15–31.

Naesens M, Kuypers DR, Sarwal M. (2009). Calcineurin inhibitor nephrotoxicity. Clin J Am Soc Nephrol. **4**: 481–508.

Newton R, Leigh R, Giembycz MA. (2010). Pharmacological strategies for improving the efficacy and therapeutic ratio of glucocorticoids in inflammatory lung diseases. Pharmacol Ther. **125**: 286–327.

Nishikawa T Miyahara E, Kurauchi K, et al. (2015). Mechanisms of fatal cardiotoxicity following high-dose cyclophosphamide therapy and a method for its prevention. PLoS One. **10**: e0131394.

Nixon A, Ogden L, Woywodt A, et al. (2017). Infectious complications of rituximab therapy in renal disease Clin Kidney J. **10**: 455–60.

Ochoa R, Bejarano PA, Glück S, et al. (2012). Pneumonitis and pulmonary fibrosis in a patient receiving adjuvant docetaxel and cyclophosphamide for stage 3 breast cancer: A case report and literature review. J Med Case Rep. **6**: 413.

Oh YJ, An JN, Kim CT. (2015). Circulating tumor necrosis factor α receptors predict the outcomes of human IgA nephropathy: A prospective cohort study. PLoS One. **10**: e0132826.

Ohashi T, Uchida K, Uchida S, et al. (2011). Dexamethasone increases the phosphorylation of nephrin in cultured podocytes. Clin Exp. Nephrol. **15**: 688–93.

Øzbay LA, Smidt K, Mortensen DM, et al. (2011). Cyclosporin and tacrolimus impair insulin secretion and transcriptional regulation in INS-1E beta-cells. Br J Pharmacol. **162**: 136–46.

Patel R, Williams-Dautovich J, Cummins CL. (2014). Minireview: New molecular mediators of glucocorticoid receptor activity in metabolic tissues. Mol Endocrinol. **28**: 999–1011.

Peckett AJ, Wright DC, Riddell MC. (2011). The effects of glucocorticoids on adipose tissue lipid metabolism. Metabolism. **60**: 1500–10.

Pedigo CE, Ducasa GM, Leclercq F, et al. (2016). Local TNF causes NFATc1-dependent cholesterol-mediated podocyte injury. J Clin Invest. **126**: 3336–50.

Penfornis A, Kury-Paulin S. (2006). Immunosuppressive drug-induced diabetes. Diabetes Metab. **32**: 539–46.

Peppa M, Krania M, Raptis SA. (2011). Hypertension and other morbidities with Cushing's syndrome associated with corticosteroids: A review. Integr Blood Press Control. **4**: 7–16.

Pereira RM, Freire de Carvalho J. (2011). Glucocorticoid-induced myopathy. Joint Bone Spine. **78**: 41–4.

Piccoli GB, Cabiddu G, Attini R. (2017). Outcomes of pregnancies after kidney transplantation: Lessons learned from CKD. A comparison of transplanted, nontransplanted chronic kidney disease patients and low-risk pregnancies: A multicenter nationwide analysis. Transplantation. **101**: 2536–44.

Piga M, Chessa E, Ibba V, et al. (2014). Biologics-induced autoimmune renal disorders in chronic inflammatory rheumatic diseases: Systematic literature review and analysis of a monocentric cohort. Autoimmun Rev. **13**: 873–9.

Podestà MA, Cucchiari D, Ponticelli C. (2015). The diverging roles of dendritic cells in kidney allotransplantation. Transplant Rev (Orlando). **29**: 114–20.

Ponticelli C. (2014). The pros and the cons of mTOR inhibitors in kidney transplantation. Expert Rev Clin Immunol. **10**: 295–305.

Ponticelli C, Altieri P, Scolari F, et al. (1998). A randomized study comparing methylprednisolone plus chlorambucil versus methylprednisolone plus cyclophosphamide in idiopathic membranous nephropathy. J Am Soc Nephrol. **9**: 440–50.

Ponticelli C, Campise R. (2005). Neurological complications in kidney transplant recipients. J Nephrol. **18**: 521–8.

Ponticelli C, Locatelli F. (2018). Glucocorticoids in the treatment of glomerular diseases: Pittfals and pearls. Clin J Am Soc Nephrol. **13**: 815–22.

Ponticelli C, Moroni G. (2015). Immunosuppression in pregnant women with systemic lupus erythematosus. Expert Rev Clin Immunol. **11**: 549–52.

Ponticelli C, Passerini P, Salvadori M, et al. (2006). A randomized pilot trial comparing methylprednisolone plus a cytotoxic agent versus synthetic adrenocorticotropic hormone in idiopathic membranous nephropathy. Am J Kidney Dis. **47**: 233–40.

Prasad B, Giebel S, Carron M, et al. (2018). Use of synthetic hormone ACTH in patients with IgA nephropathy. BMC Nephrol. **19**: 118.

Quattrocelli M, Barefield DY, Warner JL, et al. (2017). Intermittent glucocorticoid steroid dosing enhances muscle repair without eliciting muscle atrophy. J Clin Invest. **127**: 2418–32.

Ramamoorthy S, Cidlowski JA. (2016). Corticosteroids: Mechanisms of action in health and disease. Rheum Dis Clin North Am. **42**: 15–31.

Ramos-Casals M, Brito-Zerón P, Muñoz S, et al. (2007). Autoimmune diseases induced by TNF-targeted therapies: Analysis of 233 cases. Medicine (Baltimore). **86**: 242–51.

Ransom RF, Lam NG, Hallett MA, et al. (2005). Glucocorticoids protect and enhance recovery of cultured murine podocytes via actin filament stabilization. Kidney Int. **68**: 2473–83.

Rao SR, Sundararajan S, Subbarayan R, et al. (2017). Cyclosporine-A induces endoplasmic reticulum stress and influences pro-apoptotic factors in human gingival fibroblasts. Mol Cell Biochem. **429**: 179–85.

Ridruejo E, Cacchione R, Villamil AG, et al. (2007). Imatinib-induced fatal acute liver failure. World J Gastroenterol. **13**: 6608–11.

Robert N, Wong GW, Wright JM. (2010). Effect of cyclosporine on blood pressure. Cochrane Database Syst Rev. 1: CD007893. DOI: 10.1002/14651858.CD007893.pub2

Roberts RL, Barclay ML. (2015). Update on thiopurine pharmacogenetics in inflammatory bowel disease. Pharmacogenomics. **16**: 891–903.

Rodriguez-Rodriguez AE, Triñanes J, Velazquez-Garcia S, et al. (2013). The higher diabetogenic risk of tacrolimus depends on pre-existing insulin resistance. A study in obese and lean Zucker rats. Am J Transplant. **13**: 1665–75.

Rostaing L, Bunnapradist S, Grinyó JM, et al. (2016). Novel once-daily extended-release tacrolimus versus twice-daily tacrolimus in *de novo* kidney transplant recipients: Two-year results of phase 3, double-blind, randomized trial. Am J Kidney Dis. **67**: 648–59.

Saffar AS, Ashdown H, Gounni AS. (2011). The molecular mechanisms of glucocorticoids-mediated neutrophil survival. Curr Drug Targets. **12**: 556–62.

Saint-Marcoux F, Guigonis V, Decramer S, et al. (2011). Development of a Bayesian estimator for the therapeutic drug monitoring of mycophenolate mofetil in children with idiopathic nephrotic syndrome. Pharmacol Res. **63**: 423–31.

Samad F, Ruf W. (2013). Inflammation, obesity, and thrombosis. Blood. **122**: 3415–22.

Sanghavi K, Brundage RC, Miller MB, et al. (2017). Genotype-guided tacrolimus dosing in African-American kidney transplant recipients. Pharmacogenomics J. **17**: 61–8.

Santoro D, Postorino A, Costantino G, et al. (2012). Anti-TNF-α therapy in membranous glomerulonephritis. Clin Kidney J. **5**: 487–8.

Savvidaki E, Papachristou E, Kazakopoulos P, et al. (2014). Gastrointestinal disorders after renal transplantation. Transplant Proc. **46**: 3183–6.

Shang W, Ning Y, Xu X, et al. (2015). Incidence of cancer in ANCA-associated vasculitis: A meta-analysis of observational studies. PLoS One. **10**: e0126016.

Shi J, Wang L, Zhang H, et al. (2015). Glucocorticoids: Dose-related effects on osteoclast formation and function via reactive oxygen species and autophagy. Bone. **79**: 222–32.

Shi YY, Hesselink DA, van Gelder T. (2015). Pharmacokinetics and pharmacodynamics of immunosuppressive drugs in elderly kidney transplant recipients. Transplant Rev (Orlando). **29**: 224–30.

Simmonds J, Grundy N, Trompeter R, et al. (2010). Long-term steroid treatment and growth: A study in steroid-dependent nephrotic syndrome. Arch Dis Child. **95**: 146–9.

Singh JA, Wells GA, Christensen R, et al. (2011). Adverse effects of biologics: A network meta-analysis and Cochrane overview. Cochrane Database Syst Rev. CD008794. DOI: 10.1002/14651858.CD008794.pub2

Siramolpiwat S, Sakonlaya D. (2017). Clinical and histologic features of Azathioprine-induced hepatotoxicity. Scand J Gastroenterol. **52**: 876–80.

Sirvent AE, Enríquez R, Andrada E, et al. (2016). Necrotising glomerulonephritis in levamisole-contaminated cocaine use. Nefrologia. **36**: 76–8.

Smerud HK, Bárány P, Lindström K, et al. (2011). New treatment for IgA nephropathy: Enteric budesonide targeted to the ileocecal region ameliorates proteinuria. Nephrol Dial Transplant. **26**: 3237–42.

Sobiak J, Resztak M, Ostalska-Nowicka D, et al. (2015). Monitoring of mycophenolate mofetil metabolites in children with nephrotic syndrome and the proposed novel target values of pharmacokinetic parameters. Eur J Pharm Sci. **77**: 189–96.

Song G, Gao H, Yuan Z. (2013). Effect of leuprolide acetate on ovarian function after cyclophosphamide-doxorubicin-based chemotherapy in premenopausal patients with breast cancer: Results from a phase II randomized trial. Med Oncol. **30**: 667.

Song T, Rao Z, Tan Q, et al. (2016). Calcineurin inhibitors associated with posterior reversible encephalopathy syndrome in solid organ transplantation: Report of 2 cases and literature review. Medicine (Baltimore). **95**: e3173.

Snanoudj R, Royal V, Elie C, et al. (2011). Specificity of histological markers of long-term CNI nephrotoxicity in kidney-transplant recipients under low-dose cyclosporine therapy. Am J Transplant. **11**: 2635–46.

Staatz CE, Goodman LK, Tett SE. (2010). Effect of CYP3A and ABCB1 single nucleotide polymorphisms on the pharmacokinetics and pharmacodynamics of calcineurin inhibitors: Part I. Clin Pharmacokinet. **49**: 141–75.

Staatz CE, Tett SE. (2014). Pharmacology and toxicology of mycophenolate in organ transplant recipients: An update. Arch Toxicol. **88**: 1351–89.

Stahl K, Duong M, Schwarz A, et al. (2017). Kinetics of rituximab excretion into urine and peritoneal fluid in two patients with nephrotic syndrome. Case Rep Nephrol. 2017: e1372859.

Stallone G, Infante B, Pontrelli P, et al. (2011). Sirolimus and proteinuria in renal transplant patients: Evidence for a dose-dependent effect on slit diaphragm-associated proteins. Transplantation. **91**: 997–1004.

Streicher C, Djabarouti S, Xuereb F, et al. (2014). Pre-dose plasma concentration monitoring of mycophenolate mofetil in patients with autoimmune diseases. Br J Clin Pharmacol. **78**: 1419–25.

Suk HY, Zhou C, Yang TT, et al. (2013). Ablation of calcineurin Aβ reveals hyperlipidemia and signaling cross-talks with phosphodiesterases. J Biol Chem. **288**: 3477–88.

Suthanthiran M, Hojo M, Maluccio M, et al. (2009). Post-transplantation malignancy: A cell autonomous mechanism with implications for therapy. Trans Am Clin Climatol Assoc. **120**: 369–88.

Tamirou F, Husson SN, Gruson D, et al. (2017). Brief report: The Euro-lupus low-dose intravenous cyclophosphamide regimen does not impact the ovarian reserve, as measured by serum levels of anti-Müllerian hormone. Arthritis Rheumatol. **69**: 1267–71.

Tang JT, Andrews LM, van Gelder T, et al. (2016). Pharmacogenetic aspects of the use of tacrolimus in renal transplantation: Recent developments and ethnic considerations. Expert Opin Drug Metab Toxicol. **12**: 555–65.

Tedla FM, Roche-Recinos A, Brar A. (2015). Intravenous immunoglobulin in kidney transplantation. Curr Opin Organ Transplant. **20**: 630–7.

Tian J, Wang Y, Zhou X, et al. (2014). Rapamycin slows IgA nephropathy progression in the rat. Am J Nephrol. **39**: 218–29.

Tanaka H, Tsuruga K, Imaizumi T. (2015). Mizoribine in the treatment of pediatric-onset glomerular disease. World J Pediatr. **11**: 108–12.

Trachtman H, Vento S, Herreshoff E. (2015). Efficacy of galactose and adalimumab in patients with resistant focal segmental glomerulosclerosis: Report of the font clinical trial group. BMC Nephrol. **16**: 111.

Tran D, Vallée M, Collette S, et al. (2014). Conversion from twice-daily to once-daily extended-release tacrolimus in renal transplant recipients: 2-year results and review of the literature. Exp Clin Transplant. **12**: 323–7.

Trimarchi H. (2015). Abatacept and glomerular diseases: The open road for the second signal as a new target is settled down. Recent Pat Endocr Metab Immune Drug Discov. **9**: 2–14.

Tsagalis G, Psimenou E, Iliadis A, et al. (2009). Rapamycin for focal segmental glomerulosclerosis: A report of 3 cases. Am J Kidney Dis. **54**: 340–4.

Vanhove T, Annaert P, Kuypers DR. (2016). Clinical determinants of calcineurin inhibitor disposition: A mechanistic review. Pharmacogenomics. **48**: 88–112.

Veal GJ, Cole M, Chinnaswamy G, et al. (2016). Cyclophosphamide pharmacokinetics and pharmacogenetics in children with B-cell non-Hodgkin's lymphoma. Eur J Cancer. **55**: 56–64.

Vivarelli M, Colucci M, Bonanni A, et al. (2017). Ofatumumab in two pediatric nephrotic syndrome patients allergic to rituximab. Pediatr Nephrol. **32**: 181–4.

Walker BR. (2007). Glucocorticoids and cardiovascular disease. Eur J Endocrinol. **157**: 545–59.

Wallace E, Fogo AB, Schulman G. (2012). Imatinib therapy for non-infection-related type II cryoglobulinemia with membranoproliferative glomerulonephritis. Am J Kidney Dis. **59**: 122–5.

Wang-Rosenke Y, Khadzhynov D, Loof T, et al. (2013). Tyrosine kinases inhibition by imatinib slows progression in chronic anti-thy1 glomerulosclerosis of the rat. BMC Nephrol. **14**: 223.

Warry E, Hansen RJ, Gustafson DL, et al. (2011). Pharmacokinetics of cyclophosphamide after oral and intravenous administration to dogs with lymphoma. J Vet Intern Med. **25**: 903–8.

Weaver JL. (2012). Establishing the carcinogenic risk of immunomodulatory drugs. Toxicol Pathol. **40**: 267–71.

Webster AC, Woodroffe RC, Taylor RS, et al. (2005). Tacrolimus versus ciclosporin as primary immunosuppression for kidney transplant recipients: Meta-analysis and meta-regression of randomised trial data. BMJ. **331**: 810.

Weiner GJ. (2010). Rituximab: Mechanism of action. Semin Hematol. **47**: 115–23.

Wetzels JF. (2004). Cyclophosphamide-induced gonadal toxicity: A treatment dilemma in patients with lupus nephritis? Neth J Med. **62**: 347–52.

Williamson PM, Ong SL, Whitworth JA, et al. (2015). The role of sustained release isosorbide mononitrate on corticosteroid-induced hypertension in healthy human subjects. Hum Hypertens. **29**: 737–43.

Wiseman AC. (2016). Immunosuppressive medications. Clin J Am Soc Nephrol. **11**: 332–43.

Wittmann S, Daniel C, Braun A, et al. (2008). The mTOR inhibitor everolimus attenuates the time course of chronic anti-Thy1 nephritis in the rat. Nephron Exp Nephrol. **108**: e45–56.

Wu J, Zheng C, Fan Y, et al. (2014). Downregulation of microRNA-30 facilitates podocyte injury and is prevented by glucocorticoids. J Am Soc Nephrol. **25**: 92–104.

Wu L, Feng Z, Cui S, et al. (2014). Rapamycin upregulates autophagy by inhibiting the mTOR-ULK1 pathway, resulting in reduced podocyte injury. PLoS One. **8**: e63799.

Wu Q, Wang X, Nevomipova E. (2018). Mechanisms of cycloporin A nephrotoxicity: Oxidative stress, autophagy, and signalins. Food Chem Toxicol. **118**: 899–907.

Yang S, Xie L, Xue W, et al. (2013). Leflunomide plus oral prednisone in treatment of idiopathic membranous nephropathy: A retrospective clinical study of efficacy and safety. Nephrology (Carlton). **18**: 615–22.

Yilmaz B. (2016). Fulminant hepatitis B as a result of reactivation in hematologic patient after rituximab therapy. J Med Virol. **88**: 1289–90.

Yilmaz N, Emmungil H, Gucenmez S, et al. (2015). Incidence of cyclophosphamide-induced urotoxicity and protective effect of mesna in rheumatic diseases. J Rheumatol. **42**: 1664–6.

Yu CC, Fornoni A, Weins A, et al. (2013). Abatacept in B7-1-positive proteinuric kidney disease. N Engl J Med. **369**: 2416–23.

Yu H, Kistler A, Farid MH, et al. (2016). Synaptopodin limits TRPC6 podocyte surface expression and attenuates proteinuria. J Am Soc Nephrol. **27**: 3308–19.

Yuan J, Benway CJ, Bagley J, et al. (2015). MicroRNA-494 promotes cyclosporine-induced nephrotoxicity and epithelial to mesenchymal transition by inhibiting PTEN. Am J Transplant. **15**: 1682 91.

Yun H, Xie F, Delzell E, et al., (2015). Comparative risk of hospitalized infection associated with biological agents among medicare rheumatoid arthritis patients. Arthritis Rheumatol. **68**: 56–66.

Yung S, Zhang Q, Chau MK, et al. (2015). Distinct effects of mycophenolate mofetil and cyclophosphamide on renal fibrosis in NZBWF1/J mice. Autoimmunity. **48**: 471–87.

Xiang Z, Cutler AJ, Brownlie RJ, et al. (2007). FcgammaRIIb controls bone marrow plasma cell persistence and apoptosis. Nat Immunol. **8**: 419–29.

Xing K, Gu B, Zhang P, et al. (2015). Dexamethasone enhances programmed cell death 1 (PD-1) expression during T cell activation: An insight into the optimum application of glucocorticoids in anti-cancer therapy. BMC Immunol. **16**: 39.

Zaenker M, Arbach O, Helmchen U, et al. (2004). Crescentic glomerulonephritis associated with myeloperoxidase-antineutrophil-cytoplasmic antibodies: First report on the efficacy of primary anti-TNF-alpha treatment. Int J Tissue React. **26**: 85–92.

Zahran AM, Aly SS, Elsayh KI, et al. (2014). Glucocorticoid receptors expression and histopathological types in children with nephrotic syndrome. Ren Fail. **36**: 1067–72.

Zaroulis CK, Chairopoulos K, Sachanas SP, et al. (2014). Assessment of bortezomib-induced peripheral neuropathy in multiple myeloma by the reduced Total Neuropathy Score. Leuk Lymphoma. **55**: 2277–83.

Zea AH, Stewart T, Ascani J, et al. (2016). Activation of the IL-2 receptor in podocytes: A potential mechanism for podocyte injury in idiopathic nephrotic syndrome? PLoS One. **11**(7): e0157907.

Zhang B, Shi W, Ma J, et al. (2012). The calcineurin–NFAT pathway allows for urokinase receptor-mediated beta3 integrin signaling to cause podocyte injury. J Mol Med. **90**: 1407–20.

Zhang J, Pippin JW, Krofft RD, et al. (2013). Podocyte repopulation by renal progenitor cells following glucocorticoids treatment in experimental FSGS. Am J Physiol Renal Physiol. **304**: F1375–89.

Zhong W, Oguljahan B, Xiao Y. (2014). Serum and glucocorticoid-regulated kinase 1 promotes vascular smooth muscle cell proliferation via regulation of β-catenin dynamics. Cell Signal. **26**: 2765–72.

Zhou AY, Ryeom S. (2014). Cyclosporin A promotes tumor angiogenesis in a calcineurin-independent manner by increasing mitochondrial reactive oxygen species. Mol Cancer Res. **12**: 1663–76.

Chapter 4

Minimal change disease

Claudio Ponticelli, Richard J Glassock,
and Rosanna Coppo

Introduction and overview

Definition

Minimal change disease (MCD) is chiefly characterized clinically by episodes of nephrotic syndrome (NS)—presenting with massive proteinuria, hypoalbuminaemia, hyperlipidaemia, and generalized oedema. Morphologically, it is characterized by no or only minimal glomerular abnormalities in a renal biopsy examined by light microscopy and immunofluorescence, while there is diffuse effacement of the podocyte foot process by electron microscopy. MCD is the most common cause of NS in children, but it may also develop at any age, including in the elderly.

Pathology

Glomerular size and architecture are almost normal on light microscopy (see Plate 1). Mild changes, including a slight increase in mesangial matrix and mesangial hypercellularity, may be seen. The glomerular basement membranes (GBMs) are thin and delicate and glomerulosclerosis is absent, except that which is predicted by age of the subject. No immunoglobulin or complement deposits can be seen at immunofluorescence. However, a few patients may show scanty or more well-developed IgM mesangial deposits. The only abnormality regularly seen in the kidney is at the ultrastructural level. It consists of a diffuse effacement of the foot processes of the podocytes. However, this finding is not pathognomonic for only MCD as it can also be seen in other glomerular diseases with NS, including the unaffected (by light microscopy) glomeruli in the lesion of focal and segmental glomerulosclerosis (FSGS).

A differential diagnosis between MCD and early stages of FSGS can be difficult. The lesion of FSGS is, by definition, characterized by focal and segmental sclerosing glomerular lesions detectable by light microscopy. However, in the early stages, lesions of FSGS can be seen only in a few juxtamedullary glomeruli in the core of the biopsy and not in more superficial renal tissue samples. Since FSGS shows effacement of foot processes of epithelial cells foot processes on electron microscopy even in glomeruli apparently unaffected by the sclerosing lesions by light microscopy, and mesangial IgM or complement deposition (usually focal and segmental in distribution) at immunofluorescence, some biopsies initially classified as MCD may, in fact, have been FSGS from the start (see Plate 2), due to sampling error. However, some ultrastructural features may allow us to distinguish between MCD and FSGS even before scarring of glomeruli appears. Larger (hypertrophic) glomeruli have been detected in FSGS in comparison to MCD, and low birth weight has been included among the responsible mechanisms (Hodgin et al., 2009; Ikezumi et al., 2013). In MCD, podocyte injury is limited to foot process effacement and podocyte number remains normal, while in FSGS, foot process width and subendothelial widening are increased and podocyte injury may cause podocyte detachment and apoptosis, thereby initiating an injury cascade that results in the segmental scar characteristic of FSGS (Barisoni, 2012).

However, the 'evolution' of MCD to a lesion of FSGS has been observed on serial renal biopsies in individual patients. This has led some investigators to consider MCD and FSGS as two different phenotypic expressions of a unique and related entity in which common pathophysiological mechanisms operate with different intensity. On the other hand, whether this represents a true 'transformation' from one 'disease' to another cannot be confirmed due to the limitations of a purely morphological approach. The current trend considers MCD and FSGS as distinct and separate entities, largely on the basis of clinical behaviour, including responsiveness to therapy (discussed later in the chapter). To date no consistently reliable serum or urine biomarker has been shown to unequivocally separate MCD and FSGS into unique entities.

Pathogenesis

Today MCD is considered to be a podocytopathy, meaning that it results from anatomical or functional abnormalities of podocytes that lead to an abnormal permeability of the glomerular barrier. The podocyte is a highly specialized and terminally differentiated visceral epithelial cell that forms the outermost layer of the glomerular capillary loop. The molecular components of the podocyte and slit diaphragm play a critical role in the maintenance of the functional integrity of the glomerular filtration barrier. Interdigitating podocytes from neighbouring cells produce the elaborate slit diaphragm that is composed of nephrin and other specialized proteins. Podocin helps regulate trafficking of nephrin to the slit diaphragm. Proteins α-actinin-4 and INF2 play important roles in the maintenance of the actin cytoskeleton, whereas integrins help anchor the podocytes to the GBM (Pollak et al., 2014). The structural integrity of podocyte foot processes and slit diaphragms, as well as the GBM charge guarantee that molecules greater than 42 A° or 200 kDa are not filtered in the pre-urine. In this event, podocytes play the major role, even though a disruption of filtered protein retrieval by tubular cells seems to be also relevant in allowing a minimal physiological urinary protein loss (Russo et al., 2013).

The pathophysiology of MCD is still poorly elucidated. Years ago, Shalhoub (1974) postulated that MCD could be caused by the episodic production of an abnormal clone of T-cells releasing a circulating chemical mediator toxic to GBM or podocytes. This hypothesis was supported by some clinical observations, including:

i. the lack of evidence of humoral antibody response;

ii. the occurrence of MCD with Hodgkin lymphomas and malignant thymoma, in which there is a disorder of T-cell immunity;

iii. the spontaneous remission of NS in children affected by measles, a viral disease associated with suppression of T-cell response: and

iv. the association of MCD with atopic allergy, in which disorder Th2 cells are upregulated.

Several humoral factors have been supposed to cause podocyte injury and to alter the glomerular permeability in patients with MCD, including vascular endothelial growth factors and hemopexin. However, in spite of intensive research the existence and the identity of the putative factor(s) has remained elusive.

Recent attention has been focused on cardiotrophin-like cytokine factor-1 (CLCF-1), a member of IL-6 family that exerts multiple functions. In vitro and in vivo studies in rats showed that CLCF-1 increases phosphorylation of STAT3 in multiple cell types, activates podocytes leading to formation of lamellipodia and decrease in basal stress fibres, and increases glomerular permeability to albumin, leading to albuminuria (Savin et al., 2015).

Another mediator of MCD could be the costimulatory protein B7, also called CD80, which is expressed on the surface of antigen-presenting-cells, mainly mature dendritic cells, B cells, and macrophages. Normally, podocytes do not express this protein. However, B7.1 may be expressed on podocytes of patients with MCD, suggesting that its upregulation may contribute to the pathogenesis of proteinuria by disrupting the glomerular filter (Reiser et al., 2004). According to Shimada and colleagues (2011), the initial hit of MCD would be the overexpression of B7.1(CD80) on the podocyte. This would result in an alteration in shape with actin rearrangement that alters glomerular permeability and causes proteinuria. The increased CD80 expression may result from either direct binding of the podocyte by cytokines from activated Th1–Th17 cells or by activation of podocyte toll-like receptors by viral products or allergens. In normal circumstances, CD80 is only transiently expressed and proteinuria is minimal due to rapid autoregulatory response by circulating T regulatory cells or by the podocyte itself, probably due to the expression of factors, such as CTLA-4, IL-10, and TGF-β that downregulate the podocyte CD80 response. In MCD, however, there is a defect in CD80 podocyte autoregulation. This results in persistent CD80 expression and persistent proteinuria. To confirm this hypothesis, podocytes contain several costimulatory molecules necessary for activating the adaptive immunity and urinary CD80 can be significantly increased in MCD patients in relapse compared with those in remission (Ishimoto et al., 2013; Cara Fuentes et al., 2014).

Other factors may concur to increase the permeability of the glomerular barrier in MCD. A critical role might be played by a hyposialylated form of angiopoietin-like protein 4 (ANGPTL4). This glycoprotein is a potent inhibitor of serum triglyceride (TG) clearance, causing elevation of serum TG levels via inhibition of the enzyme lipoprotein lipase. ANGPTL4 may be sialylated or hyposialylated (without sialic acid residues). An upregulation of hyposialylated form of ANGPTL4 secreted by podocytes can induce in rats nephrotic-range and selective proteinuria, loss of GBM charge and foot process effacement, i.e. the morphological and clinical manifestations of human MCD. Instead, a sialylated circulating form of ANGPTL4, mostly secreted from skeletal muscle, heart, and adipose tissue, reduces proteinuria while causing hypertriglyceridaemia (Clement et al., 2015). However, another study could not identify ANGPTL4 in glomeruli of patients with MCD. Urinary levels were elevated not only in MCD but also in case of massive proteinuria due to other glomerular diseases. This data would suggest that elevated urinary ANGPTL4 levels are not specific of MCD but reflect the degree of proteinuria (Cara-Fuentes et al., 2017). Angiotensin II and Kruppel-like factors (KLFs) may also play a role. In cultured human podocytes, angiotensin II reduced the expression of KLF4 on podocytes and caused decreased nephrin expression. These effects were inhibited by angiotensin receptor blockers (Hayashi et al., 2015).

In summary, it is evident that in MCD the NS is consequent to dysfunction of the podocytes. However, the pathogenetic mechanisms leading to the development of MCD remain speculative. It is possible that MCD represents the phenotypic expression of different mechanisms that may operate synergistically or contribute separately to increase the permeability of the glomerular barrier to albumin (Figure 4.1).

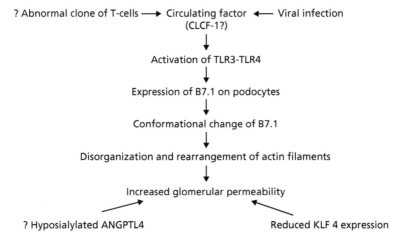

Figure 4.1 A unifying mechanistic interpretation of MCD.
A circulating factor (cardiotrophin-like cytokine factor-1?) perhaps produced by an aberrant clone of T-cells or a viral infection may stimulate the overexpression of IL-13 and the production of TLR3 or TLR4. These sentinels of the innate immunity may stimulate the production of NF-κB which, in turn, over-regulates the expression of the adhesion protein B7.1 (CD80) on podocytes. A conformational change in B7.1 would be responsible for actin cytoskeleton rearrangement, foot process effacement, and increased permeability of the glomerular barrier. Alternatively, or synergistically, a poor expression of Kruppel–like factor 4 (KLF) may reduce the production of nephrin, an essential component of slit diaphragm, so facilitating the passage of anionic proteins through the glomerular barrier. It might be also possible that a form of angiopoietin-like protein 4 (ANGPTL4) poor in sialic acid may reduce the negative charge of the GBM, although this mechanism seems to be not specific for MCD.

Aetiology

Although MCD is usually idiopathic in nature, cases occurring in association with tumours, extra-renal diseases or secondary to drugs, infection, or atopy have been reported (Glassock, 2003; see Table 4.1). MCD is frequently associated with classic Hodgkin's lymphoma. Of interest, the expression of c-MAF inducing protein, which can impair podocyte signalling and induce heavy proteinuria (Zhang et al., 2010), was found to be upregulated in lymphomatous tissues and kidney biopsy samples of patients with Hodgkin's lymphoma, suggesting a possible role in inducing both disorders (Audard et al., 2010). The association with non-Hodgkin's lymphoma is rare, preferentially occurring in cases originating from B cells (Kofman et al., 2014). Sometimes patients with thymoma or leukaemia may develop MCD or, vice versa, these tumours may develop in patients with MCD. The association of MCD with other malignancies

Table 4.1 Possible causes of secondary MCD.

Tumours	Infection	Other diseases	Drugs	Atopic agents
Lymphoma	Syphilis	Diabetes	Interferon α /β	Bee stings
Thymoma	HIV	Obesity	NSAID	Vaccination
Leukaemia	Schistosoma	SLE	Lithium	Pollen
Mesothelioma	Mycoplasma	Allogenic stem cell transplantation	Penicillamine	Dairy products
Carcinomas	Ehrlichiosis	Dermatitis herpetiform	Trimethadione Paramethadione	House dust
Nephroblastoma	Echinococcus	Kimura disease	Gold salts	Pork
Waldenstrom			Methimazole	Poison
Mycosis fungoides			Ampicillin, cefixime, rifampicin	
Chordoma			Anti-VEGF agents	

HIV = Human immunodeficiency virus; SLE = Systemic lupus erythematosus; NSAID = Non-steroidal anti-inflammatory drugs; VEGF = Vascular endothelial growth factor

is possible but very rare. Occasional cases of MCD following allogeneic hemo-poietic stem cell transplantation have been reported (Hashimura et al., 2009; Wong et al., 2016).

Several drugs may precipitate an MCD. Among them, non-steroidal anti-inflammatory drugs (NSAIDs), lithium, and some antimicrobials (ampicillin, rifampicin, cefixime) are the drugs more frequently involved (Glassock, 2003). Most frequently the NS caused by these drugs is associated with an acute inter-stitial nephritis and acute kidney injury, but some cases may exhibit only the lesion of MCD. NS usually reverses completely after discontinuation of the offending drug. Drug-induced MCD should always be considered in the dif-ferential diagnosis in view of the wide use of these agents (Radhakrishnan and Perazella, 2015).

MCD may often develop after trivial infections or vaccination. However, the causal relationship between infection and MCD has been rarely established. About 20 per cent of patients who develop MCD have a history of bronchial asthma, contact dermatitis, or allergy to milk or other foods. Significantly in-creased levels of IgE have been detected in association with relapsing MCD (Tan et al., 2011). Recent evidence suggests that dysfunction in regulatory T-cells may be induced by short chain fatty acids produced by gut microbiota. On this basis, it has been hypothesized that an aberrant microbiota in the gut resulting in defective induction of regulatory T-cells may be involved in the aetiology of idiopathic NS in children (Kaneko et al., 2017).

However, evidence that MCD is a type of allergic disorder or can be induced by a specific allergen is weak. An adolescent with marked hyperimmunoglobulinaemia E due to a mutation of the signal transducer and activator of transcription 3 gene (STAT3) developed MCD and repeated episodes of NS, suggesting that mutation of STAT3 may have altered TH1/TH2 balance (Miyazaki et al., 2011). MCD may also be superimposed to other renal diseases, particularly IgA nephropathy (Shen et al., 2015), lupus nephritis (Moysés-Neto et al., 2011), or insulin-dependent diabetes (Moysés-Neto et al., 2012).

Clinical presentation and features

Clinically, MCD is characterized by a 'full blown' NS with urinary protein excretion ranging between three and 20 grams or more per day in adults (protein/creatinine ratio >3 mg/mg), without 'nephritic' signs or symptoms. In children NS is defined by proteinuria >40 mg/m^2/hour or >50 mg/kg/day or protein/creatinine ratio >3.0 mg/mg and albuminemia <2.5 g/dl.

The onset of NS is typically abrupt rather than insidious, and patients may often be able to identify the day at which their disease was first manifest. In children 80 per cent of the cases occur before the age of six years, with the peak incidence being between the ages of two to four years. Most cases of NS developing before the age of two years are congenital and genetic forms. In these children, pure MCD is uncommon, most of them are steroid-resistant, and in many cases renal biopsy shows the histological features of FSGS or mesangial proliferation (Trautmann et al., 2015; Ranganathan, 2016). The incidence of MCD declines after the age of 12 years. Severe hypo-albuminaemia, sometimes out of proportion to the degree of proteinuria, and marked hypercholesterolaemia are common. Proteinuria is typically 'selective', with heavy loss of low molecular weight albumin while proteins of higher molecular weight are retained. Facial oedema is often the major presenting symptom in children. Fluid retention increases, rapidly or gradually, often leading to a frank anasarca with impressive oedema of legs, external genitals, and the peri-orbital area. Ascites and bilateral pleural effusions can develop, but pericardial effusions are exceedingly rare. Blood pressure is usually within normal values, but it may be elevated in some African-American children with smaller lumen and thicker walls of renal arterioles than white children (Rostand et al., 2005). In adults with MCD and NS, the circadian rhythm of blood pressure is often disrupted, either as a consequence of hypo-albuminaemia (Ando and Yasuda, 2016) or altered sodium handling (Haruhara et al., 2017). Blood pressure rhythm tends to normalize after remission. On the other hand, hypovolaemia, postural hypotension, and even shock may sometimes occur as a consequence of sudden, massive loss of albumin in the urine and/or excessive administration of diuretics. Persistent microscopic haematuria is uncommon, although occasional positive tests occur in about one-third of cases; however, gross haematuria is exceptional. Renal function is usually normal at presentation but, especially in children and in elderly subjects, acute kidney injury (AKI) may be the presenting syndrome. Risk factors for AKI include steroid-resistant NS, infection, and nephrotoxic medication exposure (Rheault et al., 2015).

During the height of disease manifestations marked depression of serum IgG levels, normal C3 and C4 levels and elevation of IgM and fibrinogen levels are characteristic of MCD. These disturbances in the serum protein composition lead to marked elevation of the erythrocyte sedimentation rate, even in the absence of inflammation. Moreover, in patients with severe NS, the increased plasma viscosity and the elevated levels of fibrinogen and lipoproteins combined with very low levels of serum albumin and urinary loss of antithrombin III may favour the development of venous thromboembolism and may require prophylactic anticoagulation (see Chapter 2).

As mentioned, it may be difficult to distinguish at presentation whether the patient is affected by a true MCD or by a FSGS. Particularly in adults, the general outcome and response to therapy are usually quite different for patients with MCD and those with FSGS. However, some exception exists, and MCD unresponsive to treatment and progressing to renal failure have been reported. In children, it is generally thought that the clinical significance of the distinction is not clearly defined and it remains controversial, even though MCD, mesangial proliferative nephropathy, IgM nephropathy, and FSGS are readily distinguished on biopsy. Some biomarkers may allow differentiation between MCD and FSGS. A significant increase in urinary CD80, normalized to urinary creatinine, was found in patients with MCD in relapse compared to those in remission or those with FSGS (Garin et al., 2010). Serum soluble urokinase-type plasminogen activator receptor (suPAR) levels have been found to be higher in children with FSGS than in those with MCD (Cara Fuentes et al., 2014), but this is likely due to differences in glomerular filtration rate (GFR) between the two disorders, since higher suPAR level is associated with decline in the GFR independently of the nature of kidney disease (Hayek et al., 2015).

In children it is a common clinical practice to consider the response to steroid more relevant for the outcome than the histological features, which range as a continuum from no lesion or minimal glomerular damage to diffuse mesangial proliferation and focal and segmental sclerosis (Vivarelli et al., 2017). Hence, idiopathic NS in children is often considered as a single entity which includes steroid-responsive and steroid-resistant cases. Steroid-resistant patients usually have a poorer outcome than steroid-sensitive patients. On the other hand, it is true that in children, steroid-resistant NS and genetically conditioned NS are mostly FSGS. Thus, we follow current practice and treat these two lesions having distinctive clinical entities separately. This is in agreement with recent data that support the hypothesis that idiopathic MCD and primary FSGS are two different diseases, with MCD most likely a functional dysfunction of podocytes, while FSGS affects the structure of the podocytes (Nagata, 2016).

Epidemiology

The annual incidence of glomerular diseases in children has been a steady at 5–10 cases/100,000 population the peak incidence ranging between two and eight years of age (Grenbaum, 2012). The exact prevalence is not known, but on the basis of disease evolution and average age of onset, it can be estimated at approximately 10–50 cases per 100,000 children (Vivarelli et al., 2017).

Among the primary glomerular diseases, MCD accounts for over 75 per cent of cases of NS in children (1–3 per 100,000 children younger than 16 years of age). In adults, MCD accounts for 10–15 per cent of primary NS. There is a male/female ratio of 2:1 in children. Male preponderance is also observed in adults.

The disease is ubiquitous, but it occurs more frequently in peoples of Asian (Far East, Southeast Asia, or the Indian subcontinent) and Arabian origin than in Caucasian subjects, while it seems to be rare but with a more severe outcome in Black children. The estimated incidence rate in children ranges between 0.23–2.8/100 000/year in Caucasian children, 2.4/100 000/year in Hispanic children, 3.4/100 000/year in Afro-Caribbean children, 7.2–11.6/100 000/year in Arabian children, and 6.2–15.6/100 000/year in Asian (see above) children who resided in the UK (McGrogan et al., 2011).

There are some data indicating that over the last decade there has been an increase in the ratio between FSGS and MCD in children and adults (see Chapter 1). In the US, the ethnicity does not seem to influence the incidence of NS, while it is likely to have an impact on the distribution of histological lesions, as African-American children have more frequently FSGS and steroid-resistant NS.

Natural history

The few studies conducted in the pre-glucocorticoid era indicated that spontaneous remissions were not uncommon (estimated at between 30 and 40 per cent), but these often were delayed, occurring only after many months or several years of observation. Today most patients are given glucocorticoids or other effective drugs soon after the diagnosis has been made, so the available data can provide information only on treated patients.

For the great majority of patients with MCD the clinical course is character-ized by an initial remission induced by glucocorticoid therapy. Remission may be followed by relapses of NS, which may occur without apparent cause or after infections or allergic reactions. About 30–35 per cent of children who respond to initial therapy do not ever have any relapses, 10–20 per cent have infrequent relapses, and 45–60 per cent have early relapses while tapering steroids or less than three months after steroid withdrawal and become frequent relapsers or steroid dependent (see definitions in Table 4.2). Studies from the 1980s re-ported that no more than 10 per cent of children had additional relapses in

Table 4.2 Definitions used to describe nephrotic syndrome (NS), responses, and relapses in patients with minimal change disease.

NS	In children, proteinuria >40 mg/m²/hour or >50 mg/kg/day or protein/creatinine ratio >3.0 mg/mg. Hypo-albuminaemia (<2.5 g/dl) and hypercholesterolaemia. In adults, proteinuria >3.5 g/day (protein/creatinine ratio >3.5 mg/mg), without 'nephritic' signs or symptoms. Hypo-albuminaemia (<2.5 g/dl) and hypercholesterolaemia.
Complete remission	Proteinuria lower than 4 mg/m²/day in children or lower than 0.2 g/day in adults for three consecutive days.
Partial remission	Proteinuria between 4 and 40 mg/m²/day in children or between 0.21 and 3.5 g/day in adults for three consecutive days.
Relapse of proteinuria	Proteinuria exceeding 4 mg/m²/day in children or 0.2 g/day in adults for at least one week, in patients who were in complete remission.
Relapse of nephrotic syndrome	Proteinuria exceeding 40 mg/m²/day in children or 3.5 g/day in adults for at least one week, in patients who were in complete or partial remission.
Frequent relapsers	Patients with two or more episodes of the NS in six months or three or more episodes of the NS in 12 months.
Steroid-dependent NS	Reappearance of the NS within two weeks after reduction or discontinuation of glucocorticoids.
Steroid-resistant NS	Children who do not respond to an eight-week course with glucocorticoids. Longer treatments are needed to define steroid resistance in adults.

adulthood, but more recent surveys indicated that frequently relapsing and steroid-dependent MCD that originates in childhood can persist after puberty in 27–42 per cent of patients (Niaudet, 2009).

The prognosis for preservation of renal function is usually excellent if patients continue to respond to glucocorticoids. However, frequent relapsers and steroid-dependent subjects with prolonged NS can suffer from a number of iatrogenic adverse events, including hypertension, osteoporosis, oligozoospermia, and cataract (Kyrieleis et al., 2009). AKI can occur in the course of MCD. It can be due to hypovolaemia, drug-induced interstitial nephritis, or, very rarely, acute bilateral renal vein thrombosis; it is most often caused by diuretics or haemodynamic factors. In children, oliguria and AKI are mainly caused by intravascular volume depletion and promptly regress with correction of hypovolaemia or after successful glucocorticoid therapy. The development of AKI is seen much more commonly in adults over the age of 40 years, and is most frequently reversible, although a few instances of permanent ESRD have been described. In a retrospective study on 95 adults with MCD, AKI occurred in 24 patients; they tended to be older and hypertensive with lower serum albumin and more proteinuria than those without AKI. At follow-up, patients with an episode of AKI had higher serum creatinine levels than those without AKI. Four patients progressed to ESRD. These patients were less likely to have responded to steroids and more likely to have FSGS on repeat renal biopsy (Waldman et al., 2007).

Apart from renal failure, patients with MCD are exposed to infections, such as bacterial peritonitis, cellulitis, septicaemia, pneumonia, and meningitis (all usually related to encapsulated organisms, e.g. pneumococci). Thrombotic complications are also frequent. In a series of 188 children with the diagnosis of NS, 17 children (9.0 per cent) developed thrombo-embolic complications. Among the screened risk factors, high factor VIII level (64.7 per cent) followed by decreased antithrombin III level (29.4 per cent) were the leading factors (Tavil et al., 2015). Venous thrombo-embolism can also occur in adults with MCD, the hypercoagulable state being more severe in patients with superimposed AKI (Huang et al., 2016). Cerebral complications, including convulsions, hypertensive encephalopathy, and cerebral thrombosis (sagittal vein thrombosis) can also occur. However, due to the rapid response of NS to therapy and low frequency of events, a prophylactic anticoagulation is not recommended (Rankin et al., 2017).

The most frequent causes of death in adults and in elderly patients are related to NS per se (e.g. cardiovascular disease, pulmonary embolism, renal failure) or to its treatment (infections, malignancy), particularly when glucocorticoid, calcineurin inhibitors, or cytotoxic drugs are used at high doses and for prolonged periods. Death is particularly frequent in patients with renal dysfunction and in those untreated or refractory to treatment (Szeto et al., 2015).

Prognostic factors

Presentation

Patients without oedema and identified by chance proteinuria tend to have less relapse than symptomatic patients (see also Table 4.3). This is a quite uncommon presentation for MCD. The magnitude of the proteinuria at the time of presentation does not predict the subsequent response rate.

Age

The response to glucocorticoids is both lower in frequency and slower to develop in adults than in children with MCD. Moreover, older patients are

Table 4.3 Factors that may influence the prognosis and the response to treatment in patients with MCD.

Factors	Prognostic impact
Age	*Children* have a high rate of rapid response to GC but high risk of relapses. *Adults* have a slower and lower response to GC but lower risk of relapses.
Ethnicity	*Black* and *Caucasian* patients with MCD are less sensitive to GC than *Asian** patients.
Low birth weight (LBW)	Patients with LBW show often frequent relapses or steroid resistance.
Genetic factors	Monogenic mutations of genes encoding podocyte proteins are often associated with steroid resistance.
Response to treatment	Patients who respond to GC usually do not progress to ESRD.
Duration of initial treatment	Full-dose GC should be given for at least 8–12 weeks. Treatment should be longer in adults who may have a late response, while the advantage of prolonged initial treatment in children is debated.
Duration of response	Patients with remission lasting less than one year have low rate of relapses.
Relapses	Patients with *early relapses* have high probability of becoming *frequent relapsers* or *steroid-dependent*.
Glomerular lesions	Whether deposits of IgM or mesangial proliferation are associated with poor prognosis is still debated. Glomerular hypertrophy might be an initial sign of FSGS.

GC = glucocorticoids; * = Far East, Southeast Asia, or the Indian subcontinent.

significantly more vulnerable to severe infection, diabetes, and cataract as compared with younger patients (Tse et al., 2003; Shinzawa et al., 2013). Among children, those under six years of age have a faster response, those between ages one and 11 years without hypertension or haematuria have good chances for benefits of steroid therapy, while in adults, those aged over 40 years tend to respond more slowly but have fewer relapses than younger patients (Lee et al., 2016a). While progression to chronic renal failure is quite exceptional in children, it may occur in patients older than 60 years of age. On the other hand, the risk of relapses is inversely correlated with age, being higher in patients whose NS started before age six than in older children and adolescents.

Ethnicity

African-American children with MCD tend to develop hypertension and chronic renal disease in the long term. Such changes have been referred to the smaller lumens and thicker walls of renal arterioles in comparison with white children (Rostand et al., 2005). The steroid resistance is particularly elevated in African-American patients (Kim et al., 2006). However, it is possible that some of these steroid-resistant subjects could be affected by APOL1 nephropathy (Herymann et al., 2017). A high prevalence of FSGS 'misdiagnosed' as MCD in the original biopsy sample can be considered in steroid-resistant patients.

Low birth weight (LBW)

Patients with LBW who develop NS are often steroid-resistant (Teeninga et al., 2008) and frequently show a lesion of FSGS at renal biopsy (Hodgin, 2009). In patients with LBW and FSGS, the number of podocytes per glomerulus is significantly lower as compared to that observed in patients with LBW and MCD, suggesting that LBW may be a predisposing factor to podocytopenia (Ikezumi et al., 2013).

Genetic influence

Rare cases of familial steroid-sensitive NS have been described. Transmission was compatible with an autosomal recessive or autosomal dominant inheritance, suggesting that familial steroid-sensitive NS is a monogenic trait. These patients respond to glucocorticoids or immunosuppressive drugs (Dorval et al., 2018). Reports on the association between HLA antigens and MCD are variable. However, the many discrepancies between reports often due to racial and ethnic differences do not allow to draw any firm conclusion from available studies at present.

Mutations in *NPHS1* or *NPHS2* genes coding respectively for nephrin and podocin may frequently occur in sporadic NS. Single mutations or variants in *NPHS1* and *NPHS2* do not modify the outcome of primary NS (Caridi et al., 2009). However, patients with homozygous or compound heterozygous mutations commonly present with steroid-resistant NS before the age of six years and rapidly progress to ESRD (Tryggvason et al., 2006; Bouchireb et al., 2014). The response to steroids may be influenced by genetic regulation of multidrug resistance gene-1 (MDR-1) gene expression. Several studies reported that that MDR1 *C3435T* or *G2677T/A* gene polymorphisms in various combinations can increase the risk of steroid resistance in children with idiopathic NS (Choi et al., 2011; Jafar et al., 2011; Youssef et al., 2013; Dhandapani et al., 2015). The rate of detection of a genetic basis for MCD progressively declines with age, being extremely frequent in the first years of age and lower than 20 per cent in adolescents (Lipska et al., 2013).

Response to glucocorticoids

Glucocorticoids represent the drug of choice for the initial treatment of MCD. A good long-term prognosis is generally observed in MCD with steroid-sensitive NS. These patients do not progress to renal failure and most achieve a persisting remission. However, patient and kidney survival rates are poor in rare cases of MCD with steroid-resistant NS, most of which eventually show an underlying FSGS at repeated biopsy.

A number of factors can influence the response to glucocorticoids. Apart from MDR-1 gene polymorphisms, the mRNA expression of glucocorticoid receptors is significantly lower in late responders than in early responders (Han et al., 2008; Zahran et al., 2014). The high number of glucocorticoid receptor isoforms may also explain the different sensitivity to glucocorticoids (Ramamoorthy and Cidlowski, 2016). A recent report of the Podonet Registry showed that the ten-year renal survival was 43 per cent in steroid-resistant children (Trautmann et al., 2017).

Duration of initial treatment

There is agreement that steroid treatment should be administered for at least eight weeks in responders, but there are conflicting views on whether the initial treatment should be prolonged beyond eight weeks. In children, a retrospective cohort study of the Southwest Pediatric Nephrology Study Group (SPNSG) reported that prolongation of the steroid treatment for the initial episode of steroid-sensitive NS may have a beneficial effect, but at the cost of increased side effects (Lande et al., 2004). A Korean study reported that children receiving initially long-term therapy showed significantly lower relapse rates during the first year than those receiving short therapy (Baek et al., 2015). However, a Japanese multicentre randomized controlled trial (RCT) showed that a two-month prednisolone therapy for steroid-sensitive NS was not inferior to six-month therapy (Yoshikawa et al., 2015) and a meta-analysis of RCTs concluded that there was no significant difference in the risk for frequent relapses between prednisone given for two or three months and longer durations (Hahn et al., 2015). These data would indicate that there is no benefit of increasing the duration of prednisone beyond two or three months in the initial episode of steroid-sensitive NS in children. On the other hand, in adults the response may be slower than in children and short treatment duration can be ineffective or can increase the risk of relapses (Lee, Yoo, et al., 2016). Therefore, it is suggested to prolong treatment up to six or more months, if well tolerated, in adults who do not show remission.

Duration of remission

The longer the remission (the relapse-free interval) the better the prognosis. After one year of remission relapses are uncommon. However, occasionally relapses may occur after 20 or more years.

Spontaneous versus treatment induced remission

Limited data (from the pre-steroid treatment era) suggest that a spontaneous remission is followed by a longer relapse-free interval that in treatment induced remissions, but in the absence of prospective controlled observations this is difficult to verify.

Relapses

An early relapse, occurring within six months after remission, is often followed by a frequent relapsing course. The number of relapses during the first six months following a standard glucocorticoid regimen is highly predictive of the subsequent clinical course. Relapse-free survival rates increases with the use of calcineurin inhibitors or Rituximab (RTX).

Glomerular lesions

Glomerular hypertrophy on morphometric analysis is a risk factor for relapses (Lee, Yoo, et al., 2016) and is a predictor of evolution from MCD to FSGS on serial renal biopsy. It has therefore a bad prognostic significance. Whether *mesangial hypercellularity* is associated with a decreased response to glucocorticoids, steroid-dependency, and poorer prognosis or does not have any impact on these variables is still a matter of controversy. Some patients with otherwise typical MCD may show *mesangial IgM deposition* with or without a slight increase in mesangial matrix. Children with IgM deposits at immuno-fluorescence may often result to have steroid-dependent or steroid-resistant NS (Swartz et al., 2009). However, the response to cyclophosphamide (Geier et al., 2012) or cyclosporine (Kanemoto et al., 2013) was independent of the presence or absence of IgM deposits in children with MCD. The presence of *mesangial deposits of IgG* is usually considered to be nonspecific. The presence of *tip lesions* in otherwise normal glomeruli at light microscopy has been considered as a distinct entity within MCD/FSGS spectrum (Stokes et al., 2004). These lesions however do not influence a response to steroids similar to what observed in patients with classic MCD.

Qualitative aspects of proteinuria

Selective glomerular proteinuria is the increased excretion of more than 300 mg medium-sized negatively charged proteins such as albumin in a 24-h urine collection. Most patients with MCD have highly selective proteinuria, with low levels of urinary excretion of higher molecular weight proteins such as IgM or IgG. If non-selective proteinuria is present this should raise the suspicion that a lesion of FSGS is present and that non-response to steroid treatment is more likely. A study of urinary proteomic profiles reported that several proteins were found to be linked to the major clinical symptoms of NS. Among them, the slit diaphragm P-cadherin appeared to be reduced in urine during NS (Andersen et al., 2012). Low levels of apolipoprotein A1 were significantly associated with steroid resistance in children with idiopathic NS (Suresh et al., 2016).

Specific treatment

Goals and objectives of treatment

The three main objectives in treating MCD are:

i. To induce a complete remission of the NS as soon as possible in order to prevent the severe complications related to the nephrotic state.

ii. To avoid relapses of NS.

iii. To minimize short- and long-term iatrogenic side-effects of therapy (such as growth retardation, cosmetic and psychological effects, or infection) in a disease which can run a long relapsing and remitting course.

Several drugs, used alone or in combination with others, and overall therapeutic strategies may be used to achieve these objectives in the majority of patients.

Glucocorticoids

Glucocorticoids are universally considered as the drug class of choice for the initial treatment of MCD in both children and adults. Although this dogmatic statement is not based on the scanty evidence from prospective RCTs, the common clinical experience confirms the efficacy of synthetic glucocorticoids in most cases of MCD. These agents not only can exert well-known anti-inflammatory and immunosuppressive effects, but can also stabilize actin filaments in podocytes and prevent podocyte motility, thus explaining their antiproteinuric activity in NS (see Chapter 3).

Initial regimen

Children

Approximately 95 per cent of children with 'true' MCD can obtain a complete disappearance of proteinuria with high-dose oral predniso(lo)ne, while the rate of response is lower with lower doses. To reduce the side-effects, glucocorticoids with short half-life (prednisone, prednisolone, methylprednisolone, deflazacort) should be administered in a single dosage between 7 and 9 a.m. to mimic the circadian rhythm of cortisol. The once-a-day and then alternate-day schedule is usually well tolerated and couples the advantages of a high response rate with those of a relatively long therapy, which may prevent relapses. The risk of adrenocortical-pituitary-hypothalamic axis deficiency upon abrupt discontinuance of therapy is strongly reduced if the glucocorticoids have been administered on a once-a-day morning or alternate-day morning dosage regimen (see Chapter 3).

The Kidney Disease: Improving Global Outcomes (KDIGO) guidelines (2012) recommend that, for the initial treatment, oral prednisone or prednisolone should be administered for at least 12 weeks. Some investigators recommend body surface area (BSA)-based prednisone dosing for children that leads to higher cumulative doses than body weight (BW)-based dosing. However, in children with MCD, clinical outcomes with BW-based dosing are equivalent to BSA dosing-related outcomes, although cumulative prednisolone doses are lower in the former (Raman et al., 2016). Prednisone should be given as a single daily dose starting at 60 mg/m²/day or 2 mg/kg/day to a maximum of 80 mg/day. It is also recommended that daily oral prednisone should be given for at least four weeks, followed by alternate-day oral medication as a single daily dose starting at 40 mg/m² or 1.5 mg/kg (maximum 40 mg on alternate days) to be continued for two to six months.

Complete remission of proteinuria occurs in about half of children within one week, in 75 per cent within two weeks, and in approximately 90 per cent within four weeks. The major problem in children is represented by the risk of relapse. The abrupt discontinuance of glucocorticoids after obtaining remission favours early relapses. However, as pointed out above, the recommendation to administer initial steroid treatment for three months or longer to reduce the risk of relapses may be challenged since a Cochrane meta-analysis reported no difference in the risk of frequent relapses between children who received an eight-week or a 12-week initial treatment with prednisone (Hahn et al., 2015).

Adults

The KDIGO guidelines recommend that the initial dose of predniso(lo)ne should be 1 mg/kg/per day (80 mg/day maximum) or alternate-days single dose of 2 mg/kg (maximum 120 mg). If well tolerated, the initial high-dose should be continued for at least four weeks if complete remission is achieved, and for a maximum period of 16 weeks if complete remission is not achieved. Some clinicians prefer to administer glucocorticoids every other day from the outset of initial therapy to reduce side effects. However, in a retrospective study no difference in the rate of remissions, the risk of relapses, and side effects was found between adults treated with an initial prednisone dosage of 1 mg/kg on the daily regimen and approximately 2 mg/kg on alternate day (Waldman et al., 2007). As with children, the glucocorticoid dosage should always be administered in the morning between 7 and 9 a.m. Very differently from children, only 50–60 per cent of adults become free of proteinuria within eight weeks of therapy, regardless of the schedule of administration. However, if glucocorticoid therapy is continued for 16 weeks or more, complete remission of proteinuria may be obtained in about 80–85 per cent of adults with MCD (Shinzawa et al., 2013; Hogan and Radhakhrisnan, 2013). It is difficult to establish whether this slower response is due to a genuine lower sensitivity of adults to glucocorticoids, or to the fact that the effective doses of glucocorticoids given to adults are proportionally lower than those given to children. Alternatively, the sensitivity of podocyte to the local effects of glucocorticoids may differ between children and adults. In adults, the duration of initial treatment influences the subsequent risk of relapses (Lee, Yoo, et al., 2016).

Treatment of infrequent relapses

Relapses are usually as responsive to glucocorticoids as the initial episode of NS. The duration of treatment of relapses does not seem to influence the subsequent rate of additional relapses. Spontaneous remission can occur within 4–14 days after onset of a relapse, but it is impossible to predict in advance which patients will remit spontaneously and which will not. Some clinicians recommend starting treatment of relapses early if proteinuria > 2–3 g/day (2–3 g/g protein/creatinine on spot urine samples, 3+ to 4+ on dipstick) persists for three consecutive days, in order to prevent a full-blown NS. Others prefer to wait seven to ten days to avoid a useless glucocorticoid therapy in those patients who may remit spontaneously.

For children with infrequent relapses treatment is with prednisone 60 mg/m^2 per day until the urine is protein-free for three consecutive days; this is followed by four weeks of alternate-day prednisone at a dose of 40 mg/every other day. A similar regimen, with lower doses of prednisone (1 mg/kg per day for the relapse and then 0.8 mg/kg every other day for four weeks), may be used in adults.

Other protocols suggest to adopt the same protocol used for the initial treatment in children with infrequent relapses who have been steroid-free for months or years. A re-biopsy in patients with infrequent relapses is not necessary if patients continue to respond to glucocorticoids.

Treatment of frequently relapsing/steroid-dependent patients

As pointed out in Table 4.2, those patients with two or more relapses of NS in 6 months or 3 or more episodes of NS in 12 months are defined as frequent relapsers, while patients showing a reappearance of NS within two weeks after reduction or discontinuation of glucocorticoids are called steroid-dependent patients.

The management of frequent relapsers and steroid-dependent patients represents a challenge for the clinician. These patients usually remain steroid-responsive but repeated courses of high-dose glucocorticoids may induce severe hypercortisolism (exogenous Cushing syndrome) and even an increased risk of life-threatening complications. Some strategies may be adopted to reduce the toxicity of prolonged glucocorticoid treatment. One such strategy is a six-month course of alternate-day therapy or a treatment based on three intravenous (IV) pulses of high-dose methylprednisolone followed by oral prednisone at moderate doses (30 mg/m^2 in children, 0.5 mg/kg in adults, gradually tapered). The two somewhat opposing strategies more frequently adopted are:

i. to wait for relapse (which will almost certainly occur) and then treat it as described previously; or

ii. to use continuous 'prophylaxis' with low-dose prednisone (usually less than or equal to 0.5 mg/kg every other day).

In children, the 2012 KDIGO guidelines suggested to treat frequent relapsers or steroid-dependent patients with daily oral prednisone until the child has been in complete remission for 3 days, followed by alternate-day prednisone in the lowest possible dose to maintain remission. However, these suggestions have a low level of evidence and have been challenged by two recent randomized controlled trials. In a Dutch RCT, 150 children who responded to a three-month course of prednisolone were assigned to either three months of prednisolone followed by three months of placebo (n=74) or six months of prednisolone (n=76). After a median follow-up of 47 months, relapses occurred in 77 per cent of patients who received three months of prednisolone and 80 per cent of patients who received six months of prednisolone (Teeninga et al., 2013). In an Indian multicentre RCT, 181 children received 12 weeks of standard therapy for a first episode of NS and were then randomized to alternate-day prednisolone in tapering doses for three months or placebo. Relapses occurred in 66.7 vs. 70.2 per cent and frequent relapses in 48.6 vs. 53.7 per cent, respectively (Sinha et al., 2015). Thus, prolonging initial steroid treatment from three to six months does not seem to favourably impact on the course of MCD in childhood.

In adults, a systematic review and meta-analysis of RCTs showed that patients treated with short courses of methylprednisolone pulses and low-dose oral prednisone responded more quickly and showed fewer adverse events than patients receiving oral steroids. The complete remission rate and relapse rate were similar in both groups (Zhao et al., 2015).

Although some patients may tolerate the continuous or frequent use of glucocorticoids without side-effects others develop important steroid toxicity. The longer is the treatment the higher is the risk of severe toxicity. Apart from many other steroid-related complications, in children these treatments can cause a significant growth retardation. Thus, alternative treatments designed to reduce the overall exposure to the adverse effects of glucocorticoids are required in many patients with frequent relapses or steroid-dependence, as is discussed below.

Cyclophosphamide

The efficacy of daily oral cyclophosphamide in preventing relapses of the NS has been known for more than 30 years and proven by suitably designed randomized clinical trials, mostly carried out in children with doses of 2- 2.5 mg/kg/day for 8-12 weeks. A systematic review of RCTs or quasi RCTs in children confirmed that cyclophosphamide significantly reduced the risk of relapse at six to 12 months (RR 0.43) and 12 to 24 months (RR 0.20) compared with prednisone alone. There was no significant difference at one year between IV and oral cyclophosphamide (Pravitsitthikul et al., 2013). In a study, more than 50 per cent of children with steroid-sensitive IgM-positive MCD remained relapse-free after four years from cyclophosphamide treatment (Geier et al., 2012).

Less information about the overall efficacy and safety of cyclophosphamide-based regimens is available in adults. After treatment with cyclophosphamide, the cumulative rate of sustained remissions may range from 50 to 78 per cent. Several factors can influence the response to cyclophosphamide:

i. An important variable is the duration of cyclophosphamide treatment. Only few patients enter a complete remission with a four-week treatment. For those patients who do not respond to a course of eight weeks, treatment may be prolonged to 12 weeks.

ii. Steroid-sensitive patients usually have an excellent rate of response to cyclophosphamide, independently of kidney histopathology, while in general, steroid-resistant children do not respond to an eight-week therapy with cyclophosphamide.

iii. Frequently relapsing patients have a higher rate of sustained remission than steroid-dependent patients. About 70 per cent of frequently relapsing children versus less than 30 per cent of steroid-dependent children with MCD treated with eight weeks of oral daily cyclophosphamide maintain stable remission. Prolonging cyclophosphamide administration for 12 weeks may increase the probability of remission.

iv. The age at onset of MCD correlates inversely with relapse rate. In adults the risk of relapse seems to be lower than in children.

The major problem with the use of cyclophosphamide concerns its toxicity. Side-effects of this agent have been detailed elsewhere in this book (see Chapter 3). In a meta-analysis on 1,504 children treated with oral daily cyclophosphamide or chlorambucil for MCD, the *fatality* rate of the treatment was approximately 1 per cent (Latta et al., 2001). *Malignancies* were observed in 14 children (0.9 per cent) after high doses of either drug. The four most important side effects of cyclophosphamide are bladder toxicity (haemorrhagic cystitis, induction of transitional cell metaplasia, and neoplasia), bone marrow toxicity (agranulocytosis, pancytopenia), gonadal toxicity (premature ovarian failure, oligo/azoospermia), and oncogenicity (induction of lymphomas and leukaemias). *Bladder toxicity* is quite rare (but always possible!) with the oral doses and duration used in MCD. To reduce the risk further, it is advisable to put patients into remission first using glucocorticoids and then to give cyclophosphamide only after diuresis has been induced. Forced hydration and sodium 2-mercaptoethanesulphonate (MESNA) should be prescribed if cyclophosphamide is administered intravenously. *Bone marrow toxicity* depends on the dose used. Leukopenia may occur in about one-third of patients. At a daily dose not exceeding 2 mg/kg every 24 hours for 8–12 weeks leukopenia may develop but it is usually reversible by decreasing the doses. Pancytopenia is rare at conventional doses of oral cyclophosphamide. The risk of azoospermia is related to the *cumulative* dosage of cyclophosphamide. In a meta-analysis study, no safe threshold for a cumulative amount of cyclophosphamide was found in males, but there was a marked increase in the risk of oligo/azoospermia with higher cumulative doses (Latta et al., 2001). Thus, dosages not higher than 2 mg/kg/day for 12 weeks should be recommended. Moreover, the cumulative dose of cyclophosphamide should not exceed 200–250 mg/kg. Females rarely develop gonadal toxicity with the above recommended dose and duration of oral cyclophosphamide. The *oncogenic risk* also depends on the cumulative dosage. Transitional cell carcinoma of the bladder or uro-epithelial tract or acute myelogenous leukaemia both have an increased incidence in patients who were given several grams of cyclophosphamide over many months (see Chapter 3). In the meta-analysis of Latta and colleagues (2001), the few cases of malignancies (0.9 per cent) were observed in children treated with high doses of either cyclophosphamide or chlorambucil. The oncogenic risk using two to three months of therapy is low. An impairment of T-helper cells can occur in patients treated with cyclophosphamide. The immune function reverts to normal within 6–12 months in patients treated for eight weeks.

In summary, an 8–12-week course of cyclophosphamide at a dose of 2 mg/kg/day (<200 mg/kg as a cumulative dose) is generally well tolerated both in the short and long term. Further subsequent courses, however, can increase the risk of gonadal toxicity, neoplasia, and prolonged immune dysfunction, and should be avoided whenever possible. To be on the safe side, leuprolide may be administered to females during cytotoxic treatment, and sperm banking may be recommended to males requiring more than one course of cyclophosphamide. IV pulses of cyclophosphamide may also reduce the cumulative dosage of this agent, but the experience in MCD is limited.

It should be reminded that both cyclophosphamide and chlorambucil are contra-indicated in pregnancy and all sexually active females receiving the drug should have a negative pregnancy test before starting the agent and be advised to use at least two contraceptive measures during its use or to entirely avoid intercourse while receiving the drug. Caution should be recommended with the use of alkylating agents in very young children with no prior history of varicella or who have negative anti-varicella antibody tests.

Chlorambucil

Good results have been reported with oral daily chlorambucil, although there is considerably less experience with this agent than with cyclophosphamide. The dosage more frequently used in patients with MCD is 0.2 mg/kg/day for eight weeks, but to be safe it is probably better to administer doses of 0.10–0.15 mg/kg/day. In the systematic review of Cochrane Renal Group's Specialised Register, chlorambucil significantly reduced the risk of relapses up to 24 months in comparison with prednisone alone. There was no significant difference in relapse risk at two years between chlorambucil and cyclophosphamide (Pravitsitthikul et al., 2013).

It is likely that oral daily chlorambucil has a lower bladder toxicity and a higher risk for azoospermia and other severe adverse events than cyclophosphamide. In the meta-analysis of Latta and colleagues (2001), severe infections were more frequent in children treated with chlorambucil than in those treated with cyclophosphamide (6.8 versus 1.5 per cent) and seizures occurred in 3.6 per cent of patients given chlorambucil versus none with cyclophosphamide. To prevent disquieting side-effects, we suggest not exceeding a cumulative dosage of 10–15 mg/kg with chlorambucil. The leukaemogenic effect of chlorambucil is related to the cumulative dosage of the drug (see Chapter 3), but the risk with the doses usually employed in MCD should be low.

In summary, an eight-week course of chlorambucil is relatively safe. However, there is a substantial risk for azoospermia and the drug should be used with great caution in males with MCD. The dose should not exceed 0.2 mg/kg/day. Probably, a dose of 0.15 mg/kg/day is equally effective and certainly less toxic. More prolonged or repeated courses should be discouraged as they entail an increased risk of long-term side-effects. The same precautions in sexually active females pertain to chlorambucil use. For reasons of toxicity, alkylating agents are used much less frequently nowadays for recurrently relapsing or steroid dependent MCD.

Cyclosporine (CsA)

CsA has potent immunosuppressive properties that reflect its ability to block the transcription of cytokine genes in activated T-cells. Moreover, CsA may protect the dephosphorylation of synaptopodin by calcineurin, thus protecting the podocyte function and the integrity of glomerular barrier (Faul et al., 2008). Finally, CsA can prevent intrapodocyte TRPC6 channel localization and activity, which contributes to podocyte dysfunction and proteinuria (Yu et al., 2016). Thus, CsA may exert beneficial effects on proteinuria via a purely local basis, independent of any disease-modulating, systemic immunosuppressive effects. This may explain, in part, why relapses are so common when CsA is discontinued. The efficacy of CsA in obtaining complete remission and in reducing the risk of relapse in children with steroid-sensitive MCD was reported more than 30 years ago and was confirmed by a large number of studies, including RCTs. A systematic review of RCTs reported that CsA was as effective as alkylating agents and significantly more effective than steroids alone in preventing relapses. However, the effects of CsA were not sustained once treatment was stopped (Pravitsitthikul et al., 2013). Good results with CsA have also been reported in adults with MCD, particularly when the drug was associated with prednisone (Meyrier, 1994; Eguchi et al., 2010; Fujiwara et al., 2015), but once again, in most patients, proteinuria relapsed when CsA was stopped or even when the doses were reduced.

The rapid recurrence of NS following cessation of CsA therapy led to the concept of 'cyclosporine-dependency', and the prospect of indefinite patient exposure to a potentially nephrotoxic drug. However, a long duration of un-interrupted treatment followed by progressive and very slow tapering of drug dose may maintain remission even after interruption of CsA therapy in some patients. Some of these lasting 'effects' may be spontaneous remissions in nature. In a number of cases, durable remission may also be maintained with low doses of CsA, i.e. 1.5–2 mg/kg/day (Meyrier et al., 1994; Inoue et al., 2013). Some investigators feel that therapeutic drug monitoring is necessary during CsA therapy and suggest that trough blood levels between 60 and 80 ng/ml are protective, while doses <40 ng/ml are not effective (Ishikura, 2008). If blood levels are monitored, one should take into account that the required CsA dose to reach a certain blood level would vary according to age but would be significantly higher for the younger children. In a study, the dose-normalized C_{max} and AUC values were significantly lower in children less than five years of age than in older children (Ushijima et al., 2012). In our experience with adults, we usually do not monitor the blood levels of CsA, but make sporadic checks to verify adherence to prescription.

The long-term use of CsA in patients with MCD may be complicated by adverse events which are time- and dose-dependent. Hypertrichosis, gingival hyperplasia, hyperlipidaemia, glucose intolerance, and arterial hypertension are the most frequent side-effects of CsA. However, the most common and severe complication with long-term use of CsA is nephrotoxicity. The potential risk of long-term CsA therapy to induce chronic renal failure in patients with MCD has been discussed controversially. When high doses of CsA were used in the past, most patients showed irreversible decrease in GFR associated with the so-called CsA nephropathy, characterized by arteriolar changes, glomerular sclerosis, interstitial fibrosis, and tubular atrophy. Today, after the introduction of CsA micro-emulsion (Neoral, Novartis Basel), the doses used in MCD rarely exceed 100 mg/m^2 in children and 4 mg/kg in adults. With such a dosage, side-effects are mild and reversible. These doses are further reduced when remission is obtained. Such a strategy is often effective for preventing relapses and protecting renal function. If the above-mentioned dosages are respected, CsA-related nephrotoxicity is rare and usually mild in patients with MCD. In a series of 20 children with steroid-dependent MCD, CsA was given in mean for five years. GFR decreased within three months, from 137 to 130 ml/min and remained stable at 126 ml/min at latest follow-up. No sign of CsA toxicity was seen at renal biopsy (Kranz et al., 2008). However, one cannot exclude that a long duration of therapy may increase the risk for nephrotoxicity. Thus, a workshop of experts suggests that it is prudent to perform regular renal biopsies in patients receiving long-term (i.e. >2 years) CsA therapy (Cattran et al., 2007). The changes in GFR induced by CsA, coupled with its tubular toxicity, can also cause reduced reabsorption of magnesium and hypomagnesaemia. Severe magnesium deficiency may cause neuromuscular irritability, hypokalaemia, and cardiac arrhythmias. It has also been reported that in experimental animals CsA-induced hypomagnesaemia can upregulate fibrogenic molecules and favour the development of interstitial fibrosis (Miura et al., 2002). Another common complication of CsA is hyperuricemia, which is caused by decreased renal urate clearance. Gout can frequently occur not only in adults, but also in paediatric renal transplant recipients and may represent a prognostic marker of poor renal outcome (Fidan et al., 2015).

In summary, CsA is effective and reasonably safe in maintaining remission in multirelapsing or steroid-dependent patients, both adults and children. This agent can be considered as an alternative to glucocorticoids and alkylating agents for treating difficult-to-manage patients. When using CsA (Neoral) we suggest initial doses no greater than 100 mg/m^2/day in children or 4 mg/kg/day in adults, preferably associated with low-dose prednisone. At these dosages the drug is well tolerated and does not cause severe renal damage. The main disadvantage is represented by the need for prolonged treatment. It is likely that many responders can maintain remission also with low doses (around 2 mg/kg/day in adults and less than 100 mg/m$^{2/}$day in children), which reduces further the risks of renal toxicity and of other side-effects. Some patients may maintain remission after stopping CsA, provided that treatment was prolonged for two years or more.

Tacrolimus (TAC)

Like CsA, TAC is a potent inhibitor of calcineurin that blocks both T-lymphocyte signal transduction and IL-2 transcription. In a model of MCD, TAC exerted a protective effect against proteinuria and glomerular barrier disruption by promoting podocyte repair and reduced glomerular and urinary angiopoietin-like protein 4 expression (Li et al., 2015). A number of studies reported that TAC, either given alone or associated with small doses of prednisone, may obtain a quick remission of NS and maintain remission when given as monotherapy in MCD. Steroid-resistant patients were less likely to respond with a complete remission, but encouraging results have been reported when TAC was associated with oral prednisone and ACE-inhibitors (Li et al., 2009; Fan et al., 2013). The results seem to be particularly good in Chinese and Japanese patients;

however, relapses are frequent after interruption of TAC, even when the doses are lowered gradually (Gulati et al., 2008; Li et al., 2008; Roberti and Vyas, 2010; Wang et al., 2012; Bock et al., 2013; Yang et al., 2016).

In an RCT, 41 patients between the ages of one and 18 years with steroid-resistant NS were randomly assigned to TAC (0.1–0.2 mg/kg/day) or CsA (5–6 mg/kg/day) plus oral prednisone and enalapril for one year. After 12 months of therapy, complete or partial remission occurred in 85 per cent of patients treated with TAC and in 75 per cent of those treated with CsA. The proportion of patients who experienced relapse was significantly greater in those receiving CsA compared with TAC. The drug had to be stopped because of nephrotoxicity in 4.7 per cent of patients in the TAC group and in 10 per cent in the CsA group (Choudhry et al., 2009).

In summary, TAC, like CsA, is very effective in maintaining remission in steroid-dependent patients, but relapses are frequent after discontinuation of the drug. In patients with MCD, TAC may be given at doses of 0.1 mg/kg/day, which may be gradually tapered in responders. The risk of nephrotoxicity is presumably low at these dosages, but serum creatinine levels should be regularly checked. The side effects of TAC are similar to those observed with CsA, although glucose intolerance is more frequent with TAC. Gingival hyperplasia and hypertrichosis do not occur with TAC, but a few patients may develop alopecia. It is not known if regular monitoring of plasma trough or peak TAC levels is needed to provide optimum results in terms of safety and/or efficacy, but such assays would increase the overall cost of such treatment.

Azathioprine

It is difficult to assess the role of oral azathioprine in patients with MCD. From the few old observational and controlled studies performed one might conclude that short-term treatment of MCD with azathioprine is of little benefit, while long-term administration may obtain remission in at least some patients. It is probably better to reserve the long-term use of azathioprine as adjuvant therapy for the very few patients who do not respond to conventional or newer treatments.

Mycophenolic acid (MPA) derivatives

A number of non-controlled studies reported that mycophenolate mofetil (MMF) may be of benefit in the treatment of children and adults with steroid-sensitive or steroid-dependent MCD (Bagga et al., 2003; Sepe et al., 2008; Siu et al., 2008; Koukoulaki and Goumenos, 2010; Sandoval et al., 2017), although most children relapse after withdrawal of the drug (Dehoux et al., 2016).

A few randomized trials are available. A Dutch multicentre RCT compared the results of MMF (1200 mg/m^2/day) to that of CsA (4–5 mg/kg/day) in 24 children with frequently relapsing NS and a histological diagnosis of MCD. Two of the 12 patients in the MMF group discontinued the drug. Seven patients in the MMF group and 11 of the 12 patients in the CsA group remained in complete remission during the study period of 12 months. Relapse rate in the MMF group was 0.83/year compared to 0.08/year in the CsA group. None of the patients reported diarrhoea. Evaluation of the changes from the baseline GFR showed an overall significant difference in favour of MMF over the treatment period (Dorrensteijn et al., 2008). A similar RCT in Germany compared the efficacy and safety of a one-year treatment with MMF (target plasma trough level of 1.5–2.5 µg/ml) or CsA (target trough level of 80–100 ng/ml) in 60 children with frequently relapsing NS. No relapse occurred in 85 per cent of patients during CsA therapy and in 64 per cent of patients during MMF therapy, the difference being at borderline significance. The time without relapse was significantly longer with CsA than with MMF during the first year, but not during the second year. There were no significant differences between groups with respect to blood pressure, growth, lipid levels, or adverse events. However, estimated GFR increased significantly with MMF compared with CsA (Gellermann et al., 2013). Another prospective study compared the efficacy of MMF with that of CsA as maintenance therapy after a single infusion of RTX. Of 29 patients with persistent steroid-dependent NS despite the use of CsA and/or MMF, 13 continued CsA therapy, maintaining a two-hour post-dose CsA level at 400–500 ng/ml, and 16 were treated with MMF, maintaining a pre-dose level of 2–5 µg/ml of mycophenolic acid. The median duration of CsA and MMF treatment was 18 and 19 months, respectively. Treatment failure occurred more frequently in the MMF group (7/16) than in the CsA group (2/13). The rate of sustained remission was also significantly higher in the CsA group than in the MMF group (Fujimaga et al., 2013). These RCTs suggest that, in comparison with CsA, MMF can have a better renal safety profile but exposes the patient with MCD to an increased risk of relapses. The role of therapeutic drug monitoring is still controversial. Some investigators recommended that MPA target AUC should exceed 45–60 mg h/l to ensure the safe and effective treatment in children with NS (Sobiak et al., 2015; Tellier et al., 2016).

In summary, oral mycophenolate salts may be considered as a useful adjunctive therapy in difficult patients with frequently relapsing MCD who have developed steroid-toxicity and who refuse treatment with cyclophosphamide or chlorambucil (on account of fears of side effects) or who have some contraindication for their use (such as a history of bladder cancer or prior herpes zoster). Mycophenolate may also be used as sequential maintenance treatment to prolong remission after RTX, to improve renal function in CsA-treated patients showing a decline in eGFR (Gellermann et al., 2012), or may be used in multidrug therapies together with prednisone and TAC or CsA for treatment of steroid resistant NS. We suggest starting MMF with a daily dose of 30 mg/kg/day in children (2 g/day in adults) to be maintained until complete remission is obtained, followed by 20–25 mg/kg/day (1.5 g/day in adults) for two months and then 15 mg/kg/day (1 g/day in adults). Treatment may be continued for more than two years if well tolerated. MMF withdrawal after one to two years of treatment can be followed by relapse in 68 per cent of the cases. The enteric coated mycophenolate sodium (MS) may also be used, but fewer data are available on efficacy and safety. The utility of monitoring the plasma level of mycophenolic acid for optimizing efficacy and safety of MMF or MS therapy of MCD is still debated. An advantage of MMF or MS is that they do not integrate into DNA and do not have any pro-oncogenic effect.

Mizoribine (MZB)

MZB is an imidazole nucleoside which exerts its activity through selective inhibition of inosine monophosphate synthetase and guanosine monophosphate synthetase, resulting in the complete inhibition of guanine nucleotide synthesis. MZB has been used successfully in a small number of Japanese patients with MCD (Aizawa-Yashiro et al., 2011; Tanaka et al., 2015).

Rituximab (RTX)

After anecdotal reports showed the possibility of inducing remission with RTX in transplant recipients with recurrence of NS (Nozu et al., 2005), and in patients with steroid-dependent NS (Francois et al., 2007), an increasing number of reports pointed out the successful use of RTX on steroid-dependent and frequently relapsing patients with MCD. Sustained remission may last for some months after RTX, but in most patients relapses of NS occur after CD19-cell recovery, requiring further administrations of RTX. A systematic review of uncontrolled studies in children recruited 211 patients with steroid-dependent NS (ten studies) and 90 patients with steroid-resistant NS (five studies), treated with variable doses of RTX. Patients were followed-up for 54 months. Response rates were >50 per cent in steroid-dependent NS and <25 per cent in steroid-resistant NS. RTX was poorly effective in patients who did not respond to a combination of steroids and calcineurin inhibitors (Ravani et al., 2016). However, these studies included both resistant and dependent forms of the disease, some patients became resistant after an initial response, and the doses of RTX varied from one to ten single or multiple courses of RTX—375 mg/m^2. To better evaluate the impact of RTX on relapses of NS, an RCT of 28 children with a mean age of seven years with steroid-dependent NS were randomly assigned to continue prednisone alone for one month (control) or to add a single IV infusion of RTX (375 mg/m²). Prednisone was tapered in both groups after one month. Three-month proteinuria was 42 per cent lower in the RTX group. All but one child in the control group relapsed within six months while median time to relapse in the RTX group was 18 months. In the RTX group, nausea and skin rash during infusion were common; transient acute arthritis occurred in one child (Ravani et al., 2015). A Japanese multicentre double-blind randomized trial assigned 52 CsA-treated children with frequent relapses or steroid dependence to receive RTX 375 mg/m² or placebo. The relapse rate was significantly lower in the RTX than in the placebo group and the time to relapse was significantly longer in the RTX than in the placebo group. Daily steroid dose after randomization was significantly lower in the RTX than in the placebo group (Iijima et al., 2017).

Good results with RTX have also been reported in adults with MCD. In a study, 17 adults with steroid-dependent MCD were treated with RTX. After the first course of RTX, 11 patients (65 per cent) did not relapse after a mean follow-up of 26.7 months and nine of them were able to come off all immunosuppressive drugs and steroids during follow-up. Six patients relapsed at least once after a mean time of 11.9 months, but their immunosuppressive drug treatment could be stopped or markedly reduced during this time (Munyentwali et al., 2013). In a prospective cohort study, single-dose infusions of RTX, at a dose of 375 mg/m² of body surface area, were administered at intervals of six months for a period of 24 months. A significant reduction in the total number of relapses was observed during the 24-month period after the first RTX infusion as compared with that during the 24-month period before the first RTX infusion (108 vs. 8). Complete remission was maintained in all patients from 12 to 24 months after the first RTX infusion (Iwabuchi et al., 2014). In a multicentre study, 41 adults with MCD received RTX. Complete remissions were obtained for 25 patients and partial remission for another seven patients (overall response 78 per cent). After a follow-up of 39 months relapses occurred in 18 responders (56 per cent). Among them, 17 received a second course of RTX, 13 had a complete response, and four a partial remission (Guitard et al., 2014). In another multicentre study, ten children and 20 adults with a diagnosis of either MCD or FSGS who were in steroid-induced remission were given one or two doses of RTX 375 mg/m.² The median number of relapses dropped from 2.5 per year to 0.5 per year and steroids could be withdrawn in 18 patients (Ruggenenti et al., 2014). Ten adolescents and adults (mean age 26 years) with immune suppression dependent MCD were treated with two doses of RTX (375 mg/m²). Maintenance immunosuppressive medication was stopped. After a mean follow-up of 43 months, three patients had four relapses, successfully retreated with RTX, after induction therapy with prednisone 60 mg/day. RTX was well tolerated and no infectious complications were recorded (Dekkers et al., 2015). In a large study, 54 adults with steroid-dependent MCD received four single-dose six-monthly infusions of RTX (375 mg/m^2 per dose) and were followed up to 24 months. Compared to the baseline the prednisone dose was significantly lower, the bone density was significantly higher and blood pressure was significantly lower at 24 months. There were no severe adverse effects of RTX. However, mild infusion reactions occurred in 31 patients (57 per cent). The frequency of the infusion reactions decreased significantly with every successive infusion (Miyabe et al., 2016). Relapses after RTX seem to be correlated with reconstitution of memory B-cells (Colucci et al., 2016).

In the quoted studies, patients treated with RTX did not experience disquieting side effects, apart from the reactions to the first infusion. The mid-term safety of RTX was confirmed by a report in children with MCD followed over a period of 9 years (Bonanni et al., 2018). However, rare cases of lethal sepsis (Fabrizi et al., 2015), multifocal leukoencephalopathy (Berger et al., 2014) and late neutropenia with fatal outcome (Aquiar-Bujanda et al., 2015) referable to RTX have been reported in patients with primary glomerulonephritis or other diseases already immunosuppressed with other drugs.

In summary, RTX can provide a time off of steroids or low cumulative steroid and CNI dose to minimize toxic effects. A drawback that may prevent its extensive use in patients with MCD is represented by the high economic cost and the occurrence of infusion-related reactions needing medical assistance. Moreover, relapses may be delayed but not eliminated, meaning that RTX administration should be repeated several times to the same child. Its use appears to be safe in the short and mid term, but we do not have information about the possible side effects in the long term. Further studies comparing the long-term effects and safety of RTX with other effective drugs will be able to better define the role of this important biological agent in MCD and other glomerular diseases.

Levamisole

A number of studies reported that oral levamisole at doses ranging from 2.5 mg/kg twice weekly to 2.5 mg/kg/day allows complete or partial steroid-sparing in many children with frequently relapsing MCD, although this beneficial effect disappeared when the drug was stopped. A systematic review of the available controlled trials found that levamisole was more effective than steroids alone in reducing the risk of relapses at six and 12 months, but the effects were not sustained once treatment was stopped (Hodson et al., 2008). A randomized trial in 99 children with steroid sensitive NS and frequent relapses showed that the time to relapse was significantly increased in the levamisole compared to the placebo group. After 12 months of treatment, 6 per cent of placebo patients vs. 26 per cent of levamisole patients were still in remission (Gruppen et al., 2018). The mechanisms of action of levamisole in MCD are still poorly defined but recent investigations showed that in immortalized human podocytes, levamisole can induce expression and activate signalling of glucocorticoid receptor. Furthermore, levamisole may protect against podocyte injury in a puromycin aminonucleoside -treated cell model (Jiang et al., 2015).

The clinical impression is that the drug may be helpful in milder cases of MCD. It is possible that higher doses and more prolonged courses might obtain better results but there are no solid data supporting this hypothesis. The drug is usually well tolerated, with the exception of neutropenia and of cutaneous lesions which may occur in some patients. Exceptional cases of granulomatous interstitial nephritis and vasculitis have also been reported (Pinto et al., 2013). The clinical interest with this drug is vanishing as it is no commercially available any more in many Western countries.

Interleukin 2 (IL2)

In animal models of NS, T regulators can revert proteinuria and reduce renal lesions. Since IL2 upregulates T regulators, it might be effective also in human NS. Bonanni and colleagues (2015) treated five nephrotic patients with six monthly cycles of low-dose IL2. No effect on proteinuria or renal function was seen.

ACTH

Intramuscular administration of natural ACTH was one of the earliest treatments used for managing MCD in children. Acthar Gel has been recently used as a primary or second-line treatment in a few patients with MCD. Most of them responded with complete or partial remission (Filippone et al., 2016; Madan et al., 2016). A recent review of five studies including 89 patients, predominantly children, reported a sustained proteinuria response in 71 per cent of patients after long-term ACTH treatment (Lieberman and Pavlova-Wolf, 2017).

Treatment of steroid-resistant nephrotic syndrome

Overall about 10 per cent of all patients with an initial histological diagnosis of MCD (about 5–7 per cent of children and 10–12 per cent of adults) do not respond to glucocorticoids given in conventional dosages and duration as outlined earlier. Most of these cases may show lesions of FSGS on further renal biopsies or are carriers of podocyte gene mutations (Joshi et al., 2013; Lovric et al., 2016). The clinical impression is that in these patients the adjunctive use of oral cyclophosphamide does not show any important benefit. Most of these cases had FSGS on further renal biopsies.

Discordant results have been reported with CsA in uncontrolled studies. Some investigators reported good rates of remission, particularly when CsA was associated with IV methylprednisolone pulse therapy, while other studies could not find any benefit with CsA either alone or associated with glucocorticoids. A multicentre prospective study in Japan reported the five-year outcomes in 35 children with steroid-resistant NS treated with CsA and steroids. Of these patients, 23 cases were classified as MCD, five as diffuse mesangial proliferation (MesPGN), and seven as FSGS. Renal survival at five years was 94.3 per cent. Patient status was complete remission in 31 (88.6 per cent) (MCD/MesPGN: 25; FSGS: 6); partial remission in one (FSGS); and non-remission in three (MCD/MesPGN), including chronic kidney disease and ESRD in one each. Response to CsA at four months predicted five-year outcome (Hamasaki et al., 2013). A cross-sectional and longitudinal multicentre study in Germany reported that 79 per cent of 82 children with non-genetic NS resistant to 2.5 months of glucocorticoid therapy responded to CsA within six months (60 per cent complete remission and 19 per cent partial remission). Most patients with complete remission maintained normal renal function in the long term. Among CsA-treated patients, 69 per cent showed FSGS and 23 per cent showed MCD at biopsy. Instead, only 3 per cent of children with genetic steroid-resistant NS experienced a complete remission and 16 per cent of patients experienced a partial remission after CsA therapy (Büscher et al., 2016).

Good results have also been reported with TAC in children. In a study of 16 children with steroid-resistant NS, 15 went into complete remission after a median of 120 days of therapy with TAC and prednisone. Nine children were able to stop steroids, while the others were on tapering doses. However, 47 per cent had relapses, and most of them were steroid-responsive (Butani and Ramsamooj, 2009). In a multicentre RCT, children with steroid-resistant NS were randomized to receive TAC for 12 months or six-monthly infusions of IV cyclophosphamide. In both groups, patients were given equal amounts of alternate-day prednisolone. Complete remission was significantly higher with TAC (52.4 per cent) than with cyclophosphamide (14.8 per cent). Sustained remission at 12 months was significantly higher with TAC than cyclophosphamide. Treatment withdrawal chiefly due to systemic infections, was higher with cyclophosphamide (Gulati et al., 2012). In another study, 13 of 33 children with steroid-resistant NS entered remission, after treatment for 12 months with TAC. The mean time to achieve remission was 4.0±3.2 months. After remission half of the patients relapsed (Yang et al., 2016). To better evaluate the benefits and harms of different interventions used in children with steroid-resistant idiopathic NS, 19 RCTs have been reviewed. The analysis demonstrated that calcineurin inhibitors increase the likelihood of complete or partial remission compared with placebo/no treatment or cyclophosphamide. For other regimens assessed, it remains uncertain whether the interventions alter outcomes (Hodson et al., 2016). TAC is also effective in adults with steroid resistant NS. In a Chinese multicentre trial, 14 adults with steroid-resistant MCD or mesangial proliferative glomerulonephritis (MesPGN) were enrolled and treated with TAC plus prednisone for 12 months. Complete or partial response was obtained in six of the eight patients with MCD, and four of the six patients with MesPGN. One patient with MesPGN experienced relapses during the subsequent six months of follow-up. Adverse events included infection, hand tremor, diarrhoea, and acute reversible or persistent nephrotoxicity (Fan et al., 2013). In a randomized trial, 119 Chinese adults with MCD received glucocorticoids or TAC (0.05 mg/kg) after a pulse of intravenous methylprednisolone. Complete remission occurred in 96.2 per cent of patients, with the probability being the same in the two arms of the study. Additionally, the risk of relapse was similar. Seven adverse events in the glucocorticoid group and two adverse events in the TAC group were serious (Li et al., 2017). In a prospective study, 45 steroid-resistant children were treated with CNI either TAC- or CSA-based on a 1:1 allocation. After six months of treatment, 16/23 (69.5 per cent) patients on CSA achieved remission and 18/22 (81.8 per cent) on TAC achieved remission. The five-year estimated renal survival (doubling of serum creatinine as event) in CSA group was 33 per cent and in TACc group was 79 per cent (Prasad et al., 2018).

The response to RTX in children with steroid-resistant NS seems to be highly variable. It should be noted, however, that serum half-life of RTX can be extremely short, due to excessive urinary losses in patients with NS and nonselective proteinuria (Councilman et al., 2015). Bagga and colleagues (2003) reported the successful use of RTX in two patients with MCD and steroid-resistant NS. In another series of four children, all patients failed to achieve sustained remission after a single dose of RTX, despite complete B-cell depletion (Kari et al., 2011). In a larger study, only five of 24 children achieved complete remission, but four of them had frequent relapses that required MMF administration (Basu et al., 2015). An association between RTX and high-dose methylprednisolone pulses obtained complete remission in 7/10 children with steroid resistant NS, but at a price of serious side-effects (Kamei et al., 2014). Anecdotal cases of success with RTX in adults with refractory steroid-unresponsive NS have been reported (Bruchfeld et al., 2014; Janardan et al., 2014; Brown et al., 2017).

In summary, the results of treatment in the uncommonly seen steroid-resistant nephrotic patients with MCD are often disappointing but variable. The difference may be accounted for by the fact that some series considered only patients who maintained a histological picture of MCD, while most other papers also included patients who developed FSGS later. It is also possible that the diagnosis of MCD was incorrect in the patients included as steroid resistant, most likely due to the under-diagnosis of FSGS from a 'sampling error' in the original diagnostic renal biopsy. Moreover, the definition of steroid resistance varied considerably in the different studies, introducing another bias which makes it difficult to assess the effects of treatment. Finally, even when the same drug was used, the doses and durations of treatment varied considerably. For all these reasons, a reappraisal of the overall effectiveness of any form of treatment in so-called steroid-resistant MCD is impossible at present. The use of angiotensin-converting enzyme inhibitors and angiotensin receptor blockers is recommended as these drugs not only allow to reduce proteinuria but may also be protective on renal function. Statins are also recommended not only to reduce lipid levels, but also because they may have a protective role against cardiovascular disease and may even reduce proteinuria. Most children (Selewski et al., 2016) and adults (Aggarwal et al., 2016) with NS have 25(OH)D deficiency. Administration of vitamin D is recommended not only to prevent bone disease, but also to exploit its antiproteinuric effects (Humalda et al., 2015). Oral or IV administration of N-acetyl-D-mannosamine, a naturally occurring precursor of sialic acid, can improve sialylation of angiopoietin-like protein 4 in vivo, and reduces proteinuria by over 40 per cent in different experimental models of NS (Chugh et al., 2014). Some phase 1–2 clinical trials with pilot studies to evaluate the safety and efficacy of N-acetyl-D-mannosamine, abatacept (a fusion protein that prevents the costimulation by binding to CD80 and CD86 so preventing their binding to CD 28) and retinoids (which may prevent proteinuria by protecting the podocytes from injury in an experimental model of MCD) in different diseases are under evaluation (Ravani et al., 2017).

Practical recommendations

Congenital NS, which develops soon after birth, is due to mutations of genes encoding for podocyte proteins. Mutation screening is therefore necessary in children with NS under one to two years of age, while it is not recommended over this age. Among the many genes with reported mutations, abnormalities in NPHS2, WT1, and NPHS1 were most commonly identified in the PodoNet registry (Trautmann et al., 2015).

Although MCD is idiopathic in the large majority of cases, a careful medical history is important to exclude the cases secondary to drug exposure, allergies, or other diseases, especially in adolescents and adults. Clinical examination is also important. An underlying lymphoma should be suspected in patients with adenopathy, fever, sweating, and/or pruritus.

Idiopathic MCD may develop a spontaneous remission (in up to 40 per cent of cases) but it usually takes months (or even years), thus exposing the patient to the undesirable and potentially dangerous effects of an untreated nephrotic state. A simple measure which may be effective in a few children is search and elimination of allergens (cow's milk) in those with a strong history of allergies. However, most patients will remain nephrotic. In the face of the potential risks of prolonged, full-blown NS, including venous thrombo-embolism, we recommend an aggressive approach in line with Glassock (1993):

i. Prolonged heavy proteinuria may result, of itself, in irreversible glomerular lesions.

ii. Hyperlipidaemia, hyperfibrinogememia, and serum protein deficiencies have undesirable and potentially harmful effects (such as favouring thrombosis or atherogenesis).

iii. The side-effects of aggressive therapy are minimal, controllable, and reversible when the treatment is brief and the dosage not excessive.

While in favour of aggressive treatment not only in children, but also in older patients with NS, we recommend a 'wait-and-see' policy for the few patients with symptomless proteinuria, unless they develop full NS.

Initial treatment

Although the influence of initial treatment duration on the rate of subsequent relapses is still a matter of discussion, we suggest prolonged administration of glucocorticoids as a first approach.

In *children*, we start with 60 mg/m²/day (or 2 mg/kg/day) of prednisone (or equivalent doses of another analogue) as a single dose given between 7 and 9 a.m. for four weeks. This treatment may be prolonged for two additional weeks in the rare cases of no remission. After remission, the child is switched to alternate-day prednisone, 40 mg/m² or 2 mg/kg every 48 hours for at least eight weeks, with subsequent tapering off of prednisone by 5–10 mg/m² (0.5 mg/kg) per 48 hours every two weeks. We conscientiously avoid the rapid discontinuance of steroid therapy as it may precipitate a relapse. Alternate-day administration of the dosage may be preferred since it may reduce the severity of side effects of more prolonged therapy. In children with steroid toxicity we reduce the dosage of prednisone or the time of administration after complete remission.

We treat *adults* with prednisone, 1 mg/kg/day as a single dose between 7 and 9 a.m. There is no objection to initiating therapy with alternate day regimen of

2 mg/kg every other day (maximum dosage 150 mg every other day), although there is no evidence that this regimen actually reduces the risk of side effects in comparison with single-morning daily treatment in adults (Waldman et al., 2007). Initial treatment is given for at least six weeks, or until complete remission. In case of early response with disappearance of proteinuria, we continue prednisone at a dose of 1.6 mg/kg every 48 hours, and reduce the dose by 0.2 to 0.4 mg/kg per 48 hours every fortnight until complete discontinuation. In case of poor response, we continue the initial treatment for at least six to eight weeks. Then, we switch the patient to alternate-day prednisone, 1.6 mg/kg per 48 hours. If there is no remission after three to four months of therapy, we give alternate day prednisone in decreasing doses for a total of six to eight months (if tolerated) before considering an adult to be steroid resistant. In patients older than 65 years of age who are at major risk for iatrogenic side-effects and are less prone to relapses, we taper off the prednisone more rapidly. This schedule is not rigid, but is tailored to an individual patient's needs. We reduce the glucocorticoid doses or stop treatment earlier if any sign of severe hypercortisolism or any steroid-related complication occurs.

Independently of age, for patients who may have contra-indications to high-dose prednisone (e.g. diabetes mellitus, massive obesity, overt cardiovascular disease, severe dyslipidaemia, peripheral obliterative vascular disease, psychiatric disorders, osteoporosis) we start treatment with cyclophosphamide, 2 mg/kg/day for 8–12 weeks, or chlorambucil, 0.15 mg/kg/day for eight weeks. The white blood cell (WBC) count is checked every one or two weeks. If it is below 5,000/mm^3 the dosage of either cyclophosphamide or chlorambucil is reduced by 50 per cent. If the WBC count is below 3,000/mm^3, the drug is temporarily withdrawn. Usually lymphopenia precedes total leucopoenia, so a differential count is useful. We do not repeat treatment with alkylating agents in case of further relapse and in order to avoid cumulative doses >200–300 mg/kg that may expose patients to long-term severe adverse events.

As an alternative to cytotoxic drugs, CsA or TAC, MMF or RTX may be used for *primary* therapy of MCD in patients at high risk of complications from steroids or alkylating agents or in patients who refuse cytotoxic agents if they or their doctors are concerned about adverse effects.

Infrequent relapses

Relapses may be triggered by infectious episodes or even immunizations and sometimes spontaneously remit after infection has been treated and cured. Whether to treat the relapse immediately in order to prevent the complications of a full NS, or whether to wait for a spontaneous remission in order to avoid unnecessary glucocorticoid administration is debatable. We prefer to wait for

7–10 days before starting prednisone, but if severe proteinuria with intractable oedema is present or appears, we recommend starting treatment earlier. The standard therapy consists of 60 mg/m^2/day (or 2 mg/kg/day) for children and of 1 mg/kg/day for adults. This dosage is given until the urine is protein free for three consecutive days. Then we give prednisone every other day for four weeks, at a dose of 40 mg/m^2 per 48 hours for children and of 0.75 mg/kg per 48 hours for adults. The maximum duration of prednisone for patients who do not respond early is similar to that of the first episode.

Frequently relapsing and steroid-dependent patients

If *frequently relapsing* and *steroid-dependent* patients have no sign of hypercorticism, they can be treated with glucocorticoids again. However, instead of high-dose oral prednisone we prefer to administer three pulses of IV methylprednisolone (10–15 mg/kg each) followed by oral prednisone 0.5 mg/kg/day until remission. Both RCT (Ponticelli et al., 1980) and retrospective studies (Fukudome et al., 2012; Shinzawa et al., 2014; Zhao et al., 2015) reported that such a schedule can obtain a more rapid remission and seems to expose the patient to fewer side-effects than high-dose prednisone. After remission, we continue prednisone 0.5 mg/kg/day for two to four weeks and then switch to alternate-day prednisone (1 mg/kg per 48 hours). We reduce the dose by 0.1 mg/kg per 48 hours trying to identify the minimal effective dose. Clearly at low dosages, prolonged glucocorticoid therapy usually does not pose any particular problem. Repeat administrations of IV methylprednisolone pulses followed by alternate-day prednisone are well tolerated by other patients.

However, a number of patients develop signs of hypercorticism and others, psychologically depressed by the frequent relapses, ask for a 'more powerful' drug. A short course of an alkylating agent, which is usually well tolerated and can obtain a sustained remission in a number of patients, has been the preferred alternative option in the past. Today, however, this treatment is rarely used in the US for the initial treatment of frequently relapsing MCD. In young males, oral cyclophosphamide is preferable to chlorambucil because it is less gonadotoxic. When using cyclophosphamide, it is better not to exceed a dose of 2 mg/kg/day. With chlorambucil, the dose should not exceed 0.15 mg/kg/day. Since the duration of treatment influences the response, cytotoxic therapy may be extended to 12 weeks in steroid-dependent patients and in frequent relapsers. With a dose of 2 mg/kg/day, the cumulative dosage of cyclophosphamide is 168 mg/kg, which is below the estimated threshold of gonadal toxicity in males (200–250 mg/kg). The cumulative dose of chlorambucil with daily dose of 0.15 mg/kg would be 12.6 mg/kg, an amount which could result in azoospermia in a few male patients, since the estimated threshold of testicular toxicity is between 10 and 20 mg/kg (the ovary seems to be more resistant). Thus, when using chlorambucil it is safer to limit the period of treatment to eight weeks. If the NS relapses, in our opinion the patient should not be treated again with alkylating agents, since their toxicity is cumulative.

If alkylating agents are not used or in case of relapses after a cycle with either cytotoxic drug, we again give glucocorticoids to obtain remission and then we prescribe cyclosporine Neoral or tacrolimus.

CsA is administered at a dose of 100–125 mg/m^2/day in children under six years of age, 100 mg/m^2/day for children between six and 16 years and 4 mg/kg/day for patients over 16 years. We check through whole-blood levels, after two for four weeks initially and then every two to three months, both to verify the compliance of the patient and to keep blood levels below an arbitrary threshold of 120 ng/ml, as assessed by the monoclonal assay or with the high-performance liquid chromatography (HPLC) method. If the patient remains in remission, CsA may be reduced after 6–12 months by 25 per cent every two months, to determine the minimal effective dose. If a patient maintains remission with CsA doses of 2–2.5 mg/kg/day or less, therapy may be continued for years with low risk of side-effects. However, these patients should be regularly monitored and some authorities recommend they receive a renal biopsy every two to three years to check for histological evidence of nephrotoxicity (Cattran et al., 2007). In the other cases, we prefer to stop CsA gradually after two years. TAC is given at an initial dose of 0.1 mg/kg/day and in patients with remission we gradually reduce the dose to 0.05 mg/kg/day. Like for CsA, we check blood levels after two to four weeks and every two to three months thereafter.

If patients continue to have frequent relapses of NS, the best option is represented by RTX. Its use may allow to reduce or avoid the use of prednisone or calcineurin inhibitors for many weeks or months. On the basis of the experience with this drug it is better first to induce remission with glucocorticoids and then administer RTX in order to maintain a stable remission. In case of further relapses, administration of RTX may be repeated several times, apparently without serious adverse events, but we cannot verify the safety of repeated courses in the very long term (Figure 4.2).

If RTX cannot be used, different drugs (including glucocorticoids, mycophenolic acid, or cytotoxic agents if not already used) may be rotated. If the patient relapses, we treat again with glucocorticoids for 6–12 months and then again with a calcineurin inhibitor for a further one to two years in order to prevent the potential toxicity of prolonged administration of either drug. Before beginning a second course of CsA or TAC, we advise a renal biopsy,

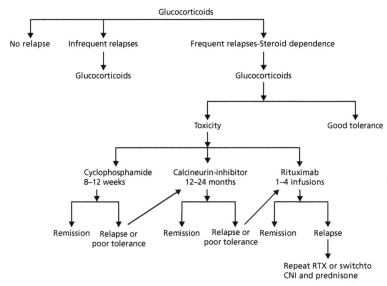

Figure 4.2 Possible therapeutic approaches in frequent relapsers and steroid-dependent patients with MCD. Rituximab may be repeated several times in case of relapses.

which may detect the presence of CNI -related lesions. For those patients who develop hypertrichosis, CsA may be replaced by TAC.

Steroid-resistant patients

Patients with a histologic 'diagnosis' of MCD who do not respond to a sufficiently prolonged course of high-dose glucocorticoids (orally and/or intravenously), as mentioned, almost always show, sooner or later, FSGS in a more careful examination of the original renal biopsy or upon a repeat renal biopsy, and should be treated accordingly. In the very few cases showing only minimal abnormalities at the initial or repeat renal biopsy, an attempt at therapy with CsA, TAC, or either drug combined with prednisone and mycophenolic acid may be tried. RTX was helpful in sporadic cases, but probably the definition of steroid-resistance was inappropriate in those patients. Indeed, RTX proved to be ineffective in true steroid-resistant patients. Repeat renal biopsies are almost never indicated in patients who display an initial pathological diagnosis of MCD and who pursue a glucocorticoid treatment-responsive, though relapsing, course. Even if a lesion of FSGS is discovered in such repeat biopsies, the course of treatment recommended would not be altered as a result of this finding.

Transplantation

Occasional cases of *de novo* MCD in renal transplants meeting strict clinical–pathologic criteria for this diagnosis have been reported, sometimes after ABO-incompatible kidney transplantation (Mochizuchi et al., 2012). NS is the usual presentation (Zafarmand et al., 2002; Nongnuch et al., 2014), but reversible AKI may also occur. The disease develops early after transplantation, usually within four months. Steroids, ACE-inhibitors, and angiotensin receptor blockers have been used. A sustained remission of proteinuria can be achieved in most cases within a year, but some patients may enter remission only after three or more years (Zafarmand et al., 2002). Theoretically, MCD may recur in the transplanted kidney, but because typical MCD so rarely produces renal failure, the opportunity to observe such a recurrence is exceedingly uncommon.

References

Aggarwal A, Yadav AK, Ramachandran R, et al. (2016). Bioavailable vitamin D levels are reduced and correlate with bone mineral density and markers of mineral metabolism in adults with nephrotic syndrome. Nephrology (Carlton). 21: 483–9.

Aguiar-Bujanda D, Blanco-Sánchez MJ, Hernández-Sosa M, et al. (2015). Late-onset neutropenia after rituximab-containing therapy for non-Hodgkin lymphoma. Clin Lymphoma Myeloma Leuk. 15: 761–5.

Aizawa-Yashiro T, Tsuruga K, Watanabe S, et al. (2011). Novel multidrug therapy for children with cyclosporine-resistant or -intolerant nephrotic syndrome. Pediatr Nephrol. 26: 1255–61.

Andersen RF, Palmfeldt J, Jespersen B, et al. (2012). Plasma and urine proteomic profiles in childhood idiopathic nephrotic syndrome. Proteomics Clin Appl. 6: 382–93.

Ando D, Yosuda G. (2016). Blood pressure rhythm is changed by improvement in hypoalbuminemia and massive proteinuria in patients with minimal change nephrotic syndrome. Cardiorenal Med. 6: 209–15.

Audard V, Zhang SY, Copie-Bergman C, et al. (2010). Occurrence of minimal change nephrotic syndrome in classical Hodgkin lymphoma is closely related to the induction of c-mip in Hodgkin-Reed Sternberg cells and podocytes. Blood. 115: 3756–62.

Baek HS, Park KS, Kang HG, et al. (2015). Initial steroid regimen in idiopathic nephrotic syndrome can be shortened based on duration to first remission. Korean J Pediatr. 58: 206–10.

Bagga A, Hari P, Moudgil A, et al. (2003). Mycophenolate mofetil and prednisolone therapy in children with steroid-dependent nephrotic syndrome. Am J Kidney Dis. 42: 1114–20.

Barisoni L. (2012). Podocyte biology in segmental sclerosis and progressive glomerular injury. Adv Chronic Kidney Dis. 19: 76–83.

Basu B, Mahapatra TK, Mondal N. (2015). Mycophenolate mofetil following rituximab in children with steroid-resistant nephrotic syndrome. Pediatrics. 136: e132–9.

Berger JR, Neltner J, Smith C, et al. (2014). Posterior reversible encephalopathy syndrome masquerading as progressive multifocal leukoencephalopathy in rituximab treated neuromyelitis optica. Mult Scler Relat Disord. 3: 728–31.

Bock ME, Cohn RA, Ali FN. (2013). Treatment of childhood nephrotic syndrome with long-term, low-dose tacrolimus. Clin Nephrol. **79**: 432–8.

Bonanni A, Bertelli R, Rossi R, et al. (2015). A pilot study of IL2 in drug-resistant idiopathic nephrotic syndrome. PLoS One. **10**: e0138343.

Bonanni A, Calatroni M, D'Alessandro M, et al. (2018). Adverse events linked with the use of chimeric and humanized anti-CD20 antibodies in children with idiopathic nephrotic syndrome. Br J Clin Pharmacol. **84**: 1238–49.

Bouchireb K, Boyer O, Gribouval O, et al. (2014). NPHS2 mutations in steroid-resistant nephrotic syndrome: A mutation update and the associated phenotypic spectrum. Hum Mutat. **35**: 178–86.

Brown LC, Jobson MA, Payan Schober F, et al. (2017). The evolving role of rituximab in adult minimal change glomerulopathy. Am J Nephrol. **45**: 365–72.

Bruchfeld A, Benedek S, Hilderman M, et al. (2014). Rituximab for minimal change disease in adults: Long-term follow-up. Nephrol Dial Transplant. **29**: 851–6.

Büscher AK, Beck BB, Melk A, et al. (2016). Rapid response to cyclosporin A and favorable renal outcome in nongenetic versus genetic steroid-resistant nephrotic syndrome. Clin J Am Soc Nephrol. **11**: 245–53.

Butani L, Ramsamooj R. (2009). Experience with tacrolimus in children with steroid-resistant nephrotic syndrome. Pediatr Nephrol. **24**: 1517–23.

Cara-Fuentes G, Segarra A, Silva-Sanchez C, et al. (2017). Angiopoietin-like-4 and minimal change disease. PLoS One.**12**: e0176198.

Cara-Fuentes G, Wei C, Segarra A, et al. (2014). CD80 and suPAR in patients with minimal change disease and focal segmental glomerulosclerosis: Diagnostic and pathogenic significance. Pediatr Nephrol. **29**: 1363–71.

Caridi G, Gigante M, Ravani P, et al. (2009). Clinical features and long-term outcome of nephrotic syndrome associated with heterozygous NPHS1 and NPHS2 mutations. Clin J Am Soc Nephrol. **4**: 1065–72.

Cattran DC, Alexopoulos E, Heering P, et al. (2007). Cyclosporin in idiopathic glomerular disease associated with the nephrotic syndrome: Workshop recommendations. Kidney International. **72**: 1429–47.

Choi HJ, Cho HY, Ro H, et al. (2011). Polymorphisms of the MDR1 and MIF genes in children with nephrotic syndrome. Pediatr Nephrol. **26**: 1981–8.

Choudhry S, Bagga A, Hari P, et al. (2009). Efficacy and safety of tacrolimus versus cyclosporine in children with steroid-resistant nephrotic syndrome: A randomized controlled trial. Am J Kidney Dis. **53**: 760–9.

Chugh SS, Macé C, Clement LC, et al. (2014). Angiopoietin-like 4 based therapeutics for proteinuria and kidney disease. Front Pharmacol. **5**: 23.

Clement LC, Macé C, Del Nogal Avila M, et al. (2015). The proteinuria-hypertriglyceridemia connection as a basis for novel therapeutics for nephrotic syndrome. Transl Res. **165**: 499–504.

Colucci M, Carsetti R, Cascioli S, et al. (2016). B-cell reconstitution after rituximab treatment in idiopathic nephrotic syndrome. J Am Soc Nephrol. **27**: 1211–22.

Counsilman CE, Jol-van der Zijde CM, Stevens J, et al. (2015). Pharmacokinetics of rituximab in a pediatric patient with therapy-resistant nephrotic syndrome. Pediatr Nephrol. **30**: 1367–70.

Dehoux L, Hogan J, Dossier C, et al. (2016). Mycophenolate mofetil in steroid-dependent idiopathic nephrotic syndrome. Pediatr Nephrol. **31**: 2095–101.

Dekkers MJ, Groothoff JW, Zietse R, et al. (2015). A series of patients with minimal change nephropathy treated with rituximab during adolescence and adulthood. BMC Res Notes. **8**: 266.

Dhandapani MC, Venkatesan V, Rengaswamy NB, et al. (2015). Association of ACE and MDR1 gene polymorphisms with steroid resistance in children with idiopathic nephrotic syndrome. Genet Test Mol Biomarkers. **19**: 454–6.

Dorresteijn EM, Kist-van Holthe JE, Levtchenko EN, et al. (2008). Mycophenolate mofetil versus cyclosporine for remission maintenance in nephrotic syndrome. Pediatr Nephrol. **23**: 2013–20.

Dorval G, Gribouval O, Martinez-Barquero V, et al. (2018). Clinical and genetic heterogeneity in familial steroid-sensitive nephrotic syndrome. Ped Nephrol. **33**: 473–83.

Eguchi A, Takei T, Yoshida T, et al. (2010). Combined cyclosporine and prednisolone therapy in adult patients with the first relapse of minimal-change nephrotic syndrome. Nephrol Dial Transplant. **25**: 124–9.

Fabrizi F, Cresseri D, Fogazzi GB, et al. (2015). Rituximab therapy for primary glomerulonephritis: Report on two cases. World J Clin Cases. **16**: 736–42.

Fan L, Liu Q, Liao Y, et al. (2013). Tacrolimus is an alternative therapy option for the treatment of adult steroid-resistant nephrotic syndrome: A prospective, multicenter clinical trial. Int Urol Nephrol. **45**: 459–68.

Faul C, Donnelly M, Merscher-Gomez S, et al. (2008). The actin cytoskeleton of kidney podocytes is a direct target of the antiproteinuric effect of cyclosporine A. Nat Med. **14**: 931–8.

Fidan C, Kantar A, Baskin E, et al. (2015). Effects of hyperuricemia on renal function in pediatric renal transplant recipients. Exp Clin Transplant. **13**: 247–50.

Filippone EJ, Dopson SJ, Rivers DM, et al. (2016). Adrenocorticotropic hormone analog use for podocytopathies. Int Med Case Rep J. **9**: 125–33.

François H, Daugas E, Bensman A, et al. (2007). Unexpected efficacy of rituximab in multirelapsing minimal change nephrotic syndrome in the adult: First case report and pathophysiological considerations. Am J Kidney Dis. **49**: 158–61.

Fujinaga S, Someya T, Watanabe T, et al. (2013). Cyclosporine versus mycophenolate mofetil for maintenance of remission of steroid-dependent nephrotic syndrome after a single infusion of rituximab. Eur J Pediatr. **172**: 513–18.

Fujiwara A, Hirawa N, Kobayashi Y, et al. (2015). Efficacy of cyclosporine combination therapy for new-onset minimal change nephrotic syndrome in adults. Clin Exp Nephrol. **19**: 240–6.

Fukudome K, Fujimoto S, Sato Y, et al. (2012). Comparison of the effects of intravenous methylprednisolone pulse versus oral prednisolone therapies on the first attack of minimal-change nephrotic syndrome in adults. Nephrology (Carlton). **17**: 263–8.

Garin EH, Mu W, Arthur JM, et al. (2010). Urinary CD80 is elevated in minimal change disease but not in focal segmental glomerulosclerosis. Kidney Int. **78**: 296–302.

Geier P, Roushdi A, Skálová S, et al. (2012). Is cyclophosphamide effective in patients with IgM-positive minimal change disease? Pediatr Nephrol. **27**: 2227–31.

Gellermann J, Ehrich JH, Querfeld U, et al. (2012). Sequential maintenance therapy with cyclosporin A and mycophenolate mofetil for sustained remission of childhood steroid-resistant nephrotic syndrome. Nephrol Dial Transplant. **27**: 1970–8.

Gellermann J, Weber L, Pape L, et al. (2013). Mycophenolate mofetil versus cyclosporin A in children with frequently relapsing nephrotic syndrome. J Am Soc Nephrol. **24**: 1689–97.

Glassock RJ. (2003). Secondary minimal change disease. Nephrol Dial Transplant. **18**: S52–8.

Greenbaum LA, Benndorf R, Smoyer WE. (2012). Childhood nephrotic syndrome-current and future therapies. Nat Rev Nephrol. **8**: 445–58.

Gruppen MP, Bouts AH, Jansen-van der Weide MC, et al. (2018). A randomized with steroid-sensitive idiopathic nephrotic syndrome clinical trial indicates that levamisole increases the time to relapse in children. Kidney Int. **93**: 510–18.

Guitard J, Hebral AL, Fakhouri F, et al. (2014). Rituximab for minimal-change nephrotic syndrome in adulthood: Predictive factors for response, long-term outcomes and tolerance. Nephrol Dial Transplant. **29**: 2084–91.

Gulati A, Prasad N, Sharma RK, et al. (2008). Tacrolimus: A new therapy for steroid-resistant nephrotic syndrome in children. Nephrol Dial Transplant. **23**: 910–13.

Gulati A, Sinha A, Gupta A, et al. (2012). Treatment with tacrolimus and prednisolone is preferable to intravenous cyclophosphamide as the initial therapy for children with steroid-resistant nephrotic syndrome. Kidney Int. **82**: 1130–5.

Hahn D, Hodson EM, Willis NS, et al. (2015). Corticosteroid therapy for nephrotic syndrome in children. Cochrane Database Syst Rev. **18**(3): CD001533. DOI: 10.1002/14651858.CD001533.pub5.

Hamasaki Y, Yoshikawa N, Nakazato H, et al. (2013). Prospective 5-year follow-up of cyclosporine treatment in children with steroid-resistant nephrosis. Pediatr Nephrol. **28**: 765–71.

Han SH, Park SY, Li JJ, et al. (2008). Glomerular glucocorticoid receptor expression is reduced in late responders to steroids in adult-onset minimal change disease. Nephrol Dial Transplant. **23**: 169–75.

Haruhara K, Tsuboi N, Koike K, et al. (2017). Circadian blood pressure abnormalities in patients with primary nephrotic syndrome. Clin Exp Hypertens. **39**: 155–9.

Hashimura Y, Nozu K, Kanegane H, et al. (2009). Minimal change nephrotic syndrome associated with immune dysregulation, polyendocrinopathy, enteropathy, X-limked syndrome. Pediatr Nephrol. **24**: 1181–6.

Hayashi K, Sasamura H, Nakamura M, et al. (2015). Renin-angiotensin blockade resets podocyte epigenome through Kruppel-like Factor 4 and attenuates proteinuria. Kidney Int. **88**: 745–53.

Hayek SS, Sever S, Ko YA, et al. (2015). Soluble urokinase receptor and chronic kidney disease. N Engl J Med. **373**: 1916–25.

Heymann J, Winkler CA, Hoek M, et al. (2017). Therapeutics for APOL1 nephropathies: Putting out the fire in the podocyte. Nephrol Dial Transplant. **32**: i65–70.

Hodgin JB, Rasoulpour M, Markowitz GM, et al. (2009). Very low birth weight is a risk factor for secondary focal segmental glomerulosclerosis. Clin J Am Soc Nephrol **4**: 71–6.

Hodson EM, Wong SC, Willis NS, et al. (2016). Interventions for idiopathic steroid-resistant nephrotic syndrome in children. Cochrane Database Syst Rev. **10**: CD003594.

Hogan J, Radhakrishnan J. (2013). The treatment of minimal change disease in adults. J Am Soc Nephrol. **24**: 702–11.

Huang MJ, Wei RB, Su TY, et al. (2016). Impact of acute kidney injury on coagulation in adult minimal change nephropathy. Medicine (Baltimore). **95**: e5366.

Humalda JK, Goldsmith DJ, Thadhani R, et al. (2015). Vitamin D analogues to target residual proteinuria: Potential impact on cardiorenal outcomes. Nephrol Dial Transplant. **30**: 1988–94.

Iijima K, Sako M, Nozu K, et al. (2017). Rituximab for nephrotic syndrome in children. Clin Exp Nephrol. **21**: 193–202.

Ikezumi Y, Suzuki T, Karasawa T, et al. (2013). Low birthweight and premature birth are risk factors for podocytopenia and focal segmental glomerulosclerosis. Am J Nephrol. **38**: 149–57.

Inoue M, Yumura W, Morishita Y, et al. (2013). Patients with adult minimal change nephrotic syndrome treated with long-term cyclosporine did not experience a reduction in their eGFR. Clin Nephrol. **79**: 101–6.

Ishikura K, Ikeda M, Hattori S, et al. (2008). Effective and safe treatment with cyclosporine in nephrotic children: A prospective, randomized multicenter trial. Kidney Int. **73**: 1167–73.

Ishimoto T, Shimada M, Gabriela G, et al. (2013). Toll-like receptor 3 ligand, polyIC, induces proteinuria and glomerular CD80, and increases urinary CD80 in mice. Nephrol Dial Transplant. **28**: 1439–46.

Iwabuchi Y, Takei T, Moriyama T, et al. (2014). Long-term prognosis of adult patients with steroid-dependent minimal change nephrotic syndrome following rituximab treatment. Medicine (Baltimore). **93**(29): e300.

Jafar T, Prasad N, Agarwal V, et al. (2011). MDR-1 gene polymorphisms in steroid-responsive versus steroid-resistant nephrotic syndrome in children. Nephrol Dial Transplant. **26**: 3968–74.

Janardan J, Ooi K, Menahem S. (2014). Sustained complete remission of steroid- and cyclophosphamide-resistant minimal-change disease with a single course of rituximab therapy. Clin Kidney J. **7**: 293–5.

Jiang L, Dasgupta I, Hurcombe JA, et al. (2015). Levamisole in steroid-sensitive nephrotic syndrome: Usefulness in adult patients and laboratory insights into mechanisms of action via direct action on the kidney podocyte. Clin Sci (Lond). **128**: 883–93.

Joshi S, Andersen R, Jespersen B, et al. (2013). Genetics of steroid-resistant nephrotic syndrome: A review of mutation spectrum and suggested approach for genetic testing. Acta Paediatr. **102**: 844–56.

Kamei K, Okada M, Sato M, et al. (2014). Rituximab treatment combined with methylprednisolone pulse therapy and immunosuppressants for childhood steroid-resistant nephrotic syndrome. Pediatr Nephrol. **29**: 1181–7.

Kaneko K, Tsuji S, Kimata T. (2017). Role of gut microbiota in idiopathic nephrotic syndrome in children. Med Hypotheses. **108**: 35–7.

Kanemoto K, Ito H, Anzai M, et al. (2013). Clinical significance of IgM and C1q deposition in the mesangium in pediatric idiopathic nephrotic syndrome. J Nephrol. **26**: 306–14.

Kari JA, El-Morshedy SM, El-Desoky S, et al. (2011). Rituximab for refractory cases of childhood nephrotic syndrome. Pediatr Nephrol. **26**: 733–7.

KDIGO. (2012). Clinical Practice Guideline for Glomerulonephritis. Kidney Int. **2S**: 1–274.

Kim JS, Bellew CA, Silverstein DM, et al. (2006). High incidence of initial and late steroid resistance in childhood nephrotic syndrome. Kidney Int. **68**: 1275–81.

Kofman T, Zhang SY, Copie-Bergman C, et al. (2014). Minimal change nephrotic syndrome associated with non-Hodgkin lymphoid disorders: A retrospective study of 18 cases. Medicine (Baltimore). **93**: 350–8.

Koukoulaki M, Goumenos DS. (2010). The accumulated experience with the use of mycophenolate mofetil in primary glomerulonephritis. Expert Opin Investig Drugs. **19**: 673–87.

Kranz B, Vester U, Büscher R, et al. (2008). Cyclosporine-A-induced nephrotoxicity in children with minimal-change nephrotic syndrome: Long-term treatment up to 10 years. Pediatric Nephrology. **23**: 581–6.

Kyrieleis HA, Löwik MM, Pronk I, et al. (2009). Long-term outcome of biopsy-proven, frequently relapsing minimal-change nephrotic syndrome in children. Clin J Am Soc Nephrol. **4**: 1593–600.

Lande MB, Gullion C, Hogg RJ, et al. (2004). Long versus standard initial steroid therapy for children with the nephrotic syndrome: A report from the Southwest Pediatric Nephrology Study Group. Pediatr Nephrol. **18**: 342–6.

Latta K, von Schnakenburg C, Ehrich JH. (2001). A meta-analysis of cytotoxic treatment for frequently relapsing nephrotic syndrome in children. Pediatr Nephrol. **16**: 271–82.

Lee H, Yoo KD, Oh YK. (2016). Predictors of relapse in adult-onset nephrotic minimal change disease. Medicine (Baltimore). **95**: e3179.

Lee SW, Yu MY, Baek SH, et al. (2016). Glomerular hypertrophy is a risk factor for relapse in minimal change disease patients. Nephron. **132**: 43–50.

Li JS, Chen X, Peng L, et al. (2015). Angiopoietin-like-4, a potential target of tacrolimus, predicts earlier podocyte injury in minimal change disease. PLoS One. **10**: e0137049.

Li X, Li H, Chen J, et al. (2008). Tacrolimus as a steroid-sparing agent for adults with steroid-dependent minimal change nephrotic syndrome. Nephrol Dial Transplant. **23**: 1919 25.

Li X, Li H, Ye H, et al. (2009). Tacrolimus therapy in adults with steroid- and cyclophosphamide-resistant nephrotic syndrome and normal or mildly reduced GFR. Am J Kidney Dis. **54**: 51–8.

Li X, Liu Z, Wang L, et al. (2017). Tacrolimus monotherapy after intravenous methylprednisolone in adults with minimal change nephrotic syndrome. J Am Soc Nephrol. **28**: 1286–95.

Lieberman KV, Pavlova-Wolf A. (2017). Adrenocorticotropic hormone therapy for the treatment of idiopathic nephrotic syndrome in children and young adults: A systematic review of early clinical studies with contemporary relevance. J Nephrol. **30**: 35–44.

Lipska BS, Iatropoulos P, Maranta R, et al. (2013). Genetic screening in adolescents with steroid-resistant nephrotic syndrome. Kidney Int. **84**: 206–13.

Lovric S, Ashraf S, Tan W, et al. (2016). Genetic testing in steroid-resistant nephrotic syndrome: When and how? Nephrol Dial Transplant. **31**: 1813–21.

Madan A, Mijovic-Das S, Stankovic A, et al. (2016). Acthar gel in the treatment of nephrotic syndrome: A multicenter retrospective case series. BMC Nephrol. **31**: 37.

McGrogan A, Franssen CFM, de Vries CS. (2011). The incidence of primary glomerulonephritis worldwide: A systematic review of the literature. Nephrol Dial Transplant. **26**: 414–43.

Meyrier A, Noel H, Auriche P, et al. (1994). Long-term renal tolerance of cyclosporin A treatment in adult idiopathic nephrotic syndrome. Kidney International. **45**: 1446–56.

Miura K, Nakatani T, Asai T, et al. (2002). Role of hypomagnesemia in chronic cyclosporine nephropathy. Transplantation. **73**: 340–7.

Miyabe Y, Takei T, Iwabuchi Y, et al. (2016). Amelioration of the adverse effects of prednisolone by rituximab treatment in adults with steroid-dependent minimal-change nephrotic syndrome. Clin Exp Nephrol. **20**: 103–10.

Miyazaki K, Miyazawa T, Sugimoto K, et al. (2011). An adolescent with marked hyperimmunoglobulinemia E showing minimal change nephrotic syndrome and a STAT3 gene mutation. Clin Nephrol. **75**: 369–73.

Mochizuki Y, Iwata T, Nishikido M, et al. (2012). *De novo* minimal change disease after ABO-incompatible kidney transplantation. Clin Transplant. **26**: 81–5.

Moysés-Neto M, Costa RS, Rodrigues FF, et al. (2011). Minimal change disease: A variant of lupus nephritis. NDT Plus. **4**: 20–2.

Moysés-Neto M, Silva GE, Costa RS, et al. (2012). Minimal change disease associated with type 1 and type 2 diabetes mellitus. Arq Bras Endocrinol Metabol. **56**: 331–5.

Munyentwali H, Bouachi K, Audard V, et al. (2013). Rituximab is an efficient and safe treatment in adults with steroid-dependent minimal change disease. Kidney Int. **83**: 511–16.

Nagata M. (2016). Podocyte injury and its consequences. Kidney Int. **89**: 1221–30.

Niaudet P. (2009). Long-term outcome of children with steroid-sensitive idiopathic nephrotic syndrome. Clin J Am Soc Nephrol. **4**: 1547–8.

Nongnuch A, Assanatham M, Sumethkul V, et al. (2014). Early post-transplant nephrotic range proteinuria as a presenting feature of minimal change disease and acute T-cell-mediated rejection. Transplant Proc. **46**: 290–4.

Nozu K, Iijima K, Fujisawa M, et al. (2005). Rituximab treatment for post-transplant lymphoproliferative disorder (PTLD) induces complete remission of recurrent nephrotic syndrome. Pediatr Nephrol. **20**: 1660–3.

Pinto B, Dhir V, Krishnan S, et al. (2013). Leflunomide-induced DRESS syndrome with renal involvement and vasculitis. Clin Rheumatol. **32**: 689–93.

Pollak MR, Quaggin SE, Hoenig MP, et al. (2014). The glomerulus: the sphere of influence. Clin J Am Soc Nephrol. **9**: 1461–9.

Ponticelli C, Imbasciati E, Case N, et al. (1980). Intravenous methylprednisolone in minimal change nephrotic syndrome. Br Med J. **280**: 685.

Prasad N, Manjunath R, Rangaswamy D, et al. (2018). Efficacy and safety of cyclosporine versus tacrolimus in steroid and cyclophosphamide resistant nephrotic syndrome: A prospective study. Indian J Nephrol. **28**: 46–52.

Pravitsitthikul N, Willis NS, Hodson EM, et al. (2013). Non-corticosteroid immunosuppressive medications for steroid-sensitive nephrotic syndrome in children. Cochrane Database Syst Rev. **10**: CD002290.

Radhakrishnan J, Perazella MA. (2015). Drug-induced glomerular disease: Attention required! Clin J Am Soc Nephrol. **10**: 1287–90.

Ramamoorthy S, Cidlowski JA. (2016). Corticosteroids: Mechanisms of action in health and disease. Rheum Dis Clin North Am. **42**: 15–31.

Raman V, Krishnamurthy S, Harichandrakumar KT. (2016). Body weight-based prednisolone versus body surface area-based prednisolone regimen for induction of remission in children with nephrotic syndrome: A randomized, open-label, equivalence clinical trial. Pediatr Nephrol. **31**: 595–604.

Ranganathan S. (2016). Pathology of podocytopathies causing nephrotic syndrome in children. Front Pediatr. **4**: 32.

Rankin AJ, McQuarrie EP, Fox JG, et al. (2017). Venous thromboembolism in primary nephrotic syndrome—Is the risk high enough to justify prophylactic anticoagulation? Nephron. **135**: 39–45.

Ravani P, Bertelli E, Gill S, et al. (2017). Clinical trials in minimal change disease. Nephrol Dial Transplant. **32**: i7–i13.

Ravani P, Bonanni A, Rossi R, et al. (2016). Anti-CD20 antibodies for idiopathic nephrotic syndrome in children. Clin J Am Soc Nephrol. **11**: 710–20.

Ravani P, Rossi R, Bonanni A, et al. (2015). Rituximab in children with steroid-dependent nephrotic syndrome: A multicenter, open-label, noninferiority, randomized controlled trial. J Am Soc Nephrol. **26**: 2259–66.

Reiser J, von Gersdorff G, Loos M, et al. (2004). Induction of B7-1 in podocytes is associated with nephrotic syndrome. J Clin Invest. **113**: 1390–7.

Rheault MN, Zhang L, Selewski DT, et al. (2015). AKI in children hospitalized with nephrotic syndrome. Clin J Am Soc Nephrol. **10**: 2110–18.

Roberti I, Vyas S. (2010). Long-term outcome of children with steroid-resistant nephrotic syndrome treated with tacrolimus. Pediatr Nephrol. **25**: 1117–24.

Rostand SG, Cross SK, Kirk KA, et al. (2005). Racial differences in renal arteriolar structure in children with minimal change nephropathy. Kidney Int. **68**: 1154–60.

Ruggenenti P, Ruggiero B, Cravedi P, et al. (2014). Rituximab in steroid-dependent or frequently relapsing idiopathic nephrotic syndrome. J Am Soc Nephrol. **25**: 850–63.

Russo LM, Srivatsan S, Seaman M, et al. (2013). Albuminuria associated with CD2AP knockout mice is primarily due to dysfunction of the renal degradation pathway processing of filtered albumin. FEBS Lett. **587**: 3738–41.

Sandoval D, Poveda R, Draibe J, et al. (2017). Efficacy of mycophenolate treatment in adults with steroid-dependent/frequently relapsing idiopathic nephrotic syndrome. Clin Kidney J. **10**: 632–8.

Savin VJ, Sharma M, Zhou J, et al. (2015). Renal and hematological effects of CLCF-1, a B-cell-stimulating cytokine of the IL-6 family. J Immunol Res. 2015: 714964. DOI: 10.1155/2015/714964.

Selewski DT, Chen A, Shatat IF, et al. (2016). Vitamin D in incident nephrotic syndrome: A Midwest Pediatric Nephrology Consortium study. Pediatr Nephrol. **31**(3): 465–72.

Sepe V, Libetta C, Giuliano MG, et al. (2008). Mycophenolate mofetil in primary glomerulopathies. Kidney International. **73**: 154–62.

Shalhoub TJ. (1974). Pathogenesis of lipoid nephrosis: A disorder of T-cell function. The Lancet. **2**: 556–60.

Shen H, Gu W, Mao J, et al. (2015). Clinical characteristics of concomitant nephrotic IgA nephropathy and minimal change disease in children. Nephron. **130**: 21–8.

Shimada M, Araya C, Rivard C, et al. (2011). Minimal change disease: A 'two-hit' podocyte immune disorder? Pediatr Nephr. **26**: 645–9.

Shinzawa M, Yamamoto R, Nagasawa Y, et al. (2013). Age and prediction of remission and relapse of proteinuria and corticosteroid-related adverse events in adult-onset minimal-change disease: A retrospective cohort study. Clin Exp Nephrol. **17**: 839–47.

Shinzawa M, Yamamoto R, Nagasawa Y, et al. (2014). Comparison of methylprednisolone plus prednisolone with prednisolone alone as initial treatment in adult-onset minimal change disease: A retrospective cohort study. Clin J Am Soc Nephrol. **9**: 1040–8.

Sinha A, Saha A, Kumar M, et al. (2015). Extending initial prednisolone treatment in a randomized control trial from 3 to 6 months did not significantly influence the course of illness in children with steroid-sensitive nephrotic syndrome. Kidney Int. **87**: 217–24.

Siu YP, Tong MK, Leung K, et al. (2008). The use of enteric-coated mycophenolate sodium in the treatment of relapsing and steroid-dependent minimal change disease. J Nephrol. **21**: 127–31.

Sobiak J, Resztak M, Ostalska-Nowicka D, et al. (2015). Monitoring of mycophenolate mofetil metabolites in children with nephrotic syndrome and the proposed novel target values of pharmacokinetic parameters. Eur J Pharm Sci. **77**: 189–96.

Stokes MB, Markowitz GS, Lin J, et al. (2004). Glomerular tip lesion: A distinct entity within the minimal change disease/focal segmental glomerulosclerosis spectrum. Kidney International. **65**: 1690–702.

Suresh CP, Saha A, Kaur M, et al. (2016). Differentially expressed urinary biomarkers in children with idiopathic nephrotic syndrome. Clin Exp Nephrol. **20**: 273–83.

Swartz SJ, Eldin KW, Hicks MJ, et al. (2009). Minimal change disease with IgM+ immunofluorescence: A subtype of nephrotic syndrome. Pediatr Nephrol. **24**: 1187–92.

Szeto CC, Lai FM, Chow KM, et al. (2015). Long-term outcome of biopsy-proven minimal change nephropathy in Chinese adults. Am J Kidney Dis. **65**: 710–18.

Tan Y, Yan D, Fan J, et al. (2011). Elevated levels of immunoglobulin E may indicate steroid resistance or relapse in adult primary nephrotic syndrome, especially in minimal change nephrotic syndrome. J Int Med Res. **39**: 2307–13.

Tanaka H, Tsuruga K, Imaizumi T. (2015). Mizoribine in the treatment of pediatric-onset glomerular disease. World J Pediatr. **11**: 108–12.

Tavil B, Kara F, Topaloglu R, et al. (2015). Case series of thromboembolic complications in childhood nephrotic syndrome: Hacettepe experience. Clin Exp Nephrol. **19**: 506–13.

Teeninga N, Kist-van Holthe JE, van Rijswijk N, et al. (2013). Extending prednisolone treatment does not reduce relapses in childhood nephrotic syndrome. J Am Soc Nephrol. **24**: 149–59.

Teeninga N, Schreuder MF, Bökenkamp A, et al. (2008). Influence of low birth weight on minimal change nephrotic syndrome in children, including a meta-analysis. Nephrol Dial Transplant. **23**: 1615–20.

Tellier S, Dallocchio A, Guigonis V, et al. (2016). Mycophenolic acid pharmacokinetics and relapse in children with steroid-dependent idiopathic nephrotic syndrome. Clin J Am Soc Nephrol. **11**: 1777–82.

Trautmann A, Bodria M, Ozaltin F, et al. (2015). Spectrum of steroid-resistant and congenital nephrotic syndrome in children: The PodoNet registry cohort. Clin J Am Soc Nephrol. **10**: 592–600.

Trautmann A, Schnaidt S, Lipska-Ziętkiewicz B, et al. (2017). Long-term outcome of steroid-resistant nephritic syndrome in children. J Am Soc Nephrol. **28**: 3055–65.

Tryggvason K, Patrakka J, Wartiovaara J. (2006). Hereditary proteinuria syndromes and mechanisms of proteinuria. N Engl J Med. **354**: 1387–401.

Tse KC, Lam MF, Yip PS, et al. (2003). Idiopathic minimal change nephrotic syndrome in older adults: steroid responsiveness and pattern of relapses. Nephrol Dial Transplant. **18**: 1316–20.

Ushijima K, Uemura O, Yamada T. (2012). Age effect on whole blood cyclosporine concentrations following oral administration in children with nephrotic syndrome. Eur J Pediatr. **171**: 663–8.

Vivarelli M, Massella L, Ruggiero B, et al. (2017). Minimal change disease. Clin J Am Soc Nephrol. **12**: 332–45.

Waldman M, Crew RJ, Valeri A, et al. (2007). Adult minimal-change disease: Clinical characteristics, treatment, and outcomes. Clin J Am Soc Nephrol. **2**: 445–53.

Wang W, Xia Y, Mao J, et al. (2012). Treatment of tacrolimus or cyclosporine A in children with idiopathic nephrotic syndrome. Pediatr Nephrol. **27**: 2073–9.

Wong E, Lasica M, He SZ, et al. (2016). Nephrotic syndrome as a complication of chronic graft-versus-host disease after allogeneic haemopoietic stem cell transplantation. Intern Med J. **46**: 737–41.

Yang EM, Lee ST, Choi HJ, et al. (2016). Tacrolimus for children with refractory nephrotic syndrome: A one-year prospective, multicenter, and open-label study of Tacrobell®, a generic formula. World J Pediatr. **12**: 60–5.

Yoshikawa N, Nakanishi K, Sako M, et al. (2015). A multicenter randomized trial indicates initial prednisolone treatment for childhood nephrotic syndrome for two months is not inferior to six-month treatment. Kidney Int. **87**: 225–32.

Youssef DM, Attia TA, El-Shal AS, et al. (2013). Multi-drug resistance-1 gene polymorphisms in nephrotic syndrome: Impact on susceptibility and response to steroids. Gene. **530**: 201–7.

Yu H, Kistler A, Farid MII, et al. (2016). Synaptopodin limits TRPC6 podocyte surface expression and attenuates proteinuria. J Am Soc Nephrol. **27**: 3308–19.

Zafarmand AA, Baranowska-Daca E, Ly PC, et al. (2002). *De novo* minimal change disease associated with reversible post-transplant nephrotic syndrome. A report of five cases and review of the literature. Clin Transplant. **16**: 350–61.

Zahran AM, Aly SS, Elsayh KI, et al. (2014). Glucocorticoid receptors expression and histopathological types in children with nephrotic syndrome. Ren Fail. **36**: 1067–72.

Zhang SY, Kamal M, Dahan K, et al. (2010). c-mip impairs podocyte proximal signaling and induces heavy proteinuria. Sci Signal. **3**: ra39.

Zhao L, Cheng J, Zhou J, et al. (2015). Enhanced steroid therapy in adult minimal change nephrotic syndrome: A systematic review and meta-analysis. Intern Med. **54**: 2101–8.

Chapter 5

Focal and segmental glomerular sclerosis

Claudio Ponticelli, Richard J Glassock, and Francesco Scolari

Introduction and overview

Definition

Focal and segmental glomerular sclerosis (FSGS) is not a single disease. Rather, it is a generic lesion having a variety of morphological variants and underlying aetiologies and pathogenesis. The histological term is used to indicate that, some, but not all, glomeruli (focal) have a partial sclerosis of the tuft (segmental). It is absolutely crucial to recognize that these lesions may complicate a number of other renal diseases, and may be caused by a number of different factors, including hemodynamic changes, infections, neoplasia, drug exposure, genetic mutations, metabolic disorders, or prior inflammation. A diagnosis of primary (idiopathic) FSGS is arrived at when other known causes have been excluded. Since the histopathologic lesion of FSGS is pathogenetically heterogeneous, it is not reasonable to categorize it as a disease diagnosis; nevertheless, its discovery in a renal biopsy of a patient with the 'full blown' nephrotic syndrome (marked proteinuria and hypoalbuminaemia) in the absence of any known cause or associated condition does have important connotations with respect to response to treatment and to long-term outcome. This justifies a categorization of such a clinical-pathological condition under the term of primary (or idiopathic) FSGS. Obviously, such a categorization is a 'diagnosis of exclusion', and its accuracy depends on the vigour of the search for secondary causes. Also, the lesion of FSGS must be distinguished from the lesion of focal and global glomerulosclerosis (FGGS), which is a normal consequence of aging and is very distinct in terms of pathogenesis, management and outcome compared to the lesion of FSGS. These two lesions may co-exist in the same biopsy, depending on the age of the subject. Patients with the primary form of FSGS typically have proteinuria in the nephrotic range (>3.5 g/day in an adult), accompanied by hypo-albuminaemia and the constellation of signs and symptoms of the nephrotic syndrome (NS), and arterial hypertension. A distinct minority of patients may have only asymptomatic non-nephrotic proteinuria (and normal serum albumin levels) and these patients usually do not progress to end-stage renal disease (ESRD). However, the natural course of the FSGS lesion is ominous in most patients with NS. Fortunately, numerous observational (mostly uncontrolled) studies have shown that about 50–60 per cent of patients may respond (in terms of reduced proteinuria) completely or partially to prolonged glucocorticoid therapy or other 'immunosuppressive' treatments and may have a fair outcome in the long term (Rosenberg and Kopp, 2017).

Pathology

At light microscopy the lesions of FSGS initially affect only a few glomeruli and are characterized by sclerosis (collapse and solidification) limited to a portion of the glomerulus. More often the initial sclerotic lesions are distributed at the periphery of otherwise normal glomeruli, sometimes they may be located either at hilum or at the tip of the tuft. Glomeruli unaffected by sclerosis may appear quite normal by light microscopy. The percentage of glomeruli affected is quite variable, but juxta-medullary glomeruli may be preferentially affected at least initially. If only small numbers of glomeruli are affected with the sclerosing lesion, the process of FSGS may go undetected, particularly when the number of glomeruli in the specimen is small (e.g. fewer than ten glomeruli), and the biopsy sample contains only superficial glomeruli. However, in the absence of classic sclerosis the infiltration of foam cells in the glomerular segment should raise the suspicion of FSGS (D'Agati et al., 2011). Varying degrees of FGGS can be observed depending on the age of the patient. Immunofluorescence studies may be negative but IgM and C3 deposits are commonly found in the areas of sclerosis. On electron microscopy there is always diffuse (>80 per cent) effacement of the foot processes of podocytes, in all glomeruli and no or only scanty electron dense deposits in the mesangium, if the patient has NS at the time the biopsy is performed.

A working proposal for subclassification of the lesions of FSGS, based on light microscopy observations, distinguished five mutually exclusive morphologic variants which can be applied to Primary and Secondary forms of FSGS (D'Agati, 2004; Stokes and D'Agati, 2014):

i. The common, generic form of FSGS not otherwise specified (NOS), also known as 'classic' FSGS, is characterized by segmental capillary lumen obliteration by extracellular matrix, with no collapsing, tip, cellular or perihilar lesions (Plate 3).

ii. The tip variant shows at least one glomerulus with a segmental lesion involving the outer 25 per cent of the tuft next to the proximal tubule.

iii. The cellular variant is so-called because of the segmental endocapillary hypercellularity (Plate 4).

iv. In the perihilar variant there is a perihilar hyalinosis involving >50 per cent of the glomeruli with segmental lesions (Plate 5).

v. The collapsing variant, is characterized by global collapse of glomerular capillaries of at least 20 per cent of glomeruli, marked epithelial cell pro-liferation and de-differentiation and clinically by very severe proteinuria and rapid progression to ESRD (see Plate 6). Some believe that collapsing FSGS is a separate and unique clinicopathological entity. On electron mi-croscopy of FSGS, foot process effacement is diffuse and severe in tip, cel-lular and collapsing variants, while they can be more variable in NOS and less severe in the perihilar variant (D'Agati et al., 2011; Sethi et al., 2015). Primary FSGS should be accompanied by diffuse (>80 per cent) efface-ment of the foot process of podocytes by electron microscopy.

By reviewing the biopsies of 138 subjects with apparent primary FSGS participating to a randomized trial, D'Agati and colleagues (2013) reported that the most frequent variant was the NOS in 68 per cent of patients, followed by collapsing in 12 per cent, tip in 10 per cent, perihilar in 7 per cent, and cellular in 3 per cent. However, the true clinical significance of this classification of FSGS remains uncertain. The tip lesion can also be seen in minimal change dis-ease (MCD) and has not been uniformly considered as a typical sign of FSGS (Taneda et al., 2015). On the other hand, although the tip lesion is associated with more frequent complete remission of the NS after steroids, there is an im-portant percentage of patients who develop chronic kidney disease and ESRD (Arias et al., 2011). It has also been pointed out that the collapsing variant is associated with the loss of normal podocyte markers and the expression of de-differentiation markers compared with other variants (Testagrossa et al., 2013). Moreover, the uncommon perihilar variant may be much more often seen in 'secondary' forms of FSGS, such as those seen in oligonephronic states, and the collapsing FSGS lesion may be seen more often in viral-associated (HIV) or drug-induced forms (intravenous [IV] bisphosphonate) of FSGS, particu-larly in association with high-risk alleles at the APOL1 locus in patients of West African ancestry (Kopp et al., 2015). The 'classic' pattern of FSGS is most often seen in patients presenting with the features of Primary FSGS. It is possible that the differences in morphologic subtypes of FSGS may reflect differences in aetiology, pathogenesis, prognosis, or optimal therapy (Choi, 2013).

Since histologic analysis by light microscopy carries high intra- and inter-reader variability a multicentre study, called NEPTUNE, has been organized in the US to systematically apply digital pathology review to morphologic analysis of NS using renal biopsy whole slide imaging for observation-based data collection (Barisoni et al., 2013). In a report, excellent concordance was achieved for interstitial fibrosis and tubular atrophy. Moderate-to-excellent concordance was achieved for all ultrastructural podocyte descriptors, with good-to-excellent concordance for descriptors commonly used in clinical practice, foot process effacement, and microvillous transformation. For all histologic and ultrastructural descriptors tested with sufficient observations, moderate-to-excellent concordance was seen for 31/54, i.e. 57 per cent (Barisoni et al., 2016).

As mentioned previously, the complete evaluation of renal biopsies in nephrotic patients showing FSGS by light microscopy must include electron microscopy. In Primary FSGS the foot process effacement is diffuse and generalized (>80 per cent), affecting even those glomeruli which are not affected by a sclerosing lesion. In secondary forms of FSGS, such as those occurring in oligonephronic states, the foot process effacement is less noticeable, and usually affects less than 50 per cent of the glomerular capillary surface area (De Vriese et al., 2018). Frequently the podocyte will show features of vacuolization, degeneration, hypertrophy, and detachment from the underlying glomerular basement membrane (GBM). Special studies of a research nature demonstrate that the podocyte has undergone de-differentiation to a more primitive state and has lost many cell surface antigens characteristic of the differentiated state (e.g. podocalyxin, synaptopodin). Such de-differentiation of podocytes does not usually occur in the lesion of MCD, which shares with FSGS prominent diffuse effacement of foot processes. Other ultramicroscopic findings are capillary collapse, mesangial expansion and hypercellularity, and occasionally visceral or parietal epithelial cell proliferation, giving rise to a 'pseudo-crescent' appearance. Hyalinosis and foamy podocytes are frequent features of FSGS. These lesions respectively represent the non-specific accumulation of proteins on the subendothelial side of the capillary lumen and cholesterol in podocytes.

The early histological lesions predominate in the juxtamedullary glomeruli but progressively spread to the outer cortex. The lesion starts with hyalinosis of few capillary loops then the focal and segmental hyaline changes spread in the capillary tufts. Focal areas of podocyte detachment are followed by adhesion of the denuded GBM to the parietal layer of Bowman's space ('synechia'). The process of segmental sclerosis and capillary collapse progresses to sclerosis gradually obliterating the glomeruli. The completely sclerosed glomeruli may subsequently undergo complete 'reabsorption' leaving behind non-functioning aglomerular tubules (Kriz and LeHir, 2005). The lesions that initially affect only few glomeruli progressively involve an increasing larger fraction of the glomerular population and this progression is strongly associated with a progressive form of interstitial fibrosis, tubular atrophy and vascular changes. In some cases, the lesion of FSGS can already be seen at renal biopsy at the onset of proteinuria, while in other patients, initial biopsy shows only minimal changes and a full histological picture of FSGS may be seen only in repeat biopsies.

Longitudinal observations indicating a possible evolution of MCD into FSGS led to a dispute as to whether FSGS should be considered as a separate clinicopathological entity, or as a particularly severe subset of MCD that progresses to FSGS. Obviously, until we have complete understanding of the aetiopathogenesis of both FSGS and MCD, this dispute cannot be fully resolved. It is very clear that lesions of FSGS may be so focal in the early stages that they are easily 'missed' in an initial renal biopsy, even with an adequate number of glomeruli in the sample. Some subtle features in a renal biopsy, such as focal areas of interstitial fibrosis, subtle glomerular hypertrophy, extensive podocyte vacuolization and detachment, and evidence of a de-differentiated state for podocytes, may be clues to an underlying FSGS even when biopsies fail to reveal the typical sclerosing lesions. Ultrastructural studies showed that foot process width was significantly higher in the FSGS group than that in the MCD. Percentage of GBM length showing podocyte detachment was also significantly increased in the FSGS group. However, these differences were evident in the collapsing, cellular, and NOS variants while they were less marked in patients with tip lesions (Taneda et al., 2015). At any rate, we prefer to consider MCD and FSGS as distinct, as they have different pathological features, clinical presentation, response to therapy and outcome. Recent studies have also suggested that urinary CD80 excretion is greatly elevated in relapsing MCD whereas it remains normal or only slightly elevated in FSGS (Garin et al., 2015).

Pathogenesis

Primary FSGS is now categorized as a 'podocytopathy', since there is now evidence that podocyte is the major player in its pathogenesis. This highly differentiated and specialized cell type has essential roles in maintaining the integrity of glomerular architecture, resisting endocapillary hydraulic pressure and hindering egress of proteins into the urinary space. As a fully differentiated cell the resting podocyte is unable to replicate and even the damage of a single podocyte may initiate a sequence of events eventually leading to the degeneration of the whole glomerulus. The earliest consequence of podocyte injury is represented by cytoskeleton disorganization and foot process effacement, which probably represents a protective mechanism against the risk of detachment from GBM (Kriz and Lemley, 2015). Distinct pathways of injury and repair characterize the different podocytopathies. In MCD, the podocyte injury is limited to foot process effacement while podocyte number remains normal. A more severe form of podocyte injury in FSGS may cause glomerular and podocyte hypertrophy. If the glomerular growth exceeds the capacity of podocytes to adapt and adequately cover some parts of the filtration surface podocytes may detach from GBM (Nishizono et al., 2017). In this regard, a deleterious role has been attributed to uPAR-activated plasminogen. In podocytes exposed to plasminogen there is increased production of superoxide anion that promotes endothelin-1 synthesis and increased intracellular cholesterol uptake resulting in podocyte apoptosis (Raij et al., 2016). As long as the podocyte loss is limited, restitution or repair is possible, but a large podocyte loss results in a scarring response (Lasagni et al., 2015). Experimental models showed that the focal adherence of detached podocytes to the Bowman capsule can activate parietal epithelial cells (LeHir and Kriz, 2007; Kuppe et al., 2015; Kriz, 2018). Podocytes and parietal epithelial cells have common mesenchymal progenitors; therefore, parietal epithelial cells could be a source of podocyte repopulation after podocyte injury. Activated epithelial cells produce parietal extracellular matrix and migrate to a segment of the glomerular tuft via an adhesion to denuded GBM. From this entry site, activated parietal epithelial cells displace podocytes and deposit matrix eventually leading to FSGS (Smeets et al., 2011; Lim et al., 2016; Nagata, 2016; see also Figure 5.1).

The question of what is the *primum movens* leading to podocyte injury in primary FSGS remains very unanswerable at the present time, but it appears likely that the lesion is pathogenetically heterogeneous. *Primary FSGS is not one disease, but many with a common phenotype.* The experience with kidney transplantation showed that a number of patients with FSGS may have a very rapid recurrence of proteinuria almost immediately after transplantation, suggesting that some *circulating factor* (or factors) may be responsible for an increased glomerular permeability and FSGS recurrence. Among different candidates, attention has been focused on the possible role of a *soluble urokinase-type plasminogen activator receptor* (suPAR) which is normally present in human blood in low concentrations. Urokinase plasminogen activator surface receptor (uPAR) expressed in all glomerular cells can influence cells migration, adhesion, differentiation, and proliferation through its interaction with integrins, in particular $\alpha v \beta 3$ integrins, i.e. membrane glycoproteins that link extracellular matrix to actin filaments. By this pathway, activated uPAR can regulate cytoskeletal changes, podocyte migration, and foot process effacement induced by lipopolysaccharides (Wei et al., 2008). The cleavage of uPAR and

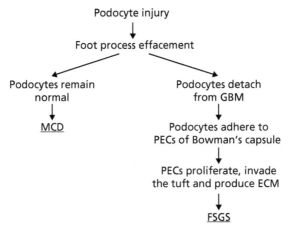

Figure 5.1 Pathogenesis of FSGS.
The intensity of injury and the reaction of podocytes can lead to foot process effacement not severe enough to modify the podocyte structure as in the case of minimal change disease (MCD) or may be so severe to cause hypertrophy and detachment of podocytes from the glomerular basement membrane (GBM). Some detached podocytes may adhere to the parietal epithelial cells (PECs) forming bridges between the tuft and Bowman's capsule. The contact activates parietal epithelial cells that proliferate, produce an extracellular matrix (ECM), and invade the glomerular tuft through the adhesion to denuded GBM, initiating a segmental sclerosis.

the following glycosylation of the cleavage fragments generate the circulating suPAR fragments, which may act on the same pathways of uPAR. Wei and colleagues (2011) reported that high levels of suPAR were detected in plasma of two-thirds of subjects with primary FSGS and high plasma concentrations of suPAR underlined an increased risk of FSGS recurrence after transplantation. Using three mouse models, they also showed that circulating suPAR activated podocyte β3 integrin in both native and grafted kidneys, with consequent disassembly of the actin cytoskeleton, foot process effacement, proteinuria and FSGS-like glomerulopathy. Further studies on two cohorts of North-American and European primary FSGS confirmed that the majority of patients with primary FSGS have increased serum suPAR levels (Wei et al., 2012). However, whether suPAR are sensitive and specific biomarkers of FSGS remains controversial. Indeed, high serum suPAR levels were found not only in primary FSGS, but also in secondary forms of FSGS (Huang et al., 2013). Other investigators reported that the plasma suPAR levels were not significantly different in children with FSGS, non-FSGS glomerular disease, and healthy controls (Bock et al., 2013). Rather, an inverse correlation between the levels of estimated glomerular filtration rate (eGFR) and serum levels of suPAR was found in adults (Meijers et al., 2014; Spinale et al., 2015) and children (Sinha et al., 2014). Finally, plasma levels of suPAR were elevated not only in patients with post-transplant recurrence of FSGS, but also in other transplant candidates (Franco Palacios et al., 2013). Thus, the measurement of suPAR in the plasma with the available enzyme-linked immunosorbent assay cannot help in diagnosing primary FSGS or its risk of recurrence after transplantation. Alternatively, McCarthy and colleauges (2010) proposed the *cardiotrophin-like cytokine factor 1* (CLCF1) as an active factor in FSGS. In isolated rat glomeruli CLCF1 activated podocytes increased glomerular albumin permeability and increased phosphorylation of STAT3 (signal transducer and activator of transcription 3) in peripheral blood cells and renal cortex. These data suggest that CLCF1 has potentially important systemic effects, may alter podocyte function and contribute to renal dysfunction and albuminuria (Savin et al., 2015).

Podocyte factors might also play a pathogenetic role. It has been reported that FSGS patients may show upregulation of the costimulatory *protein B7.1* (also called CD80) on podocytes. This abnormal podocyte expression of B7.1 would promote podocyte migration and detachment through inactivation of β1 integrin (Yu et al., 2013). However, other investigators could not find B7.1 expression in mouse podocytes treated with lipopolysaccaride, Adriamycin, or subtotal nephrectomy (Baye et al., 2016). Even in podocytes of patients with FSGS no upregulation of B7.1 was observed (Novelli et al., 2016). *CD40,* another costimulatory protein, may be variably expressed on podocyte. The upregulation might induce the production of autoantibodies. Indeed, circulating *anti-CD40 antibodies* showed a strong correlation with the risk of posttransplant recurrence of FSGS. These antibodies were particularly pathogenic in human podocyte cultures and enhanced suPAR mediated proteinuria in wild-type mice, suggesting a possible convergence of anti-CD40 pathogenic activity on suPAR-αvβ3 integrin pathway, with consequent actin cytoskeleton changes (Delville et al., 2014; Wei et al., 2015). *Krüppel-like transcription factors* (KLF) are essential regulators of mitochondrial function in podocytes. In patients with FSGS there is a low podocyte expression of KLF6 (Mallipattu et al., 2015). This reduced expression of KLF6 in podocytes is associated with a low expression of nephrin that can be reset by blocking the renin-angiotensin system, suggesting a protective role of KLF6 in injured podocytes (Hayashi et al., 2015). Furthermore, knockdown of KLF15 reduced cell survival and destabilized the actin cytoskeleton in differentiated human podocytes. Conversely, overexpression of KLF15 stabilized the actin cytoskeleton under cell stress in human podocytes (Mallipattu et al., 2017). Mutations of *connexins*, i.e. membrane-spanning proteins that allow for the formation of cell-to-cell channels and cell-to-extracellular space hemichannels might also alter the podocyte protein expression (Sala et al., 2016). *Yes-associated protein* (YAP) is a prosurvival signalling molecule and an antagonist of podocyte apoptosis. YAP silencing in murine podocytes can lead to histological features of FSGS, suggesting that factors inhibiting YAP activity may favour the development of FSGS and increase the permeability of glomerular barrier (Schwartzman et al., 2016). An interesting novel hypothesis points out the role of local *tumour necrosis factor* (TNF) and defective extrusion of free cholesterol from podocyte. Accumulation of renal lipids has been observed in several conditions, including FSGS, linking local fat to the pathogenesis of kidney disease (Wahl, 2016). Cholesterol can be captured by podocyte and its intracellular ingress/extrusion is regulated by ATP-binding cassette transporter A1 (ABCA1). Pedigo and colleagues (2016) demonstrated that in cultured human podocytes, local TNF expression caused free cholesterol-dependent apoptosis in podocytes by activating the nuclear factor of activated T-cells 1 (NFATc1). Albuminuria induced by TNF was aggravated in mice with podocyte-specific ABCA1 deficiency. ABCA1 overexpression or cholesterol depletion was sufficient to reduce albuminuria in mice with podocyte-specific NFATc1 activation. This data implicate an NFATc1/ABCA1-dependent mechanism in which local TNF is sufficient to cause free cholesterol-dependent podocyte injury.

Immunological changes may also play a role in the pathogenesis of FSGS. As mentioned previously, costimulatory proteins B7.1 or CD40 may be abnormally expressed on podocytes in some cases of FSGS. There is an increased activity of effector Th-17 cells, as shown by the abundant IL-17 staining in FSGS biopsies (Wang et al., 2013). Auto-antibodies against CD40 have been observed in kidney transplant recipients with recurrent FSGS (Delville et al., 2014), and the complement system is activated in patients with primary FSGS (Thurman et al., 2015). Anti-serum CD40 ligand antibodies have been detected in children with idiopathic NS and in adults with biopsy-proven FSGS (Doublier et al., 2017). All these data speak for the involvement of the immune system in the pathogenesis of primary FSGS (Kronbichler et al., 2016; Reggiani and Ponticelli, 2016). Finally, microRNA can also modulate FSGS (Fogo, 2015; Leierer et al., 2016). Overexpression of miRNA-193A in transgenic mice led to foot-process effacement, FSGS and dedifferentiation of podocytes with loss of expression of Wilms tumour protein (WT1), podocalyxin, and nephrin (Gebeshuber et al., 2013); miRNA-30 is reduced in patients with FSGS and injured cultured human podocytes can be rescued by exogenous miRNA-30 (Wu et al., 2014).

Finally, a role of mechanical stress originating in a disordered mesangium may be a major part of the podocytopathy seen in FSGS (Kriz, 2018).

In summary, a number of studies highlight the critical role of systemic soluble factors and the importance of podocyte response to injury. Abnormalities of the innate and adaptive immunity are also likely to participate to the pathogenesis of primary FSGS, but their role is still poorly elucidated. It is possible that these damages may favour the externalization of inactive TGFβ in form of a large latent complex from macrophages and inflammatory cells. This large complex releases the active TGFβ through the mediation of thrombospondin-1. The active TGFβ binds to its receptors and phosphorylates SMADs (small intracellular signal transducer proteins) that favour the transduction of the signalling from extracellular TGFβ to the nucleus (Kamato et al., 2013; Ponticelli and Anders, 2017). In podocytes and glomerular epithelial cells, this results in organization of collagen fibrils and extracellular matrix assembly.

Aetiology

By definition, the aetiology of primary FSGS is unknown. However, reports of cases of familial FSGS associated with mutations of genes crucial for podocyte functions suggest a potential role of subtle genetic abnormalities influencing the susceptibility to what is defined as primary FSGS. These inherited podocytopathies are most often steroid-resistant. Pathologic lesions consist of sclerosis and, more frequently, FSGS, often of the classic or NOS variant. In the renal-limited genetic forms, the genome-based defects affect assembly of podocyte structures, including slit diaphragm and actin-based cytoskeleton (Table 5.1). It is likely that targeted or whole exome sequencing and clinicopathological information will be able to reveal novel and rare gene mutations and provide possible insights into aetiopathogenesis of renal diseases with equivocal clinical and pathologic presentations (Chen and Liapis, 2015; Lovric et al., 2016). Collagen IV mutations, including *COL4A3, COL4A4, and COL4A5*, frequently underlie a steroid-resistant FSGS, particularly in patients with a positive family history (Gast et al., 2016; Braunisch et al., 2018; Hines et al., 2018). In addition to mutations affecting the structural genes for specific proteins, animal studies suggest that states of mitochondrial dysfunction and endoplasmic cellular stress due to autophagy failure may induce a 'vulnerable podocyte' phenotype eventually leading to FSGS (Kawakami et al., 2015). Among these genetic forms, particularly frequent is the APOL-1 variant, a major cause of FSGS in sub-Saharan African descents (Genovese et al., 2010) and one of the three more frequent forms of FSGS in the US (Rosenberg and Kopp, 2017).

Apart from cases potentially related to gene mutations, a number of patients with proteinuria may also show segmental sclerosing lesions that can be associated with several clinical circumstances, including other primary glomerular diseases. This has led to nosologic confusion since many authors used the term FSGS not only to indicate the classic primary form, but also any form

Table 5.1 The most frequent gene mutations leading to the development of FSGS.

Gene	Encoded Protein	Role of the encoded protein
ACTN4	α-actinin 4	The assembling of actin filaments and their binding to slit diaphragm.
TRPC6	TRPC6	Non-selective conduction of ions.
CD2AP	CD2AP	A scaffolding protein that regulates the actin cytoskeleton by interacting with synaptopodin.
APOL1	Apolipoprotein 1	Promotion of pore formation, cellular injury, and programmed cell death.
INF2	Actin-regulator protein	Regulation of actin polymerization.
NPHS1	Nephrin	A scaffolding protein that recruits nephrin and CD2AP to the lipid rafts of slit diaphragm.
NPHS2	Podocin	A major component of slit diaphragm.
ADCK4	ADCK3 protein	Altered co-enzyme Q10 biosynthesis.
WT-1	Wilms tumour protein	Urogenital system development.
LAMB2	Laminin Beta 2	An extracellular matrix protein.
COL4	Collagen IV	A collagen of the lamina densa.

of secondary segmental sclerosing lesions, including those superimposed on another primary glomerular disease process, associated with other systemic diseases, caused by functional hyperfiltration (postadaptive FSGS), triggered by massive proteinuria and/or systemic arterial hypertension, or caused by viral infection or use of nephrotoxic drugs (Table 5.2). According to the different aetiopathogenetic and clinical characteristics a new classification of FSGS has been recently proposed. This includes three forms that are most common-i.e. primary FSGS, APOL-1 FSGS, and adaptive FSGS- and three less common forms, i.e. high penetrance genetic FSGS, medication-associated FSGS, and viral FSGS (Rosenberg and Kopp, 2017).

In contradistinction to primary FSGS, these secondary forms of FSGS are associated with a much lower frequency of hypo-albuminaemia, particularly when sclerotic lesions are related to glomerular hyperfiltration, as in the case of vesico-ureteric reflux nephropathy, morbid obesity, renal hypoplasia, and re-duced renal mass (oligonephronia). Oedema is quite infrequently seen in the so-called 'secondary' forms of FSGS (De Vriese et al., 2018). The progression to renal failure is also much less frequent and usually slower in the forms secondary to glomerular hyperfiltration than in primary FSGS. Such progression,

Table 5.2 Main causes of secondary FSGS.

Adaptive (nephron loss)	Drugs-toxins	Infection
Morbid obesity	IV Bisphosphonate	HIV
Vesico-ureteral reflux	Calcineurin inhibitors	Parvovirus B19
Familial dysautonomia	Sirolimus	BK polyoma virus
Any glomerular disease	Lithium	Cytomegalovirus
Mitochondrial disease	Anabolic steroids	Pyelonephritis
Renal transplant	Addictive drugs	
Elderly	Adriamycin	
Glycogen stores	Puromycin	

if present, may be further delayed by the use of drugs interfering with the renin-angiotensin system and by weight loss in the obesity related glomerulopathy (Praga and Morales, 2006). Renal biopsy may also guide in the right diagnosis. In maladaptive FSGS the glomerular tuft may appear hypertrophic and perihilar lesion is predominant over the other variants. As mentioned previously, it bears repeating that the degree of foot process effacement at electron microscopy is a crucial clue to a primary versus secondary forms of FSGS (Sethi et al., 2015). Foot process effacement is severe and diffuse (>80 per cent) in primary FSGS while segmental foot process effacement (<80 per cent) usually speaks for a secondary FSGS. However, there are cases of FSGS secondary to HIV, IV bisphosphonates, or interferon that are characterized by a widespread diffusion of foot process effacement. The genetic forms of FSGS tend to cluster in infants, children, and young adults.

Clinical presentation and features

The clinical presentation of primary FSGS is similar at any age, although NS is more frequent in children and hypertension is more frequent in adults. The onset of proteinuria is more often insidious than abrupt, different than that observed in MCD. A full-blown NS is present in 70–90 per cent of patients with tip lesions or collapsing variant, and it is very frequently seen at presentation in patients with NOS variant, while patients with perihilar variant (most often a lesion of secondary rather than primary FSGS) often present with sub-nephrotic proteinuria. At any rate, patients who initially only have asymptomatic sub-nephrotic proteinuria may become frankly nephrotic at some time during their clinical course. Microscopic, dysmorphic haematuria is found initially in about half of the cases, while macroscopic haematuria is quite rare. In this regard, it should be outlined that a number of patients with thin basement nephropathy may eventually develop a superimposed FSGS, particularly those with a functional variant of NEPH3 (Voskarides et al., 2017). Some 30–40 per cent of patients present with arterial hypertension.

Malignant hypertension is quite uncommon. Impaired renal function may be already present at the time of clinical discovery onset in about 20–25 per cent of patients, implying steady progression even at an 'asymptomatic' stage of the disorder. Serum complement levels are normal, but lipid levels may be strikingly elevated.

Epidemiology

The incidence of a lesion of FSGS in prospective or retrospective studies ranges between 0.2/100 000/year and 1.1/100 000/year depending on geographic and ancestral factors (Mc Grogan et al., 2011), but the exact frequency of primary vs. secondary and genetic forms of FSGS cannot be ascertained by these types of epidemiologic studies. There is a small predominance of primary FSGS in males over females in adults, while primary FSGS seems to be more frequent in girls in paediatric series (Boyer et al., 2007; Borges et al., 2007). The lesion of FSGS is far more commonly encountered in Hispanic and African-Americans than in Caucasian or Chinese or Japanese populations. A disproportionally high frequency of global glomerular sclerosis has been observed in African-American black adults and children carrier of coding variants G1, G2 in the *APOL1* gene (Dummer et al., 2015; Anyaegbu et al., 2015).

In the recent decades an increased prevalence of FSGS lesion among renal biopsies performed for diagnosis of apparently idiopathic NS has been reported in different countries (Swaminatan et al., 2007; Alwahaibi et al., 2013; Golay et al., 2013; Chávez-Valencia et al., 2014; Jegateesan et al., 2016). Even in children the incidence of steroid-resistant NS and FSGS increased significantly (Filler et al., 2003; Woo et al., 2010; Kiffel et al., 2011; Banaszak and Banaszak, 2012). Familial FSGS is common in China, suggesting that genetic factors are involved in its pathogenesis (Xie and Chen, 2013). The reasons are unknown for the exceptional growth in the frequency of FSGS in many countries. It is not due to the increased use of renal biopsy for diagnosis. The involvement of a latent virus infection operating as a second hit is likely in FSGS secondary to *APOL1* mutations (Kruzel-Davila et al., 2016) but has been never proven in primary FSGS.

Natural history

Older studies reported that about two-thirds of patients with primary FSGS develop ESRD within 10–15 years from diagnosis. In a few cases, often called 'malignant' FSGS, the disease shows a rapidly progressive course associated with severe arterial hypertension, marked hyperlipidaemia and thrombotic complications. The prognosis for FSGS is better today as most patients receive an adequate symptomatic as well as specific treatment, after the demonstration that a large number of patients may benefit from glucocorticoids or other drugs, which were previously considered to be rather ineffective. Although in a single patient proteinuria may have large day-to-day or month-to-month fluctuations, spontaneous complete remission (i.e. urinary protein excretion lower than 0.2 g/day in timed urine samples or less than 0.2 urine protein/creatinine ratio in a first morning 'spot' untimed urine samples) only occurs exceptionally in untreated nephrotic patients. However, a number of patients with non-nephrotic proteinuria may maintain normal renal function over extended periods of time (Korbet, 2012; Ponticelli and Graziani, 2014).

Prognostic factors

A number of clinical and histological factors may influence the outcome of FSGS (Table 5.3). These factors need to be taken into account, both individually and collectively, in making treatment decisions.

Age

In the first year of life the NS is almost invariably caused by mutations of genes encoding podocyte proteins and is steroid resistant. With this exception, the rate of complete remission is similar in the treated children compared with the treated adults (Cattran and Rao, 1998). Whether older subjects with FSGS are susceptible to a more rapid decline of renal function is still uncertain. In normal subjects GFR begins to decline after 30–40 years of age and the decline accelerates after age 50–60 years. This decline, which is part of the normal physiologic process of cellular and organ senescence, is associated with structural changes in the kidneys, including the lesion of FGGS, but not FSGS (Hodgin et al., 2015; Glassock and Rule, 2016; Hommos et al., 2018).

Gender

A retrospective analysis of 370 patients with FSGS showed that the rate of renal function decline and outcome favoured women over men. This gender 'benefit' was mainly related to lower proteinuria and blood pressure at presentation in women and throughout follow-up (Cattran et al., 2008).

Table 5.3 Main clinical and histological prognostic factors in patients with nephrotic syndrome (NS) and a histological lesion of FSGS.

Prognostic factors	Clinical impact
Clinical parameters	
Age	In the first year of age NS is due to gene mutations and is steroid resistant. Similar prognosis for older children and adults.
Race/ethnicity	Lower response to steroids and higher risk of progression in African-Americans (*APOL1* gene).
Proteinuria (amount/ duration)	Persistent elevated proteinuria is associated with poor renal outcome.
Renal function	With the exception of kidney dysfunction related to hypovolaemia, stable increases in serum creatinine indicate poor renal prognosis.
Response to therapy	Complete remission of proteinuria is associated with excellent renal prognosis. Partial remission is also associated with good prognosis.
Histological features	
Glomerular hypertrophy	An expression of maladaptive response.
Variant	Tip lesion variant has the best renal prognosis, while collapsing variant has the worst. Not otherwise specified (NOS) is in the middle.
Tubulo-interstitial changes (T-I)	The severity of T-I changes is a marker of renal prognosis

Ancestry and ethnicity

The response to steroids is lower and the rate of progression to renal failure is higher in African-American Black than in Caucasian patients with Primary FSGS (Korbet, 2012). This difference is probably accounted for by the inclusion in FSGS of African-Americans with coding variants in the *APOL1* gene. Patients with *APOL1* G1 and G2 risk alleles more likely progress to ESRD than their counterparts with zero or one risk allele (Foster et al., 2013; Dummer et al., 2015). However, APOL1 risk genotype did not influence proteinuria responses to therapy (Kopp et al., 2015).

Proteinuria

The level of proteinuria at presentation has very little diagnostic significance but can have prognostic importance (Gipson et al., 2016). Patients with primary FSGS and persisting nephrotic-range proteinuria in spite of therapy have a very poor prognosis, particularly when urine protein excretion exceeds 10 g/day (Korbet, 2012). The length of exposure to proteinuria is even more important than the current proteinuria value. Time-varying proteinuria, calculated from any instantaneous value at any given time point, has been considered as the ideal metric to capture the risk of a 50 per cent reduction in eGFR or ESRD (Barbour et al., 2015). The prognostic significance of proteinuria may be explained by the fact that proteinuria may be directly involved in mechanisms favouring the progression of renal diseases. Exposure of the tubule to excess amounts of protein and the necessity for augmenting protein reabsorption can be a direct cause of phenotypic alteration in tubular behaviour that can drive the formation of interstitial fibrosis, capillary rarefaction, and potentially glomerulosclerosis (Grgic et al., 2012).

Also, the quality of urine protein excretion may have some prognostic significance. In a retrospective study on patients with FSGS and NS, fractional excretion of IgG and α2-macroglobulin have been found to be powerful predictors of outcome and responsiveness to steroids and cyclophosphamide (Bazzi et al., 2013). Analysing urinary proteome might represent a promising approach to identify patients who respond to steroids. A study demonstrated that apolipoprotein A-1 and Matrix-remodelling protein 8 were over- and under-represented, respectively, in steroid sensitive compared to steroid resistant urine samples (Kalantari et al., 2014).

Renal function

There is agreement that impaired renal function at presentation generally indicates a poor prognosis. However, in assessing renal function in a nephrotic patient one should be aware of the fact that an increase in serum creatinine level does not necessarily reflect an already established chronic renal insufficiency. In a number of patients, the serum creatinine level may increase temporarily because of hypovolaemia, either caused by profound hypo-albuminaemia or by diuretic therapy, and can completely reverse after hypovolaemia has been corrected. However, in other cases, objective signs of hypovolaemia cannot be documented. In these cases, the glomerular ultrafiltration coefficient may be reduced by as much as 50 per cent, suggesting that severe reduction in GFR may result from interaction between acute ischemic tissue injury and pre-existing intrinsic renal abnormalities or that diffuse foot process effacement may result in reduced hydraulic conductivity at the single nephron level. It is also worth remembering that the GFR as estimated from endogenous creatinine clearance or formulas predicting GFR from serum creatinine concentrations may overestimate the true GFR by 10–15 per cent due to the tubular secretion of creatinine.

Response to therapy

The response to therapy is considered by nearly all clinicians and investigators to be the *best* single clinical indicator of eventual outcome, even more important than the initial histological picture. Children with FSGS who do not achieve partial or complete remission have a 50 per cent risk of progression to ESRD within five years, whereas those who enter complete remission have a five-year kidney survival rate of 90 per cent (Sethna and Gibson, 2012). Most adults who respond completely to glucocorticoid therapy maintain normal renal function over time (even when steroid-responsive relapses subsequently occur), while steroid-resistant patients often progress to ESRD (Korbet, 2012; Ponticelli and Graziani, 2014). While there is also general agreement that a complete remission of proteinuria (usually defined by a daily proteinuria ≤200 mg) is associated with an excellent outcome in the long term, a partial remission (defined by 40 per cent proteinuria reduction and proteinuria <1.5 g/g) is also a reliable predictor of good long-term renal survival (Troost et al., 2018).

Spontaneous remission

Although spontaneous complete remission of proteinuria is very exceptional, partial remission may occur in some patients with primary FSGS. Spontaneous complete or partial remissions are usually associated with a significant improvement in the overall natural history of FSGS, both in terms of progression to ESRD and of NS-related complications.

Arterial hypertension

Arterial hypertension can contribute to the development of renal failure in FSGS. As autoregulation of glomerular pressure in FSGS is disturbed, the increment in systemic blood pressure leads to the rise in glomerular pressure, which results in glomerular capillary wall stretch, endothelial damage, and a rise in protein glomerular filtration (Ljutić and Kes, 2003).

Hyperlipidaemia

Elevation of plasma lipids and an abnormal partition of the lipid fractions is highly prevalent in nephrotic patients and may be involved in the pathogenesis of FSGS (Wahl et al., 2016). There is now experimental evidence that the incapacity of podocyte to extrude free cholesterol can cause podocyte injury and proteinuria (Pedigo et al., 2016). HMG coA-reductase inhibitors ('statins') and non-statin ezetimibe may affect the expression of inflammatory elements, curtail oxidative stress, and enhance endothelial function. These effects can probably reduce the risk of cardiovascular events in patients with kidney disease, since in the general population every 1 mmol/l (~40 mg/dl) reduction in LDL cholesterol (LDL-C) can result in a 22 per cent decrease in CVD events (Stein and Raal, 2015). However, there is no evidence that statins can alter the outcome of patients with FSGS.

suPAR levels

Independently of the nature of renal disease, an elevated level of suPAR is associated with an accelerated decline in the eGFR (Hayek et al., 2015). High serum levels of suPAR and low levels of uPAR may be indicators of progression in clinical subjects and animal models of FSGS (Chen et al., 2016).

Vitamin D binding protein (VDBP)

In a preliminary study, concentrations of VDBP in the urine were significantly higher in patients with steroid resistant than in patients with steroid sensitive NS and normal controls. A urinary VDBP cut-off of 362 ng/ml yielded the optimal sensitivity (80 per cent) and specificity (83 per cent) to distinguish steroid-resistant from steroid-sensitive patients (Bennett et al., 2016).

Glomerular hypertrophy

Glomerular enlargement, or glomerulomegaly, is frequent and pathogenetically important in secondary forms of FSGS (particularly in those conditions associated with hyperfiltration and oligonephronia). In the early phases of idiopathic FSGS, glomeruli are enlarged both in adults and children (Hughson et al., 2002; Cho et al., 2007). These data suggest that glomerular hypertrophy might represent a compensatory change that could immediately precede a rapid decline in renal function as an expression of an adaptation to nephron loss that could itself maladaptively predispose to the future development of renal failure.

Mesangial proliferation

In a review of our own experience with FSGS, we found by multivariate analysis that the presence of superimposed mesangial proliferation was significantly and independently associated with the risk of doubling of serum creatinine over time. Patients showing mesangial proliferation at renal biopsy had a relative risk of 4.6 for doubling their serum creatinine (Ponticelli et al., 1999). Mesangial proliferation may also increase the risk of recurrent disease in the renal allograft (see '*De novo* FSGS').

Number of glomeruli affected

Diffuse and multiple segmental lesions at initial biopsy (an increased sclerosis index) and even more an increase in the percentage of globally sclerotic glomeruli in a follow-up biopsy correlate highly with the development of chronic renal failure.

Glomerular crescents

True, rather than 'pseudo', epithelial crescents are quite rare in FSGS. When present they may concur to a rapid progression of disease. When the podocyte undergoes marked dedifferentiation and proliferation it can simulate a glomerular crescent ('pseudo-crescents' of FSGS).

Histological variants

There has been controversy in the past about the prognostic significance of D'Agati and colleagues' proposed morphological variants of FSGS. However, there is now some suggestion that this classification may provide clinically useful prognostic and therapeutic information. Although few patients with tip variant may progress to ESRD, they have the lowest pathologic injury scores, baseline creatinine, and rate of progression, and highest response rate to steroid treatment. In comparison with NOS, collapsing variant presents with more severe NS and lower eGFR. Most patients with the hilar variant are steroid resistant. At three years, 47 per cent of collapsing, 20 per cent of NOS, and 7 per cent of tip variant patients reached ESRD (D'Agati et al., 2013). A favourable prognosis for patients with tip lesions and a worse outcome for patients with collapsing variants was also outlined by other studies in different countries (Kwon et al., 2014; Mungan et al., 2015; Swamalata et al., 2015). Patients with primary FSGS and IgM and C3 deposition show unfavourable therapeutic response and poor renal outcome (Zhang et al., 2016).

Tubulointerstitial changes

As in all other glomerular diseases, a very high correlation is usually found between the severity of tubulointerstitial changes (chronicity index) and the final renal outcome in FSGS. The prognosis is severe in patients showing diffuse interstitial fibrosis and tubular atrophy at renal biopsy (D'Agati et al., 2013; Mariani et al., 2018). This association merely reflects the fact that if chronic damage occurred in the past (as shown in the 'snapshot' of the renal biopsy at a particular time), it is most likely to continue into the future, all other things being equal.

Genetics

As mentioned previously, most forms of genetic FSGS have a poor prognosis. This is true not only for familial cases but also for patients with sporadic FSGS and mutations of podocin, alpha-actinin 4, and TRPC6. Anecdotal cases of response to therapy have been reported in patients with PLCE1 mutation. We also do not know whether or how single-nucleotide polymorphisms in the genes involved in hereditary forms of FSGS affect kidney function. These patients are good candidates for renal transplantation, as the risk of recurrence is very low. At present, assessment of APOL1 gene variation plays no role in determining treatment choices in African-Americans with FSGS and NS (Kopp et al., 2015).

There are different views about the prognostic significance of genetic abnormalities of the renin-angiotensin system (RAS). To evaluate the association between ACE I/D gene polymorphism and FSGS susceptibility, a meta-analysis of 12 articles was performed. Seven studies were conducted in Asians, two in

Caucasians, one in Africans, two in Arabs, and one in Jews. In Asians, there was a markedly positive association between the D allele or DD genotype and FSGS susceptibility; the II genotype played a protective role against FSGS onset. Instead, a link between ACE I/D gene polymorphism and FSGS risk was not found in Caucasians, Africans, Arabs, or Jews (Zhou et al., 2011).

Specific treatment

Goals and objectives of treatment

The aims of treatment in primary FSGS should be clearly understood at the outset of making a treatment decision and should be always balanced by an assessment of the potential risks both of specific and symptomatic therapy. The comments below refer to patients with a clinicopathologic diagnosis of primary FSGS. The over-arching principles for the goals and objectives of specific treatment are:

  i. to reverse, halt, or delay progression to ESRD;
 ii. to favour a complete or partial remission of the proteinuria in order to prevent NS-related complications; and
iii. to render the patient as asymptomatic as possible within the constraints of undesirable side-effects of therapy (e.g. to improve the overall quality of life).

Many different drugs and combinations of drugs have been and are now being used for the treatment of primary FSGS, showing that no single therapeutic approach has obtained ideal results. Any assessment of the validity of treatment is made difficult by the fact that most of the available studies are observational, retrospective and uncontrolled and therefore contain the biases and potential confounding of non-controlled trials, namely ill-defined criteria of case inclusion and exclusion, different treatments for different periods, different follow-ups, and poorly defined and heterogenous end-points. Some of the reported trials may have inadvertently included secondary or genetic forms of FSGS, thus rendering them less relevant to the issue of treatment of primary FSGS. The lack of well-designed, adequately powered, appropriately controlled, long-term prospective studies coupled with the considerable underlying morphological and pathogenetic heterogeneity of the disorder can explain many of the uncertainties about the optimum therapeutic approach to primary FSGS and the different attitudes held by nephrologists as a whole. We will attempt to sort out this confusing situation and offer our own advice regarding therapeutic approaches, adhering to the goals and objectives principles outlined here, and taking into account that the most correct and most stringent way of interpreting the available retrospective studies is that of evaluating the rate of *complete remission, rather than 'just' a diminution in urinary protein excretion.*

Glucocorticoids

Glucocorticoids have been the first agents to be used in primary FSGS. Apart from their anti-inflammatory and immunomodulating properties, these agents can directly increase podocyte regeneration by augmenting the number of podocyte progenitors (Zhang et al., 2013), promote improved podocyte function, and can prevent the downregulation of microRNA-30 that facilitates podocyte injury (Wu et al., 2014).

For many years, children and adults with biopsy-proven FSGS, often presumed to be of a primary form, received an initial treatment with prednisone for four to eight weeks—a regimen similar to that used in patients with MCD. Only 19 per cent of patients responded with a complete remission to such a treatment, and only 36 per cent had stable renal function after a mean period of six years (Schena and Cameron, 1988). As a consequence, many patients were considered to be 'steroid-resistant' and remained untreated. Further uncontrolled studies showed that adults treated with glucocorticoids for four to six months had a rate of complete or partial remissions of about 60 per cent, with complete remissions ranging between 30 and 40 per cent (Ponticelli et al., 1999; Chun et al., 2004). Among responders to glucocorticoid therapy, remissions seemed to be more stable in adults than in children. Renal function also tended to be maintained at normal levels over time in most responders. Although it is not possible to exclude an effect of selection—only patients with a good tolerance to therapy and with some improvement of proteinuria continued glucocorticoids for a long period—a review of the available studies gives the strong impression that the more aggressive and prolonged the glucocorticoid therapy, the higher the rate of response (Ponticelli and Graziani, 2014).

The KDIGO guidelines (2012) suggest administering oral prednisone at a single dose of 1 mg/kg/day (maximum 80 mg) or alternate-day 2 mg/kg (maximum 120 mg) for a minimum of four weeks to be continued for 16 weeks if well tolerated or until complete remission is achieved. Obviously, a four-week treatment duration is inadequate for a definition of 'steroid-resistant' primary FSGS. Glucocorticoids should be tapered slowly over a period of six months. However, one cannot neglect the risks of adverse events with such a treatment regimen. Not only remissions, but also the incidence and the severity of side-effects, are proportional to the intensity and duration of steroid treatment. This may represent a problem for those patients who do not show an early (i.e. by 8–12 weeks of treatment) response (the majority unfortunately!), and even more so for those patients who have frequent relapses. On the other hand, it is very difficult to identify any clinical or pathological feature that can allow to predict the response to glucocorticoids in nephrotic patients with sporadic (non-familial) FSGS (with the exception of genomic studies identifying a podocyte protein mutation in a sporadic form, as discussed previously). The value of identifying morphologic variants of FSGS for the selection of a specific treatment regimen has not yet been examined in a randomized controlled fashion. Thus, the only sure means to know whether a patient will or will not respond is to actually administer a full course (e.g. four to six months) of therapy with prednisone. Some measures should always be adopted to reduce the steroid-related morbidity that may occur with this course of treatment. These include the administration of the daily steroid dose in a single morning administration (ideally between 7 and 9 a.m.) and the possible switch from a daily to an alternate-day administration for a maintenance treatment. The patient should also be encouraged to follow physical and dietetic measures to prevent increase in body weight, diabetes, myopathy, and osteoporosis (Table 5.4). Blood pressure, lipidaemia, and glycaemia should be regularly checked and treated when necessary. In young patients without obvious cardiovascular disease, the goal blood pressure should be 120–130/75–80 mmHg (measured at home), and the use of inhibitors of angiotensin II should be preferred. However, the most important measure remains a strict control of clinical and psychological conditions by the

Table 5.4 Recommendations for the use of glucocorticoids in the treatment of FSGS.

Type of glucocorticoid (GC)	Prefer short-acting GC (prednisone, prednisolone, methylprednisolone) for oral administration.
Dosage	Start with 1 mg/kg/day of prednisone (or equivalent) in adults, 1.5 mg/kg/day in children in a single administration between 7 and 9 a.m., or give a doubled dose every other day (alternate-day regimen). Tailor the dosage according to the tolerance.
Duration of treatment	Give this dose for six to eight weeks (if well tolerated) then reduce the daily dose of 5 mg every week (or 10 mg every other day, in case of alternate-day therapy). When a daily dose of 10 mg/day (or 20 mg/48 hours) is reached, GC may be continued up to 8–12 months if well tolerated. Do not stop GC abruptly!
Dietetic measures	Low-salt (to prevent oedema/hypertension), normocaloric or mildly low-calorie diet (to prevent obesity). Use 0.8–1 g/kg/BW high biologic value proteins plus the amount of protein lost in the urine every day.
Physical activity	Encourage walking, swimming, aerobic exercise to prevent myopathy and obesity.
Monitoring	Regularly check blood pressure (ideally ≤130/80 mmHg), body weight, glycaemia, serum lipid levels.

regular monitoring of the patient by the physician and an adequate tailoring of the doses, according to the tolerance to treatment.

Cyclosporine (CsA)

CsA is a calcineurin inhibitor (CNI) that may exert potential benefits in primary FSGS through different mechanisms:

i. By inhibiting calcineurin, a complex of phosphatases, CsA prevents the dephosphorylation of NF-AT (the nuclear factor of activated T-cells) and its entrance into the nucleus where NF-AT participates in the synthesis of IL-2;

ii. The inhibited access to the nucleus of NF-AT prevents the binding of this transcription factor to the gene promoter encoding uPAR, which affects podocyte motility via activation of the β3 integrin pathway (Zhang et al., 2012);

iii. The inhibition of calcineurin can prevent the dephosphorylation of synaptopodin in podocytes, a protein critical for stabilizing the podocyte actin cytoskeleton (Faul et al., 2008);

iv. In rats with puromycin aminonucleoside-induced NS, CsA reduced proteinuria, repaired foot process effacement, and reorganized the actin cytoskeleton by upregulating expression of cofilin-1 in podocytes (Li et al., 2014);

v. The impaired cholesterol extrusion from podocytes caused by local TNF is mediated by NF-AT activation (Pedigo et al., 2016), which may be inhibited by CsA. Thus, independently of its effects on T-cells, CsA may reduce proteinuria and protect the integrity of the glomerular barrier by stabilizing the actin cytoskeleton in podocytes.

According to the 2012 KDIGO clinical guidelines, CsA remains the first-line drug for children and adults with steroid-resistant FSGS. In children with steroid-resistant NS, many observational studies report the possibility of obtaining a partial remission and, less frequently, a complete remission, with CsA (Ghiggeri et al., 2004; Heering et al., 2004; Hamasaki et al., 2013; Klaassen et al., 2015; Inaba et al., 2016, Laurin et al., 2016). A multicentre randomized trial compared CSA (at doses adjusted to achieve trough levels of 120–180 ng/ml) versus IV cyclophosphamide (500 mg/m^2 per month) in the initial therapy of children with steroid-resistant NS and histologically proven MCD, FSGS, or mesangial hypercellularity. All patients were on alternate-day prednisone therapy. After 24 weeks, no difference in complete remission was seen between patients receiving CsA (2/15, or 13 per cent) or cyclophosphamide (1/17, or

5 per cent). Partial remission was achieved by seven of the 15 (46 per cent) CsA-treated patients and two of the 15 (11 per cent) cyclophosphamide-treated patients (p <0.05). The number of adverse events was comparable between both groups (Plank et al., 2008). In adults with FSGS, an overview of randomized or quasi-randomized controlled trials reported that CsA at an initial dose of 3.5–5 mg/kg/day in combination with oral prednisolone 0.15 mg/kg/day was more likely to achieve a partial remission of the NS compared with symptomatic treatment or prednisolone alone. However, there was a probability of deterioration of kidney function due to the nephrotoxic effect of CSA in the long term (Braun et al., 2008). In a retrospective review of 458 patients with FSGS, treatment with glucocorticoids or CsA was associated with better renal survival than no immunosuppression (hazard ratio 0.49). However, CsA with or without glucocorticoids was not significantly associated with a lower likelihood of ESRD compared with glucocorticoids alone (Laurin et al., 2016). A meta-analysis of five randomized controlled trials (RCTs) including both adults and children showed that, compared to other treatments, CSA therapy resulted in a significantly greater partial remission rate, but no complete remission (Chiou et al., 2017).

The incidence of CsA side-effects in patients with FSGS is comparable to that reported in MCD. A main concern in using CsA in FSGS is that the nephrotoxic effects of the drug may accelerate the progression of renal lesions. At least in a few patients, repeat biopsies disclosed global glomerulosclerosis, tubular atrophy, interstitial fibrosis, arteriolar hyalinosis, and other signs of renal toxicity, particularly in patients with persisting elevated proteinuria (Sinha et al., 2013; Singh et al., 2015). However, the risk of CsA nephropathy is low if dosing guidelines are followed and patients are monitored regularly (Cattran et al., 2007). In patients with already reduced renal function, the nephrotoxic effects of CsA (and other CNIs) can be augmented and they should be used with great caution or not at all in such patients.

In summary, there is a high level of evidence that CsA can induce an antiproteinuric effect in about 50–60 per cent of patients with primary FSGS who have not responded to a short course of steroids. CsA may be considered as a useful alternative therapeutic approach for patients with primary FSGS who display persistent nephrotic-range proteinuria in spite of a prolonged treatment with high-dose prednisone, or for patients with severe steroid-related side-effects. In patients with a high risk of steroid-related complications it may be possible to use a CsA regimen for the initial therapy of primary FSGS and the NS.

When using CsA microemulsion (Neoral), the drug should be started at doses not greater than 100–150 mg/m^2/day in children or 4–5 mg/kg/day in adults.

Since long-term treatment (with the attendant potential risks of cumulative nephrotoxicity) is usually required, doses should be progressively reduced for maintenance, taking into account that low doses of CsA (1.5–2 mg/kg/day) are often sufficient to maintain remission, usually partial. Some physicians prefer to administer the daily dose of CsA in a single morning administration, both to simulate the circadian rhythm of cellular immunity and facilitate the adherence to prescriptions (Corbetta and Ponticelli, 2010). The association with alternate-day prednisone for the first six months (40 mg/m² per 48 hours for two months, followed by 30 mg/m² per 48 hours for two months, and then by 20 mg per 48 hours for two months in children) may significantly improve the results (Cattran et al., 2007).

We do not believe that regular monitoring of blood CsA levels is needed, but we periodically measure trough (C0) blood levels to verify the compliance to treatment and to reduce the dosage if CsA trough levels exceed 150 ng/ml. If a patient does not show any improvement within three to six months, CsA is probably ineffective and should be withdrawn. In case of complete remission, CsA may be gradually tapered off after one to two years of continuous therapy. A number of patients may subsequently relapse, but a long-term treatment with CsA reduces the probability of relapse. In case of relapse after discontinuation, CsA may be resumed and some patients may be maintained in remission by giving low-dose CsA for many years. Of course, a continuous monitoring of renal function is required in these cases. A consensus conference recommended a repeat renal biopsy after two to three years of treatment with CsA (Cattran et al., 2007), although it may be difficult even for an expert pathologist to recognize whether increasing interstitial fibrosis and glomerular scarring are attributable to drug toxicity or natural progression of FSGS (Table 5.5).

Tacrolimus (TAC)

Good results with TAC have been reported both in children (Bhimma et al., 2006; Kallash and Aviles, 2014; Kim et al., 2014; Morgan et al., 2015; Jahan et al., 2015) and in adults (Li et al., 2009; Fan et al., 2013; Ramachandran et al., 2014) with presumed primary FSGS. Some trials comparing TAC with other drugs in FSGS have also been done. In a study, 41 patients with eGFR <60 ml/min and a diagnosis of steroid-resistant MCD, FSGS, or mesangioproliferative GN were randomly assigned to treatment with alternate-day prednisone and enalapril plus TAC (0.1–0.2 mg/kg/day) or CsA (5–6 mg/kg/day). After six months of therapy, remission occurred in 18/21 (85.7 per cent) patients treated with TAC and 16/20 (80 per cent) treated with CsA. The proportion of patients who experienced relapse was greater in those receiving CsA (RR, 4.5; P=0.01). Blood cholesterol levels were lower with TAC. Nephrotoxicity necessitating

Table 5.5 Calcineurin inhibitors in FSGS.

Drug	Mechanism of action	Dosage	Recommendations
Cyclosporine (CsA)	By inhibiting calcineurin, CsA inhibits synthesis of IL-2 and prevents synaptopodin degradation by calcineurin. CsA may also protect the integrity of glomerular barrier by stabilizing the actin cytoskeleton in podocytes.	Initial dose: 4–5 mg/kg/day in adults; 100–150 mg/m2/day in children. Maintenance: 2–3 mg/kg/day in adults; 50–80 mg/m2/day in children.	The association with small doses of prednisone may improve the results. If no reduction in proteinuria within six months, CsA is probably ineffective. In responders, continue CsA for one to two years, then taper off CsA gradually.
Tacrolimus (TAC)	TAC is also an inhibitor of calcineurin and prevents the synthesis of IL-2. It is likely that TAC may exert antiproteinuric effects with mechanisms similar to those exerted by CsA.	Initial dose: 0.1–0.15 mg/kg/day in adults and children. Maintenance: 0.05 mg/kg/day in adults, 0.05–0.1 mg/kg/day in children.	The recommendations for the use of TAC are similar to those of CsA.

stoppage of TAC and CsA was seen in 4.7 per cent and 10 per cent of patients, respectively. Cosmetic side effects (hypertrichosis and gum hypertrophy) were significantly more frequent in CsA-treated patients (Choudhry et al., 2009). In a multicentre RCT, 43 children with steroid-resistant FSGS were randomized to receive TAC for 12 months or six infusions of IV cyclophosphamide every month. In both arms of the study, patients were given equal amounts of alternate-day prednisolone. Complete or partial remissions were significantly higher with TAC than with cyclophosphamide. Sustained remission at 12 months was also significantly higher with TAC. Treatment withdrawal was higher with cyclophosphamide, mainly because of systemic infections (Gulati et al., 2012).

Thus, observational studies and randomized trials show that TAC may obtain a high rate of remission. Its efficacy may be considered similar to that of CsA, although it is difficult to make a fair comparison between two drugs that are used at non-equivalent doses. In comparison with CsA, TAC does not cause aesthetic changes or gum hypertrophy. Hyperlipidaemia and hypertension occur less frequently, while the risk of diabetes is higher with TAC than CsA. On the other hand, the risk of nephrotoxicity is similar. At present, the indications and the recommendations for the use of TAC in FSGS are similar to those of CsA. It should be noted that the risk of nephrotoxicity and other major complications is mainly dose-related. We recommend that the mean dosage of TAC for maintenance should be kept ≤0.1 mg/kg/day. However, small children may require higher doses and trough (C0) blood levels ≥ 5 ng/ml.

Alkylating agents

Cyclophosphamide and (less frequently) chlorambucil have been the alkylating agents most widely used as adjunctive therapy in patients with FSGS (Box 5.1). Good results have been reported in the distant past but these were mainly anecdotal observations. The KDIGO guidelines (2012) reported that there is a moderate evidence suggesting that alkylating agents *should not be used* in children with steroid-resistant NS. In adults with FSGS, a few small-sized observational studies reported good results with oral cyclophosphamide or chlorambucil, but *only* in steroid-responsive or steroid-dependent patients, not in steroid-resistant FSGS.

A good response may be obtained when cyclophosphamide or chlorambucil, either alone or in combination with glucocorticoids, is given as a first treatment (before any knowledge is obtained regarding the potential for a response to steroids alone or for the potential for relapses). Usually, treatment should be prolonged to obtain a complete or partial remission, just as with a steroid only course of treatment (Das et al., 2009; Ren et al., 2013; Bazzi et al., 2013).

Box 5.1 Alkylating agents in FSGS

In steroid-sensitive patients either cyclophosphamide or chlorambucil may obtain a good rate of partial or complete response.

The longer is the treatment the higher is the rate of response but also the rate and severity of side effects.

In steroid-resistant patients the response to alkylating agents is poor if any.

It is suggested not to exceed a dose of 2 mg/kg/day for cyclophosphamide and 0.15 mg/kg/day for chlorambucil. The doses should be further decreased in older patients.

Check WBC regularly and halve the doses if WBC are <5,000/cmm. Stop the alkylating agent if WBC <3,000/cmm, and restart at low doses when WBC >5,000/cmm.

Do not exceed a cumulative dose of 200–300 mg/kg for cyclophosphamide and 9–10 mg/kg for chlorambucil to prevent gonadal and neoplastic effects.

The results of alkylating agents are very poor in steroid-resistant cases. Even long-term administration of cyclophosphamide may obtain a response only in very few steroid-resistant patients. It is worth noting that cumulative doses of cyclophosphamide higher than 250–300 mg/kg (or chlorambucil >9–10 mg/kg) can result in azoospermia or ovarian failure. Moreover, prolonged exposure to cyclophosphamide increases the risk of bladder toxicity or malignancy.

In summary, the available studies show that a course with alkylating agents may favourably influence the renal outcome only in nephrotic patients with primary FSGS who respond to steroids and may obtain results similar to those of glucocorticoids when given as a first-line therapy in untreated patients. In primary therapy the only advantage with these agents is a longer duration of remission. It is possible to speculate that with more long-term treatment the results may be improved. However, such prolonged therapy with alkylating agents exposes the patient to the risk of disquieting side-effects, e.g. bone-marrow toxicity, infection, gonadal toxicity, mutagenic effects, and neoplasia. The risk of severe toxicity and the limited benefits (if any) should *greatly discourage* the extensive use of long-term therapies with cyclophosphamide or chlorambucil in FSGS.

Mycophenolate

A few observational clinical studies reported that the administration of mycophenolate mofetil (MMF), either alone or associated with prednisone, may obtain short-term benefits on proteinuria in a few patients with FSGS (Senthil Nayagam et al., 2008; de Mello et al., 2010; Gargah and Lakhoua, 2011). In the US, an RCT compared the safety and efficacy of MMF combined with oral pulse dexamethasone versus cyclosporine in children and young adults with steroid-resistant FSGS (not uniformly proven to be primary FSGS due to the absence of electron microscopic findings). At 12 months, partial or complete remission was achieved in 22/66 (33.3 per cent) patients on MMF/dexamethasone, and 33/72 (45.8 per cent) on CsA. During the entire 78 weeks of the study, eight patients treated with CsA and seven with MMF/dexamethasone died or developed kidney failure (Gipson et al., 2011). Overall, the benefits of MMF/dexamethasone were fewer than those found with CsA, but this was not statistically significant, perhaps due to the underpowered nature of the study. After the trial was completed, 20 MMF/dexamethasone-treated and 22 CsA-treated patients who experienced a complete or partial remission were studied through 78 weeks. The median proteinuria in MMF/dexamethasone and in CsA-responsive patients fell by 82.7 per cent and 89.8 per cent at 52 weeks; the fall was sustained at 78 weeks (80.3 per cent, and 74.7 per cent, respectively). The mean eGFR decreased by 19.4 per cent in the CsA group and continued to fall by 2.6 per cent; instead, GFR rose by 7.0 per cent in the MMF/dexamethasone group at 52 weeks, and subsequently rose by 16.4 per cent. These data suggest that the posited favourable effects of MMF/dexamethasone on proteinuria and renal function were sustained for six months after therapy (Hogg et al., 2013). This study has been criticized for its underpowered nature and for the criteria used for enrolment of patients who may or may not have had primary FSGS. As such, it does not provide definitive information concerning the efficacy of MMF in primary FSGS. Additionally, a systematic review of three controlled and 18 uncontrolled clinical trials evaluating the use of MMF in primary FSGS patients reported that MMF is no more effective than CsA or cyclophospha-mide for promoting kidney function preservation when glucocorticoids were used as baseline treatment (Lau et al., 2013). In an open RCT, steroid-resistant children with complete or partial remission after six months of TAC therapy were randomly assigned to receive MMF (29) or to continue TAC (31); at one year, frequent relapses occurred in 16 (55.2 per cent) patients given MMF and in three (9.7 per cent) patients on TAC (Sinha et al., 2017).

In summary, the available data suggest that mycophenolate salts might obtain a reduction of proteinuria only in a small number of patients with primary FSGS, when used as a first-line treatment of FSGS. Better results may be obtained at times, but not predictably so, in a few steroid-resistant patients, if mycophenolate is associated with dexamethasone pulses (Gipson et al., 2011), CsA (Segarra-Medrano et al., 2011; Gellermann et al., 2012), or TAC plus gluco-corticoids (Kim et al., 2014). Additional studies need to be conducted to better assess the role of mycophenolate in FSGS. Furthermore, the optimal dosage of mycophenolate should be assessed, as in the few published studies, the drug has been given at different doses.

Adrenocorticotropic hormone (ACTH)

In an observational, uncontrolled trial, Hogan and colleagues (2013) admin-istered ACTH gel (Acthar*) to 24 patients with presumed primary FSGS: six steroid-dependent and 15 steroid-resistant. At the end of different periods of therapy, two patients experienced complete remission and five partial remis-sion (total responses 7/24, or 29 per cent). Two responders relapsed during a mean follow-up of 70±31 weeks. However, 33 per cent of the patients had sub-nephrotic range proteinuria and 25 per cent of the patients had normal serum albumin at enrolment, raising the concern that some may have had a secondary form of FSGS. In another study, of ten patients with FSGS treated with ACTH gel, two entered complete remission and two partial remission (Filippone et al., 2016). In a retrospective case series, 12 of 15 patients with FSGS treated with ACTH gel entered partial or complete remission (Madan et al., 2016). These studies do not provide sufficient evidence to warrant employing ACTH gel for initial treatment of primary FSGS with NS.

Sirolimus

The indications for sirolimus (Rapamycin) in primary FSGS are controversial as a number of reports on kidney transplant recipients pointed out the onset of proteinuria, sometimes in a nephrotic range, in patients who were switched from calcineurin inhibitors to sirolimus. The mechanisms responsible of proteinuria are far from being elucidated, but possible hypotheses are apoptosis of podocytes, apoptosis of epithelial tubular cells inhibiting protein reabsorption, and previous presence of proteinuria masked by the use of calcineurin inhibitors. Whatever the mechanism(s), the possible proteinuric effects associated with drug-related hyperlipidaemia do not render Sirolimus a very attractive alternative treatment for FSGS.

In spite of these reservations, low-dose treatment with rapamycin efficiently diminished disease progression in a murine FSGS model (Zschiedrich et al., 2017), and favourable results were reported by two single prospective, open-label, uncontrolled trials. In a study, 21 patients with idiopathic, steroid-resistant FSGS were given sirolimus (at doses not specified) for six months. Complete remission occurred in four patients (19 per cent) and partial remissions in eight patients (38 per cent). Among sirolimus-responsive patients, proteinuria decreased from a mean of 8.8 to 2.1 g/24 hours. In responsive patients, GFR was maintained throughout the study, whereas it tended to decrease in non-responders (Tumlin et al., 2006). In a Spanish study, 13 children, mean age of ten years, with steroid-resistant FSGS were administered sirolimus 3.6 mg/m²/day. Nine of 13 patients responded to the treatment, five with complete remission and four with partial remission. A 65 per cent reduction in proteinuria was observed in the four patients who did not respond with remission (Liern et al., 2012).

We remain concerned that in patients with FSGS, the side effects of sirolimus may exceed its potential benefits, which are still not demonstrated in a controlled trial, and do not recommend its use in FSGS. The drug is not approved for use in FSGS in the US by the United States Food and Drug Administration (USFDA) or in Europe by the European Medicines Agency (EMA).

Rituximab (RTX)

Rituximab (RTX) has been largely used in patients with MCD, while little information is available about its use in FSGS. A systematic review reported that RTX is effective in reducing the number of relapses and sparing immunosuppression in frequently relapsing and steroid-dependent NS due to MCD and

FSGS (Kronbichler et al., 2014). However, the benefit seems to be very limited or non-existent in steroid-resistant patients with underlying FSGS (Fernandez-Fresnedo et al., 2009; Ochi et al., 2012; Kronbichler and Bruchfeld, 2014; Roccatello et al., 2017). The doses used varied between 375 mg/m² per dose at weekly intervals for four to six weeks and a single dose of 1 g repeated after two weeks. No substantial adverse effects have been reported.

In an RCT, 31 children (ages 2–16 years) with idiopathic NS unresponsive to combined calcineurin-inhibitor and prednisone were randomized to continue with the same regimen or to add two doses of IV RTX (375 mg/m²). RTX did not reduce proteinuria at three months. Adjustments for previous remission and baseline proteinuria did not change the results. According to the investigators, these data do not support the addition of RTX to prednisone and calcineurin inhibitors in children with steroid-resistant idiopathic NS (Magnasco et al., 2012). In a small observational study, five children not responding to steroids obtained remission by associating RTX with cyclosporine (Suyama et al., 2016). Among children with FSGS and poor sustained remission under calcineurin inhibitors, those who had significantly low response to T-cell stimulation with mitogen had good probability of responding to RTX (Chan et al., 2016).

In summary, while RTX appears very effective in steroid-sensitive patients with idiopathic NS, independently of the histological pattern, the evidence of efficacy of RTX in steroid-resistant FSGS is low, perhaps limited to patients with poor T-cell activation. For those few steroid-resistant patients who respond to RTX, the administration of MMF has been suggested in order to reduce the risk of relapses (Basu et al., 2015).

Apheresis

A systematic review reported that *plasmapheresis* or *immunoadsorption with protein A* improved proteinuria and stabilized renal function in 44 per cent of adults with FSGS (Bosch and Wendler, 2001). However, due to the uncontrolled study design and small patient cohorts in most trials, the level of evidence of these studies is very low. Large prospective, controlled, and randomized clinical trials are needed for recommendations based on high-level evidence.

LDL-apheresis (LDL-A) is used to correct dyslipidaemia rapidly. In nephrotic patients there is hypercholesterolaemia and increased levels of LDL (see Chapter 2). Oxidized LDL are incorporated by mesangial cells with scavenger receptors, forming foam cells that, together with macrophages, cause tissue damage by expressing various inflammatory cytokines and chemokines. In 29 Japanese patients with steroid-resistant FSGS treated with LDL-A for one month or longer followed by reduced doses of glucocorticoids, the cumulative remission rate at two years was 62 per cent. The results were even better at five years with 53 per cent of patients being in complete remission and another 33 per cent in partial remission (Muso, 2014). On the basis of this study, the Japanese regulatory authorities approved the use of LDL-A in patients with FSGS. On October 2013, the USFDA approved the Liposorber LA-15 system for LDL apheresis. in children with treatment-resistant NS. This approval was recently extended to adults. A prospective multicentre Japanese study (POLARIS) demonstrated complete remission at two years in 25 per cent of the 44 patients enrolled in the study, and reported that an additional 23 per cent of patients had partial remission, defined as proteinuria <1 g/day (Muso et al., 2015). The response to LDL apheresis is poor in patients with high levels of apolipoprotein E and serum amyloid protein (Kuribayashi-Okuma et al., 2016). LDL apheresis may play a role in difficult treatment resistant cases of primary FSGS.

Miscellanea

Coppo and colleagues (2012) administered saquinavir to ten patients with idiopathic NS. Among six steroid-dependent patients, five became infrequent relapsers, while only one of four steroid-resistant patients responded to saquinavir.

Pirfenidone is an orally available antifibrotic agent that has shown benefit in clinical trials of pulmonary fibrosis, multiple sclerosis, and hepatic cirrhosis. An open-label trial evaluated the safety and efficacy of pirfenidone in 21 patients with idiopathic and postadaptive FSGS. The 18 patients who were given pirfenidone for a median of 13 months showed a median reduction of eGFR from a median of -0.61 ml/min per 1.73 m^2 during baseline period to -0.45 ml/min per 1.73m^2 after pirfenidone. Pirfenidone had no effect on blood pressure or proteinuria. Adverse events included dyspepsia, sedation, and photosensitive dermatitis (Cho et al., 2007). A larger trial with pirfenidone is under way in the US.

The Novel Therapies for Resistant Focal Segmental Glomerulosclerosis (FONT) multicentre RCT investigated the efficacy of adalimumab, a monoclonal antibody directed against TNF-α (Abkhezr et al., 2015), versus galactose, a monosaccharide that may interact with permeability factors (Savin et al., 2008), and versus standard therapy with lisinopril, losartan, and atorvastatin in patients with FSGS resistant to glucocorticoids and other immunosuppressive agents. Twenty-one subjects were assigned to one of the three study arms. None of the adalimumab-treated subjects achieved the primary outcome. We now know that it is the local, not the systemic, TNF-α that causes podocyte apoptosis. Instead, two subjects in the galactose arm and two in the standard therapy arm had a 50 per cent reduction in proteinuria without a decline in eGFR (Trachtman et al., 2015).

In animal studies, IL-2 induces T regulators and plays a transient protective effect on proteinuria induced by lipopolysaccaride. However, in children with FSGS or MCD, low-dose IL-2 given in monthly pulses modified the levels of circulating Tregs but did not lower proteinuria or affect renal function (Bonanni et al., 2015).

In experimental glomerulonephritis, treatment of cultured podocytes with connexin 43 specific blocking peptides attenuated TGF-β induced cytoskeletal and morphologic changes and apoptosis, as did treatment with the purinergic blocker suramin and connexin 43 specific antisense oligodeoxynucleotide (Kavvadas et al., 2017).

Ongoing studies are evaluating the role of new agents, including Ofatumumab, an anti-CD20 monoclonal antibody; Mizoribine, an imidazole nucleoside; Losmapimod, a P38 kinase inhibitor; Fresulimumab, an anti-TGF-β antibody; Sparsertan, an antagonist of endothelin A receptor and angiotensin receptor; and Cyclodextrin, an oligosaccharide that could favour the extrusion of cholesterol from podocytes with ABCA1 deficiency (ClinTrials.gov).

Practical recommendations

Is FSGS primary or secondary?

Before planning any treatment, the physician should always ascertain whether the lesion of FSGS found in a renal biopsy is primary (idiopathic) in its nature or secondary to other diseases, conditions, or drugs (see Table 5.2). It is important to remember how difficult it can be to establish a diagnosis of primary FSGS on renal biopsy findings alone; thus, it may prove difficult to establish in some particular instances (e.g. in the elderly, obese, hypertensive patients, in individuals with a congenitally single kidney). The secondary forms caused by maladaptive glomerular haemodynamic alterations may be distinguished by the absence of hypo-albuminaemia, hypercholesterolaemia, and oedema in spite of nephrotic levels of proteinuria (Zand et al., 2017). Renal biopsy may provide some additional clues for differential diagnosis. Four histological features may allow a correct diagnosis of segmental glomerular lesions (see also Table 5.6):

i. the proportion of glomeruli affected (i.e. whether the lesions are focal or diffuse);

ii. the position of segmental lesions within glomeruli;

iii. the size of glomeruli; and

iv. the ultrastructural features, notably the extent of foot-process effacement.

Table 5.6 Main clinical and histological features that may allow to distinguish primary from secondary FSGS.

	Primary FSGS	**Secondary FSGS**
Clinical features	Most patients have proteinuria in a nephrotic range. Hypo-albuminaemia, hyperlipidaemia, and oedema are common.	Proteinuria is often lower than 3.5 g/24 hours even in case of proteinuria >3.5 g/24 hours, hypo-albuminaemia, hypercholesterolaemia, and/or oedema are often absent.
Histological features	LM. Initially only some glomeruli are affected by segmental sclerosis. Segmental sclerosis may be located everywhere (NOS variant is the most common). The size of glomeruli is normal. EM. No electron dense deposits. Diffuse foot process effacement.	LM. Most glomeruli are affected by sclerosis. Usually sclerosis is located in the perihilar area. Glomeruli are often enlarged. EM. Sometimes there are electron dense deposits in the mesangium or subendothelium. With some exceptions, foot process effacement is often limited to <50%.

LM = light microscopy; EM = electron microscopy; NOS = not otherwise specified

In the primary (idiopathic) form of FSGS the sclerotic lesions are focally and randomly distributed, at least in the early stages of the disease. The presence of large glomeruli associated with sclerosing lesions confined to the hilus of the glomerular tuft lesions suggests haemodynamic or maladaptive changes, while the presence of Tip lesions recalls idiopathic FSGS or MCD. The presence of mesangial hypercellularity is more typical of the idiopathic form of FSGS. Electron microscopy features are crucial to distinguish between a primary versus secondary form of FSGS (Sethi et al., 2015). Extensive presence of electron dense deposits in the mesangium or subendothelial areas should indicate another primary or systemic disease. The presence of less than 50 per cent effacement of the foot-processes along the capillary surface should suggest a secondary rather than primary FSGS, with the exception of cases of FSGS secondary to HIV, interferon, or IV bisphosphonate infusion. In these forms of FSGS, the histological findings are similar to those seen in idiopathic forms, but lesions are more severe, most often of the collapsing variety, and extensive tubuloreticular structures may be found in endothelial cells. These forms progress to ESRD within a few months compared with the slower progression for idiopathic FSGS.

Which FSGS patients should be offered genetic testing?

There is agreement that genetic testing should be offered for the subjects with a familial form of FSGS in order to identify the responsible gene. This will provide additional data on a genotype/phenotype correlation and might also be clinically informative in situations where living-related donor transplant is considered. Causal mutations in four genes (*NPHS1, NPHS2, WT1, LAMB2*) explain the majority (66 per cent) of NS that present in the first year of life. Thus, whenever a NS develops in a very precocious age or in the presence of a strong family history suggesting an autosomal recessive, autosomal dominant, X-linked, or mitochondrial inheritance pattern, a genetic screening may be performed before starting treatment. Monogenic forms of FSGS are frequent and resistant to steroids and other immunosuppressive drugs (Rheault and Gbadegesin, 2016). Thus, response to corticosteroids precludes the need for genetic analysis, while in steroid-resistant cases genetic testing may be considered even in the absence of a positive family history (De Vriese et al., 2018; Wareiko et al., 2018). Clinicians cannot establish on clinical grounds whether a given sporadic (non-familial) case of FSGS is or is not inherited, since in some (nuclear) families a recessive disease will be apparent in only one child. In sporadic patients, the role of genetic testing will depend on the frequency of the different forms of inherited FSGS and on the response to specific treatment, since most (although not all) inherited podocyte diseases do not respond to any therapy.

In a child ≥2 years of age, or in an adult with nephrotic-range proteinuria and FSGS, genetic testing should not change the initial evaluation. However, it is now clear that a significant fraction (25 per cent) of sporadic FSGS resistant to steroid treatment in children or in adults younger than 25 years is due to monogenic mutations (Lovric et al., 2016). More than 50 recessive or dominant genes may cause steroid-resistant NS. Among them, *NPHS2*, encoding podocin, is the most frequent. Thus, in a young subject with new-onset NS not responding to steroids, *NPHS2* testing is warranted. However, since recessive mutation is rare in older Caucasian adults with FSGS, mutation screening is not recommended for these subjects. In patients with a clear family history of FSGS and NS, evaluation is required, regardless of age. Mutations in other genes may occur, but they are much less likely to be a cause of FSGS. In clinical practice the decision to perform the costly genetic analysis may be based on treatment decisions in difficult cases, transplantation, and genetic counselling. A possible exception is represented by African subjects with hypertension and FSGS, usually of the collapsing variant. They are often carrier of *APOL1* alleles G1 and G2, which confer protection against trypanosomal infections but increase the risk of FSGS (Chen and Liapis, 2015). However, assessment of *APOL1* variants in such patients accrues no benefits for therapeutic decision making. The type of screening will influence the results—whole genome sequencing (WGS) will identify more cases of genetic FSGS than targeted exome sequencing (TES).

Should non-nephrotic patients with FSGS be treated?

Patients with presumed primary FSGS who have sustained non-nephrotic levels of proteinuria less than 2.0 g/day usually do not progress to ESRD, are not exposed to the possible complications of the NS, and are generally asymptomatic. Therefore 'specific' treatment is not strictly necessary for these patients. Control of blood pressure however should always be vigorous, preferably using angiotensin-converting enzyme inhibitors (ACEi), angiotensin receptor blockers (ARBs), or both, in view of their benefits on proteinuria, endothelial function, and cardiac protection (see Chapter 2).

One of the most difficult areas of management of FSGS is for those patients who have persisting proteinuria between 2.0 and 3.5 g/day, do not have hypoalbuminaemia, but have mild to moderate decrease in renal function. These patients are often hypertensive and are good candidates for treatment with ACEi and/or ARB. Along with vigorous blood pressure control, these agents have been shown to be able to decrease the level of proteinuria and slow the progression of renal insufficiency in patients with FSGS (Korbet, 2012). However, RCTs specific for FSGS are lacking. ACEi and ARB appear to be of particular value for patients with FSGS secondary to conditions associated with hyperfiltration and/or reduced nephron mass and those patients with non-nephrotic primary FSGS. Since low plasma 25(OH)D is associated with higher risk of developing increased albuminuria (Keyzer et al., 2015), supplementation of 25(OH) vitamin D is recommended in patients with deficient levels of 25(OH)D. Statins are also recommended to lower lipid levels and to reduce the risk of cardiovascular disease; their efficacy in reducing proteinuria is still unproven. If proteinuria neither remits nor falls below 2.0 g/day with these measures and the overall clinical condition of the patient is favourable, we feel justified in performing a trial with glucocorticoids in a patient with subnephrotic proteinuria (2.0–3.5 g/day) to obtain a full remission of proteinuria to less than 2.0 g/day and hopefully slow the progression towards renal failure.

Should nephrotic patients with FSGS be treated with 'specific' therapy?

An aggressive approach is justified in nephrotic patients with FSGS both because spontaneous complete remission of proteinuria is very uncommon and because patients with persistent nephrotic-range proteinuria usually progress to ESRD. On the contrary, if it is possible to induce complete or partial remission, the long-term renal outcome is generally favourable. A further reason in favour of treatment is that nephrotic patients may be exposed to an increased risk of severe and even life-threatening complications, including intravascular thrombosis and cardiovascular disease. Moreover, nephrotic patients need several drugs to control oedema, hyperlipidaemia, electrolyte disorders, etc. Each of these drugs has a cost and potential side-effects.

Treatment for nephrotic patients

Even if we lack of RCTs showing the superiority of glucocorticoids over placebo in FSGS, a number of observational studies have shown that an initial short-term course with glucocorticoids is generally safe and can obtain response in at least some patients (around 20–25 per cent). Usually this first therapeutic approach consists of high-dose oral prednisone (60 mg/m^2/day for children; 1 mg/kg/day for adults) for two months, often associated with renin-angiotensin system (RAS) inhibitors. For patients who respond, the subsequent treatment may consist in a progressive tapering off along six months. However, only a relatively few patients can be anticipated to respond to this initial treatment regimen (perhaps one in four to five treated patients).

It remains quite uncertain as to what is the best course for patients who do not respond to an initial short-term course of glucocorticoids. Until recently, many clinicians preferred to stop any form of 'specific' treatment and to provide only 'symptomatic' therapy, including renin-angiotensin system (RAS) inhibition, in order not to expose patients with little chances of responding to the possible iatrogenic morbidity of continued glucocorticoid or immunosuppressive therapy. In this regard, it must be pointed out that combined treatments with low-salt diet, diuretics, hypolipidaemic drugs, renin-angiotensin system (RAS) inhibitors, and anti-thrombotic agents may keep some patients asymptomatic (including oedema free), although their influence on progression to renal failure in primary FSGS specifically is still unproven. The attitude of nephrologists toward treatment of the patients with FSGS who do not display any response at all to short-term steroid treatment has changed after the demonstration that more than 50 per cent of nephrotic patients with primary FSGS will respond to more prolonged steroid therapy or to other treatments. Thus, several different, but equally acceptable, therapeutic approaches may be used in patients who do not respond to a short-term course of glucocorticoids.

Prolonged steroid treatment

Observational, non-randomized trials provided consistent evidence that patients with FSGS who are resistant to an eight-week course with oral prednisone in high-dosage may subsequently respond to a more prolonged steroid administration. Thus, according to the 2012 KDIGO guidelines, prednisone should be given at a daily single dose of 1 mg/kg (maximum 80 mg) or alternate-day dose of 2 mg/kg (maximum 120 mg) for a minimum of four weeks up to a maximum of 16 weeks, as tolerated, or until complete remission has been achieved, followed by reduced doses for at least six months. About 50–60 per cent of patients treated in this fashion can be expected to respond with a remission (complete or partial).

However, some patients who tolerated a short-term course of glucocorticoids may develop steroid-related toxicity when treatment is prolonged (diabetes, obesity, Cushingoid appearance, infections, cataracts, bone complications, psychiatric reactions, etc.). Particularly delicate is the problem in children, in whom a prolonged administration of glucocorticoids can reduce the growth velocity and can be responsible for stature retardation. Moreover, a number of responders may develop frequent relapses or steroid dependency aggravating the problem further.

Calcineurin inhibitors (CNI)

A good therapeutic option for patients who do not respond to a short course of glucocorticoids is represented by calcineurin inhibitors (CNI). Observational and randomized controlled studies showed that CsA and TAC, especially when associated with steroids, can induce complete or partial response of proteinuria in 50–60 per cent of nephrotic patients with FSGS who were initially steroid intolerant or unresponsive. These data provide a good quality of evidence and a rationale for recommending CNI, particularly in patients at risk of complications with glucocorticoids and in children to allow a normal growth rate, and to avoid the aesthetic changes of steroids that may reduce the adherence to prescriptions.

However, some guidelines must be carefully followed with the use of CNI (see Chapter 3). In particular, patients with sustained renal insufficiency (i.e. GFR <50 ml/min), arterial hypertension, diffuse glomerular sclerosis, and/ or moderately advanced tubulo-interstitial lesions at renal biopsy should be considered poor candidates for therapy with CNI. Most patients who do not respond within six months are unlikely to remit later, but late response may occur in rare instances. In patients who respond with a partial or complete remission, CNI may be gradually tapered after 6–12 months in order to identify the minimal effective dosage. A few patients treated for two years or more may be able to maintain a stable remission after a progressive tapering of CNI to zero.

Mycophenolate salts

Mycophenolate salts are a further option in steroid- and/or CNI-intolerant patients. MMF at a dose of 2 g/day (or sodium mycophenolate at a dose of 1440 mg/day) may be given for six months and continued at half doses for another 18–24 months. The association with low-dose steroids or combination with a CNI may improve the efficacy. However, the current evidence is insufficient to place much confidence that a good result will be obtained by this strategy.

Alkylating agents

An 8–12-week course with an alkylating agent may obtain the same rate of response than a short course of high-dose prednisone and may be therefore indicated as a primary treatment in patients who have contra-indications to glucocorticoids. However, there is no evidence that cytotoxic drugs can obtain good results in patients with FSGS who do not respond to glucocorticoids and its use in steroid-resistant patients cannot be recommended.

Rituximab

Rituximab is poorly effective in steroid-resistant FSGS but might obtain some improvement in proteinuria if given in association with CNI and/or mycophenolate.

Treatment recommendation for nephrotic patients with primary FSGS

In summary, we propose the following initial regimen for nephrotic patients with FSGS (Figure 5.2). A course of eight weeks with full-dose prednisone (60 mg/m^2/day in children; 1 mg/kg/day in adults) should be offered to all nephrotic patients who do not have specific contra-indications to glucocorticoids. For responders who do not relapse, treatment should be stopped. In case of poor response but good tolerance, prednisone should be continued at tapering doses up to four to six months. Calcineurin inhibitors (CNIs) may be given initially in patients who are intolerant to glucocorticoids or at high risk for steroid-related complications. If well tolerated and effective, CNIs may be continued for one to two years, or even longer in patients who relapse after drug withdrawal. If CNIs do not obtain any improvement in proteinuria after six months, these drugs may be considered ineffective. Alternative treatments may include a 12-week course with cyclophosphamide at a dose of 2 mg/kg/day (with or without low-dose alternate day prednisone depending on the contraindications to steroids), or mycophenolate salts plus low-dose prednisone. RTX, plasmapheresis, and lipopheresis may also be used for initial treatment, but the response to these treatments is difficult to predict.

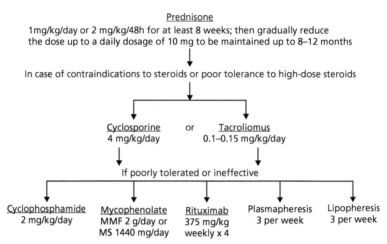

Figure 5.2 Initial treatment for patients with primary FSGS and nephrotic syndrome. In patients with contraindications or poor tolerance to glucocorticoids, cyclosporine, or tacrolimus may be proposed. Cyclophosphamide, mycophenolate, rituximab, plasmapheresis, or LDL apheresis may be attempted as initial compassionate treatments in refractory cases, but their efficacy is usually poor.

Whatever the therapeutic decision, it is mandatory that a nephrotic patient is followed carefully, so that the effectiveness and tolerance of the treatment can be checked on a regular basis. Clearly, the therapeutic choice may be modified according to the clinical outcome or the development of side-effects. A more aggressive approach from the outset may be tried in patients who develop severe, debilitating NS or progressive renal failure. On the other hand, therapy may have to be stopped or modified in patients showing iatrogenic toxicity under the assigned treatment regimen.

How to treat relapses of NS?

For patients who have frequent or infrequent relapses, one or more courses of glucocorticoids may be prescribed, the schedule being similar to that used for steroid-sensitive relapsers with MCD.

In case of steroid toxicity or intolerance, CNIs or RTX are the preferred alternative treatments. Either CsA or TAC should be administered for one to three years, if well tolerated, possibly associated with low-dose prednisone, and at the lowest effective doses.

RTX is very effective in steroid-sensitive patients and may represent an option in patients who are steroid- or CNI-dependent. However, after weeks of remission, relapses still occur, requiring further courses of RTX.

What to do with patients with primary FSGS refractory to treatment?

There is little evidence that patients who do not respond to any of the previous treatments may benefit by further therapies, and the cumulative toxicity of treatment is a growing concern. In the case of no response to the previously mentioned therapeutic regimens, the physician may choose among different options for additional therapy according to the clinical status of the patient and his/her wishes and fears:

  i. symptomatic therapy;
 ii. oral cyclosporine or tacrolimus plus low-dose alternate day steroids and MMF;
iii. Rituximab;
 iv. ACTH;
  v. Plasmapheresis or LDL apheresis.

Symptomatic therapy should be chosen in the case of a frail patient (often elderly or diabetic) particularly susceptible to the side-effects of glucocorticoids or CNI. CsA or tacrolimus associated with low-dose prednisone and mycophenolate may obtain some reduction of proteinuria even in patients refractory to glucocorticoids, but should be used with caution in patients with reduced renal function. The choice between CsA and TAC is mainly conditioned by the expected side-effects and the tolerance of the individual patients for these effects. A few patients who did not respond to CsA were reported to respond to a switch to TAC, given however at relatively high dosage.

Rituximab, ACTH, LDL apheresis, plasma exchange, and immuno-adsorption with column A have been observed to be of benefit in sporadic case reports. It is impossible to give recommendations on the basis of the scanty available data. Each treatment decision must be made on a case-by-case basis, analysing the potential (but largely unknown) benefits and the potential (and often known) risks. In making these decisions, we should always take into account the general clinical conditions of the patient and his/or her desires after an informed discussion of the benefits and risks. Written consent is often desirable when using approved drugs for off-label purposes.

What to do in patients with primary FSGS and renal insufficiency?

In general, there is not convincing evidence that any form of treatment is useful in patients who develop renal insufficiency despite treatment. CNI should not be used in these instances as they can further aggravate the kidney damage.

Cytotoxic agents are generally ineffective and poorly tolerated by patients with reduced renal function. Glucocorticoids also should be used with caution. Mycophenolate salts may be better tolerated, but there is no valuable information on their effectiveness in patients with deteriorating renal function due to progressive FSGS. Thus, in most cases, we prefer not to insist on treatments which have little chances of efficacy and a high risk of iatrogenic toxicity; rather, we maximize the symptomatic therapy with RAS inhibitors (checking serum potassium levels), statins, antiplatelet agents, and vitamin D supplements to correct the low levels of 25(OH) D in nephrotic patients (Selewski et al., 2016). However, we suggest not interrupting abruptly an immunosuppressive treatment, as this decision can accelerate the progression of renal failure in some cases. Therefore, it is better to reduce gradually the doses of the drugs used.

Transplantation

Recurrent FSGS

Patients with primary FSGS are at high risk of recurrence after renal transplantation. Approximately 20–30 per cent of patients develop recurrence of FSGS in the first allograft and 90–100 per cent have recurrence in the second allograft if a previous renal transplant failed because of FSGS recurrence (Ponticelli, 2010). Rapid progression to ESRD, higher levels of proteinuria, lower levels of serum albumin at diagnosis, an age younger than 18 years, and white ethnicity are the most powerful predictors of recurrence (Maas et al., 2013; Rudnicki, 2016). Patients with a history of non-familial, presumed primary FSGS and hypo-albuminaemia may have a risk of recurrence of FSGS lesions exceeding 70 per cent for the first renal transplant (Maas et al., 2013). Other factors include collapsing variant of FSGS and mesangial proliferative glomerulonephritis superimposed to FSGS (Table 5.7). As discussed, the familial forms of FSGS associated with recessive or dominant monogenic mutation seldom recur following transplantation, and even if a recurrence does develop it is generally mild and responsive to treatment (Vincenti and Ghiggeri, 2005). Also, patients with the sporadic variety of FSGS who also have homozygous or complex heterozygous monogenic mutations have a low recurrence rate. The results with living donation in FSGS are worse than in patients without FSGS (Baum et al., 2001). However, retrospective analyses of the US Renal Data System (Abbott et al., 2001), ERA/EDTA registry (Pippias et al., 2016), and the Australian and New Zealand registry (Francis et al., 2016) found that, despite that recurrence of FSGS was more frequent with live donors than with deceased donors, graft survival in live donor recipients was significantly better, suggesting that live donor transplantation should not be avoided in patients with FSGS.

Table 5.7 Risk of early recurrence of FSGS after transplantation.

High risk of recurrence	Low risk of recurrence
Second graft if the previous one was lost because of recurrence	Second graft without signs of recurrence in the previous graft
Children and young adults with primary FSGS	Children and young adults with congenital/familial form of NS
Pre-transplant circulating antibodies against CD40	Absence of pretransplant circulating antibodies against CD40?
Rapid progression of the original disease in the native kidney	Slow progression of the original disease in the native kidney
Low GFR, elevated proteinuria and low serum albumin at diagnosis	Non-nephrotic proteinuria, normal serum albumin at diagnosis
Mesangial proliferation or collapsing variant in the native kidney	Secondary forms of FSGS
Live donor	Deceased donor

There are two clinical presentations of recurrent FSGS after transplantation; an *early recurrence* with massive proteinuria within hours to days after implantation of the new kidney, and a *late* (more insidious) *recurrence* several months or years after transplantation. In patients with early recurrence, proteinuria, usually in a nephrotic range, may precede the development of histological lesions that develop in a median 10–18 days after transplantation. Initial biopsies may show normal-appearing glomeruli by light microscopy but diffuse foot process effacement by electron microscopy. Segmental sclerosing lesions associated with endocapillary proliferation and foam cell accumulation may occur later and progress to glomerular sclerosis and interstitial fibrosis. Fidelity of type of FSGS is usually, but not invariably, seen with recurrence of FSGS in the transplant (Fogo, 2015). Spontaneous remission of proteinuria is exceptional. Patients with early recurrence of FSGS have a high risk of graft failure. Late recurrence is rare and it is difficult to distinguish from *de novo* FSGS. The outcome is relentless but slower than in cases with early relapse.

The *pathogenesis* of recurrent FSGS is far from being established. The frequent occurrence of a rapid or even immediate relapse of proteinuria after transplantation suggests that at least some patients with FSGS have circulating factor(s) capable of altering glomerular permeability in normal grafts. However, despite an intensive research, the presence and the nature of this factor are still speculative. Use of research bio-assays for this putative permeability factor and its utility in predicting recurrence produced conflicting results. Recently, the attention of the investigators focused on the inter-podocyte connection. A role for costimulatory molecule B7-1(CD80) in podocytes as an inducible modifier of glomerular permselectivity has been suggested. Upregulation of B7-1 in podocytes may disrupt the glomerular filter and favour proteinuria (Reiser et al., 2004). It would be possible to hypothesize that ischemia-reperfusion injury may favour an overexpression of B7-1 in podocytes of the donated kidney. However, the possibility that B7.1 is expressed in human podocytes has been challenged (Novelli et al., 2016). Alternatively, it is possible that a subset of patients with FSGS may produce autoantibodies that may alter glomerular permeability. Indeed, antibodies directed against an epitope of extracellular domain of CD40, a costimulatory protein located on the membrane of antigen-presenting cell, have been isolated in sera of patients with post-transplant recurrence of FSGS (Delville et al., 2014). According to the molecular mimicry theory, the circulating antibodies of the recipient can recognize the amino acid sequences or the homologous three-dimensional crystal structure of immune-dominant epitopes of the donor, so disassembling the actin filaments, aggravating the podocyte cytoskeleton, and increasing the glomerular permeability to proteins.

The *management* of patients with recurrent FSGS and NS is difficult and not well established. RAS blockers are frequently administered to reduce proteinuria, but complete remission is exceptional (Bansal et al., 2017). Good results have been reported with high-dose CsA and steroids (Canaud et al., 2010). However, the long-term efficacy and tolerance of such a therapy remains to be established. The most commonly used therapeutic approach is represented by the use of plasmapheresis or immunoadsorption with protein A. A meta-analysis of six nonrandomized studies with 117 cases enrolled showed that plasmapheresis significantly increased the probability of complete or partial remission (Vlachopanos et al., 2015). Good results have been also reported with immuno-adsorption (Allard et al., 2018). However, these data were retrospective and anecdotal, the follow-up was variable, in many cases plasmapheresis had to be repeated for many months or years, and in spite of prolonged treatment, many patients eventually progressed to graft failure in the long term. It is also possible that not all the cases of failure have been reported.

RTX has also been used. Apart from its immunosuppressive activity, RTX can protect podocyte function and reduce proteinuria by preventing acid sphingomyelinase deregulation in podocytes (Fornoni et al., 2011). A systematic review of 39 cases of recurrent FSGS treated with RTX and plasmapheresis demonstrated complete response to therapy in 17 (43.6 per cent) patients and partial remission in eight (20.5 per cent; Araya and Dharnidharka, 2011). In a large multicentre retrospective study on 19 new cases who developed FSGS recurrence, initial treatment consisted of plasma exchanges, high doses of calcineurin inhibitors, and steroids. RTX was introduced either immediately (in six cases), or after failure of the initial treatment (ten cases), or failed attempted weaning from plasmapheresis (three cases). Nine patients (47 per cent) entered complete remission and three (16 per cent) obtained partial remission. Relapses occurred in four patients who needed further courses of RTX. Severe infections occurred in 14 of 19 patients (Garrouste et al., 2017).

Yu and colleagues (2013) reported that abatacept, a costimulatory inhibitor that target B7-1, may stabilize β1-integrin activation in podocytes and reduce proteinuria in a few patients with B7-1-positive FSGS. However, these data have not been confirmed by others (Garin et al., 2015; Delville et al., 2016; Kristensen et al., 2017). Sporadic cases of remission with ACTH (Mittal et al., 2015) have also been reported.

In summary, a genetic evaluation is advisable before transplanting a patient with FSGS, since patients with mutation of podocyte protein components have a low risk of recurrence. Conflicting reults have been reported with the use of pre-emptive plasmapheresis whenever possible, and particularly in patients receiving the kidney from a living donor and in those who lost a previous transplant from recurrence. A review of the literature reported that the risk of recurrence may be halved in patients with FSGS who received plasmapheresis before transplantation (Bosch and Wendler, 2001). A recent study reported that the incidence and time to recurrence of FSGS in the kidney allograft were not significantly different in patients that did and did not undergo prophylactic plasmapheresis (Verghese et al., 2018). After transplantation, proteinuria may herald the development of FSGS even if early biopsy does not show glomerular abnormalities at light microscopy. Patients with post-transplant proteinuria >2 g/day who have FSGS as their original disease should be treated as soon as possible with an intensive course of plasmapheresis (an exchange a day for three days, then two to three exchanges per week for the first two weeks, followed by one to two exchanges per week using 5 per cent albumin as the replacement fluid). The median number of treatments to response was nine in series (Davenport, 2001). It should be kept in mind that in some cases, prolonged plasmapheresis, even for many months, is needed before seeing complete or partial remission of proteinuria. If a complete disappearance of proteinuria is obtained, plasmapheresis treatment may be stopped. A further course of plasmapheresis may be attempted in the case of relapse of nephrotic proteinuria. If proteinuria improves but remains over 2–3 g/day, long-term plasma exchange therapy may be given at longer intervals. We also recommend the administration of high-dose RAS inhibitors and statins in order to exploit their antiproteinuric and antilipemic effects. The role of rituximab should be better elucidated by further studies, but in the absence of contra-indication a course with RTX might be attempted if plasmapheresis is of no benefit. However, the optimal doses and duration of treatment with RTX have not been established. In the few available reports the schedules varied from 375 mg/m^2 every week for four weeks to 1 g given two weeks apart, repeated at six months. The role of abatacept or ACTH requires further investigation.

De novo FSGS

De novo FSGS can occur in kidney transplant recipients. In a retrospective review of 2,599 renal allograft biopsies, 1.6 per cent of biopsies were reported as *de novo* FSGS. The majority were live related female donors with a mean age of 43.8 years. Most patients were receiving CNI (Patel et al., 2017). While *recurrent* FSGS usually presents early post-transplant as a NS, *de novo* FSGS is often detected more than 12 months after transplantation and is associated with variable amounts of proteinuria (including NS), hypertension, and progressive deterioration of renal allograft function.

The pathogenesis is probably multifactorial. Low nephron dose in the transplanted kidney, hypertension, diabetes, BK polyoma virus, parvovirus B19 infection, CNI toxicity, chronic rejection, or any other condition leading to loss of renal mass can be involved in the pathogenesis of FSGS. At light microscopy, the picture is dominated by chronic lesions with arteriolar occlusion, interstitial nephritis, striped interstitial fibrosis, tubular atrophy, and focal or global glomerular sclerosis (Ponticelli et al., 2014), and on electron microscopy the foot process effacement is less severe than in primary FSGS. Moreover, hypo-albuminaemia and oedema are less frequent and severe in *de novo* FSGS.

The prognosis is poor with a renal survival of only 40 per cent at five years after diagnosis in cases associated with chronic allograft nephropathy. Attempts to withdraw CNI, by introducing mTOR inhibitors, may obtain improvement or stabilization of renal function if the conversion is performed early, but this manoeuvre may increase the risk of rejection and result in graft failure if creatinine clearance is lower than 40 ml/min or proteinuria is more than 800 mg/day (Diekmann et al., 2004); cases of *de novo* FSGS have been reported in transplant recipients converted from CNI to high doses of Sirolimus in the presence of proteinuria (Letavernier et al., 2009). Graft failure caused by *de novo* FSGS does not represent a contra-indication to retransplant. However, efforts should be made to identify the factors responsible for FSGS and to prevent its development after re-transplantation by measures, such as minimization of CNI or antiviral prophylaxis.

References

Abbott KC, Sawyers ES, Oliver III JD, et al. (2001). Graft loss due to recurrent focal segmental glomerulosclerosis in renal transplant recipients in the United States. Am J Kidney Dis. **37**: 366–73.

Abkhezr M, Kim EY, Roshanravan H, et al. (2015). Pleiotropic signaling evoked by tumor necrosis factor in podocytes. Am J Physiol Renal Physiol. **309**: F98–108.

Allard L, Kwon T, Krid S, et al. (2018). Treatment by immunoadsorption for recurrent focal segmental glomerulosclerosis after paediatric kidney transplantation: A multicentre French cohort. Nephrol Dial Transplant. **33**: 954–63.

Alwahaibi NY, Alhabsi TA, Alrawahi SA. (2013). Pattern of glomerular diseases in Oman: A study based on light microscopy and immunofluorescence. Saudi J Kidney Dis Transpl. **24**: 387–91.

Anyaegbu EI, Shaw AS, Hruska KA, et al. (2015). Clinical phenotype of APOL1 nephropathy in young relatives of patients with end-stage renal disease. Pediatr Nephrol. **30**: 983–9.

Araya CE, Dharnidharka VR. (2011). The factors that may predict response to rituximab therapy in recurrent focal segmental glomerulosclerosis: A systematic review. J Transplant. **2011**: 374213.

Arias LF, Franco-Alzate C, Rojas SL. (2011). Tip variant of focal segmental glomerulosclerosis: Outcome and comparison to 'not otherwise specified' variant. Nephrol Dial Transplant. **26**: 2215–21.

Banaszak B, Banaszak P. (2012). The increasing incidence of initial steroid resistance in childhood nephrotic syndrome. Pediatr Nephrol. **27**: 927–32.

Bansal SB, Sethi SK, Jha P, et al. (2017). Remission of post-transplant focal segmental glomerulosclerosis with angiotensin receptor blockers. Indian J Nephrol. **27**: 154–6.

Barbour SJ, Cattran DC, Espino-Hernandez G, et al. (2015). Identifying the ideal metric of proteinuria as a predictor of renal outcome in idiopathic glomerulonephritis. Kidney Int. **88**: 1392–401.

Barisoni L, Nast CC, Jennette JC, et al. (2013). Digital pathology evaluation in the multicenter Nephrotic Syndrome Study Network (NEPTUNE). Clin J Am Soc Nephrol. **20138**: 1449–59.

Barisoni L, Troost JP, Nast C, et al. (2016). Reproducibility of the NEPTUNE descriptor-based scoring system on whole-slide images and histologic and ultrastructural digital images. Mod Pathol. **29**: 671–84.

Basu B, Mahapatra TK, Mondal N. (2015). Mycophenolate mofetil following rituximab in children with steroid-resistant nephrotic syndrome. Pediatrics. **136**: e132–9.

Baum MA, Stablein DM, Panzarino VM, et al. (2001). Loss of living donor renal allograft survival advantage in children with focal segmental glomerulosclerosis. Kidney Int. **59**: 328–33.

Baye E, Gallazzini M, Delville M, et al. (2016). The costimulatory receptor B7-1 is not induced in injured podocytes. Kidney Int. **90**: 1037–44.

Bazzi C, Rizza V, Casellato D, et al. (2013). Urinary IgG and α2-macroglobulin are powerful predictors of outcome and responsiveness to steroids and cyclophosphamide in idiopathic focal segmental glomerulosclerosis with nephrotic syndrome. Biomed Res Int. 2013: 941831

Bennett MR, Pordal A, Haffner C, et al. (2016). Urinary vitamin d-binding protein as a biomarker of steroid-resistant nephrotic syndrome. Biomark Insights. **11**: 1–6.

Bhimma R, Adhikari M, Asharam K, et al. (2006). Management of steroid-resistant focal segmental glomerulosclerosis in children using tacrolimus. Am J Nephrol. **26**: 544–51.

Bock ME, Price HE, Gallon L, et al. (2013). Serum soluble urokinase-type plasminogen activator receptor levels and idiopathic FSGS in children: A single-center report. Clin J Am Soc Nephrol. **8**: 1304–11.

Bonanni A, Bertelli R, Rossi R, et al. (2015). A pilot study of IL2 in drug-resistant idiopathic nephrotic syndrome. PLoS One. **10**: e0138343.

Borges FF, Shiraichi L, da Silva MP, et al. (2007). Is focal segmental glomerulosclerosis increasing in patients with nephrotic syndrome? Ped Nephrol. **22**: 1309–13.

Bosch T, Wendler T. (2001). Extracorporeal plasma treatment in primary and recurrent focal segmental glomerular sclerosis: A review. Ther Apher. **5**: 155–60.

Boyer O, Moulder JK, Somers MJ. (2007). Focal and segmental glomerular sclerosis in children: A longitudinal assessment. Ped Nephrol. **22**: 1159–66.

Braun N, Schmutzler F, Lange C, et al. (2008). Immunosuppressive treatment for focal segmental glomerulosclerosis in adults. Cochrane Database Syst Rev. **3**: CD003233.

Braunisch MC, Buttner-Herold M, Gunthner R, et al. (2018). Heterozygous COL4A3 variants in histologically diagnosed focal segmental glomerulosclerosis. Front Ped. **6**: 171.

Canaud G, Martinez F, Noël LH, et al. (2010). Therapeutic approach to focal and segmental glomerulosclerosis recurrence in kidney transplant recipients. Transplant Rev (Orlando). **24**: 121–8.

Cattran DC, Alexopoulos E, Heering P, et al. (2007). Cyclosporin in idiopathic glomerular disease associated with the nephrotic syndrome: Workshop recommendations. Kidney Int. **72**: 1429–47.

Cattran DC, Rao P. (1998). Long-term outcome in children and adults with classic focal segmental glomerulosclerosis. Am J Kidney Dis. **32**: 72–9.

Cattran DC, Reich HN, Beanlands HJ, et al. (2008). The impact of sex in primary glomerulonephritis. Nephrol Dial Transplant. **23**: 2247–53.

Chan CY, Liu ID, Resontoc LP, et al. (2016). T lymphocyte activation markers as predictors of responsiveness to rituximab among patients with FSGS. Clin J Am Soc Nephrol. **11**: 1360–8.

Chávez Valencia V, Orizaga de La Cruz C, Becerra Fuentes JG, et al. (2014). Epidemiology of glomerular disease in adults: A database review. Gac Med Mex. **150**: 186–93.

Chen JS, Chang LC, Wu CZ, et al. (2016). Significance of the urokinase-type plasminogen activator and its receptor in the progression of focal segmental glomerulosclerosis in clinical and mouse models. J Biomed Sci. **23**: 24. DOI: 0.1186/s12929-016-0242-7

Chen YM, Liapis H. (2015). Focal segmental glomerulosclerosis: Molecular genetics and targeted therapies. BMC Nephrol. **16**: 101.

Chiou YY, Lee YC, Chen MJ. (2017). Cyclosporine-based immunosuppressive therapy for patients with steroid-resistant focal segmental glomerulosclerosis: A meta-analysis. Curr Med Res Opin. **33**: 1389–99.

Cho ME, Smith DC, Branton MH, et al. (2007). Pirfenidone slows renal function deterioration in patients with focal segmental glomerulosclerosis. Clin J Am Soc Nephrol. **2**: 906–13.

Cho MH, Hong EH, Lee TH, et al. (2007). Pathophysiology of minimal change nephrotic syndrome and focal segmental glomerulosclerosis. Nephrology (Carlton). **12**: S11–14.

Choi MJ. (2013). Histologic classification of FSGS: Does form delineate function? Clin J Am Soc Nephrol. **8**: 344–6.

Choudhry S, Bagga A, Hari P, et al. (2009). Efficacy and safety of tacrolimus versus cyclosporine in children with steroid-resistant nephrotic syndrome: A randomized controlled trial. Am J Kidney Dis. **53**: 760–9.

Chun MJ, Korbet SM, Schwartz MM, et al. (2004), Focal segmental glomerulosclerosis in nephrotic adults: Presentation, prognosis, and response to therapy of the histologic variants. J Am Soc Nephrol. **15**: 2169–77.

Coppo R, Camilla R, Porcellini MG, et al. (2012). Saquinavir in steroid-dependent and - resistant nephrotic syndrome: A pilot study. Nephrol Dial Transplant. **27**: 1902–10.

Corbetta G, Ponticelli C. (2010). Once-a-day administration of everolimus, cyclosporine, and steroid after renal transplantation: A review of the rationale. Transplant Proc. **42**: 1303–7.

D'Agati VD, Alster JM, Jennette JC, et al. (2013). Association of histologic variants in FSGS clinical trial with presenting features and outcomes. Clin J Am Soc Nephrol. **8**: 399–406.

D'Agati VD, Fogo AB, Bruijn JA, et al. (2004). Pathologic classification of focal segmental glomerulosclerosis: A working proposal. Am J Kidney Dis. **43**: 368–82.

D'Agati VD, Kaskel FJ, Falk RJ. (2011). Focal segmental glomerulosclerosis. N Engl J Med. **365**: 2398–411.

Das U, Dakshinamurty KV, Prasad N. (2009). Ponticelli regimen in idiopathic nephrotic syndrome. Indian J Nephrol. **19**: 48–52.

Davenport RD. (2001). Apheresis treatment of recurrent focal segmental glomerulosclerosis after kidney transplantation: Re-analysis of published case-reports and case-series. J Clin Apher. **16**: 175–8.

Delville M, Baye E, Durrbach A, et al. (2016). B7-1 blockade does not improve post-transplant nephrotic syndrome caused by recurrent FSGS. J Am Soc Nephrol. **27**: 2520–7.

Delville M, Sigdel TK, Wei C, et al. (2014). A circulating antibody panel for pretransplant prediction of FSGS recurrence after kidney transplantation. Sci Transl Med. **6**: 256ra136.

de Mello VR, Rodrigues MT, Mastrocinque TH, et al. (2010). Mycophenolate mofetil in children with steroid/cyclophosphamide-resistant nephrotic syndrome. Pediatr Nephrol.**25**: 453–60.

De Vriese AS, Sethi S, Nath KA, et al. (2018). Differentiating primary, genetic, and secondary FSGS in adults: A clinicopathologic approach. Jam Soc Nephrol. **29**: 759–74.

Diekmann F, Budde K, Oppenheimer F, et al. (2004). Predictors of success in conversion from calcineurin inhibitor to sirolimus in chronic allograft dysfunction. Am J Transplant. **4**: 1869–75.

Doublier S, Zennaro C, Musante L, et al. (2017). Soluble CD40 ligand directly alters glomerular permeability and may act as a circulating permeability factor in FSGS. PLoS One. **12**: e0188045.

Dummer PD, Limou S, Rosenberg AZ, et al. (2015). APOL1 kidney disease risk variants: An evolving landscape. Semin Nephrol. **35**: 222–36.

Fan L, Liu Q, Liao Y. (2013). Tacrolimus is an alternative therapy option for the treatment of adult steroid-resistant nephrotic syndrome: A prospective, multicenter clinical trial. Int Urol Nephrol. **45**: 459–68.

Faul C, Donnelly M, Merscher-Gomez S, et al. (2008). The actin cytoskeleton of kidney podocytes is a direct target of the antiproteinuric effect of cyclosporine A. Nat Med. **14**: 931–8.

Fernandez-Fresnedo G, Segarra A, González E, et al. (2009). Rituximab treatment of adult patients with steroid-resistant focal segmental glomerulosclerosis. Clin J Am Soc Nephrol. **4**: 1317–23.

Filippone EJ, Dopson SJ, Rivers DM, et al. (2016). Adrenocorticotropic hormone analog use for podocytopathies. Int Med Case Rep J. **9**: 125–33.

Filler G, Young E, Geier P, et al. (2003). Is there really an increase in non-minimal change nephrotic syndrome in children? Am J Kidney Dis. **42**: 1107–13.

Fogo AB. (2015). Causes and pathogenesis of focal segmental glomerulosclerosis. Nat Nephrol Rev. **11**: 76–87.

Fornoni A, Sageshima J, Wei C, et al. (2011). Rituximab targets podocytes in recurrent focal segmental glomerulosclerosis. Sci Transl Med. **3**: 85ra46.

Foster MC, Coresh J, Fornage M, et al. (2013). APOL1 variants associate with increased risk of CKD among African Americans. J Am Soc Nephrol. **24**: 1484–91.

Francis A, Trnka P, McTaggart SJ. (2016). Long-term outcome of kidney transplantation in recipients with focal segmental glomerulosclerosis. Clin J Am Soc Nephrol. **7**: 2041–6.

Franco Palacios CR, Lieske JC, Wadei HM, et al. (2013). Urine but not serum soluble urokinase receptor (suPAR) may identify cases of recurrent FSGS in kidney transplant candidates. Transplantation. **96**: 394–9.

Gargah TT, Lakhoua MR. (2011). Mycophenolate mofetil in treatment of childhood steroid-resistant nephrotic syndrome. J Nephrol. **24**: 203–7.

Garin EH, Reiser J, Cara-Fuentes G, et al. (2015). Case series: CTLA4-IgG1 therapy in minimal change disease and focal segmental glomerulosclerosis. Pediatr Nephrol. **30**: 469–77.

Garrouste C, Canaud G, Buchler M, et al. (2017). Rituximab for recurrence of primary focal segmental glomerulosclerosis after kidney transplantation: Clinical outcomes. Transplantation. **101**: 649–56.

Gast C, Pengelly J, Lyon M, et al. (2016). Collagen (COLA4) mutations are the most frequent mutations underlying adult focal segmental glomerulosclerosis. Nephrol Dial Transplant. **31**: 961–70.

Gebeshuber CA, Kornauth C, Dong L, et al. (2013). Focal segmental glomerulosclerosis is induced by microRNA-193a and its downregulation of WT1. Nat Med. **19**: 481–7.

Gellermann J, Ehrich JH, Querfeld U. (2012). Sequential maintenance therapy with cyclosporin A and mycophenolate mofetil for sustained remission of childhood steroid-resistant nephrotic syndrome. Nephrol Dial Transplant. **27**: 1970–8.

Genovese G, Friedman DJ, Ross MD, et al. (2010). Association of trypanolytic ApoL1 variants with kidney disease in African Americans. Science. **329**: 841–5.

Ghiggeri GM, Catarsi P, Scolari F, et al. (2004). Cyclosporine in patients with steroid-resistant nephrotic syndrome: An open-label, non-randomized, retrospective study. Clin Ther. **26**: 1411–18.

Gipson DS, Trachtman H, Kaskel FJ, et al. (2011). Clinical trial of focal segmental glomerulosclerosis in children and young adults. Kidney Int. **80**: 868–78.

Gipson DS, Troost JP, Lafayette RA, et al. (2016). Complete remission in the nephrotic syndrome study network. Clin J Am soc Nephrol. **11**: 81–9.

Glassock RJ, Rule AD. (2016). Aging and the kidneys. Anatomy, physiology and consequences for defining chronic kidney disease. Nephron. **134**: 25–9.

Golay V, Trivedi M, Kurien AA, et al. (2013). Spectrum of nephrotic syndrome in adults: Clinicopathological study from a single center in India. Ren Fail. **35**: 487–91.

Grgic I, Campanholle G, Bijol V, et al. (2012). Targeted proximal tubule injury triggers interstitial fibrosis and glomerulosclerosis. Kidney Int. **82**: 172–83.

Gulati A, Sinha A, Gupta A, et al. (2012). Treatment with tacrolimus and prednisolone is preferable to intravenous cyclophosphamide as the initial therapy for children with steroid-resistant nephrotic syndrome. Kidney Int. **82**: 1130–5.

Hamasaki Y, Yoshikawa N, Nakazato H, et al. (2013). Prospective 5-year follow-up of cyclosporine treatment in children with steroid-resistant nephrosis. Pediatr Nephrol. **28**: 765–71.

Hayashi K, Sasamura H, Nakamura M. (2015). Renin-angiotensin blockade resets podocyte epigenome through Kruppel-like factor 4 and attenuates proteinuria. Kidney Int. **88**: 745–53.

Hayek SS, Sever S, Ko YA, et al. (2015). Soluble urokinase receptor and chronic kidney disease. N Engl J Med. **373**: 1916–25.

Heering P, Braun N, Mullejans R, et al. (2004). Cyclosporine A and chlorambucil in the treatment of idiopathic focal segmental glomerulosclerosis. Am J Kidney Dis. **43**: 10–18.

Hines SL, Agarwal A, Ghandour M, et al. (2018). Novel variants in *COL4A4* and *COL4A5* are rare causes of FSGS in two unrelated families. Hum Genome Var. **5**: 15.

Hodgin JB, Bitzer M, Wickman L, et al. (2015). Glomerular aging and focal global glomerulosclerosis: A podometric perspective. JASN. **26**: 3162–78.

Hogan J, Bomback AS, Mehta K, et al. (2013). Treatment of Idiopathic FSGS with adrenocorticotropic hormone gel. Clin J Am Soc Nephrol. **8**: 2072–81.

Hogg RJ, Friedman A, Greene T, et al. (2013). Renal function and proteinuria after successful immunosuppressive therapies in patients with FSGS. Clin J Am Soc Nephrol. **8**: 211–18.

Hommos MS, Zeng C, Liu Z, et al. (2018). Global glomerulosclerosis with nephrotic syndrome: The clinical importance of age adjustment. Kidney Int. **93**: 1175–82.

Huang J, Liu G, Zhang Y-M, et al. (2013). Plasma soluble urokinase receptor levels are increased but do not distinguish primary from secondary focal segmental glomerulosclerosis. Kidney Int. **84**: 366–72.

Hughson MD, Johnson K, Young RJ, et al. (2002). Glomerular size and glomerulosclerosis: Relationships to disease categories, glomerular solidification, and ischemic obsolescence. Am J Kidney Dis. **39**: 679–88.

Inaba A, Hamasaki Y, Ishikura K, et al. (2016). Long-term outcome of idiopathic steroid-resistant nephrotic syndrome in children. Pediatr Nephrol. **31**: 425–34.

Jahan A, Prabha R, Chaturvedi S, et al. (2015). Clinical efficacy and pharmacokinetics of tacrolimus in children with steroid-resistant nephrotic syndrome. Pediatr Nephrol. **30**: 1961–7.

Jegatheesan D, Nath K, Reyaldeen R, et al. (2016). Epidemiology of biopsy-proven glomerulonephritis in Queensland adults. Nephrology (Carlton). **21**: 28–34.

Kalantari S, Nafar M, Rutishauser D, et al. (2014). Predictive urinary biomarkers for steroid-resistant and steroid-sensitive focal segmental glomerulosclerosis using high resolution mass spectrometry and multivariate statistical analysis. BMC Nephrol. **15**: 141.

Kallash M, Aviles D. (2014). Efficacy of tacrolimus in the treatment of children with focal segmental glomerulosclerosis. World J Pediatr. **10**: 151–4.

Kamato D, Burch ML, Piva TJ, et al. (2013). Transforming growth factor-β signalling: Role and consequences of Smad linker region phosphorylation. Cell Signal. **25**: 2017–24.

Kavvadas P, Abed A, Poulain C, et al. (2017). Decreased expression of connexin 43 blunts the progression of experimental GN. J Am Soc Nephrol. **28**: 2915–30.

Kawakami T, Gomez IG, Ren S, et al. (2015). Deficient autophagy results in mitochondrial dysfunction and FSGS. J Am Soc Nephrol. **26**: 1040–52.

KDIGO. (2012). Clinical Practice Guideline for Glomerulonephritis. Kidney Int. **2S**: 1–274.

Keyzer CA, Lambers-Heerspink HJ, Joosten MM, et al. (2015). Plasma vitamin D level and change in albuminuria and eGFR according to sodium intake. Clin J Am Soc Nephrol. **10**: 2119–27.

Kiffel J, Rahimzada Y, Trachtman H. (2011). Focal segmental glomerulosclerosis and chronic kidney disease in pediatric patients. Adv Chronic Kidney Dis. **18**: 332–8.

Kim J, Patnaik N, Chorny N, et al. (2014). Second-line immunosuppressive treatment of childhood nephrotic syndrome: A single-center experience. Nephron Extra. **4**: 8–17.

Klaassen I, Özgören B, Sadowski CE, et al. (2015). Response to cyclosporine in steroid-resistant nephrotic syndrome: Discontinuation is possible. Pediatr Nephrol. **30**: 1477–83.

Kopp JB, Winkler CA, Zhao X, et al. (2015). Clinical features and histology of apolipoprotein L1-associated nephropathy in the FSGS clinical trial. J Am Soc Nephrol. **26**: 1443–8.

Korbet SM. (2012). Treatment of FSGS in adults. J Am Soc Nephrol. **23**: 1769–76.

Kristensen T, Ivarsen P, Povlsen JV. (2017). Unsuccessful treatment with abatacept in recurrent focal segmental glomerulosclerosis after kidney transplantation. Case Rep Nephrol Dial. **7**: 1–5.

Kriz W. (2018). Maintenance and breakdown of glomerular tuft architecture. J Am Soc Nephrol. **29**: 1075–7.

Kriz W, LeHir M. (2005). Pathways to nephron loss starting from glomerular diseases-insights from animal models. Kidney Int. **67**: 404–19.

Kriz W, Lemley KV. (2015). A potential role for mechanical forces in the detachment of podocytes and the progression of CKD. J Am Soc Nephrol. **26**: 258–69.

Kronbichler A, Bruchfeld A. (2014). Rituximab in adult minimal change disease and focal segmental glomerulosclerosis. Nephron Clin Pract. **128**: 277–82.

Kronbichler A, Kerschbaum J, Fernandez-Fresnedo G, et al. (2014). Rituximab treatment for relapsing minimal change disease and focal segmental glomerulosclerosis: A systematic review. Am J Nephrol. **39**: 322–30.

Kronbichler A, Leierer J, Oh J, et al. (2016). Immunologic changes implicated in the pathogenesis of focal segmental glomerulosclerosis. Biomed Res Int. **2016**: 2150451.

Kruzel-Davila E, Wasser WG, Aviram S, et al. (2016). APOL1 nephropathy: From gene to mechanisms of kidney injury. Nephrol Dial Transplant. **31**: 349–58.

Kuppe C, Gröne HJ, Ostendorf T, et al. (2015). Common histological patterns in glomerular epithelial cells in secondary focal segmental glomerulosclerosis. Kidney Int. **88**: 990–8.

Kuribayashi-Okuma E, Shibata S, Arai S, et al. (2016). Proteomics approach identifies factors associated with the response to low-density lipoprotein apheresis therapy in patients with steroid-resistant nephrotic syndrome. Ther Apher Dial. **20**: 174–82.

Kwon YE, Han SH, Kie JH, et al. (2014). Clinical features and outcomes of focal segmental glomerulosclerosis pathologic variants in Korean adult patients. BMC Nephrol. **15**: 52.

Lasagni L, Angelotti ML, Ronconi E, et al. (2015). Podocyte regeneration driven by renal progenitors determines glomerular disease remission and can be pharmacologically enhanced. Stem Cell Reports. **11**: 248–63.

Lau EW, Ma PH, Wu X, et al. (2013). Mycophenolate mofetil for primary focal segmental glomerulosclerosis: Systematic review. Ren Fail. **35**: 914–29.

Laurin LP, Gasim AM, Poulton CJ, et al. (2016). Treatment with glucocorticoids or calcineurin inhibitors in primary FSGS. Clin J Am Soc Nephrol. **11**: 386–94.

LeHir M, Kriz W. (2007). New insights into structural patterns encountered in glomerulosclerosis. Curr Opin Nephrol Hypertens. **16**: 184–91.

Leierer J, Mayer G, Kronbichler A. (2016). Primary focal segmental glomerulosclerosis: miRNA and targeted therapies. Eur J Clin Invest. **46**: 954–64.

Letavernier E, Bruneval P, Vandermeersch S, et al. (2009). Sirolimus interacts with pathways essential for podocyte integrity. Nephrol Dial Transplant. **24**: 630–8.

Li X, Li H, Ye H, et al. (2009). Tacrolimus therapy in adults with steroid- and cyclophosphamide-resistant nephrotic syndrome and normal or mildly reduced GFR. Am J Kidney Dis. **54**: 51–8.

Li X, Zhang X, Li X, et al. (2014). Cyclosporine A protects podocytes via stabilization of cofilin-1 expression in the unphosphorylated state. Exp Biol Med (Maywood). **239**: 922–36.

Liern M, De Reyes V, Fayad A, et al. (2012). Use of sirolimus in patients with primary steroid-resistant nephrotic syndrome. Nefrologia. **32**: 321–8.

Lim BJ, Yang JW, Do WS, et al. (2016). Pathogenesis of focal segmental glomerulosclerosis. J Pathol Transl Med. **50**: 405–410.

Ljutić D, Kesl P. (2003). The role of arterial hypertension in the progression of non-diabetic glomerular diseases. Nephrol Dial Transplant .**18**: v28–v30.

Lovric S, Ashraf S, Tan W, et al. (2016). Genetic testing in steroid-resistant nephritic syndrome: When and how? Nephrol Dial Transplant .31: 1813–21.

Maas RJ, Deegens JK, van den Brand JA, et al. (2013). A retrospective study of focal segmental glomerulosclerosis: Clinical criteria can identify patients at high risk for recurrent disease after first renal transplantation. BMC Nephrol. 14: 47.

Madan A, Mijovic-Das S, Stankovic A, et al. (2016). Acthar gel in the treatment of nephrotic syndrome: A multicentre retrospective case series. BMC Nephrol. 17: 37.

Magnasco A, Ravani P, Edefonti A, et al. (2012). Rituximab in children with resistant idiopathic nephrotic syndrome. J Am Soc Nephrol. 23: 1117–24.

Mallipattu SK, Guo Y, Revelo MP, et al. (2017). Krüppel-Like factor 15 mediates glucocorticoid-induced restoration of podocyte differentiation markers. J Am Soc Nephrol. 28: 166–84.

Mallipattu, SK, Horne SJ, D'Agati V, et al. (2015). Krüppel-like factor 6 regulates mitochondrial function in the kidney. J Clin Invest. 125: 1347–61.

Marcos-Palacios CRF, Lieske JC, Wadei HM, et al. (2013). Urine but not serum soluble urokinase receptor (suPAR) may identify cases of recurrent FSGS in kidney transplant candidates. Transplantation. 96: 394–9.

Mariani LH, Martini S, Barisoni L, et al. (2018). Interstitial fibrosis scored on whole-slide digital imaging of kidney biopsies is a predictor of outcome in proteinuric glomerulopathies. Nephrol Dial Transplant. 33: 310–18.

McCarthy ET, Sharma M, Savin VJ. (2010). Circulating permeability factors in idiopathic nephrotic syndrome and focal segmental glomerulosclerosis. Clin J Am Soc Nephrol. 5: 2115–21.

McGrogan A, Franssen CFM, de Vries C. (2011). The incidence of primary glomerulonephritis worldwide: A systematic review of the literature. Nephrol Dial Transplant. 26: 414–43.

Meijers B, Maas RJ, Sprangers B, et al. (2014). The soluble urokinase receptor is not a clinical marker for focal segmental glomerulosclerosis. Kidney Int. 85: 636–40.

Mittal T, Dedhia P, Roy-Chaudhury P, et al. (2015). Complete remission of post-transplantation recurrence of focal segmental glomerulosclerosis with the use of adrenocorticotrophic hormone gel: Case 4eport. Transplant Proc. 47: 2219–22.

Morgan C, Sis B, Pinsk M, et al. (2011). Renal interstitial fibrosis in children treated with FK506 for nephrotic syndrome. Nephrol Dial Transplant. 26: 2860–5.

Mungan S, Turkmen E, Aydin MC, et al. (2015). Tip lesion variant of primary focal and segmental glomerulosclerosis: Clinicopathological analysis of 20 cases. Ren Fail. 37: 858–65.

Muso E. (2014). Beneficial effect of LDL-apheresis in refractory nephrotic syndrome. Clin Exp Nephrol. 18: 286–90.

Muso E, Mune M, Hirano T, et al. (2015). Immediate therapeutic efficacy of low-density lipoprotein apheresis for drug-resistant nephrotic syndrome: Evidence from the short-term results from the POLARIS Study. Clin Exp Nephrol. 19: 379–86.

Nagata M. (2016). Podocyte injury and its consequences. Kidney Int. 89: 1221–30.

Nishizono R, Kikuchi M, Wang Su Q, et al. (2017). FSGS as an adaptive response to growth-induced podocyte stress. J Am Soc Nephrol. 28: 2931–45.

Novelli R, Gagliardini E, Ruggiero B, et al. (2016). Any value of podocyte B7-1 as a biomarker in human MCD and FSGS? Am J Physiol Renal Physiol. **310**: F335–41.

Ochi A, Takei T, Nakayama K, et al. (2012). Rituximab treatment for adult patients with focal segmental glomerulosclerosis. Intern Med. **51**: 759–62.

Patel RD, Vanikar AV, Nigam LA, et al. (2017). *De Novo* focal segmental glomerulosclerosis in renal allograft-histological presentation and clinical correlation: Single centre experience. J Clin Diagn Res. **11**: EC39–42.

Pedigo CE, Ducasa GM, Leclercq F, et al. (2016). Local TNF causes NFATc1-dependent cholesterol-mediated podocyte injury. J Clin Invest. **126**: 3336–50.

Pippias M, Stel VS, Aresté-Fosalba N, et al. (2016). Long-term kidney transplant outcomes in primary glomerulonephritis: Analysis from the ERA-EDTA Registry. Transplantation. **100**: 1955–62.

Plank C, Kalb V, Hinkes B, et al. (2008). Cyclosporin A is superior to cyclophosphamide in children with steroid-resistant nephrotic syndrome: A randomized controlled multicentre trial by the Arbeitsgemeinschaft für Pädiatrische Nephrologie. Ped Nephrol. **23**: 1483–93.

Ponticelli C. (2010). Recurrence of focal segmental glomerular sclerosis (FSGS) after renal transplantation. Nephrol Dial Transplant. **25**: 25–31.

Ponticelli C, Anders JA. (2017). Thrombospondin immune regulation and the kidney. Nephrol Dial Transplant. **32**: 1084–9.

Ponticelli C, Graziani G. (2014). Current and emerging treatments for focal and segmental glomerulosclerosis in adults. Expert Rev Clin Immunol. **9**: 251–61.

Ponticelli C, Moroni G, Glassock RJ. (2010). *De novo* glomerular diseases after renal transplantation. Clin J Am Soc Nephrol. **5**: 2363–72.

Ponticelli C, Villa M, Banfi G, et al. (1999). Can prolonged treatment improve the prognosis in adults with focal segmental glomerulosclerosis? Am J Kidney Dis. **34**: 618–25.

Praga M, Morales E. (2006). Obesity, proteinuria and progression of renal failure. Curr Opin Nephrol Hypertension. **15**: 481–6.

Raij L, Tian R, Wong JS, et al. (2016). Podocyte injury: The role of proteinuria, urinary plasminogen, and oxidative stress. Am J Physiol Renal Physiol. **311**: F1308–17.

Ramachandran R, Kumar V, Rathi M, et al. (2014). Tacrolimus therapy in adult-onset steroid-resistant nephrotic syndrome due to a focal segmental glomerulosclerosis: Single-center experience. Nephrol Dial Transplant. **29**: 1918–24.

Reggiani F, Ponticelli C. (2016). Focal segmental glomerular sclerosis: Do not overlook the role of immune response. J Nephrol. **29**: 525–34.

Reiser J, von Gersdorff G, Loos M, et al. (2004). Induction of B7-1 in podocytes is associated with nephrotic syndrome. J Clin Invest. **113**: 1390–7.

Ren H, Shen P, Li X, et al. (2013). Tacrolimus versus cyclophosphamide in steroid-dependent or steroid-resistant focal segmental glomerulosclerosis: A randomized controlled trial. Am J Nephrol. **37**: 84–90.

Rheault MN, Gbadegesin RA. (2016). The genetics of nephrotic syndrome. J Pediatr Genet. **5**: 15–24.

Roccatello D, Sciascia S, Rossi D, et al. (2017). High-dose rituximab ineffective for focal segmental glomerulosclerosis: A long-term observational study. Am J Nephrol. **46**: 108–13.

Rosenberg AZ, Kopp JB. (2017). Focal segmental glomerulosclerosis. Clin J Am Soc Nephrol. **12**: 502–17.

Rudnicki M. (2016). FSGS recurrence in adults after renal transplantation. Biomed Res Int. **2016**: 3295618.

Sakamoto K, Ueno T, Kobayashi N, et al. (2014). The direction and role of phenotypic transition between podocytes and parietal epithelial cells in focal segmental glomerulosclerosis. Am J Physiol Renal Physiol. **306**: F98–104.

Sala G, Badalamenti S, Ponticelli C. (2016). The renal connexome and possible roles of connexins in kidney diseases. Am J Kidney Dis. **67**: 677–87.

Savin VJ, McCarthy ET, Sharma R, et al. (2008). Galactose binds to focal segmental glomerulosclerosis permeability factor and inhibits its activity. Transl Res. **151**: 288–92.

Savin VJ, Sharma M, Zhou J, et al. (2015). Renal and hematological effects of CLCF-1, a B-Cell-stimulating cytokine of the IL-6 Family. J Immunol Res. **2015**: 714964.

Schena PF, Cameron JS. (1988). Treatment of proteinuric idiopathic glomerulonephritis in adults: A retrospective study. Am J Med. **85**: 315–26.

Schwartzman M, Reginensi A, Wong JS, et al. (2016). Podocyte-specific deletion of yes-associated protein causes FSGS and progressive renal failure. J Am Soc Nephrol. **27**: 216–26.

Segarra Medrano A, Vila Presas J, Pou Clavé L, et al. (2011). Efficacy and safety of combined cyclosporin A and mycophenolate mofetil therapy in patients with cyclosporin-resistant focal segmental glomerulosclerosis. Nefrologia. **31**: 286–91.

Selewski DT, Chen A, Shatat IF, et al. (2016). Vitamin D in incident nephrotic syndrome: A Midwest Pediatric Nephrology Consortium study. Pediatr Nephrol. **31**: 465–72.

Senthil Nayagam L, Ganguli A, Rathi M, et al. (2008). Mycophenolate mofetil or standard therapy for membranous nephropathy and focal segmental glomerulosclerosis: A pilot study. Nephrol Dial Transplant. **23**: 1926–30.

Sethi S, Glassock RJ, Fervenza FC. (2015). Focal segmental glomerulosclerosis: Towards a better understanding for the practicing nephrologist. Nephrol Dial Transplant. **30**: 375–84.

Sethna CB, Gibson DS. (2012). Treatment of FSGS in children. Adv Chronic Kidney Dis. **21**: 194–9.

Singh L, Singh G, Sharma A, et al. (2015). A comparative study on renal biopsy before and after long-term calcineurin inhibitors therapy: An insight for pathogenesis of its toxicity. Hum Pathol. **46**: 34–9.

Sinha A, Bajpai J, Saini S, et al. (2014). Serum-soluble urokinase receptor levels do not distinguish focal segmental glomerulosclerosis from other causes of nephrotic syndrome in children. Kidney Int. **85**: 649–58.

Sinha A, Gupta A, Kalaivani M, et al. (2017). Mycophenolate mofetil is inferior to tacrolimus in sustaining a remission in children with idiopathic steroid-resistant nephrotic syndrome. Kidney Int. **92**: 248–57.

Sinha A, Sharma A, Mehta A, et al. (2013). Calcineurin inhibitor induced nephrotoxicity in steroid resistant nephrotic syndrome. Indian J Nephrol. **23**: 41–6.

Smeets B, Kuppe C, Sicking EM. (2011). Parietal epithelial cells participate in the formation of sclerotic lesions in focal segmental glomerulosclerosis. J Am Soc Nephrol. **22**: 1262–74.

Spinale JM, Mariani LH, Kapoor S, et al. (2015). A reassessment of soluble urokinase-type plasminogen activator receptor in glomerular disease. Kidney Int. **87**: 564–74.

Stein EA, Raal FJ. (2015). Lipid-lowering drug therapy for CVD prevention: Looking into the future. Curr Cardiol Rep. **17**: 104.

Stokes MB, D'Agati VD. (2014). Morphologic variants of focal segmental glomerulosclerosis and their significance. Adv Chronic Kidney Dis. **21**: 400–7.

Suyama K, Kawasaki Y, Miyazaki K, et al. (2016). Rituximab and low-dose cyclosporine combination therapy for steroid-resistant focal segmental glomerulosclerosis. Pediatr Int. **58**: 219–23.

Swaminathan S, Leung N, Lager DJ, et al. (2007). Changing incidence of glomerular disease in Olmsted County, Minnesota: A 30-year renal biopsy study. Clin J Am Soc Nephrol. **1**: 483–7.

Swarnalatha G, Ram R, Ismal KM. (2015). Focal and segmental glomerulosclerosis: Does prognosis vary with the variants? Saudi J Kidney Dis Transpl. **26**: 173–81.

Taneda S, Honda K, Ohno M, et al. (2015). Podocyte and endothelial injury in focal segmental glomerulosclerosis: An ultrastructural analysis. Virchows Arch. **467**: 449–58.

Testagrossa L, Azevedo Neto R, Resende A, et al. (2013). Immunohistochemical expression of podocyte markers in the variants of focal segmental glomerulosclerosis. Nephrol Dial Transplant. **28**: 91–8.

Thurman JM, Wong M, Renner B, et al. (2015). Complement activation in patients with focal segmental glomerulosclerosis. PLoS One. **10**: e0136558.

Trachtman H, Vento S, Herreshoff E, et al. (2015). Efficacy of galactose and adalimumab in patients with resistant focal segmental glomerulosclerosis: Report of the FONT clinical trial group. BMC Nephrol. **16**: 111.

Troost JP, Trachtman H, Nachman PH, et al. (2018). An outcomes-based definition of proteinuria remission in focal segmental glomerulosclerosis. Clin J Am Soc Nephrol. **13**: 414–21.

Tumlin JA, Miller D, Near M, et al. (2006). A prospective, open-label trial of sirolimus in the treatment of focal segmental glomerulosclerosis. Clin J Am Soc Nephrol. **1**: 109–16.

Verghese PS, Rheault MN, Jackson S, et al. (2018). The effects of peri-transplant plasmapheresis in the prevention of recurrent FSGS. Pediatr Transplant. **22**: e13154.

Vincenti F, Ghiggeri GM. (2005). New insights into the pathogenesis and the therapy of recurrent focal glomerulosclerosis. Am J Transplant. **5**: 1179–85.

Vlachopanos G, Georgalis A, Gakiopoulou H. (2015). Plasma exchange for the recurrence of primary focal segmental glomerulosclerosis in adult renal transplant recipients: A meta-analysis. J Transplant. **2015**: 639628.

Voskarides K, Stefanou C, Pieri M, et al. (2017). A functional variant in NEPH3 gene confers high risk of renal failure in primary hematuric glomerulopathies. Evidence for predisposition to microalbuminuria in the general population. PLoS One. **12**: e0174274.

Wahl P, Ducasa GM, Fornoni A. (2016). Systemic and renal lipids in kidney disease development and progression. Am J Physiol Renal Physiol. **310**: F433–45.

Wang L, Li Q, Wang L, et al. (2013). The role of Th17/IL-17 in the pathogenesis of primary nephrotic syndrome in children. Kidney Blood Press Res. **37**: 332–45.

Wareiko JK, Fan W, Daga A, et al. (2018). Whole exome sequencing of patients with steroid-resistant nephrotic syndrome. Clin J Am Soc Nephrol. **13**: 53–62.

Wei C, El Hindi S, Li J, et al. (2011). Circulating urokinase receptor as a cause of focal segmental glomerulosclerosis. Nat Med. **17**: 952–60.

Wei C, Möller CC, Altintas MM, et al. (2008). Modification of kidney barrier function by the urokinase receptor. Nat Med. **14**: 55–63.

Wei C, Sigdel TK, Sarwal MM, et al. (2015). Circulating CD40 autoantibody and suPAR synergy drives glomerular injury. Ann Transl Med. **3**: 300.

Wei C, Trachtman H, Li J, et al. (2012). Circulating suPAR in two cohorts of primary FSGS. J Am Soc Nephrol. **23**: 2051–9.

Woo KT, Chan CM, Mooi CY, et al. (2010). The changing pattern of primary glomerulonephritis in Singapore and other countries over the past 3 decades. Clin Nephrol. **74**: 372–83.

Wu J, Zheng C, Fan Y, et al. (2014). Downregulation of microRNA-30 facilitates podocyte injury and is prevented by glucocorticoids. J Am Soc Nephrol. **25**: 92–104.

Xie J, Chen N. (2013). Primary glomerulonephritis in mainland China: An overview. Contrib Nephrol. **181**: 1–11.

Yu C-C, Fornoni A, Weins A, et al. (2013). Abatacept in B7-1–positive proteinuric kidney disease. N Engl J Med. **369**: 2416–23.

Zand L, Glassock RJ, De Vries AS, Sethi S, Fervenza F (2017). What are missing in the clinical trials of focal segmental glomerulosclerosis? Nephrol Dial Transplant. **32**: 14–21.

Zhang B, Shi W, Ma J, et al. (2012). The calcineurin–NFAT pathway allows for urokinase receptor-mediated beta3 integrin signaling to cause podocyte injury. J Mol Med. **90**: 1407–20.

Zhang J, Pippin JW, Krofft RD, et al. (2013). Podocyte repopulation by renal progenitor cells following glucocorticoids treatment in experimental FSGS. Am J Physiol Renal Physiol. **304**: F1375–89.

Zhang YM, Gu QH, Huang J, et al. (2016). Clinical significance of IgM and C3 glomerular deposition in primary focal segmental glomerulosclerosis. Clin J Am Soc Nephrol. **11**: 1582–9.

Zhou TB, Qin YH, Su LN, et al. (2011). The association between angiotensin-converting enzyme insertion/deletion gene variant and risk of focal segmental glomerulosclerosis: A systematic review and meta-analysis. J Renin Angiotensin Aldosterone Syst. **12**: 624–33.

Zschiedrich S, Bork T, Liang W, et al. (2017). Targeting mTOR signaling can prevent the progression of FSGS. J Am Soc Nephrol. **28**: 2144–57.

Chapter 6

Membranous nephropathy

Claudio Ponticelli, Richard J Glassock,
and Patrizia Passerini

Introduction and overview

Definition

Primary membranous nephropathy (MN) is an auto-immune glomerular disease which is characterized histologically by uniform thickening of the glomerular capillary due to the presence of sub-epithelial immune complexes. The lesion of MN should be regarded as a pattern of injury as it is not always possible to distinguish a primary from secondary form of MN by light or electron morphology alone. MN is a frequent cause of nephrotic syndrome (NS) in adults. It may have a tendency for spontaneous remission in some subjects while other patients show persistent proteinuria and slow progression to end-stage renal disease (ESRD). Those patients with severe and un-remitting NS may also suffer from disabling and even life-threatening extra-renal complications, such as thrombo-embolic events and cardiovascular disease.

Pathology

At the level of light microscopy, the lesion of primary MN may show a spectrum of abnormalities of the glomerular capillary wall caused by subepithelial deposits of immune complexes. These changes are diffuse to all glomeruli, and involve the whole glomerulus. Thus, a single glomerulus in a renal biopsy specimen is sufficient to make a distinction of the pattern of injury of MN with precision, but this is not always reliably diagnostic of a primary versus a secondary disorder. Immunofluorescence microscopy studies of phospholipase A2 receptor (PLA2R) expression and immunoglobulin subclass (IgG 1,2,3,4) deposition may aid in the morphological identification of likely primary MN (see later). Usually in cases of primary MN there is little or no associated cellular proliferation, although some mesangial hypercellularity may be detectable using quantitative morphometry, and very rarely a crescentic lesion may be superimposed on a lesion of MN. Four pathologic stages of glomerular lesions have been described by Ehrenreich and Churg (1968):

Stage 1 refers to the presence of sub-epithelial deposits without any alteration in GBM morphology or thickness which may be seen in the earliest stages detectable only on electron microscopy. At this stage the light microscopy (PAS and haematoxylin and eosin stains) may be normal but the deposits may be seen with special stains (Mallory Trichrome, see Plate 7);

Stage 2 is characterized by projections of basement membrane-like material ('spikes') that protrude from the external surface of GBM in between the deposits. These abnormalities of GBM can also be seen at light microscopy with Periodic Acid-Silver methenamine staining (Jones stain);

Stage 3 shows the deposits surrounded by basement membrane-like material ('domes') and incorporated into the GBM, which appears irregularly thickened (Plate 8);

Stage 4 shows the deposits becoming electron lucent and undergoing 'reabsorption'. They are reabsorbed into the GBM, which may assume a 'bubbly' or 'swiss-cheese' appearance and be quite remarkably and irregularly thickened. At all stages, the changes of GBM may also be associated with podocyte foot process effacement on electron microscopy.

By immunofluorescence microscopic examination there are granular subepithelial deposits of IgG (mainly IgG4 in the primary MN) and C3, with lesser amounts of IgM or IgA and uncommonly C1q, suggesting that complement is not activated by the classical pathway. Co-deposition of Mannose binding lectin C3d, C4d, and the C5b-C9 membrane attack complex strongly suggests an 'immunologically' active disease (Ma et al., 2013). Fibrinogen stains are usually negative. In the more advanced phases, focal and segmental glomerulosclerosis, progressive interstitial fibrosis, and tubular changes are seen.

Generally, MN is a *diffuse* and *global* glomerular disease. However, cases of *segmental* MN that show IgG deposits in a portion of the glomerulus have been reported in Japanese children. In this variant of MN, there is segmental thickening of the GBM, with spike formation at light microscopy, and mesangial electron-dense deposits are frequently seen on electron microscopy (Obana et al., 2006). Of note, C1q deposits are more frequent and intense than in classic MN (Segawa et al., 2010). It is still unclear whether segmental MN should be considered a separate glomerular disease entity, as it displays a child predominance distinctive from the typical primary MN. Rare cases of MN stage 3 or 4 with low serum levels of C3 have also been described in children. In these cases, hypocomplementemia was caused by C3 nephritic factor, an antibody directed against C3 convertase (C3bBb) of the alternative pathway of complement, which stabilizes this enzyme (Niel et al., 2015). A rare association of MN with IgA nephropathy has been reported particularly in Japanese and Chinese subjects (Kobayashi et al., 2015; Chen et al., 2018). In a study, the serum anti-PLA2R was detected as positive in all of the patients (Hu et al., 2016).

In a number of cases MN may be secondary to lupus, cancer, drug reaction, or infectious disease (Table 6.1). Differentiation of the primary from secondary forms of MN may be difficult. Some histologic features may help in the

Table 6.1 Causes of secondary membranous nephropathy.

Infections	Auto-immune Disorders	
Hepatitis B or C	SLE	RA
Enterococcal endocarditis	Dermatomyositis	Systemic sclerosis
Filariasis	Biliary cirrhosis	Ankylosing spondylitis
Hydatid disease	Mixed connective tissue disease	Thyroiditis
Influenza		
Leprosy	Miscellaneous Disorders	
Quartan malaria	Diabetes	Primary biliary cirrhosis
Schistosomiasis	Sarcoidosis	Renal transplantation
Streptococcal infections	IgG4 disease	Bone marrow transplantation
Syphilis	Crohn's disease	Sickle cell disease
	Dermatitis herpetiformis	Sjogren's syndrome
Neoplasia	Guillain-Barré syndrome	Systemic mastocytosis
Carcinomas	Multiple sclerosis	Temporal arteritis
Hodgkin's disease	Myasthenia gravis	Periaortic fibrosis
Melanoma	Myelodysplasia	
Mesothelioma		
Non-Hodgkin's lymphoma	*Drugs and Nutrients*	
Pheochromocytoma	NSAIDs	Mercury compounds
Retroperitoneal sarcoma	Captopril	Penicillamine
Benign tumours	Gold	Probenecid
	Lithium	Sulindac
	Trimethadione	Thiola
	Levodopa	Cow milk

differential diagnosis. Atypical features, such as mesangial proliferation and/or a wide spectrum of different immunoglobulin and complement component deposits at immunofluorescence, suggest that the disease may be secondary. The features which suggest a lupus-related MN include 'full-house' deposits of IgG, IgM, IgA, C3, and C1q by immunofluorescence, tubulo-reticular structures in endothelial cells, electron-dense deposits in mesangial or sub-endothelial areas, and prominent deposition of IgG1 and IgG2 (instead of IgG4). Most patients with an underlying malignancy show glomerular deposits of IgG2 at immunofluorescence, while IgG4 deposits are absent (Lonnbro-Widgren et al., 2015). The number of inflammatory cells infiltrating the glomeruli has also been found to be significantly higher in patients with cancer-associated MN. The best cut-off value for distinguishing malignancy-related cases from controls was eight cells per glomerulus, with a specificity of 75 per cent and a sensitivity of 92 per cent (Lefaucher et al., 2006). Very importantly, in most (80–85 per cent) cases of primary MN epitopes of the PLA2R protein are hyperexpressed in glomeruli in a pattern similar to the IgG deposits (Hoxha et al., 2012; Beck, 2017) using direct immunofluorescence microscopy of frozen tissue or paraffin-immunofluorescence of pronase digested specimens. Such deposits of IgG and PLA2R antigen may persist for long periods (weeks, months) after the immune activity of the disease has waned (Ronco and Debiec, 2010). In normal glomeruli such glomerular expression of PLA2R antigen, uniquely on the podocyte cell surface, is minimal. In some instances of apparent secondary MN (most notably sarcoidosis and hepatitis B viral infection, HBV) hyperexpression of PLA2R antigen can be observed and rarely in cancer-associated MN as well. But in the absence of clinical evidence of these disorders, PLA2R hyperexpression can generally be regarded as indicating a primary form of MN. More uncertain is the meaning of thrombospondin 7A (see 'Pathogenesis').

Electron microscopy can reveal deposits of varying electron density and shape confined to the subepithelial space of glomeruli or incorporated into irregular projections of GBM-like material ('spikes and domes'). Mesangial electron deposits should be absent or scanty in primary MN. The electron-density of the deposits and the presence of C3/C4 proteins at immunofluorescence may be signs of 'active' formation of in situ immune deposits and an indirect feature of the activity of the disease. Electron lucent deposits are a sign of immunologically inactive disease. In secondary MN, these electron-dense deposits can also be located in subendothelial or mesangial sites (Table 6.2). In immunologically quiescent and advanced disease these deposits acquire a more lucent appearance. Extensive, almost universal, effacements of podocyte foot processes are commonly observed when nephrotic-range proteinuria is present. Extensive subepithelial electron-dense deposit formation without

Table 6.2 Differences between primary and secondary MN at renal biopsy.

	Primary MN	**Secondary MN**
Light microscopy	Endocapillary proliferation absent or mild.	Endocapillary proliferation may be seen in cases secondary to SLE or cancer.
Light microscopy	No inflammatory cells infiltration.	Inflammatory cells infiltration in MN associated with cancer or SLE.
Immunofluorescence	IgG4 deposits predominant.	IgG 1-3 deposits frequent.
Immunofluorescence	Deposits of other Ig rare and mild.	IgA, IgM, C1q deposits in SLE.
Immunofluorescence	Staining with PLA2R usually positive.	Staining with PLA2R usually negative.
Electron microscopy	Subepithelial electron-dense deposits.	Subepithelial and subendothelial or mesangial deposits. Tubulo-reticular inclusions in SLE.

accompanying granular IgG deposition by standard immunofluorescence microscopy may be due to hidden antigenic determinants of monoclonal IgG deposition that can be revealed by pronase digestion of tissue sections (Larsen et al., 2014). In patients with MN due to systemic lupus erythematosus (SLE) endothelial cell inclusions of a tubuloreticular nature ('interferon-fingerprints') and concomitant subendothelial electron dense deposits can be seen (Sam et al., 2015).

Pathogenesis

Studies in Heymann nephritis, a murine experimental model of MN, supported the hypothesis that in MN there is an in situ formation of immune complexes as a consequence of a reaction between a circulating antibody and either an antigen planted in the subepithelial position on the podocyte membrane surface or an intrinsic glomerular antigen in the same location. This in situ reaction could produce proteinuria in a complement–dependent and T-cell-dependent fashion (reviewed in Glassock, 2012).

Importantly, Debiec and Ronco (2002) have demonstrated that in a rare form of congenital human MN the disease is caused by in situ immune complex formation induced by binding of circulating antibodies to a planted podocytic antigen. These investigators described the case of a mother genetically deficient in neutral endopeptidase (NEP) who bore a child in which NEP was present. They showed that the mother formed anti-NEP antibodies that crossed the placenta and produced MN in the newborn by reacting with NEP in the podocyte.

However, antibodies to NEP were not found to be responsible for the initiation of MN in adults, except very rarely.

In a landmark study, Beck and colleagues (2009) demonstrated that circulating auto-antibodies to epitopes expressed on the podocyte membrane associated muscle-type phospholipase-A2 receptor 1 (PLA2R1) were present in about 80 per cent of adults with primary MN. Instead, circulating anti-PLA2R1 antibodies are not usually detectable in secondary MN, with the possible exception of a few cases associated with carcinoma (Qin et al., 2011), sarcoidosis (Stehlé et al., 2015), hepatitis B (Xie et al., 2015), or biliary cirrhosis (Dauvergne et al., 2015). Kidney biopsy specimen staining for PLA2R1 show >90 per cent specificity and about an 80 per cent sensitivity for the diagnosis of primary MN (Francis et al., 2016). The immunodominant epitope of PLA2R1 has been discovered to be an N-terminal cysteine-rich ricin domain of PLA2R1 (Fresquet et al., 2015) which is located within the three terminal domains of PLA2R1, namely cysteine-rich ricin, fibronectin-like type II, and C-type lectin-like domain 1 (Kao et al., 2015). In Caucasian patients with MN a strong interaction was found between the HLA-DQA1 allele and the most common variant of PLA2R1. When variants or polymorphisms are present at both sites the risk of primary MN is augmented almost eighty- to a hundredfold (Stanescu et al., 2011; Saeed et al., 2014). Recently, the focus shifted to the HLA–DRB locus. An independent and strong association between the HLA-DRB1*15:01 and HLA-DRB3*02:02 alleles and PLA2R-related MN has been found in the Chinese population (Le et al., 2017). It is not clear, however, if these haplotypes are equally important in other populations, or if additional variants were missed because of power or coverage limitations (Madkova and Kiryluk, 2017).

At any rate, PLA2R is not the only antigen involved in the pathogenesis of primary MN. Circulating antibodies against thrombospondin type-1 domain-containing 7A (THSD7A), a protein colocalized with nephrin on the podocyte, were detected in 10 per cent of the Caucasian patients with primary MN who had no antibodies against PLA2R1 (Tomas et al., 2014) and in 2 per cent of Chinese patients with apparently primary MN (Wang et al., 2017). These antibodies have been proven to be pathogenic (Hoxha et al., 2016; Tomas et al., 2016; Anders and Ponticelli, 2016). At immunohistochemical analysis an enhanced granular expression of THSD7A was detected in 9 per cent of Japanese patients with primary MN (Iwakura et al., 2015). Anti-THSD7A and anti- PLA2R antibodies are not mutually exclusive (Larsen et al., 2016). Cases with the presence of both antibodies have been reported (Wang et al., 2017). Of concern, the THSD7A-associated MN may be associated with malignancy (Beck et al., 2017). Other circulating antibodies can coexist with anti-PLA2R1 antibodies (Murtas and Ghiggeri, 2016). These antibodies are directed against intracellular podocyte enzymes, such as superoxide dismutase, alpha-enolase, or aldose reductase (Prunotto et al., 2010; Bruschi et al., 2011). Circulating anti-α-enolase antibodies may be detected in about 70 per cent of patients with MN but the absence of α-enolase from subepithelial immune deposits suggests that these antibodies do not contribute directly to immune-deposit formation (Kimura et al., 2017). It is possible to speculate that these antibodies are either a result of intermolecular epitope spreading or are generated by the podocyte damage caused by auto-antibodies against PLA2R1 or THSD7A.

In summary, primary MN is an auto-immune disease in which circulating antibodies (mainly IgG4) are directed against podocyte membrane expressed proteins. As suggested by Couser and Johnson (2014), it is possible that a genetic predisposition would operate as a *first hit* and that a *second hit*, probably a viral attack or other unidentified factors, may induce a conformational change in the transmembrane M-type of PLA2R1 or, more rarely, in the matricellular THSD7A. The molecular patterns of modified PLA2R1 or THSD7A are recognized as danger signals by toll-like receptors that induce or amplify the inflammatory response. In the inflammatory milieu, dendritic cells (DCs) become mature and after intercepting the antigen, migrate to lymph nodes where they present the antigen to specific T-cell receptors. Activated T-cells proliferate and under the influence of DCs differentiate into TH1 and TH17. These effector T-cells can directly cause glomerular injury and can activate B-cells to produce plasma cells and antibodies against the protein recognized as a foreign antigen. The binding of antibodies (again, mainly IgG4) with their target leads to in situ formation of subepithelial immune deposits, which further aggravate podocyte injury through an increased production of reactive oxygen species, cytokines, and chemokines (Ponticelli and Glassock, 2014). An important role is played by complement activation and formation of the membrane-attack complex C5b-C9. As IgG4 are the only immunoglobulins unable to activate complement through the classical pathway, it is likely that in MN the lectin-binding mannan pathway (Bally et al., 2016) and alternative pathways are involved (Luo et al., 2018). However, alternative and even classical pathways may also be involved in a few cases (Reddy et al., 2017; Couser, 2017). The final result would consist of in derangement of actin cytoskeleton, loss of permselectivity of the glomerular barrier, and proteinuria (Figure 6.1). Similar mechanisms are probably operating in some secondary MN in which the antigen may be represented by a molecular element of viral hepatitis, nucleosomes in case of SLE, oncogenic antigens, or THSD7A, a glycoprotein that may either favour or suppress oncogenesis.

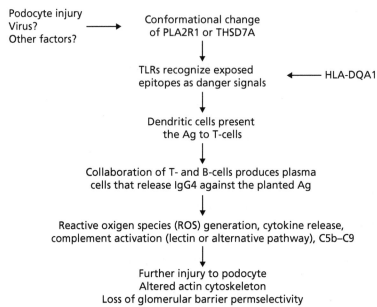

Figure 6.1 A schematic representation of possible pathogenesis of primary MN. In predisposed patients (carriers of HLA-DQA1 allele) an injury possibly caused by a virus producing conformational changes in PALA2R. The revealed epitopes are recognized as danger signals by toll-like receptors with activation of innate immunity and inflammation. In the inflammatory environment the dendritic cells capture the antigen, migrate, and present the antigen to immunocompetent cells. The collaboration T-cell/B-cell elicits the production of auto-antibodies and formation of immune complexes *in situ* that trigger inflammation, complement activation, and ROS generation. These factors cause further injury, an altered cytoskeleton, foot process effacement, and loss of glomerular barrier permselectivity.

Aetiology

The *primum movens* initiating the pathogenetic events described is still unknown, although a role for genetic factors and viral infection cannot be ruled out. Instead, a number of aetiological factors have been recognized as being responsible for secondary MN (see Table 6.1). The pathogenesis of these secondary forms has not been clearly defined. *Helicobacter pylori* antigens, viral antigens, tumour antigens, nucleosomes, and thyroglobulin have been detected in the subepithelial deposits, but there is no real proof that these antigens are pathogenic. MN is frequently associated with HBV or HCV hepatitis, particularly in children and in patients from Eastern Europe, sub-Saharan Africa, and Asia (Bhimma and Coovadia, 2004; Lai and Lai, 2006). The pathogenesis of HBV-related MN is likely to be immune complex mediated (Gupta and Quigg,

2015). An aetiological role of hepatitis Be antigen (HBeAg) may be suggested. HBeAg is found in two forms of 19,000 and 300,000 Daltons. Theoretically, the small molecular weight antigen might pass through the GBM and localize in the subepithelial area, eliciting the formation of antibodies. However, there is currently little evidence to support this hypothesis. The presence of the HCV antigen in the glomeruli has been demonstrated in a few patients but was not confirmed by other studies. The possibility that HCV triggers MN via an auto-immune mechanism cannot be ruled out. A number of other infections affecting the immune system may also be associated with MN.

MN may frequently occur in SLE and other auto-immune diseases in which synthesis of auto-antibodies, rheumatoid factor, and antismooth muscle antibodies can concur to the development of MN. Particularly frequent in our experience was the association with thyroiditis.

MN may also complicate systemic diseases such as diabetes mellitus, sarcoidosis, or IgG4-related disease (IgG4-RD). This is a protean systemic disease characterized by high serum levels of IgG4. IgG4-RD can affect many organs causing lymphoplasmacytic infiltrations that lead to swelling and enlargement of the affected organ. Kidney involvement is characterized by a tubulo-interstitial nephritis. MN and other glomerulopathies with or without the presence of tubulo-interstitial nephritis have also been described in IgG4RD (Stylianou et al., 2014; Acevedo Ribò et al., 2016).

The most worrying association of MN is with cancer. Carcinoma of solid organs are the most frequent type of cancer associated with MN. A systematic review and meta-analysis of cohort studies in Caucasian patients reported an estimated prevalence of cancer in 10 per cent of patients with MN. Lung and prostate cancer were the most frequent tumours, followed by haematologic malignancies, colorectal cancer, breast cancer, and stomach and oesophageal cancer. The mean age of MN patients with cancer was 67 + 7 years (Leeaphorn et al., 2014). In patients with MN secondary to carcinomas, the tumour may be an important source of antigens that can provoke the production of specific antibodies. However, the presence of tumour antigens and their corresponding antibodies in patients with paraneoplastic glomerulopathies does not necessarily mean that they are involved in the initial pathogenic process. In some cases, these components can be passively deposited because of increased glomerular permeability to proteins as a result of the initial insult. Alternatively, it is possible that immune perturbations in cancer patients make them prone to developing immune-complex nephritis through the production of antibodies against tumour or self-antigens. Recently, a causal relationship between simultaneous expression of THSD7A in a gallbladder carcinoma and in MN has been described in a woman. Moreover, out of 25 patients with MN and circulating anti- THSD7A antibodies, seven had a malignant tumour (Hoxha et al., 2016). As shown by Timmermans and colleagues (2013), patients with anti-PLA2R-negative MN are at much higher risk of having a cancer-related form of MN compared to patients with anti-PLA2R positive MN.

Finally, a number of drugs, including non-steroidal anti-inflammatory drugs (NSAIDs), penicillamine, gold, or others heavy metals (such as mercury) may cause MN with NS. Usually the disease resolves spontaneously when the drug is withdrawn. A particular and rare form of secondary MN is caused in children by cow's milk. High levels of cationic circulating anti-bovine serum albumin (BSA) antibodies, of IgG1 and IgG4 subclasses, may be detected in these cases, and BSA may be recognized in subepithelial immune deposits. These data suggest that in a few children with MN, cationic BSA introduced with cow's milk may result in pathogenic MN if it passes the intestinal barrier. Once in the blood, BSA may bind to the anionic glomerular capillary wall, be reached by antibodies, and cause in situ formation of immune complexes (Debiec et al., 2011).

Clinical presentation and features

MN is one of the most common causes of NS in adults, while it is rare in children. Secondary forms of MN only account for 20–25 per cent of MN in adults whereas secondary forms account for over 75 per cent of cases of MN in children. The distribution of primary versus secondary MN in the population is influenced by geography and the prevalence of endemic infectious diseases, especially hepatitis B.

Proteinuria is the hallmark of the disease. Usually proteinuria is non-selective and can often be associated with microscopic (dysmorphic) haematuria. About 70–80 per cent of patients referred to nephrologists because of MN have a full-blown NS at presentation, i.e. proteinuria ≥3.5 g/day associated with hypo-albuminaemia, hypercholesterolaemia, and various degrees of oedema. However, other patients may be asymptomatic and are discovered to be affected by the disease only at routine check-up visits or by incidental urinalyses. Renal dysfunction may be present at clinical onset in many cases, particularly if the diagnosis has been delayed. Few patients with severe NS may develop thromboembolic complications near to the clinical onset of the disease and these events may be the main reason for discovery of MN.

The clinical presentation of MN is similar in older and younger patients, although elderly patients more often present with a lower glomerular filtration rate (GFR), in part due to the physiological decline in GFR in advancing age (Hommos et al., 2017). Arterial hypertension is seen more often in older patients.

In cases of secondary MN, the clinical presentation is quite variable. Apart the signs and symptoms of NS when present, the clinical features may be dominated by the presence of an underlying disease, as in the case of malignancies, viral-associated liver diseases, SLE, etc. Around 10–20 per cent of patients with lupus nephritis may show a MN lesion at renal biopsy. Sometimes, SLE may present with proteinuria and abnormal urine sediment as the sole disease manifestation, antedating other clinical features and even immunological markers of the disease by years. These patients show an apparent Primary MN at presentation as the clinical or serological features of SLE are absent. Atypical findings on renal biopsy may suggest the secondary nature of MN.

MN associated with underlying malignancies is more common in older patients and in children. It is difficult to separate a MN secondary to malignancy from a Primary MN on the basis of renal histology alone, but in a number of cases an accurate evaluation of findings at light microscopy, immunofluorescence and electron microscopy may allow to distinguish primary from secondary forms. PLA2R antigen hyper-expression along the capillary wall and the presence of circulating anti-PLA2R auto-antibody also play for a diagnosis of primary MN (see Table 6.2). In approximately half of patients the neoplasia is recognized at the time of renal biopsy but proteinuria may antedate by months or years the clinical signs and symptoms of an underlying carcinoma. (Lefaucher et al., 2006). Of note, of 49 patients with MN screened by positron emission tomography/computed tomography, five (10.2 per cent) resulted to have an occult malignancy (Feng et al., 2016). Other studies reported that up to 28 per cent of patients with MN positive for THSD7A had a malignant tumour (Hoxha et al., 2016; Ren et al., 2018), suggesting an aggressive research for an underlying cancer in patients with MN and anti-THSD7A antibodies. The presence of anaemia, which is rarely associated with primary MN, may raise the suspicion of an underlying haematologic malignancy or a gastrointestinal cancer. The most frequent types of carcinomas in patients with MN are located in the lung and prostate. The frequency of malignancy increases with age to as high as 20–25 per cent after age 60 years (Lefaucher et al., 2006). Thus, the evaluation of an adult with MN should include a diligent work-up, especially if the patient is aged ≥50 years and biopsy does not show hyperexpression of PLA2R antigen along the capillary wall. This includes a number of invasive and noninvasive procedures to detect possible solid organ tumours (Table 6.3), and a bone marrow aspiration in case of persistent severe anaemia not caused by gastrointestinal bleeding.

In patients with rheumatoid arthritis (RA), MN may be triggered by the use of gold salts, NSAID, or penicillamine, but in a number of cases no aetiological agent may be found, suggesting a possible role for a common

Table 6.3 Suggested check-up for solid organ cancer in a patient with MN.

Cancer	Young Adult	Old Adult
Lung	Chest X-ray	Computed tomography
Prostate	Rectal digital examination	Ultrasonography Prostate biopsy
Colorectal	Faecal occult blood. If positive or in the presence of anaemia or unexplained weight loss, colonoscopy is recommended	Colonoscopy
Breast	Physical examination	Mammography
Stomach	Faecal occult blood. If positive or in the presence of anaemia or unexplained weight loss, gastroscopy is recommended	Gastroscopy
Kidney	Ultrasonography Malignant cells in the urine	Computed tomography Malignant cells in the urine
Uterus	Gynaecologic examination	Colposcopy

genetic background. While the finding of diabetes is more common among patients with MN it is not well established whether this association is of a causal nature. It may be fortuitous and related to a common genetically based predisposition.

Younger patients with hepatitis B-associated MN and those with smaller burden of subepithelial immune deposits may have spontaneous remission of proteinuria. Instead, spontaneous remission is rare in adults with MN due to HBV infection and some of them may eventually progress to ESRD. However, antiviral treatment alone or in combination with tacrolimus may obtain remission of proteinuria in a number of patients (Yang et al., 2016; Wang et al., 2016). MN may also be associated with malaria, trypanosomiasis, leprosy, or other infections particularly frequent in tropical areas. However, the true incidence of MN secondary to infection in tropical countries is unknown at the present.

The number of drugs potentially triggering MN is continuously increasing. Proteinuria may appear rapidly after the drug is begun and usually disappears after its withdrawal. In other cases, MN may develop months or up to several years after treatment. In these patients the recovery of the disease after withdrawal of the offending drug may take a long time, roughly related to the length of the exposure to the drug. The exposure to substances such as solvents and hydrocarbons may also favour the development or progression of MN, but this remains as a highly controversial issue.

Epidemiology

Primary MN has an incidence of 12 cases per million population per year in adults, and while it is very rare in children, its incidence ranges between 0.002 and 0.009 per million population (McGrogan et al., 2011). Most textbooks still report that primary MN has a peak incidence between 40 and 60 years. Nevertheless, the more liberal policy of renal biopsy in older patients has shown that the disease is more frequent than expected in the elderly. MN is more frequent in men, with a predominance of males over females, at a 2:1 ratio (Hogan et al., 1995).

The current view is that primary MN on worldwide basis is largely prevailing over secondary MN. However, this estimate should probably be reassessed if one takes into account also the cases of MN in tropical areas, where an indefinite number of cases of MN is associated with endemic infections. On the other hand, the increasing number and use of drugs that may cause MN will probably decrease the ratio of primary to secondary MN also in Western countries. The association between MN and malignant neoplasia is well known. In about 10 per cent of patients with MN, a malignancy may be discovered at the time of renal biopsy or within a year thereafter (Lefaucher et al., 2006).

Natural history

A number of untreated patients with MN may enter a partial or even a complete remission of proteinuria. In a retrospective, multicentre study of 328 Spanish individuals with primary MN and NS treated with conservative therapy (renin-angiotensin system inhibition, diuretics, statins), 'spontaneous' complete (52 patients) or partial remission (52 patients) occurred in 104 (32 per cent) patients. Proteinuria progressively declined after diagnosis until remission of disease at 14.7 ± 11.4 months. Although spontaneous remission was more frequent with lower levels of baseline proteinuria, it also occurred in patients with massive proteinuria. Most patients who entered spontaneous remission had a decrease in proteinuria >50 per cent from baseline during the first year (Polanco et al., 2010). Spontaneous remission is much more common in patients with apparent primary MN and negative or low titre of circulating anti-PLA2 R antibody (Timmermans et al., 2015). In a study, 67 of 128 (52 per cent) patients with MN entered spontaneous partial remission, in mean after 20 months. Relapse occurred in 31 per cent of patients after remission and was significantly associated with severe renal failure. Cumulative incidence of adverse events at 15 years after first presentation included death (14 per cent), ESRD (28 per cent), and relapse (40 per cent) (Kanigicherla et al., 2016). Rarely, spontaneous remission of proteinuria may occur even in patients with renal function deterioration. Out of 11 such patients, serum creatinine remained stable or even improved in nine, while in two patients NS relapsed and renal function rapidly decreased (Polanco et al., 2012). Apart from patients with spontaneous remission, the natural course of primary MN may be characterized by persisting proteinuria fluctuating in a nephrotic range and may slowly progress to ESRD over many years.

However, it is difficult to assess the true percentage of patients with any of these possible outcomes in the absence of any treatment because most of the few relevant studies had too a short follow-up and included both nephrotic and non-nephrotic patients. Studies with follow-ups of ten years or more clearly showed that the probability of renal survival largely depends on the length of follow-up. In a randomized controlled trial on Italian patients with biopsy-proven primary MN and NS at presentation, only 5 per cent of patients assigned to symptomatic treatment were in complete remission and another 28 per cent were in partial remission (33 per cent in total) after ten years of follow-up. However, 40 per cent of patients receiving only symptomatic therapy entered ESRD or died within ten years from randomization (Ponticelli et al., 1995). In a systematic review including all studies reported up to 1994, Hogan and colleagues (1995) found that the renal survival of patients with MN averaged about around 50 per cent at 14 years. DuBuf-Vereijken and colleagues (2005) also analysed the reports published during the previous 25 years. They excluded patients with a follow-up of less than three years and attributed a 100 per cent renal survival rate to non-nephrotic patients. Overall, nearly 50 per cent of the patients with MN and NS developed renal function deterioration and were probably destined to enter ESRD in the long term. Thus, it is quite incorrect to assume that MN is a benign disease, not requiring any specific therapy, at least in Caucasian patients. It should be noted that many observational studies have shown that MN progresses to ESRD at a much lower frequency in Asian patients (Shiiki et al., 2004), who are also more susceptible to the antiproteinuric effects of steroid therapy (see 'Specific treatment').

Apart from renal function deterioration, MN may also expose patients to the adverse clinical consequences of the NS per se (see also Chapter 2). NS is associated with several disorders of haemostasis, including excessive platelet activation, impaired fibrinolysis, increased serum levels of procoagulant factors such as factor VIII, factor V, factor XIII, fibrinogen, plasminogen activator inhibitor, and decreased levels of anticoagulant factors, such as anti-thrombin III, free protein S, and vitamin B6, which are lost in the urine, having a low molecular weight. The risk of thrombotic events may be further aggravated by low levels of serum albumin (<2.5 g/dl) and endothelial dysfunction as well as by haemodynamic characteristics that favour thrombosis, such as the tendency toward hypovolaemia and haemoconcentration. As a consequence, deep vein thrombosis and renal vein thrombosis are frequent in MN. A prospective study reported the development of venous thrombo-embolism in 36 per cent of patients with MN and NS (Li et al., 2012). These patients are also at high risk of developing a pulmonary embolism, although it may often remain asymptomatic (Zhang et al., 2014). The risk of thrombotic complications is particularly elevated in older patients and in those with a serum albumin level below 2.5 g/dl. This heightened risk of thrombosis in MN with NS has led to suggest that prophylactic anticoagulation is indicated at least in some cases. According to Markov decision analysis, the benefit-to-risk ratios of anticoagulation increase with worsening hypo-albuminaemia from 4.5:1 for an albumin under 3 g/dl to 13.1:1 for an albumin under 2 g/dl in patients at low bleeding risk. Patients at intermediate bleeding risk with an albumin under 2 g/dl have a moderately favourable benefit-to-risk ratio (under 5:1). Patients at high bleeding risk are unlikely to benefit from prophylactic anticoagulation regardless of albuminaemia. From these data, a decision tree programme may be constructed to aid decision making (Lee et al., 2014). However, its application to individual patients is not easy. Indeed, many factors bear on the risk of thrombo-embolic events and/or serious bleeding (Glassock, 2014). Less frequently, arterial thrombosis can also occur, the risk being associated with the degree of hypo-albuminaemia. In patients with serum albumin <2.5 g/dl low aspirin may be prescribed to prevent arterial thrombosis (Hofstra and Wetzels, 2016).

It is now agreed that hyperlipidaemia represents a risk factor for survival and for thrombo-embolic events. Most nephrotic patients also show hyperlipidaemia and a highly pro-atherogenic lipid profile with hypercholesterolaemia, hypertriglyceridaemia, and an increase in LDL, IDL, and VLDL lipoproteins, while HDL levels are normal or reduced. An increase in lipoprotein (a) level and low levels of serum albumin (<2.5 g/dl) further aggravate the atherosclerotic risk of nephrotic patients with MN. Another important risk factor for cardiovascular events is renal dysfunction, which has been demonstrated to be a powerful independent predictor of fatal and non-fatal cardiovascular events in the general population and in patients who have already suffered from a myocardial infarction. In patients with chronic kidney disease the risk of cardiovascular events increases when GFR declines (Herzog et al., 2011). A retrospective study reported that the risk of cardiovascular events in patients with MN was similar to that of patients with ESRD, the risk being higher in older patients, diabetics, those with previous cardiac complications, and in patients with prolonged exposure to NS (Lee et al., 2016).

In summary, although MN is often (erroneously in our view) considered as a benign renal disease, the few studies examining the very long-term outcome (ten to twenty years) speak against this optimistic concept. On the other hand, it is likely that at present the long-term prognosis of the disease is improving since a prior nihilist attitude of not treating patients with MN has now changed. Today, most high-risk patients with MN are receiving a regimen of specific treatment that may consistently alter the natural course of the disease and also receive the benefits of improved symptomatic and preventive treatment (see Chapter 2) based on statins, ACE-inhibitors, angiotensin-receptor blockers (ARBs), diuretics, low-dose aspirin, and/or prophylactic anticoagulation. This more aggressive approach has considerably improved the outcome when compared to the recent past, so allowing the prevention of more severe complications of NS and to improve the long-term prognosis of MN.

Prognostic factors

(See Table 6.4)

Age

MN in children is a rare but serious disease. Newborns with MN caused by anti-NEP antibodies present manifestations of NS often associate with impaired hypertension and renal failure severe enough to require dialysis (Vivarelli et al., 2015). In children with primary MN, about 50 per cent may show signs of progression to renal failure in the long term (Chen et al., 2007). Thrombotic complications are also quite frequent in children.

The prognosis of elderly patients with MN is not very different from that of younger adults (Yamaguchi et al., 2014). However, older patients often have

Table 6.4 Main prognostic factors in patients with primary membranous nephropathy.

Favourable outcome	Poor outcome	Significance
Complete/partial remission	Persisting nephrotic proteinuria	Strong
No tubulointerstitial lesions	Severe tubulointerstitial lesions	Strong
Normal eGFR	Low eGFR (confirmed)	Strong
Low titre of anti-PLA2R antibodies	High titre of anti-PLA2R antibodies	Moderate
Low excretion of low MW proteins	High excretion of low MW proteins	Moderate
Female gender	Male gender	Mild-moderate
No association HLA-DQA1/PLA2R	Association HLA-DQA1 / PLA2R	Mild-moderate

MW = molecular weight

higher than normal levels of serum creatinine at presentation and increased risk of developing renal insufficiency, infection, and vascular thrombosis than younger adults. Moreover, elderly patients are more vulnerable to the consequences of NS and have a poorer tolerance than younger adults to treatments. Thus, the dosage of symptomatic and immunosuppressive drugs should be tailored to age (Ponticelli et al., 2015).

Gender

There is general agreement that in MN women fare better than men. This view has been substantiated by a systematic review showing that female gender is associated with better probability of spontaneous remission and slower rate of progression (Cattran et al., 2008). The outcome of repeated pregnancies in women with MN is good, with 90 per cent live births. Repeated pregnancies do not influence the course of MN (Malik et al., 2002).

Ancestry (racial and ethnic origin)

The disease seems to run a more favourable course in the Asian than in the Caucasian population. A large Japanese study involving 949 patients with biopsy-proven MN showed renal survival rates of 90.3 per cent at ten years and 81.1 per cent at 15 years after diagnosis (Shiiki et al., 2004).

Proteinuria

The magnitude and the persistence of proteinuria impacts on the eventual outcome of MN. Cattran and colleagues (1997) elaborated a prediction model for risk of progression in MN, based on the severity of proteinuria over a six-month observation, and validated the results on a large pool of Canadian, Italian, and Finnish patients. According to this model, a subject with MN, normal serum creatinine, and proteinuria <4 g/day over six months has only 6 per cent probability of progressing to chronic renal insufficiency at 52 months, while a patient with abnormal or deteriorating serum creatinine and/or proteinuria >8 g/day over six months has 72 per cent probability of entering renal insufficiency, and patients with normal or nearly normal serum creatinine and variable amounts of proteinuria over six months have *intermediate* risks of progression. Further studies reported that time-varying proteinuria was the best metric to account for the prognostic effects of proteinuria in MN, especially earlier in the disease course (Barbour et al., 2015).

The quality of proteinuria may also provide additional prognostic information. Van den Brand and colleagues (2012) reported that a spot urine sample showing elevation in the urinary excretion of Beta2 microglobulin and α1 microglobulin may have a similar accuracy in predicting prognosis in MN to the risk score proposed by Cattran and colleagues (1997). Even a fractional excretion of IgG ≥0.02 may predict an increased risk of kidney failure and lower chance of remission (Bazzi et al., 2014). However, other investigators reported that quantification of low-, medium-, and high-molecular-weight urinary proteins does not correlate with long-term outcomes (Irazabal et al., 2013).

Remission

Patients entering complete remission (<0.2 or <0.3 g/day with normal renal function) can maintain stable renal function in the long term (Ponticelli and Passerini, 2010; Thompson et al., 2015). Also, partial remission may predict a fair outcome (Troyanov et al., 2004), but relapses of NS are frequent and the long-term outcome depends on the treatment used to obtain remission. Although the longer the remission, the better the long-term outcome, patients with remission durations as short as three months had improved renal prognosis compared with patients who relapsed (Cattran et al., 2017).

Renal insufficiency

There is a general consensus that increased serum creatinine levels (>1.4 mg/dl) at presentation presages the later development of ESRD. However, in a number of cases with severe NS, renal insufficiency may be functional and reversible, being caused by a hypovolaemia related to severe hypo-albuminemia, excessive dosage of diuretics, or drug-associated acute interstitial nephritis. A further concern is represented by a lack of standard calibration in serum creatinine assays across laboratories. On the other hand, one should take into account that estimated GFR overestimates true GFR when hypo-albuminaemia is present.

Glomerular lesions

There is no convincing evidence that the stage of glomerular lesions is consistently predictive of the future of progression (or remissions). Whether a superimposed focal segmental glomerulosclerosis (FSGS) is a discriminative parameter with independent prognostic value has been a matter of discussion. In a study, the risk of renal failure was almost equally distributed between patients with or without superimposed FSGS (Heeringa et al., 2007), but other papers reported that segmental glomerular sclerosis was associated with renal function decline (Chen et al., 2014; Morita et al., 2015).

Tubulo-interstitial lesions

A number of multivariate analyses reported a positive correlation between the severity of tubulo-interstitial lesions (interstitial fibrosis and tubular atrophy) and the deterioration of renal function (Rocha et al., 2004; Chen et al., 2014; Zhang et al., 2016).

Anti-PLA2R antibodies

High titres of PLA2R1-antibodies are associated with decreased rates of response to treatment while low levels of antibodies are associated with high rate of spontaneous remission (Hoxha et al., 2014; Kim et al., 2015; Ruggenenti et al., 2015; Timmermans et al., 2015; Qin et al., 2016; Song et al., 2018). Decrease in the anti-PLA2R titre correlates with response to therapy and often occurs earlier than the reduction in proteinuria (Radice et al., 2016; Ramachandran et al., 2016b; Wei et al., 2016). In patients whose MN is associated with the anti-PLA2R antibody, the possibility of reducing or maintaining a lower level of immunosuppression on either the disappearance or percent change in its titre is exciting but needs to be proven (Cattran and Brenchley, 2017). It has also been reported that PLA2R epitope spreading at baseline is associated with a reduced probability of spontaneous remission (Seitz Polski et al., 2018). On the other hand, spontaneous remission is significantly more frequent in patients who are anti-PLA2R antibody seronegative (Timmermans et al., 2015; Wu et al., 2018).

HLA alleles

HLA-DQA1 and PLA2R1 genotype combination adjusted for baseline proteinuria may strongly predict renal function decline and response to immunosuppressive therapy (Bullich et al., 2014).

Tumour necrosis factor alpha (TNFα).

TNFα is a pleiotropic cytokine with pro-inflammatory and immunoregulatory properties. Its actions are mediated by TNF receptors (TNFR). A retrospective study demonstrated that eGFR and proteinuria tended to worsen when the levels of circulating TNFR increased, suggesting that TNFR blood levels at the time of initial diagnosis could predict renal progression in patients with MN (Lee et al., 2014).

Treatment

Goals and objectives of treatment

The primary goals of treatment in MN are:

i. to avoid or minimize the adverse consequences of NS;

ii. to prevent the possible progression to renal failure; and

iii. to improve the quality of life and to prolong life-expectancy.

While there is a general agreement on the use of symptomatic therapy in patients with MN (see Chapter 2), there is still controversy on whether it is better to start specific therapy early, or to delay therapy until some marker predictive of a likely poor outcome develops. This is essentially a risk stratification man-oeuvre in which only those destined to have a poor outcome, based on clinical characteristics and biomarker profile, are treated initially, based on the presup-position that a delay in treatment will not adversely affect the responsiveness to therapy as compared to early treatment. This approach tends to neglect the adverse consequences of more prolonged exposure to the nephrotic state per se in those patients allocated to a delayed treatment strategy. The next sections present the arguments for an early start versus a delayed treatment strategy in primary MN with NS at presentation.

A number of drugs are now available for and have been evaluated in the treat-ment of MN. Glucocorticoids, alkylating agents, calcineurin inhibitors (CNI), rituximab (RTX), mycophenolate salts (MMF and MPS), and ACTH (synthetic and natural) have received the greatest attention.

Specific treatment

Glucocorticoids

In the past, oral administration of glucocorticoids has been a frequently recom-mended treatment approach in MN. The results of retrospective uncontrolled studies have been inconsistent and controversial, mainly because the inclusion criteria, the doses of glucocorticoids, and the duration of treatment were ex-tremely variable in the different studies. A meta-analysis of four randomized, open-label, controlled trials concluded that the probability of obtaining com-plete remission at three years and the actuarial renal survival at five years were almost identical in patients who received symptomatic therapy and in those treated with prednisone (Hogan et al., 1995). The studies included in this meta-analysis can be criticized as they employed prednisone either short term or at moderate doses, or both. One cannot exclude a better efficacy of glucocortic-oids when given at high doses and for prolonged periods, but these approaches may result in severe side effects.

In summary, the available controlled trials have not shown a clear benefit of glucocorticoids over symptomatic therapy in MN. It is possible that a population of steroid-sensitive patients with MN does exist but they are in a quite small minority (probably around 5–10 per cent), and cannot readily be distinguished from early spontaneously remitting patients. Accordingly, the concept of steroid-resistant MN should be considered a misnomer and it is disappointing to see continued reference in published papers claiming the success of treatments in 'steroid-resistant' MN, when the existence of such an 'entity' is in such serious doubt. On the other hand, if the use of glucocorticoids alone is probably ineffective, in combination with other immunosuppressive drugs steroids may exert synergistic or additive anti-inflammatory, immunomodulating, and 'renal' effects that reinforce the therapeutic activity of these associations.

It should be pointed out, however, that if glucocorticoids are of little benefit in Caucasian patients with MN, they may be effective in other ethnicities. In a large retrospective and uncontrolled Japanese study, the renal survival rate in patients who had received a four-week course of steroid therapy was significantly higher than in patients on supportive therapy alone (Shiiki et al., 2004). The results of this study are subject to a great deal of confounding, and the results should be interpreted with great caution.

Alkylating agents

The 2012 KDIGO guidelines for glomerulonephritis suggested that continuous daily therapy with oral alkylating agents might be effective but can be associated with greater risk of toxicity, particularly when administered for more than six months. Cyclophosphamide has been the agent most frequently used. A Cochrane review reported that combined glucocorticoids and alkylating agents significantly reduced death or risk of ESRD and increased the probability of complete or partial remission. On the other hand, this combined regimen was associated with a significantly higher risk of discontinuation or hospitalization due to adverse effects (Chen et al., 2013). However, it is difficult to draw any conclusion from that review as it considered all together papers with different criteria of inclusion and exclusion, different dosages and duration of treatments with alkylating agents, different doses and duration of steroids, and different follow-ups from nine to 120 months.

In a retrospective analysis, 124 patients with MN and deteriorating renal function or untreatable NS received a treatment predominantly consisting of daily cyclophosphamide combined with steroids. In most patients, cyclophosphamide was given for 12 months, at a dose of 1.5 mg/kg/day. At ten years, 3 per cent of patients entered renal replacement therapy and 10 per cent died. Complete remission rates were 38 per cent at five years and another 45 per cent of patients had partial remission after five years. Serious adverse events occurred in 23 per cent of patients. The most notable complications were infection (17 per cent), leukopenia (18 per cent), and cardiovascular events (13 per cent) (van den Brand et al., 2014a). Cancer incidence was 21.2 per 1000 person-years in treated patients compared with 4.6 per 1000 person-years in patients who did not receive cyclophosphamide (van den Brand et al., 2014b). A few observational studies reported the efficacy of intravenous (IV) pulses of cyclophosphamide and oral glucocorticoids in patients with primary MN (Mathrani et al., 2017; Kanigicherla et al., 2018).

In summary, the use of daily oral cyclophosphamide in association with prednisone may be justified only in patients with MN and full-blown NS. However,
we recommend that the doses should not exceed 2 mg/kg/day for three months
or 1 mg/kg/day for six months to prevent malignancy or gonadal toxicity.

Only few studies reported the results with daily oral chlorambucil in MN.
This drug was used initially in the cyclical therapy alternating glucocorticoids with a cytotoxic agent (see 'Alternating glucocorticoids and cytotoxic
drugs (cyclical therapy)') or in association with steroids. In a Polish study, low-
dose chlorambucil (4 mg/day) was given for six months together with three
methylprednisolone pulses and oral prednisone, 1 mg/kg/day for eight weeks,
followed by gradual tapering up to six months. Out of 32 patients with MN and
NS, complete remission was obtained in 14 patients (47.3 per cent) and partial
remission in 16 patients (50 per cent). No side effects were observed with the
exception of glucose intolerance after steroid pulses in four subjects (Idasiak-
Piechocka et al., 2009).

Alternating glucocorticoids and cytotoxic drugs (cyclical therapy)

An Italian multicentre prospective randomized trial assessed the long-term
efficacy and safety of a treatment consisting of three consecutive cycles of a
two-month therapy. Treatment began with 1 g pulse of IV methylprednisolone
(MP) repeated for three consecutive days, followed by oral prednisolone 0.5
mg/kg/day (or oral methylprednisolone 0.4 mg/kg/day) for one month; then
the steroid was stopped and oral chlorambucil (initial dosage 0.2 mg/kg/day)
was given daily for one month, followed by a month with MP and oral prednisone, another month with chlorambucil, and again steroids for one month,
followed by chlorambucil for another month. Thus, the cyclical therapy lasted
six months, three with steroids and three with chlorambucil. Eighty-one nephrotic adults with biopsy-proven primary MN were randomized to receive either
supportive treatment or the cyclical therapy. The two groups were homogenous
at randomization. Patients were followed for ten years. The probability of surviving at ten years without developing ESRD was significantly better in patients
given cyclical MP and chlorambucil than in controls (92 per cent versus 60
per cent). The probability of having a remission (complete plus partial) of NS
as a *first event* was significantly higher in treated patients (83 per cent versus
38 per cent; p = 0.0038); about half of remissions occurred *after* the termination of treatment, and thus treatment resistance cannot be reliably determined
at the end of a six-month course of treatment. Some patients had a relapse of
proteinuria so that at ten years, 40.5 per cent of patients were still in complete
remission and 21.5 per cent in partial remission. The slope of the reciprocal of
plasma creatinine with time, expressed in mg/dl, was significantly better after

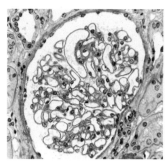

Plate 1 Minimal change disease. Light microscopy: the glomerulus is unremarkable; capillary lumina are patent, capillary walls are single contoured and there is no increase in cellularity (periodic acid-Schiff stain)

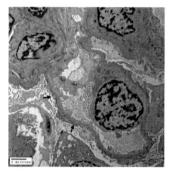

Plate 2 Minimal change disease. Electron microscopy: glomerular capillaries with complete effacement of the processes of podocytes (arrows). Note microvillous transformation of the free surfaces of these cells. Basement membranes are normal.

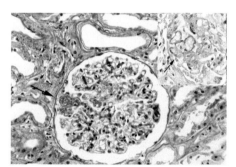

Plate 3 Focal segmental glomerulosclerosis ('classic' variant). Small area of capillary collapse and sclerosis at the periphery of an otherwise normal tuft (arrow) (AFOG stain × 63).

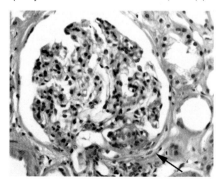

Plate 4 Focal segmental glomerulosclerosis ('tip' variant). Few collapsed capillaries adhere to swollen epithelial cells of the tubular pole of the glomerulus. (AFOG stain × 63).

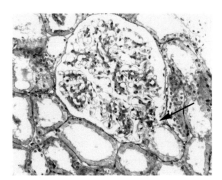

Plate 5 Focal segmental glomerulosclerosis ('hilar' variant). The area of glomerular sclerosis is adjacent to the vascular pole (arrow) (AFOG stain × 63)

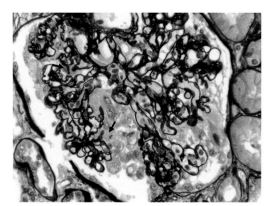

Plate 6 Focal and segmental glomerulosclerosis, collapsing type. Light microscopy: in this glomerulus, clusters of podocytes are enlarged, coarsely vacuolated and contain protein reabsorption droplets; mitotic figures are in several cells (arrows). Capillary walls in association.

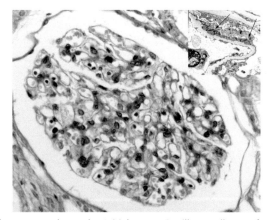

Plate 7 Membranous nephropathy. Initial stage. Capillary walls are of normal thickness (AFOG stain × 63). Insert: electron microscopy shows fine granular electrondense deposits in sub-epithelial position (arrows) (× 9100)

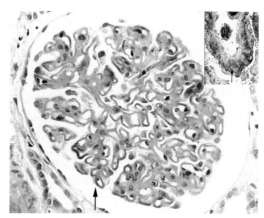

Plate 8 Membranous nephropathy. Later stage. Diffuse homogeneous thickening of capillary walls with coalescent granular (red) parietal deposits (AFOG stain × 63). Insert. sub-epithelial electrondense deposits are surrounded and partially covered by projections of newly formed basement membrane ('spikes') (× 7500).

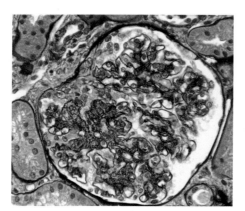

Plate 9 IgA nephropathy. Light microcopy: glomerulus with segmental increase in cellularity involving several mesangial regions. Capillary walls are single contoured. (periodic acid-methenamine silver stain).

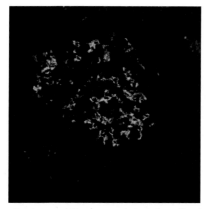

Plate 10 IgA nephropathy. Immunofluorescence: IgA deposits throughout mesangial regions of all lobules.

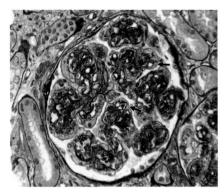

Plate 11 Membranoproliferative glomerulonephritis. Light microscopy: the glomerulus has pronounced lobular architecture with increase in mesangial cellularity, leukocytes in some capillary lumina and many double-contoured capillary walls (arrows) (periodic acid-methenamine silver stain).

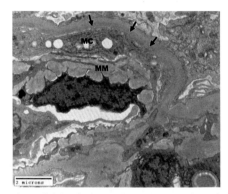

Plate 12 C3 Glomerulonephritis. Electron Microscopy: portion of glomerular capillary with thick wall because of interposition of mesangial cells (MC) and mesangial matrix (MM) between endothelial cell, the nucleus of which nearly fills the capillary lumen, and electron dense deposits (arrows) beneath the basement membrane.

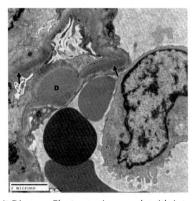

Plate 13 Dense Deposit Disease. Electron micrograph with intramembranous elongated densities in several capillary walls (arrows); there is also a subepithelial hump shaped deposit (D).

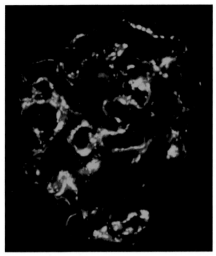

Plate 14 C3 Glomerulonephriis. Immunofluoresence microscopy. Note the mesangial and peripheral capillary loop deposits of C3 (Courtesy of Gabriella Moroni).

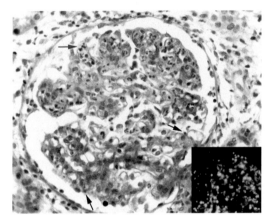

Plate 15 Acute post-infectious glomerulonephritis. Diffuse intracapillary hypercellularity with some small 'hump-like' deposit (black arrows) and polymorphs in the lumina (red arrow) (AFOG (aniline fucsin and orange G) stain × 63)). Insert: diffuse granular deposition of C3 ('starry sky') at immunofluorescence (× 50).

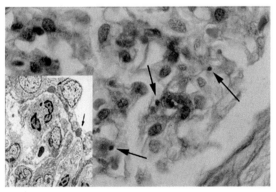

Plate 16 Acute post-infectious glomerulonephritis. 'Hump like' deposits in sub-epithelial position (arrows). (AFOG stain × 100). Insert. ovalar electrondense sub-epithelial deposits at electron microscopy (arrows) (× 9500).

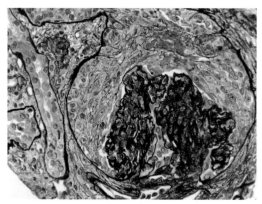

Plate 17 Crescentic glomerulonephritis. Light microscopy: glomerulus with extensive fresh crescent with cells and fibrin filling the urinary space and associated with compression and distortion of the capillary tufts (periodic acid-methenamine silver stain).

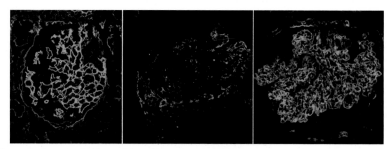

Plate 18 Crescentic glomerulonephritis. Immunofluorescence: this composite figure indicates the typical immunofluorescence patterns associated with crescentic glomerulonephritis: A: linear IgG in all capillary walls, indicative of anti-glomerular basement membrane disease. B: glomerulus with sparse and widely scattered granular deposits of C3, indicative of pauci-immune crescentic glomerulonephritis. C: widespread granular deposits of C3 in mesangial regions and capillary walls, indicative of immune complex glomerulonephritis.

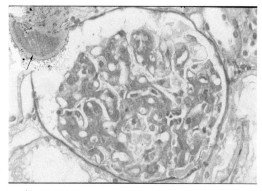

Plate 19 Collagenofibrotic glomerulopathy. Electron microscopy: the mesangium is replaced by collagen fibrils; some display defined periodicity and many are curved or frayed and are in irregularly-shaped bundles. The inset discloses these findings at higher magnification.

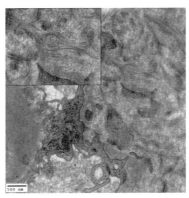

Plate 20 Collagenofibrotic glomerulopathy. Light microscopy: the glomeruli have widened mesangial regions with lighter staining material which is also present in the subendothelial aspects of capillary walls. Basement membranes are preserved (arrows) (periodic acid-Schiff stain).

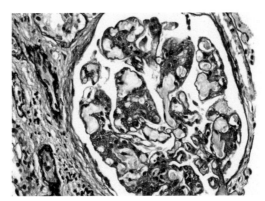

Plate 21 Lipoprotein glomerulopathy. Light microscopy: capillary lumina are filled with pale staining amorphous material forming 'thrombi.' There is widening and mild increase in cellularity of mesangial regions. Some capillary walls are double contoured (periodic acid-Schiff stain).

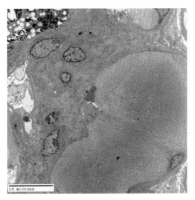

Plate 22 Lipoprotein glomerulopathy. Electron microscopy: glomerular capillary is filled with a mass of granular and finely vacuolated material.

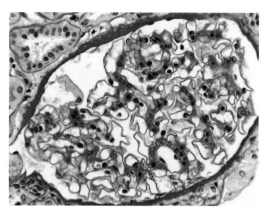

Plate 23 Mesangial proliferative glomerulonephritis. Glomerulus with mild widening of mesangial regions and mild increase in mesangial cellularity; there are no other abnormalities (periodic acid-Schiff stain).

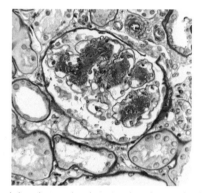

Plate 24 Idiopathic nodular glomerulosclerosis. The glomerulus has nodular appearance with increase in mesangial matrix and variable but mild increase in cellularity. Capillary basement membranes are of normal thickness and capillary lumina are patent. Note that there are no insudative lesions (hyalinosis) in the arterioles adjacent to the glomerulus (periodic acid-Schiff stain).

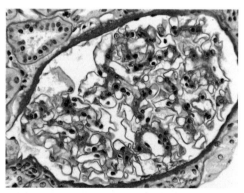

Plate 25 Fibrillary glomerulonephritis. Mesangisal areas and capillary walls are expanded by acellular material (PAS stain × 63). Insert: electron microscopy shows accumulation of non-branching, randomly arranged fibrils (× 16500)

ten years in treated patients (from 1.0 to 0.84) than in controls (from 1.0 to 0.51; p = 0.035). Among treated patients, one died of myocardial infarction and two entered dialysis; instead, three patients died and nine entered dialysis among controls. Four patients had to stop treatment because of reversible side-effects. In the long-term one treated patient developed diabetes and another one became obese (Ponticelli et al., 1995). The main defect of this study is that it was unblinded, and that it compared a combination of drugs to non-specific therapy (which did not include ACE inhibitors in all subjects, since the antiproteinuric effect of these agents was discovered after the trial was started). In another randomized controlled trial, cyclical therapy obtained a significantly higher rate of responses at two years and a significantly lower slope of reciprocal of serum creatinine decline in comparison to a therapy with MP alone (Ponticelli et al., 1992). In a third trial, patients who received cyclical therapy with cyclophosphamide (2 mg/kg/day) or chlorambucil showed a similar benefit and rate of side effects, although numerically lower, with cyclophosphamide (Ponticelli et al., 1998). A review of the three Italian trials showed that three patients among those who received chlorambucil (662 patient-years of follow-up) developed cancer, a ratio of 4.5/1,000 patient-years similar to the 4.3/1,000 patient-years observed in male Caucasian subjects examined in the same period of time (Ponticelli et al., 1998). Thus, no oncogenic effect was found when chlorambucil was used at a cumulative dosage of ≤18 mg/kg. However, we now feel that good results can also be obtained if chlorambucil is given at doses of 0.1 mg/kg/day, a dosage that can further reduce the risk of adverse events and malignancy.

Good results with cyclical therapy have also been reported by a long-term Indian randomized trial. Jha and colleagues (2007) compared the effect of a six-month course of alternating prednisolone and oral cyclophosphamide with supportive treatment in 93 adults with NS caused by MN. Patients were followed up for a median of 11 years. Data were analysed on an intention-to-treat basis. Of the 47 patients who received the cyclical therapy, 34 (72 per cent) achieved complete (15) or partial (19) remission compared with 16 remissions (five complete, 11 partial) in the 46 controls (35 per cent; p <0.01). The ten-year dialysis-free survival was 89 per cent in the experimental group and 65 per cent in control group (p = 0.016), and the likelihood of survival without death, dialysis, and doubling of serum creatinine were 79 per cent and 44 per cent, respectively (p = 0.0006). At ten years, hypertension, hypercholesterol-aemia, and oedema were significantly less frequent in treated patients than in controls. Serious infection occurred in 15 per cent of treated patients versus 24 per cent of untreated controls. Also, the quality of life index was significantly better in patients who received treatment. In another study, cyclical therapy with cyclophosphamide and steroids obtained remission in eight out of ten patients with MN who proved to be resistant or have relapse of NS after tacrolimus (Ramachandran et al., 2016c). Taken all together the results of these randomized trials, it appears that the cyclical treatment alternating steroids and alkylating agents (most commonly oral cyclophosphamide) can obtain a high rate of remission (Table 6.5).

Various schedules of cyclical therapy have also been used in patients with an already established renal insufficiency. A number of small-sized, nonrandomized studies reported that treatment obtained reduction of proteinuria and improvement or stabilization of renal function. However, in most patients, serum creatinine did not return to normal values. Moreover, the administration of glucocorticoids and cytotoxic agents to patients with renal insufficiency considerably increased the risk of side effects. In a British randomized trial, 108 patients with mean creatinine clearance of 50 ml/min were assigned to supportive therapy (38) or standard doses of prednisolone and chlorambucil (33), or standard doses of cyclosporine (37). Most patients had a further decline in renal function. Risk of further 20 per cent decline in creatinine clearance was significantly lower in the prednisolone and chlorambucil group (58 per cent) than in cyclosporine (81 per cent) or supportive therapy (84 per cent) (p = 0.003). Serious adverse events were frequent in all three groups but were higher in the prednisolone and chlorambucil group than in the supportive care group (Howman et al., 2013). This study has been criticized because cyclosporine was given at doses of 5 mg/kg/day and chlorambucil at doses of 0.2 mg/kg/day, while the doses of these drugs should be substantially reduced in patients with renal insufficiency. Moreover, it is very

Table 6.5 First event results with the use of cyclical therapy (steroids alternated with an alkylating agent for six months) in patients with primary MN. Results of randomized controlled trials.

Authors	Patients	Complete remission	Partial remission
Ponticelli et al., 1989	42	24	10
Ponticelli et al., 1992	41	14	13
Ahmed et al., 1994	10	5	3
Ponticelli et al., 1998	87	28	48
Jha et al., 2007	47	15	19
Ramachandran et al., 2016a	35	20	10
TOTAL	262	106 (40.4%)	103 (39.3%)

likely that the monitoring of patients and modifications of treatment were absolutely inadequate, if one considers the nature and severity of adverse events (Ponticelli and Glassock, 2013).

In conclusion, cyclical therapy may increase the probability of remission and protect renal function in patients with MN and full-blown NS. This treatment may also slow the rate of progression and improve proteinuria in some patients with declining renal function, but in these instances cytotoxic agents should be used at lower doses. Careful monitoring of blood count is needed to prevent severe haematologic side effects. Regimens using IV cyclophosphamide are not consistently effective and this route of administration is not generally recommended. Cyclical regimens that omit the IV administration of high-dose glucocorticoids have not been studied in randomized trials.

Calcineurin inhibitors (CNI)

Cyclosporine (CsA)

A number of observational studies reported a favourable antiproteinuric effect of CsA in MN. Taken together, the available data showed that CsA may achieve remission (complete or partial) of NS in about 66 per cent of patients (Table 6.6). The addition of small doses of prednisone may increase

Table 6.6 First event results with the use of cyclosporine or tacrolimus (in *italics*) in MN.

Author	Patients	Complete remission	Partial remission
Meyrier, 1992	73	14	18
Rostoker, 1993	15	4	7
Fritsche, 1999	41	14	12
Cattran et al., 2001	28	2	19
Alexopoulos, 2006	51	26	17
Kalliakmani, 2010	32	18	10
Tao, 2011	51	12	17
Coban et al., 2014	23	8	8
Chen, 2010	*39*	*11*	*22*
Caro, 2015	122	42	58
Ramachandran, 2016	35	15	8
Qin et al., 2017	408	92	156
TOTAL	918	259 (28.2%)	372 (40.5%)

the probability of remission. Reduction of proteinuria usually occurs within three to four months of starting therapy. However, in about one-third of patients with MN, remission may occur after six months or later (Fritsche et al., 1999). Most responders show a relapse of NS after interruption of treatment or even after reduction of CsA doses. Thus, many patients need to continue CsA, at low doses, for a long period of time. Whether such a policy may prevent the nephrotoxicity of CsA is still a matter of discussion. Goumenos (2008) reported remission of NS in >80 per cent of MN patients. Repeat renal biopsies showed no signs of CsA nephrotoxicity, but chronic histological lesions worsened with time, even in cases with remission. Kalliakmani and colleagues (2010) treated 32 nephrotic patients with prednisolone and CsA who had well-preserved renal function. Complete remission of NS was observed in 18 patients (56 per cent) and partial remission in ten patients (31 per cent) after 12 months of treatment (total response rate of 87 per cent). Relapses were observed in 39 per cent of patients, with complete remission and in 60 per cent of patients with partial remission. Multiple relapses occurred in 25 per cent of patients, who showed gradual unresponsiveness to CsA and decline of renal function. Among these patients, more than 50 per cent of renal biopsies showed a progression of the stage of the disease and a worsened glomerulosclerosis and tubulo-interstitial injury, without the typical features of CsA nephrotoxicity. On the other hand, it has also been reported that patients in remission receiving long-term CsA may maintain stable renal function (Alexopoulos et al., 2006; Tao et al., 2011). Of note, patients with MN who do not respond to CNI have low levels of serum amyloid A1, while patients with normal or subnormal levels are likely to achieve complete remission under CNI (Yu et al., 2018).

In summary, there is evidence that CsA may obtain remission of proteinuria in a substantial number of nephrotic patients with MN and normal or near normal baseline levels of renal function, although the rate of remission varies in different studies. However, little information is available on whether CsA therapy may be protective or harmful on renal function in the long term. The risk of nephrotoxicity is low if guidelines on CsA dosing and monitoring are followed (see Chapter 3). No head-to-head comparisons of CsA therapy with the standard cyclical alkylating agent–prednisone therapy regimen have been conducted to date. An ongoing multicentre randomized controlled trial (MENTOR) is comparing CsA with RTX in MN (Fervenza et al., 2015). Preliminary data reported at the 2018 meeting of the American Society of Nephrology showed that RTX was superior to CsA in maintaining remission at 24 months.

Tacrolimus (TAC)

A number of observational studies reported a good rate of remissions (more frequently partial) with TAC in MN (Table 6.6). However, relapses of protein-uria were frequent after interruption of TAC. A Spanish multicentre study re-ported the results of monotherapy with TAC in 122 patients with MN, NS, and stable renal function. Duration of treatment was 17.6 ± 7.2 months, including a full-dose and a tapering period. TAC was administered at a mean dose of 0.05 mg/kg/day. After 18 months of treatment, 102 (84 per cent) patients responded. Among responders, 42 per cent achieved complete remission and 58 per cent partial remission. The amount of proteinuria at baseline predicted remission— the lower the baseline proteinuria, the higher the probability of remission. Only ten patients (8 per cent) received concomitantly glucocorticoids. Almost half (44 per cent) of the responders relapsed (Caro et al., 2015). A Chinese study reported the outcome of 408 consecutive patients with MN and nephrotic syn-drome who were treated with tacrolimus. The cumulative partial or complete remission after tacrolimus therapy were 50 per cent at six months and 67 per cent at 24 months. The cumulative complete remission rates were 4 per cent and 23 per cent, respectively. A relapse occurred in 101 of the 271 (37.3 per cent) patients with partial or complete remission (Qin et al., 2017).

A controlled trial reported a very high percentage of remission in patients assigned to TAC in comparison with untreated controls after 18 months of therapy (94 per cent versus 35 per cent) but relapse of NS occurred in approxi-mately half of patients after TAC withdrawal (Praga et al., 2007). In a Chinese multicentre trial, 73 patients with nephrotic MN were randomized to TAC plus prednisone for nine months, or cyclophosphamide plus prednisone for four months. Remission was reached earlier with TAC but at 12 months the remission rate was comparable in the two groups. Patients receiving TAC were more likely to develop diabetes, infection, and hypertension (Chen et al., 2010). A single-centre randomized trial compared the effects of TAC plus prednisone versus a cyclical therapy with cyclophosphamide alternated with steroids in 70 patients with MN and persistent NS or with complications of NS. Intention-to-treat analysis showed that remissions at the end of 12 months (71 per cent with TAC versus 77 per cent with cyclical therapy) were comparable. Patients on cyclophosphamide had a significantly higher risk of amenorrhea while those on TAC had a greater risk of reversible nephrotoxicity (Ramachandran et al., 2016a).

In summary, TAC is a useful therapeutic option for nephrotic patients and well-preserved renal function. The majority of patients will experience a remis-sion with a significant reduction in the risk for deteriorating renal function, but a high relapse rate can be expected when therapy is discontinued, just as with CsA. It is still to be demonstrated if the addition of prednisone or mycophenolate may improve the therapeutic index of monotherapy with TAC.

Adrenocorticotrophic hormone (ACTH)

Berg and colleagues (1999) reported that synthetic ACTH (synacthen) administered intramuscularly twice per week for one year improved lipoprotein profile and obtained complete remission of proteinuria in three patients and partial remission in 2/5 patients with MN. In a further study, Berg and Arnadottir (2004) reported that all the 15 patients treated with synthetic ACTH 0.75–1 mg twice weekly for nine months obtained remission of NS as a first event. After a follow-up of 18–30 months, 14 patients were still in remission. A small randomized controlled trial compared the six-month regimen based on steroids alternated to an alkylating agent with intramuscular synthetic ACTH given at a dose of 1 mg twice a week for one year (Ponticelli et al., 2006). In the first group, 15 of 16 participants entered complete or partial remission as a first event, versus 14 of 16 in the second group. Median proteinuria decreased from 5.1 g/day to 2.1 g/day in the first group and from 6.0 g/day to 0.3 g/day in the ACTH group. No important side effects were seen in participants assigned to ACTH. However, in our experience, out of the trial, one elderly patient had vertebral collapse and another developed diabetes. Therefore, caution with ACTH therapy should be used, particularly in elderly subjects. The efficacy of synthetic ACTH has been confirmed by other observational studies (Lorusso et al., 2015; Goldsmith and Hammad, 2015). In a retrospective study, 17 patients were treated with synthetic ACTH for nine months. Four patients entered complete remission and seven a partial remission. These results were inferior to those observed in historical controls given oral cyclophosphamide for one year (van de Logt et al., 2015).

In the United States, the effects of a natural ACTH gel formulation, which has a longer chain of amino acids, have been evaluated in 11 nephrotic individuals with MN treated with gel ACTH; two participants entered complete remission and seven a partial remission, while two patients failed to respond, resulting in an 81 per cent overall response rate (Bomback et al., 2011). In another study, 20 patients with MN and NS received a subcutaneous dose of 40 or 80 IU twice weekly. At 12 months, there was a significant improvement in proteinuria in the entire cohort, decreasing in mean from 9.1 g/day to 3.9 g/day with significant improvements in serum albumin as well as total and LDL cholesterol. There was a trend toward better outcomes among patients who received greater cumulative doses. No significant adverse effects were documented (Hladunewich et al., 2014).

It has been hypothesized that the mechanism responsible for the beneficial effect of ACTH probably rests on activation of melanocortin receptor-1 (MCR-1) which is co-localized with synaptopodin in podocytes. MCR-1 might interfere with catalase and RHO-1 protein activity, so regulating cytoskeleton and preventing podocyte apoptosis (Elvin et al., 2016). However, although all MCRs may be activated by ACTH, the main melanocortin receptor for ACTH is MCR-2. In addition, it has been demonstrated that in MCR1 null mice, melanostimulating hormone could reduce proteinuria and protect podocytes from lipopolysaccharide injury, via a MCR1-independent mechanism (Qiao et al., 2016). It is possible that the effects of ACTH may be modulated by β-defensins, a new class of melanocortin ligands that may cross talk between MCRs and the immune system.

In summary, the data on the use of ACTH in MN are still limited. The available information rests on small-sized studies, with short-term follow-up. Side effects mainly consist of tanning, obesity, and aggravation of Type 2 diabetes. However, other steroid-like adverse events may occur, particularly in older subjects. The benefits and risks of ACTH in patients with MN and impaired renal function are largely unknown. In the US, the natural ACTH gel (Acthar gel) is approved by the FDA for induction of remission in NS due to primary renal disease, in the absence of uraemia. However, the cost of a single vial of Acthar gel is more than US$34,000.

Purine synthesis inhibitors

Azathioprine

No adequately powered, randomized controlled trials of azathioprine in MN have ever been conducted, although retrospective observational studies have suggested a small benefit. The drug is not recommended by KDIGO for treatment of MN.

Mycophenolate

Uncontrolled observational studies involving small numbers of patients reported the possibility of reducing proteinuria with mycophenolate mofetil (MMF), usually associated with glucocorticoids, in nephrotic patients with MN and normal renal function. The data, however, are scarce and conflicting: the doses used ranged from 0.5 to 2 g/day for three to seven months. Proteinuria decreased in many patients, but very few of them ever attained a complete remission. Mean serum creatinine tended to remain stable but the follow-ups were very short. Side effects of MMF were infrequent and generally mild. Relapses following discontinuation of treatment were common and the impact of MMF on circulating levels of anti-PLA2R antibody in primary MN is very poorly understood. In a retrospective study, MMF given 1 g twice daily for 12 months was compared to cyclophosphamide given 1.5 mg/kg/day for 12 months. Both groups also received intermittent MP and alternate-day prednisone. Cumulative incidence of remission (66 per cent vs. 72 per cent) and side effects (75 per cent vs. 69 per cent) were similar, but the risk of relapse was greater in MMF (38 per cent) than in cyclophosphamide (13 per cent) patients (Branten et al., 2007).

Three small-sized randomized trials evaluating the role of MMF associated with steroids have been performed. A prospective, controlled, open-label study randomized 20 patients with MN to be given MMF and prednisolone for six months or a modified cyclical regimen (steroids alternated with chlorambucil). Remission (complete or partial) rates were 63.6 per cent in the MMF group and 66.7 per cent in the cyclical treatment group. Serum creatinine and creatinine clearance remained stable during a mean follow up of 15 months. Two patients on MMF and one on cyclical therapy showed relapse of NS. Chlorambucil resulted in more leukopenia compared with MMF (Chan et al., 2007). Senthyl Nayagam and colleagues (2008) compared the efficacy of MMF with cyclical therapy in 21 nephrotic adults with MN. Of the 11 participants randomized to receive MMF (2 g/day for six months) along with oral prednisolone (0.5 mg/kg/day for two to three months), seven (64 per cent) entered complete or partial remission versus 8/10 (80 per cent) assigned to a six-month regimen of steroids alternated with cyclophosphamide every other month. Another controlled trial randomized 36 patients with primary MN to receive MMF at a dose 2 g/day for one year or symptomatic therapy. At 12 months, there was no difference between the two groups in decrease of mean proteinuria or in the rate of complete and partial remissions. Serious adverse effects were observed in 4/19 (20 per cent) patients receiving MMF (Dussol et al., 2008).

MMF with steroids has also been used in children with MN and declining renal function as 'rescue' therapy. In a small observational study, MMF obtained reduction of proteinuria >50 per cent over the baseline in three patients, while the fourth child progressed to ESRD (Bhimma et al., 2013).

It is possible to attribute some role for MMF in improving proteinuria, at least over the short term; however, complete remissions are rare, relapses are very frequent, and the follow-ups are all short-term. A single small controlled trial of MMF monotherapy has shown disappointing results, while good results have been reported when MMF was associated with glucocorticoids. On the basis of these few data it seems premature to recommend the use of mycophenolate salts in the management of MN, except perhaps for those who are intolerant to other more established regimens and who still have full-blown NS or as rescue therapy in cyclophosphamide-intolerant patients. When using mycophenolate, the drug should be associated with steroids to increase its efficacy in MN. However, the optimal doses and length of treatment of MMF and steroids has not yet been determined. Neither MMF nor sodium mycophenolate (Myfortic®) are approved for use in MN by the Food and Drug Administration (FDA) in the US or by the European Medical Agency (EMA).

Mizoribine

Mizoribine is an immunosuppressive drug with characteristics similar to Azathioprine. The drug has been mainly used in Japan. An observational study in 13 patients with MN and nephrotic-range proteinuria showed that Mizoribine at an initial dose of 150 mg/day, associated with prednisone (20 mg/day) could significantly reduce proteinuria in a number of observational Japanese studies (Matsumoto et al., 2013; Ito et al., 2015; Wang et al., 2016; Saito et al., 2017).

Intravenous immunoglobulins (IVIg)

A few anecdotal uncontrolled reports suggested a possible benefit of high-dose IVIg therapy in MN (Floccari et al., 2008; Tran et al., 2015). However, a number of questions remain unanswered regarding IVIg therapy. It is unclear how long a patient should be treated before considering her/him as a non-responder and which is the optimal dosage. No information is available about the long-term outcome of these patients. It is still unknown whether the potential response to treatment is influenced by the exact preparations of IVIg, which may differ for each batch, and for other features such as quantity and type of anti-idiotypic antibodies or IgA concentration. Finally, sucrose-stabilized formulations of IVIg should be avoided as they may cause respiratory distress and reduced renal function. At present, there is little evidence supporting the use of IVIg in primary MN.

Rituximab (RTX)

The efficacy of RTX was initially tested in nine patients with MN. RTX was given at a dose of 375 mg/m² every week for four weeks. Proteinuria decreased from a mean of 8.6 ± 1.4 g/day to 3.8 ± 0.8 g/day after four weeks and remained stable around these levels (Remuzzi et al., 2002). After this pilot study other observational studies reported the results with RTX in MN. In an open-label trial, 15 patients with severe NS were enrolled. RTX was given two weeks apart and, at six months, patients who remained proteinuric were given a second course of treatment. Proteinuria significantly decreased by about half at 12 months. Full remission was achieved in two patients, and partial remission in six patients (Fervenza et al., 2008). In a multicentre study, RTX, 375 mg/m² every week for four weeks was administered to 20 patients with MN and proteinuria >5 g/day (Fervenza et al., 2010). Treatment was repeated after six months. Two patients did not respond to the first course and 18 patients completed the treatment. Proteinuria decreased from 11.9 to 2.0 g/day. At the last visit, four patents were in complete remission (20 per cent), 12 in partial remission (60 per cent), one patient had limited response, and one relapsed. Beck and colleagues (2011) investigated whether levels of anti-PLA2R antibodies correlated with the response to RTX. In 25 out of 35 patients with MN, anti-PLA2R antibodies were detected. In 17 patients, antibodies disappeared after RTX. Five of them achieved complete remission and ten partial remission at two years. None of the eight patients with persisting elevated levels of anti-PLA2R antibodies entered remission at one year and three had partial remission at two years. A multicentre study in France reported the outcome of patients treated with RTX for primary MN. At 12 months, complete remission was achieved in 6/23 (26 per cent) patients and partial remission in 13 patients (overall renal response = 82.6 per cent). Three patients suffered a relapse of NS 27–50 months after treatment. At univariate analysis an eGFR <45 ml/min/1.73 m^2 was an independent factor that predicted lack of response to RTX. Anti-PLA2R antibodies became negative in all the five responders with available follow-up sera (Michel et al., 2011). Soukiyyeh and colleagues (2015) treated 25 patients with MN and NS and obtained complete remission in ten and partial remission in seven (total 68 per cent). The largest uncontrolled series was that of Ruggenenti and colleagues (2015). Out of 132 patients with MN treated with RTX and followed in mean for 30 months, 84 patients responded (63.6 per cent), 43 achieved complete remission (32.6 per cent), and 41 partial remission (31.0 per cent). Among responders, 25 had a relapse of NS, the risk being higher for those who achieved partial remission (50 per cent versus 30 per cent). Although the response was similar in patients with positive or negative anti-PLA2R antibodies, re-emergence of circulating antibodies predicted disease relapse. It is worth noting that prior treatment with an immunosuppressive agent has no appreciable effect on the response rate to RTX. Most observational studies reported a good tolerance for RTX. However, in a previous paper by Ruggenenti (2012), out of 100 patients treated with RTX, eight died or progressed to ESRD. Another eight patients had serious cardiovascular events. It is difficult to know whether these complications were related to NS, to previous treatments, to RTX, or to a combination of these factors.

In a randomized controlled trial, 75 patients with biopsy-proven MN were assigned to six-month therapy with antiproteinuric treatment alone or antiproteinuric treatment plus RTX, 375 mg/m^2 on days 1 and 8. There was no difference in remission rates at six months. During the observational phase, remission rates 24 of 37 (64.9 per cent) patients in RTX group versus 13 of 38 (34.2 per cent) controls had complete or partial remission (p<0.01). Eight serious adverse events occurred in each group. The median time for remission was seven months. Positivity and titre of anti-PLAR antibodies predicted the response to treatment (Dahan et al., 2017). In another study, patients who clinically responded to RTX had a significantly lower percentage of Tregs at baseline compared to non-responders and a significantly increased percentage at day eight (Rosenzwajg et al., 2017).

Finally, RTX has also been used in combination with plasmapheresis or cyclophosphamide and steroids. A patient with MN refractory to RAS inhibitors and CNI rapidly responded to plasmapheresis and RTX (Wen et al., 2014). In another study, plasmapheresis against albumin, IVIgs, and RTX were given to ten patients with MN and proteinuria >10 g/day. Partial remission was observed in 90 per cent of patients (Muller-Deile et al., 2015). In a small observational study, patients with MN received a combination treatment regimen. Cyclophosphamide was administered orally at 2.5 mg/kg/day for one week, then 1.5 mg/kg/day for seven weeks. Prednisone was initiated at 60 mg/day, tapered to 15 mg/day by four weeks, and then slowly tapered to complete a six-month course. Concurrently, RTX was initiated with two 1000 mg IV doses separated by approximately two weeks. Then, 1000 mg of RTX were administered every four months for two years. Among 15 patients, 93 per cent achieved complete remission at a median time of 13 months. Three patients experienced reversible serious side effects, severe neutropenia and viral infection in two patients, and altered mental status in the third patient (Cortazar et al., 2017). Most studies reported that RTX is well tolerated, with the exception of infusion reactions. However, a retrospective review of 98 patients who received RTX in eight French nephrology departments reported an infection rate of 21.6 per 100 patient/years, and a risk of death of 5 per cent within 12 months from RTX infusion (Trivin et al., 2017). Thus, it is recommended the use of low-dose trimethoprim-sulfamethoxazole to avoid opportunistic infection (Jiang et al., 2015).

In summary, the available studies show that RTX, when given alone or with short-term steroids, can induce remission in at least 60 per cent of patients with MN (Table 6.7). The response is more frequent in patients showing decline or disappearance of anti-PLA2R antibodies. However, some points should be clarified before RTX may be considered as a standard of care therapy for MN:

   i. As shown in Tables 6.5–6.7, there is no published, randomized and controlled evidence that the efficacy of RTX alone in MN is superior to that of other treatments. This deficiency will be overcome once the MENTOR

Table 6.7 First event results with the use of rituximab in patients with primary MN.

Authors	Patients	Complete remission	Partial remission
Fervenza et al., 2010	20	4	12
Beck et al., 2011	25	5	13
Michel et al., 2011	23	6	13
Souqiyyeh et al., 2015	25	10	7
Ruggenenti et al., 2015	132	43	48
Roccatello et al., 2016	17	14	1
Dahan et al., 2017	37	7	17
Moroni et al., 2017	34	5	10
TOTAL	313	94 (30.0%)	121 (38.6%)

trial is published in a peer-reviewed journal, but only for a comparison of RTX to CsA, not cyclical alkylating steroid therapy.

ii. Little information is yet available on the long-term results (beyond 24–36 months), which will be particularly important for a disease which runs a long course and for a treatment that has marked and prolonged interference with the immune system.

iii. The optimal doses and the duration of treatment, including the use of maintenance dosing of RTX, are not well established. Poor responses have been reported with the use of low doses of RTX (Moroni et al., 2017).

iv. RTX seems to be ineffective in patients with reduced renal function or tubulo-interstitial changes at renal biopsy, but a threshold for these parameters that indicates futility of RTX treatment is not well established.

v. It is still uncertain whether a combination therapy of RTX with CNI or other cytotoxic drugs (e.g. MMF) may improve the long-term efficacy without increasing toxicity. Hopefully, ongoing trials in the US and in Europe will be able to better define the role and the indications for this expensive drug in MN (see clinicaltrials.gov).

Practical recommendations

Before deciding whether, when, and how to treat a patient with MN, the clinician should always attempt to establish if the disease is primary or secondary in its pathogenesis, if the patient is oligosymptomatic or symptomatically affected by a NS, if his/her renal function is normal or deteriorating, and should clearly consider the potential risks and benefits of the different possible treatments, particularly in the case of elderly or frail patients. The role of using serology (anti-PLA2R antibody levels in the assessment of when (and how) to treat apparently primary MN is in a state of evolution, but the evidence is pointing in the direction that serology can help in both treatment decision making and prognostication. Conservative (symptomatic) treatment of primary MN is similar to that used in primary GN and is outlined in Chapter 2. Unfortunately, RAS inhibition may be very ineffective in lowering proteinuria or inducing a partial remission of NS in patients with primary MN and very marked proteinuria (>10 g/day) and the long-term benefits and risks of RAS inhibition have not been examined in RCT in primary MN. Modest effects on inducing 'spontaneous remission' were noted by Polanco and colleagues (2010).

Is MN primary or secondary?

In some 10 per cent of patients, depending upon age, MN is associated with malignancy (Leeaphorn et al., 2014). Often the neoplasia is recognized at the time of renal biopsy, but in 20 per cent of cases proteinuria may antedate the initial manifestations of an underlying cancer by months or even years. Carcinomas of the lung, prostate, colon, rectum, breast, stomach, and kidney are the most frequent neoplasias, but Hodgkin's disease, non-Hodgkin's lymphoma, and chronic lymphocytic leukaemia may also be associated with MN. As mentioned, it is difficult to unequivocally differentiate the primary MN from cancer-associated disease at renal biopsy. Extensive mesangial and/or subendothelial deposits, a high number of inflammatory cells infiltrating the glomerulus, the lack of IgG4 dominance in the deposits, and absence of PLA2R glomerular staining suggest the possibility of an underlying carcinoma in high-risk older patients, especially in smokers (see Table 6.1). How extensive should be the investigation for detecting an 'occult' underlying cancer in a patient with MN is still a matter of debate. At least in heavy smokers and in the elderly patients, however, an extensive investigation is advisable, since some 20–25 per cent of MN patients aged over 60 have an underlying malignancy (Lefaucher et al., 2006). Thus, especially in these patients and in those with circulating anti-THSD7A antibodies, in addition to a thorough history and physical examination, a chest radiogram (preferably a computed tomography because of its higher sensitivity in detecting small lung neoplasms), a digital rectal exam of the prostate, a thorough breast examination and mammography in women, and renal ultrasonography (usually already done in connection with a renal biopsy) are suggested. A gastroscopy and a colonoscopy (or at the very least a stool occult blood examination) can also be done in older patients or in the presence of upper gastrointestinal symptoms, early satiety, unexplained weight loss, or iron-deficiency anaemia (see Table 6.3). Bone marrow aspiration and computed tomography are recommended in patients with severe anaemia not justified by evident or occult bleeding. Moreover, patients should be closely followed as neoplasia may be undetectable on initial screening. The possibility that the surgical removal or successful chemotherapy of the cancer can result in a complete remission of MN is well established.

In a number of patients MN can be secondary to drugs or toxic agents (see Table 6.2). Sometimes the drug exposure can be overlooked, leading to the misdiagnosis of primary MN. In drug-induced MN, proteinuria usually remits after the removal of the offending agent. Although MN can develop in patients with RA who have never received any arthritis modulating therapy, it more often occurs, in this setting, after NSAIDs (especially meclofenamate congeners) or penicillamine and can be reversible after the drug has been stopped. Both topical (e.g. ammoniated mercury creams) as well as systemically administered agents have been associated with the occurrence of MN.

The infection most frequently associated with MN is HBV. Many patients are asymptomatic but nearly all patients have hepatitis B surface antigenemia at the time of diagnosis. Hepatitis B-viral DNA and hepatitis B antigen, indicating active viral replication, are frequently found. An association between MN and HCV has also been reported. Therefore, patients with MN should be investigated for a possible association with both HBV and HCV infection. Liver disease may be very mild and consist only of transaminitis in many cases. The use of glucocorticoids or RTX in hepatitis B/C viral-associated MN is contraindicated as it can reactivate viral replication. Antiviral therapy may obtain remission of MN (Lin et al., 2013; Gupta and Quigg, 2015; Mozessohn et al., 2015). Tenofovir, entecavir, telbivudine, and lamivudine are currently used for treating HBV infection. In many cases these agents may obtain HBeAg clearance and remission of proteinuria (Yang et al., 2016). Tacrolimus combined with entecavir rapidly and effectively induced partial or complete remission of HBV-MN in a series of Chinese adults (Wang et al., 2016). The treatment of HCV completely changed after the development of multiple direct-acting antivirals (DAAs). There are four classes of DAAs: 3/4A (NS3/4A) protease inhibitors, NS5B nucleoside polymerase inhibitors, NS5B non-nucleoside polymerase inhibitors, and NS5A inhibitors. Combining two DAA regimens with different mechanisms may allow for shorter treatment durations that are effective across multiple genotypes (Lawitz et al., 2017).

Should non-nephrotic patients with MN be treated?

Almost all patients with subnephrotic proteinuria (usually fewer than 3.5–4.0 g/ day) and primary MN do not need 'specific' treatment and can be managed very effectively by conservative means (see also Chapter 2) with follow-up measurement of urine protein excretion and renal function. The risk of developing renal failure is minimal for these patients, unless they evolve into a full-blown NS. Moreover, since non-nephrotic patients are nearly always asymptomatic and normo-albuminaemic, they are not exposed to the potential harmful consequences of the NS. Ideally, blood pressure should be kept ≤130/85 mmHg. In some cases, the administration of an ACE inhibitor or an ARB may obtain a further reduction and even the disappearance of proteinuria. Statins are also recommended in case of hyperlipidaemia resistant to dietary measures. Low-dose aspirin may be prescribed to prevent cardiovascular or thrombo-embolic disease, although there is no clear-cut evidence that patients with non-nephrotic proteinuria and mild hypo-albuminaemia have any increased risk of cardiovascular or thrombo-embolic events after adjustment for other traditional risk factors (e.g. age, smoking, diabetes, hypertension). The risk of developing ESRD is minimal if any for patients who remain non-nephrotic over time. Nevertheless, it is mandatory that these patients are regularly followed, as a number of them may develop a full-blown NS sooner or later.

Should nephrotic patients with MN be treated and when?

(See Table 6.8)

Table 6.8 The pros and cons of an early initial treatment in patients with primary MN and nephrotic syndrome (NS).

	PROs	CONs
Elderly age	The response is similar to that of younger adults. Elderly patients are more susceptible to the complications of NS.	The older the patient the higher the risk of iatrogenic morbidity. Elderly kidneys are more susceptible to renal toxicity of CNI.
Female gender	The response to treatment is similar or even better in women than in men.	The natural course of primary MN is more favourable in females. Thus, in women, it is better to wait and see.
Nephrotic syndrome	The risk of complications and renal failure is higher in patients with NS than in those with asymptomatic proteinuria.	A number of patients with NS may enter spontaneous remission and can avoid the potential toxicity of treatment.
Renal function	Treatment may halt the progression and improve proteinuria even in patients with reduced GFR. Thus, it is better not to wait until GFR deteriorates before starting treatment.	In most cases renal function does not improve and side effects are more frequent and severe in patients with renal dysfunction.

While there is agreement for a 'wait-and-see' policy in non-nephrotic patients with MN, there are different attitudes for those who present with NS. At the two extremes, some clinicians prefer an early treatment at the time of presentation or shortly thereafter, independently of the age and sex of patients, while others use symptomatic measures only unless or until renal functional deterioration occurs or a 'disabling' NS develops. The partisans of the first choice argue that waiting to treat until renal insufficiency develops may be too late, since even a moderate increase of serum creatinine may reflect an underlying development of irreversible histological lesions that markedly reduce the chances of a beneficial response to treatment. Moreover, an early treatment can prevent, in responders, the potential complications of a severe and protracted NS. Those who are against an early treatment argue that some 40–50 per cent of patients, particularly if of female gender, would receive an unnecessary treatment since they will not develop ESRD or the ill-effects of NS, even after protracted follow-up.

Unfortunately, it is not easy to recognize at the time of initial presentation which patient will have an uncomplicated, favourable evolution and a spontaneous remission and which patient is destined to develop renal failure, a thrombo-embolic event, or cardiovascular disease. Even the role of renal biopsy is limited. It can predict a high risk of progression in patients with interstitial fibrosis and glomerular sclerosis but it cannot provide prognostic clues when performed in the initial phases of MN. Some investigators reported that high levels of circulating anti-PLA2R antibodies are usually associated with an unfavourable outcome (Kim et al., 2015), while low levels may predict spontaneous remission (Beck et al., 2011; Kim et al., 2015). Thus, low baseline and decreasing anti-PLA2R antibody levels can favour a conservative therapy while high baseline or increasing anti-PLA2R antibody levels should encourage prompt initiation of immunosuppressive therapy. Such an approach may be used in patients with circulating anti-PLA2R antibodies (about 60 per cent to 70 per cent). Moreover, re-emergence of or increase in antibody titres usually precedes a clinical relapse (De Vriese et al., 2017). However, it should be noted that there are several methods to assess anti-PLA2R antibodies, including indirect immunofluorescence (IIF), ELISA, Western blot, ALBIA, laser bead assay, and luciferase immunoprecipitation. In clinical practice, the ELISA test is the most suitable for follow-up measurements, whereas the laser bead immunoassay is a more sensitive technique for the detection of PLA2R antibodies. The definition of PLA2R positivity is another issue. The manufacturer's definition for PLA2R antibody positivity of the commercial ELISA assay is >14 RU/ml, while it has been proposed that any titre >2 RU/ml may be considered positive (Timmermans et al., 2015). Thus, an area of uncertainty remains even when the course of MN is monitored by anti-PLA2R antibodies. What threshold should be used to define 'negative' and 'positive' anti-PLA2R antibody and precisely how the results of anti-PLA2R antibody testing should influence treatment decisions are critical questions requiring randomized, prospective trials.

In summary, whatever the decision, there is a risk of over-treating an intrinsically 'benign' condition or to inappropriately avoid an effective therapy in a 'dangerous' disease. At the individual patient level this is a delicate balance affected by many imponderables. A compromise could be an immediate treatment for adults with severe, symptomatic NS (usually patients with proteinuria exceeding 10 g/day, or with plasma albumin levels lower than 2 g/dl) and high titre of anti-PLA2R antibody levels (by ELISA method), while postponing the treatment by six months or so, in order to 'risk stratify' the relatively symptom-free patients, depending on serial values of urinary protein excretion (possibly including urinary β2 microglobulin and α1 microglobulin) creatinine clearance (or eGFR), and anti-PLA2 antibody levels (by ELISA). Low or declining levels (>50 per cent from baseline) probably indicate a high likelihood of a remission in the next two to four months and might be used as a rationale to delay specific therapy (DeVriese et al., 2017).

What might be initial treatment for nephrotic patients with MN?

(See Table 6.9)

The KDIGO guidelines (2012) recommended that initial therapy should consist of a six-month course of alternating oral and IV corticosteroids with oral alkylating agents, cyclophosphamide being preferred to chlorambucil. Such a cyclical therapy is being used by several renal units, but many other nephrologists prefer alternative treatments, being concerned about the oncogenic, gonadotoxic, and bladder injurious effects of alkylating agents. The oncogenic risk is mainly related to the cumulative dose of the cytotoxic drug, since the DNA repair can correct the damage induced by low-dose of cytotoxic drugs. When alkylating agents are given for no longer than three months, the oncogenic risk does not exceed that of age-matched general population (Ponticelli et al., 1998; Jha et al., 2007). Alkylating agents can also cause irreversible azoospermia. This risk is more elevated with chlorambucil than with cyclophosphamide. Giving a cumulative dose of cyclophosphamide of 180 mg/kg (i.e. 2 mg/kg/day for three months) should keep the patient under the threshold of gonadal toxicity, which is generally estimated to be around 200–300 mg/kg. At any rate, young males might be encouraged to deposit their semen in a sperm bank before starting therapy. The ovary is more resistant to cytotoxic drugs but, to be on the safe side, fertile women could receive leuprolide therapy to induce gonadal arrest and decrease gonadal injury due

Table 6.9 Advantages and drawbacks of the treatments more frequently used in primary MN with nephrotic syndrome.

Treatment	Advantages	Drawbacks
Alkylating agents plus steroids	Can favour remission and protect renal function in the long-term.	No randomized trials. Risk of cancer or gonadal toxicity with prolonged use of cytotoxic drugs.
Cyclical therapy (Alkylating agents alternated with steroids)	Can favour remission and protect renal function in the long-term. Confirmed by randomized trials with ten-year follow-up. The risk of cancer is minimal.	A few patients do not tolerate treatment. Risk of gonadal toxicity in repeated treatments.
Calcineurin inhibitors	Can reduce proteinuria and favour remission.	Frequent relapses, potential nephrotoxicity, and hypertension.
Mycophenolate	Can obtain remission in association with steroids. Poor efficacy when given alone.	Small-sized studies. No information about long-term results.
ACTH	High rate of remission.	Small-sized studies. No information about long-term results. High cost with gel formulation.
Rituximab	High rate of remission.	Small-sized studies. No information about long-term results. High cost.
IV immunoglobulins	May favour remission.	Anecdotal studies. No information about long-term results. High cost.

to alkylating drugs. Alternatively, the cumulative dose of the alkylating agent may be decreased to protect gonadal function. Bone marrow toxicity may be prevented by monitoring blood cells every week during administration of the alkylating agent and by halving the dose if leucocytes are lower than 5,000/mm^3 or withdrawing the drug if they are below 3,000/mm^3. A higher incidence of side-effects with this regimen may occur in patients with an already-established renal insufficiency. It is well known that the bone marrow of patients with renal dysfunction is more vulnerable to the toxic effects of alkylating agents; moreover, these patients are more susceptible to infections. Therefore, it is highly recommended not to exceed daily doses of 0.1 mg/kg when using chlorambucil and 1.5 mg/kg when using cyclophosphamide in patients with a serum creatinine ≥ 2.0 mg/dl or a creatinine clearance ≤ 60 ml/

min. Bladder toxicity is seldom of concern with oral dosing of short duration (Ponticelli et al., 2018).

In case of poor response, intolerance, or contraindication to this regimen, the KDIGO guidelines of 2012 suggest CNI as an alternative option, as they may obtain a high initial rate of remission in patients with MN and NS, comparable to the overall response rate seen with combined MP and alkylating agents, but usually with inferior results for complete remissions. However, a prolonged administration and the association of CNI with moderate doses of glucocorticoids may improve the probability of complete remission. The main problem with CNI therapy is that, in most responders, proteinuria increases when the drug is stopped. The risk of relapse is particularly elevated when CNI are withdrawn abruptly and/or after short-term treatment. Moreover, in spite of clinical remission repeat biopsies may show histological progression of MN, although typical features of CsA toxicity are not observed (Kalliakmani et al., 2010; Goumenos et al., 2008). To reduce the risk of relapse the recommendation is to continue CsA for at least three to four months after complete remission is obtained (Cattran et al., 2007). For patients with partial remission CsA should be continued at full doses for at least one to two years and then maintained at non-toxic serum levels indefinitely so long as serum creatinine concentration remains stable, if the patient has failed to respond to other treatments. Similar recommendations may be adopted with the use of TAC. Impressive results have been reported in patients with MN, even with very low doses of TAC (Caro et al., 2015). However, TAC should be avoided in obese patients with glucose intolerance and in patients with overt diabetes mellitus because of its diabetogenic effect. We suggest to start with doses not exceeding 4 mg/kg/day for CsA and 0.1 mg/kg/day for TAC. The time of response is unpredictable but if no change in proteinuria occurs after six months of treatment the chances of remission are low. In case of remission, most often partial, the initial doses may be gradually reduced in order to catch the minimal dose that may maintain proteinuria in an asymptomatic range. For maintenance treatment we suggest keeping trough blood levels between 50 and 100 ng/ml for CsA and between 3 and 6 ng/ml for TAC. The 2012 KDIGO recommendations are undergoing revision and new recommendations are due to appear in the summer of 2019.

In the last few years RTX is increasingly being used as initial therapy for MN. RTX can obtain response (more often partial remission) in a substantial fraction (60 per cent or more) of patients with MN and no serious adverse events occur, at least in the short term. However, the cost of the drug is quite high and it is unclear if RTX may actually offer in MN results better or at least comparable to those obtained with steroid–cytotoxic regimens or with CNI. No head-to-head comparisons of RTX with these more standard-of-care approaches have yet been published, but the MENTOR trial has preliminarily reported superior results with RTX compared to CsA at 24 months. No comparator trials of RTX vs. cyclical therapy have yet been conducted. A retrospective study compared RTX versus combined steroid and cyclophosphamide. Although the cumulative incidence of partial remission was lower in the RTX group, rates of complete remission and the composite renal end point did not differ significantly between groups. Serious adverse events were significantly more frequent in combined steroid–cyclophosphamide (Van den Brand et al., 2017). However, the study was retrospective, one group of participants given cyclophosphamide was followed in the Netherlands and the other group treated with RTX was followed in Italy, in different periods. More important, cyclophosphamide was used every day for six to 12 months together with prednisone. Such a schedule is completely different from that used in cyclical therapy, in which the alkylating agent and steroids were given alternatively every other month for a cumulative period of three months each. A decision-analytic model estimated the cost-effectiveness of RTX versus the cyclical therapy from the perspective of the National Health Service in the UK. At one year post-treatment, RTX therapy dominated. At five years post-treatment, RTX therapy was cheaper than the cyclical regimen, but at a loss of 0.014 quality-adjusted life years (QALYs) with an incremental cost-effectiveness ratio. Over a lifetime, RTX remained the cheaper option but with reduced QALYs (Hamilton et al., 2018). The paper is statistically incontrovertible. However, there are important limitations:

i. The analysis compared the data reported by an RCT made in India (Jha et al., 2007) with those reported by a retrospective observational study made in Italy (Ruggenenti et al., 2012);

ii. The RCT was reported in 2007 and the observational study was published five years later; and

iii. Patients enrolled in the RCT were followed for ten years while in the Ruggenenti et al. study (2012), the median follow-up was 29 months.

Hopefully, ongoing randomized trials such as MENTOR (see 'Cyclosporine (CsA)' and RI-CYCLO will better clarify the initial effectiveness, relapse rate, requirement for repeated administrations, and the long-term efficacy of RTX compared to other regimens in primary MN (see Clinical Trials.gov).

A further option is the administration of synthetic or natural ACTH. The reported results so far are good, but all based on uncontrolled trials. However, the number of patients who received this treatment was too small and the follow-up was too short to recommend ACTH as a first-line treatment for MN. The results should be substantiated by further trials. ACTH may be suggested for those patients who are intolerant or do not respond to other treatments.

The place of MMF and sodium mycophenolate in the therapy of MN is still very poorly defined. Only few small randomized trials with short-term follow-up are available. On the basis of these trials and personal experience it seems that the association of mycophenolate with steroids may favour a complete or partial remission. In a handful of patients resistant or intolerant to other treatments we have observed a good rate of remission when these agents were given together with moderate doses of prednisone. Relapse shortly following suspension of mycophenolate therapy are very common, if not universal. In order to prevent relapses in responders or to achieve late responses treatment may be continued for two or more years by halving the initial doses. However, well-designed randomized trials with an adequate number of participants and follow-up are needed to better assess the effectiveness, dosage, duration of treatment, as well as the role of potential association with steroids for mycophenolate salts in MN.

In summary, on the basis of the available data we feel that either cyclical therapy or RTX should be considered for the initial treatment of primary MN. Cyclical therapy has the advantage of being validated by randomized controlled trials showing its efficacy in achieving remissions and protecting renal function in the long term. However, treatment lasts six months and serious side effects may occur, although they are unusual and reversible in most cases. RTX is also likely to be effective in reducing proteinuria, and is usually quite well tolerated, at least over the short term. However, the response occurs after some months, and little information is available about its long-term efficacy and safety.

Whatever treatment is chosen, for patients who show remission and then re-lapse of NS a second course of treatment can be given, since the tolerance and probability of response to re-treatment are similar to those observed after the first course. However, we recommend *not to prescribe a third course* of cyclical therapy in case of further relapses. In the case of refusal, intolerance, or poor re-sponse, one may switch from cyclical therapy to RTX, or vice versa. Lack of effi-cacy with one regimen does not translate to a lack of efficacy of treatment with drugs of another class. Multidrug-resistant forms of primary MN are distinctly uncommon. A second option may consist of either cyclosporine or tacrolimus. An advantage of the TAC regimen rests on the possibility of obtaining a high rate of remissions while using very low doses and the lack of need for con-comitant steroid administration. In case of response, CNI treatment should be prolonged for one to two years or even longer at the minimal effective doses if the drug is well tolerated. Short-term therapy with a CNI (<6–12 months) will frequently be accompanied by a relapse when the drug is stopped.

In case of failure of these treatments, synthetic ACTH may be given at a dose of 1 mg twice a week for one year or natural ACTH gel in twice weekly doses of 80 units for about six months (cumulative dose about 4000 units). Alternatively, mycophenolate salts plus steroids (IV or orally) may be tried. It is common experience that a few patients who did not respond to usual therapies may develop remission with other treatments potentially less active. It is still unclear if these unexpected remissions reflect different subjective sensitivity, late responses, or spontaneous remission. If patients do not respond to any of these treatments a compassionate therapy with plasmapheresis, RTX, and/or IVIg may be attempted (Muller-Deile et al., 2015), although caution should be used to avoid the risks of overimmunosuppression in patients who received different treatments (Figure 6.2).

In spite of the abundant controlled evidence speaking against the utility of monotherapy with oral glucocorticoids, a number of patients with MN are still given high-dose glucocorticoids for initial treatment, perhaps because of some lingering doubts that some patients may in fact be 'steroid-responsive'. Although a few patients may 'respond' to initial monotherapy with oral glucocorticoids, these may, in fact, be 'spontaneous' remissions. These patients may have frequent relapses that require further courses of steroid treatment with the risk of developing iatrogenic morbidity. Therefore, *we do not recommend short (three to four months) courses of daily oral steroid monotherapy for initial treatment of primary MN*, with the possible exception of Asian patients, who seem to respond better than Caucasian subjects to steroid monotherapy.

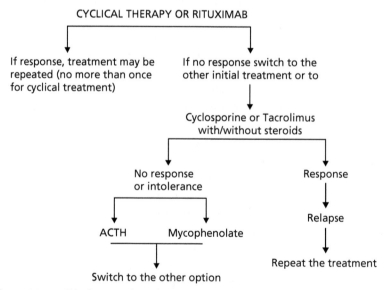

Figure 6.2 Possible therapeutic options in patients with primary MN and nephrotic syndrome.

What to do in patients with MN and declining renal function?

Treatment of superimposed renal complications

Before deciding whether or not to treat patients with declining renal function, every effort should be made to recognize and appropriately handle any complication superimposed on the original disease. The three most frequently superimposed causes of deterioration of renal function in MN are represented by acute drug-associated interstitial nephritis (most often due to diuretics), acute bilateral renal vein thrombosis, and extracapillary (crescentic) glomerulonephritis.

Acute hypersensitivity interstitial nephritis can be suspected by a rapidly progressive renal insufficiency often, but not always, associated with rash, fever, eosinophilia, and/or eosinophiluria in patients taking diuretic agents, antibiotics, allopurinol, or NSAIDs. Renal biopsy is often necessary to confirm the diagnosis. Stopping the administration of the responsible drug and an early course of high-dose oral prednisone (1 mg/kg/day) can obtain the complete recovery of renal function in most of these instances.

Renal vein thrombosis (RVT) can occur in 22 per cent to 52 per cent of patients with MN (Radhakrishnan, 2012). Clotting abnormalities, increased blood viscosity, and depletion of intravascular volume are probably predisposing factors. Hypo-albuminaemia, particularly <2.8 g/dl, is the most significant independent predictor of venous thrombotic risk (Loniaki et al., 2012). Acute bilateral RVT causing AKI is very uncommon, with chronic RVT being predominant. Chronic RVT is insidious, usually discovered incidentally, or may be detected when searching the cause of pulmonary embolism. However, clinically apparent venous thrombo-embolic events may occur in about 7 per cent of patients with MN (Loniaki et al., 2012). The current opinion is that chronic RVT (unilateral or bilateral) has little influence on proteinuria or renal function, but it can be responsible for pulmonary embolism. However, even if the deleterious role of chronic RVT on kidney function is still under discussion, there is clear evidence that an acute bilateral RVT can precipitate a sudden, often irreversible, deterioration of renal function. The diagnosis is suspected by the sudden onset of flank pain and macroscopic haematuria and can be confirmed by a positive test for D-dimer, a fibrin degradation product, echocolour Doppler scan, renal venography, magnetic resonance, or spiral computed tomography imaging. A prompt and correct diagnosis is of utmost importance in these symptomatic patients as early administration of fibrinolytic agents can obtain recovery of renal function in oligo-anuric patients.

The development of an *extracapillary (crescentic) glomerulonephritis* superimposed on MN is an exceptional but well-recognized possibility (Basford et al., 2011). Whenever the steady evolution of MN is interrupted by a rapidly progressive course, such a complication should be considered. A sudden increase in dysmorphic erythrocytes and leukocytes in the urine sediment can signal the development of proliferative glomerular lesions in patients with a rapidly progressive course. The correct diagnosis can be obtained by a renal biopsy. Either (or both) ANCA and anti-GBM auto-antibody pathogenetic mechanisms may be responsible for this occurrence in MN. Treatment of these cases does not differ from that of rapidly progressive (crescentic) glomerulonephritis and includes IV high-dose methylprednisolone pulses, cytotoxic agents, and/or RTX. The prognosis is variable. The disease may respond to therapy, but most patients develop a long-term decline in GFR (Rodriguez et al., 2014).

Treatment of patients with steady progression and renal insufficiency

Patients with renal insufficiency and MN are more exposed to the risk of side-effects caused by glucocorticoids, cytotoxic drugs, or CNI. Thus, treatment should be limited to those cases having actual and reasonable chances of improving. Although there are neither controlled nor uncontrolled studies that attempt to correlate response to therapy with levels of serum creatinine or the histological picture, it appears from the available data that no patient with MN has ever responded to therapy when his/her plasma creatinine exceeded 400 μmol/l (4.5 mg/dl) on a chronic progressive basis (e.g. rapidly progressive or acute kidney injury supervening in cases of MN).

Patients with atrophic and hyperechogenic kidneys at ultrasonography and/ or those with very extensive glomerular sclerosis and severe chronic tubulo-interstitial changes at renal biopsy are also very unlikely to respond to any 'specific' treatment. Absence of C5b-C9 from urine, or very low serum levels of anti-PLA2R antibodies (in patients previously positive) may be a sign of 'inactive' disease. Therefore, patients with these characteristics should logically be excluded from attempts at 'rescue' treatment as such management is unlikely to obtain any sustained improvement but can cause considerable iatrogenic morbidity.

Which treatment should be tried in patients with declining renal function who have not yet reached an irreversible stage? Even in 'responders' the effects of high-dose glucocorticoids (given orally or IV) seem to be transient and not sustainable. Evidence of efficacy and safety for use of CNI in patients with MN and deteriorating renal function is completely lacking. We strongly discourage the use of CNI in patients with severe interstitial fibrosis and/or with stable or declining values of estimated GFR <40 ml/min. A slower deterioration of renal function may be obtained by a six-month treatment alternating MP and either cyclophosphamide or chlorambucil every other month. However, side-effects may be frequent in patients with renal insufficiency when alkylating agents are used at standard doses (Howman et al., 2013). It is strongly recommended to halve the doses of IV MP and alkylating agents when they are used in patients with chronic renal disease and to further reduce the doses if eGFR levels are <30 ml/min. There is little experience with RTX, but the available studies seem to indicate that it is ineffective when eGFR is <45 ml/min (Michel et al., 2011). There is little information about ACTH, IVIg, or RTX as 'rescue' treatments in patients with progressive MN.

On the basis of the available reports, we suggest the following options for patients with slowly progressive renal insufficiency. Patients showing a steady increase in plasma creatinine to >400 μmol/l (4.5 mg/dl) or those with a considerable reduction of kidney size at ultrasonography should be treated with symptomatic therapy alone (see Chapter 2). In the absence of contraindications, a renal biopsy should be carefully considered in patients with less marked renal insufficiency or in those with a sudden onset of a rapidly progressive course. If severe glomerular sclerosis and tubulo-interstitial changes are seen, any form of treatment is probably useless. If these lesions are not advanced and if fresh deposition of immune complexes (electron-dense deposits combined with strongly positive IgG and C3 deposition) is found, a specific treatment may be tried, especially if PLA2R-antibody test is positive. RTX may be useful if the eGFR ranges around 50 ml/min (Busch et al., 2013), but it is ineffective for low levels of eGFR especially if associated with severe tubulointerstitial damage (Ruggenenti et al., 2006). When choosing between a six-month course of MP and an alkylating agent, we recommend maintaining three courses of IV MP pulses at doses of 0.5/g each and reducing the doses of chlorambucil to 0.05–0.1 mg/kg/day or cyclophosphamide to 1.0–1.5 mg/kg/day. As an alternative option, one may consider prolonged treatment (about 12 months) with low-dose prednisone (10–15 mg per day or double doses every other day) and cyclophosphamide (1.0–1.5 mg/kg/day) for six months or mycophenolate (MMF 1 g/day or sodium mycophenolate 720 mg/day) for 12–24 months. Whether occasional addition of MP pulses may improve the response to the latter treatment is still unclear and remains untested. Patients with advanced diseases, stable but nephrotic range proteinuria who are consistently negative for anti-PLA2R antibody may have 'immunologically inactive' disease and probably should not be treated with immunosuppressive agents. In summary, whether to treat patients with chronic renal insufficiency with potent immunosuppressive agents and which therapy to choose should also be decided on the basis of the totality of the clinical characteristics of the patient, including anti-PLA2R serology and the extent of chronic irreversible changes on renal biopsy. The tolerance of the chosen treatment should be very carefully monitored, and treatment should be reduced or stopped in case of serious side effects.

What treatment for elderly patients with MN?

Older patients are particularly susceptible to the thrombotic and cardiovascular complications of NS. This might justify a therapeutic trial, at least in the older patients with severe NS and/or incipient renal failure. On the other hand, if the response to treatment is similar in older and younger adults, the drugs used in MN can have specific relative contraindications in many elderly patients. Glucocorticoids can aggravate arterial hypertension, arterial occlusive disease, glucose intolerance, cardiovascular disease, and other pathological conditions that may already be present. Alkylating agents carry an increased risk of leukopenia, bladder toxicity, and infections (both bacterial and viral) in the frail, aged patient, and are contraindicated for their carcinogenic potential in patients with a previous malignancy. Calcineurin inhibitors may worsen hypertension, cause diabetes, and precipitate thrombotic complications. Moreover, elderly subjects have often reduced levels of GFR and the ageing kidney is particularly vulnerable to the nephrotoxic effects of CNI. There is little experience with synthetic ACTH, but a prolonged treatment might cause osteoporosis, diabetes, and/or hypertension. RTX seems to be well tolerated, apart from the cytokine-release syndrome after the first infusion. However, sepsis and neutropenia have been reported in a few cases. Even symptomatic therapy should be prescribed with caution in the elderly since ACE-inhibitors, ARB, NSAIDs, statins, and diuretics may precipitate a deterioration of renal function, which can be irreversible in some cases, especially if undiagnosed bilateral renal artery atheromas are present. No data are available with alternative therapies.

Once again, the decision on whether and how to treat an elderly patient should be based on the personal experience of the treating nephrologists and the clinical characteristics of the particular patient.

Transplantation

Recurrence of MN

The recurrence of MN after renal transplantation is probably more frequent than generally estimated, most cases occurring in adults (Ponticelli and Glassock, 2010). However, the true proportion of recurrence is difficult to assess as the indications for graft biopsy are extremely variable among transplant centres. Moreover, a *de novo* form of MN may develop in transplanted kidneys showing a histological pattern indistinguishable from *recurrent* MN. However, no case of *de novo* MN with PLA2R hyperexpression in glomeruli has been observed, so immunohistology is a good way of distinguishing *de novo* from *recurrent* MN. Finally, the clinical diagnosis of recurrent MN is often made late as recurrence can remain clinically silent for months to years. With these difficulties in mind, the rate of MN recurrence may be estimated to range between 30 per cent and 45 per cent in adults (Moroni et al., 2010; Sprangers, 2010; Cosio and Cattran, 2016) and around 30 per cent in children (Cochat et al., 2009).

Recurrence is usually diagnosed between the second and third year after transplantation. No histological factor seems to reliably predict the risk of recurrence. However, elevated anti-PLA2R antibody levels may predict an increased risk of post-transplantation recurrence of MN (Seitz-Polski et al., 2014; Quintana et al., 2015; Gupta et al., 2016; Xipell et al., 2018). The initial clinical manifestations of recurrent MN may be mild or absent and in a number of cases recurrence may be detected only by 'protocol' renal biopsies (Dabade et al., 2008; El-Zoghby et al., 2009). On the other hand, the risk of recurrence increases over time. In a study, the diagnosis of recurrent MN, based on protocol or clinical biopsies, was 18.9 per cent at one year and 45.4 per cent at three years (Cosio and Cattran, 2016). There is no contraindication to living donation to patients with MN, although recurrent MN may be more common in living donor transplantation (Andresdottir and Wetzels, 2012). An analysis of ERA/EDTA registry reported that the graft survival at 15 years in patients with MN was significantly better for transplants from a living donor than in transplants from deceased donors (Pippias et al., 2016).

Recurrent disease is probably caused by the reaction of circulating IgG4 autoantibodies directed against extracellular PLA2R (Kattah et al., 2015). However, an exceptional case of circulating IgG3κ-restricted anti-PLA2R antibodies and recurrent MN has been described (Debiec et al., 2012).

Histologically, the features of recurrent MN may resemble those observed in cases of MN, although microscopic changes may be subtle initially. In some cases, however, the histology of early recurrent MN does not include subepithelial electron-dense deposits and/or glomerular C3 deposits, although GBM granular C4d deposits are prominent (Rodriguez et al., 2012). In *de novo* MN, hyperexpression of PLA2R is absent (see 'De novo MN'). In an undefined number of cases, the glomerular lesions are associated with vascular and tubulo-interstitial lesions caused by rejection, CNI toxicity, or infection. Clinically, the recurrence of MN may be heralded by the appearance of proteinuria, which may be asymptomatic or may exceed 3.5 g/day leading to signs and symptoms of NS. The outcome of recurrent MN may be as variable as in the original native disease. In a series, patients with MN recurrence had a lower ten-year graft survival in comparison with transplant recipients with nonrecurrent MN, but the difference was at borderline significance (Moroni et al., 2010).

Symptomatic treatment with diuretics, ACE-inhibitors, ARB, hypolipaemic drugs, and anticoagulants might help in reducing the signs and symptoms related to the NS. RTX has been used successfully in several cases of post-transplant MN recurrence. Complete clinical and histological remission has been reported when RTX was used in patients with mild-to-moderate protein-uria. The doses ranged from a single shot of 1 g (Spinner et al., 2015) to four weekly doses of 375 mg/m^2 (Sprangers et al., 2010). Anecdotal cases of response to cyclical therapy with steroids and cyclophosphamide have also been reported (Carneiro-Roza et al., 2006; Moroni et al., 2010).

De novo MN

Overall, recurrent and *de novo* MN are about equally common post-transplant, but a patient with MN as the original disease and post-transplant MN is over-whelmingly likely to have recurrent, rather than *de novo*, disease. *De novo* MN usually occurs many months or years after transplantation, but rare cases may occur earlier, even within three months after transplantation. Contrary to pri-mary MN, the recurrent form may develop not only in adults but also in chil-dren with similar frequency.

The histopathological findings may either be similar to those of classical MN or may be subtler, showing mesangial proliferation and/or focal segmental variation in severity, often in conjunction with the features of chronic allograft nephropathy or transplant glomerulopathy. The IgG subclass distributions are very different in recurrent and *de novo* MN in allograft kidneys. IgG4 is the dominant or co-dominant IgG subclass in capillary loop deposits in recurrent MN, while IgG1 staining is dominant in *de novo* MN (Kearney et al., 2011). PLA2R staining is also useful for differentiating a *de novo* from recurrent MN, as it is always negative in *de novo* MN (Larsen and Walker, 2013). Instead, HLA-DR expression is detectable on the podocytes in most cases of *de novo* MN (Wen et al., 2016).

The pathogenesis is unknown. In many cases, *de novo* MN develops after different types of kidney injury, e.g. rejection, viral hepatitis, or non-immune-mediated kidney diseases, suggesting that these injuries may produce an in-flammatory environment in the kidney allograft that can expose hidden podocyte-related autologous antigens and stimulate the production of circu-lating antibodies (of the IgG1 subclass) eventually leading to in situ immune complex formation, subepithelial deposits, and the morphological lesion of MN (Ponticelli and Glassock, 2012). The expression of HLA-DR antigen on podocytes might suggest an important role of alloimmune response *de novo* MN (Wen et al., 2016).

The clinical presentation may be asymptomatic or characterized by NS. A number of patients already show renal allograft dysfunction at presentation. The prognosis as well as the risk factors that may predict a poor outcome are not well established. In a paediatric series 60 per cent of children lost their graft on average after six years (Antignac et al., 1988). In adults, the prognosis of *de novo* MN may be variable. Some studies did not find different outcomes between patients with *de novo* MN and transplant recipients with other kidney diseases (Schwarz et al., 1994), while others reported that 40 per cent of patients with *de novo* MN may progress to graft failure within three years (Truong et al., 1989). Rare cases of spontaneous remission have also been reported (Okyay et al., 2012). In most cases with an unfavourable outcome, signs of antibody-mediated rejection can be seen in kidney graft biopsy (Honda et al., 2011). The treatment of *de novo* MN is elusive. There is no evidence that reinforcement of immunosuppressive treatment or introduction of new cytotoxic agents is of any benefit. There is little experience with RTX. Antiviral therapy may be effective in cases associated with HBV infection.

References

Acevedo Ribó M, Ahijado Hormigos FJ, Díaz F, et al. (2016). IgG4-related disease and idiopathic membranous nephropathy: 'The clothes do not make the man'. Clin Nephrol. 86: 345–8.

Ahmed S, Rahman M, Alam MR, et al. (1994). Methylprednisolone plus chlorambucil as compared with prednisolone alone for the treatment of idiopathic membranous nephropathy-A preliminary study. Bangladesh Ren J. 13: 51–4.

Alexopoulos E, Papagianni A, Tsamelashvili M, et al. (2006). Induction and long-term treatment with cyclosporine in membranous nephropathy with the nephrotic syndrome. Nephrol Dial Transplant. 21: 3127–32.

Anders HJ, Ponticelli C. (2016). Glomerular disease: Membranous nephropathy and the Henle-Koch postulates. Nat Rev Nephrol. 12: 447 8.

Andresdottir MB, Wetzels JF. (2012). Increased risk of recurrence of membranous nephropathy after related-donor kidney transplantation. Am J Transplant. 12: 265–6.

Antignac C, Hinglais N, Gubler MC, et al. (1988). *De novo* membranous glomerulonephritis in renal allografts in children. Clin Nephrol. 30: 1–6.

Bally S, Debiec A, Ponard D, et al. (2016). Phospholipase A2 receptor-related membranous nephropathy and mannan-binding lectin deficiency. J Am Soc Nephrol. 27: 3539–44.

Barbour SJ, Cattran DC, Espino-Hernandez G, et al. (2015). Identifying the ideal metric of proteinuria as a predictor of renal outcome in idiopathic glomerulonephritis. Kidney Int. 88: 1392–401.

Basford AW, Lewis J, Dwyer JP, et al. (2011). Membranous nephropathy with crescents. J Am Soc Nephrol. 22: 1804–8.

Bazzi C, Rizza V, Casellato D, et al. (2014). Fractional excretion of IgG in idiopathic membranous nephropathy with nephrotic syndrome: a predictive marker of risk and drug responsiveness. BMC Nephrol. **15**: 74.

Beck LH Jr. (2012). Monoclonal anti-PLA2R and recurrent membranous nephropathy: Another piece of the puzzle. J Am Soc Nephrol. **23**: 1911–13.

Beck LH Jr. (2017). PLA2R and THSD7A: Disparate paths to the same disease? J Am Soc Nephrol. **28**: 2579–89.

Beck LH Jr, Bonegio RG, Lambeau G, et al. (2009). M-type phospholipase A2 receptor as target antigen in idiopathic membranous nephropathy. N Engl J Med. **361**: 11–20.

Beck LH Jr, Fervenza FC, Beck DM, et al. (2011). Rituximab-induced depletion of anti-PLA2R autoantibodies predicts response in membranous nephropathy. J Am Soc Nephrol. **22**: 1543–50.

Berg AL, Arnadottir N. (2004). ACTH-induced improvement in the nephrotic syndrome in patients with a variety of diagnosis. Nephrol Dial Transplant. **19**: 1305–7.

Berg AL, Nilsson-Ehle P, Arnadottir M. (1999). Beneficial effects of ACTH on the serum lipoprotein profile and glomerular function in patients with membranous nephropathy. Kidney Int. **56**: 1534–43.

Bhimma R, Coovadia HM. (2004). Hepatitis B virus associated-nephropathy. Am J Nephrol. **24**: 198–211.

Bhimma R, Naicker E, Ramdial PK. (2013). Mycophenolate mofetil therapy in children with idiopathic membranous nephropathy. Clin Nephrol. **80**: 441–8.

Bomback AS, Tumlin JA, Baranski J, et al. (2011). Treatment of nephrotic syndrome with adrenocorticotropic hormone (ACTH) gel. Drug Des Devel Ther. **5**: 147–53.

van den Brand JA, van Dijk PR, Hofstra JM, et al. (2014a). Long-term outcomes in idiopathic membranous nephropathy using a restrictive treatment strategy. J Am Soc Nephrol. **25**: 150–8.

van den Brand JA, van Dijk PR, Hofstra JM, et al. (2014b). Cancer risk after cyclophosphamide treatment in idiopathic membranous nephropathy. Clin J Am Soc Nephrol. **9**: 1066–73.

van den Brand JA, Hofstra JM, Wetzels JF. (2012). Prognostic value of risk score and urinary markers in idiopathic membranous nephropathy. Clin J Am Soc Nephrol. **7**: 1242–8.

van den Brand JAJG, Ruggenenti P, Chianca A, et al. (2017). Safety of rituximab compared with steroids and cyclophosphamide for idiopathic membranous nephropathy. J Am Soc Nephrol. **28**: 2729–37.

Branten AJ, duBuf-Vereijken PW, Vervloet M, et al. (2007). Mycophenolate mofetil in idiopathic membranous nephropathy: A clinical trial with comparison to a historic control group treated with cyclophosphamide. Am J Kidney Dis. **50**: 248–56.

Bruschi M, Carnevali ML, Murtas C, et al. (2011). Direct characterization of target podocyte antigens and auto-antibodies in human membranous glomerulonephritis: Alfa-enolase and borderline antigens. J Proteomics. **74**: 2008–17.

Bullich G, Ballarín J, Oliver A, et al. (2014). HLA-DQA1 and PLA2R1 polymorphisms and risk of idiopathic membranous nephropathy. Clin J Am Soc Nephrol. **9**: 335–43.

Busch M, Ruster C, Schinkothe C, et al. (2013). Rituximab for the second- and third-line therapy of idiopathic membranous nephropathy: A prospective single center study using a new treatment strategy. Clin Nephrol. **80**: 105–13.

Carneiro-Roza F, Medina-Pestana JO, Moscoso-Solorzano G, et al. (2006). Initial response to immunosuppressive and renoprotective treatment in posttransplant glomerulonephritis. Transplant Proc. **38**: 3491–7.

Caro J, Gutiérrez-Solís E, Rojas-Rivera J, et al. (2015). Predictors of response and relapse in patients with idiopathic membranous nephropathy treated with tacrolimus. Nephrol Dial Transplant. **30**: 467–74.

Cattran DC, Alexopoulos E, Heering P, et al. (2007). Cyclosporin in idiopathic glomerular disease associated with the nephrotic syndrome: Workshop recommendations. Kidney Int. **72**: 1429–47.

Cattran DC, Appel GB, Hebert LA, et al. (2001). Cyclosporine in patients with steroid-resistant membranous nephropathy: A randomized trial. Kidney Int. **59**: 1484–90.

Cattran DC, Brenchley P. (2017). Membranous nephropathy: Thinking to the therapeutic options. Nephrol Dial Transplant. **32**: i22–i29.

Cattran DC, Kim ED, Reich H, et al. (2017). Membranous nephropathy: Quantifying remission duration on outcome. J Am Soc Nephrol. **28**: 995–1003.

Cattran DC, Pei Y, Greenwood CM, et al. (1997). Validation of a predictive model of idiopathic membranous nephropathy: Its clinical and research implications. Kidney Int. **51**: 901–7.

Cattran DC, Reich HN, Beanlands HJ, et al. (2008). The impact of sex in primary Glomerulonephritis. Nephrol Dial Transplant. **23**: 2247–53.

Chan TM, Lin AW, Tang SC, et al. (2007). Prospective controlled study on mycophenolate mofetil and prednisolone in the treatment of membranous nephropathy with nephrotic syndrome. Nephrology (Carlton). **12**: 576–81.

Chen A, Frank R, Vento S, et al. (2007). Idiopathic membranous nephropathy in pediatric patients: presentation, response to therapy, and long-term outcome. BMC Nephrol. **8**: 11.

Chen M, Li H, Li XY, et al. (2010). Tacrolimus combined with corticosteroids in treatment of nephrotic idiopathic membranous nephropathy: A multi-center randomized controlled trial. Am J Med Sci. **339**: 233–8.

Chen P, Shi SF, Qu Z, et al. (2018). Characteristics of patients with co-existing IgA nephropathy and membranous nephropathy. Ren Fail. **40**: 213–18.

Chen Y, Schieppati A, Cai G, et al. (2013). Immunosuppression for membranous nephropathy: a systematic review and meta-analysis of 36 clinical trials. Clin J Am Soc Nephrol. **8**: 787–96.

Chen Y, Tang L, Feng Z, et al. (2014). Pathological predictors of renal outcomes in nephrotic idiopathic membranous nephropathy with decreased renal function. J Nephrol. **27**: 307–16.

Coban M, Eke RN, Kizilates F, et al. (2014). Effect of steroid and cyclosporine in membranous nephropathy that is resistant to steroid and/or cytotoxic treatment. Int J Clin Exp Med. **7**: 255–61.

Cochat P, Fargue S, Mestrallet G, et al. (2009). Disease recurrence in paediatric renal transplantation. Pediatr Nephrol. **24**: 2097–108.

Cortazar FB, Leaf DE, Owens CT, et al. (2017). Combination therapy with rituximab, low-dose cyclophosphamide, and prednisone for idiopathic membranous nephropathy: A case series. BMC Nephrol. **18**: 44.

Cosio FG, Cattran DC. (2016). Recent advances in our understanding of recurrent primary glomerulonephritis after kidney transplantation. Kidney Int. **91**: 304–14.

Couser WG. (2017). Primary membranous nephropathy. Clin J Am Soc Nephrol. **12**: 983–7.

Couser WG, Johnson RJ. (2014). The etiology of glomerulonephritis: Roles of infection and autoimmunity. Kidney Int. **86**: 905–14.

Dabade TS, Grande JP, Norby SM, et al. (2008). Recurrent idiopathic membranous nephropathy after kidney transplantation: A surveillance biopsy study. Am J Transplant. **8**: 1318–22.

Dahan K, Debiec H, Plaisier E, et al. (2017). Rituximab for severe membranous nephropathy: A 6-month trial with extended follow-up. J Am Soc Nephrol. **28**: 348–58.

Dauvergne M, Moktefi A, Rabant M, et al. (2015). Membranous nephropathy associated with immunological disorder-related liver disease: A retrospective study of 10 cases. Medicine (Baltimore). **94**: e1243.

Debiec H, Guigonis V, Mougenot B, et al. (2002). Antenatal membranous glomerulonephritis due to anti-neutral endopeptidase antibodies. N Engl J Med. **346**: 2053–60.

Debiec H, Hanoy M, Francois A. (2012). Recurrent membranous nephropathy in an allograft caused by IgG3κ targeting the PLA2 receptor. J Am Soc Nephrol. **23**: 1949–54.

Debiec H, Lefeu F, Kemper MJ, et al. (2011). Early-childhood membranous nephropathy due to cationic bovine serum albumin. N Engl J Med. **364**: 2101–10.

DeVriese A, Glassock RJ, Nath KA, et al. (2017). Proposal for a serology-based approach to membranous nephropathy. J Am Soc Nephrol. **28**: 421–30.

Du Buf-Vereijken PW, Branten AJ, Wetzels JF. (2005). Idiopathic membranous nephropathy: Outline and rationale of a treatment strategy. Am J Kidney Dis. **46**: 1012–29.

Dussol B, Morange S, Burtey S, et al. (2008). Mycophenolate mofetil monotherapy in membranous nephropathy: A 1-year randomized controlled trial. Am J Kidney Dis. **52**: 699–705.

Ehrenreich T, Churg J. (1968). Pathology of membranous nephropathy. In SC Sommers (ed), *Pathology Annual*, pp. 145–86. Appleton-Century-Crofts, New York.

Elvin J, Buvall L, Lindskog Jonsson A, et al. (2016). Melanocortin 1 receptor agonist protects podocytes through catalase and RhoA activation. Am J Physiol Renal Physiol. **310**: F846–56.

El-Zoghby ZM, Grande JP, Fraile MG, et al. (2009). Recurrent idiopathic membranous nephropathy: Early diagnosis by protocol biopsies and treatment with anti-CD20 monoclonal antibodies. Am J Transplant. **9**: 2800–7.

Feng Z, Wang S, Huang Y, et al. (2016). A follow-up analysis of positron emission tomography/computed tomography in detecting hidden malignancies at the time of diagnosis of membranous nephropathy. Oncotarget. **7**: 9645–51.

Fervenza FC, Abraham RS, Erickson SB, et al. (2010). Rituximab therapy in idiopathic membranous nephropathy: A 2-year study. Clin J Am Soc Nephrol. **5**: 2188–98.

Fervenza FC, Canetta PA, Barbour SJ, et al. (2015). A multicenter randomized controlled trial of rituximab versus cyclosporine in the treatment of idiopathic membranous nephropathy (MENTOR). Nephron. **130**: 159–68.

Fervenza FC, Cosio FG, Erickson SB, et al. (2008). Rituximab treatment of idiopathic membranous nephropathy. Kidney Int. **73**: 117–25.

Floccari F, Cosentini V, Giacobbe M, et al. (2008). A case-by-case protocol of membranous nephropathy treatment with endovenous infusion of high doses of human immunoglobulins. Nephron Clin Pract. **108**: c113–20.

Francis JM, Beck LH Jr, Salant DJ. (2016). Membranous nephropathy: A journey from bench to bedside. Am J Kidney Dis. **68**: 138–47.

Fresquet M, Jowitt TA, Gummadova J, et al. (2015). Identification of a major epitope recognized by PLA2R autoantibodies in primary membranous nephropathy. J Am Soc Nephrol. **26**: 302–13.

Fritsche L, Budde K, Färber L, et al. (1999). Treatment of membranous glomerulopathy with cyclosporin A: How much patience is required? Nephrol Dial Transplant. **14**: 1036–8.

Glassock RJ. (2012). The pathogenesis of membranous nephropathy: Evolution and revolution. Curr Opin Nephrol Hypertens. **21**: 235–42.

Glassock RJ. (2014). Thrombo-prevention in membranous nephropathy: A new tool for decision making? Kidney Int. **85**: 1265–6.

Goldsmith CJ, Hammad S. (2015). A review of the re-emergence of adrenocorticotrophic hormone therapy in glomerular disease: More than a drug of last resort? Clin Kidney J. **8**: 430–2.

Goumenos DS. (2008). What have we learned from the use of ciclosporin A in the treatment of nephrotic patients with idiopathic membranous nephropathy? Expert Opin Pharmacother. **9**: 1695–704.

Gupta A, Quigg RJ. (2015). Glomerular diseases associated with hepatitis B and C. Adv Chronic Kidney Dis. **22**: 343–51.

Gupta G, Fattah H, Ayalon R, et al. (2016). Pre-transplant phospholipase A2 receptor autoantibody concentration is associated with clinically significant recurrence of membranous nephropathy post-kidney transplantation. Clin Transplant. **30**: 461–9.

Hamilton P, Kanigicherla D, Venning M, et al. (2018). Rituximab versus the modified Ponticelli regimen in the treatment of primary membranous nephropathy: A health economic model. Nephrol Dial Transplant. **33**: 2145–55.

Heeringa SF, Branten AJ, Deegens JK, et al. (2007). Focal segmental glomerulosclerosis is not a sufficient predictor of renal outcome in patients with membranous nephropathy. Nephrol Dial Transplant. **22**: 2201–7.

Herzog CA, Asinger RW, Berger AK, et al. (2011). Cardiovascular disease in chronic kidney disease. A clinical update from Kidney Disease: Improving Global Outcomes (KDIGO). Kidney Int. **80**: 572–86.

Hladunewich MA, Cattran D, Beck LH, et al. (2014). A pilot study to determine the dose and effectiveness of adrenocorticotrophic hormone (H.P. Acthar® Gel) in nephrotic syndrome due to idiopathic membranous nephropathy. Nephrol Dial Transplant. **29**: 1570–7.

Hofstra JM, Wetzels JF. (2016). Should aspirin be used for primary prevention of thrombotic events in patients with membranous nephropathy? Kidney Int. **89**: 981–3.

Hogan SL, Muller KE, Jennette JC, et al. (1995). A review of therapeutic studies of idiopathic membranous glomerulopathy. Am J Kidney Dis. **25**: 862–75.

Hommos MS, Glassock RJ, Rude AD. (2017). Structural and functional changes in human kidneys with healthy ages. J Am Soc Nephrol. **28**: 2838–44.

Honda K, Horita S, Toki D, et al. (2011). *De novo* membranous nephropathy and antibody-mediated rejection in transplanted kidney. Clin Transplant. **25**: 191–200.

Howman A, Chapman TL, Langdon MM, et al. (2013). Immunosuppression for progressive membranous nephropathy: A UK randomised controlled trial. Lancet. **381**: 744–51.

Hoxha E, Kneißler U, Stege G, et al. (2012). Enhanced expression of the M-type phospholipase A2 receptor in glomeruli correlates with serum receptor antibodies in primary membranous nephropathy. Kidney Int. **82**: 797–804.

Hoxha E, Thiele I, Zahner G, et al. (2014). Phospholipase A2 receptor autoantibodies and clinical outcome in patients with primary membranous nephropathy. J Am Soc Nephrol. **25**: 1357–66.

Hoxha E, Wiech T, Sthal PR, et al. (2016). A mechanism for cancer-associated membranous nephropathy. N Engl J Med. **374**: 1995–6.

Hu R, Xing G, Wu H, et al. (2016). Clinicopathological features of idiopathic membranous nephropathy combined with IgA nephropathy: A retrospective analysis of 9 cases. Diagn Pathol. **11**: 86.

Idasiak-Piechocka I, Oko A, Łochyńska-Bielecka K, et al. (2009). Efficacy and safety of low-dose chlorambucil in nephrotic patients with idiopathic membranous nephropathy. Kidney Blood Press Res. **32**: 263–7.

Irazabal MV, Eirin A, Lieske J, et al. (2013). Low- and high-molecular-weight urinary proteins as predictors of response to rituximab in patients with membranous nephropathy: A prospective study. Nephrol Dial Transplant. **28**: 137–46.

Ito T, Mochizuki K, Oka T, et al. (2015). Study of mizoribine therapy in elderly patients with membranous nephropathy: Comparison with patients not receiving mizoribine. Int Urol Nephrol. **47**: 131–5.

Iwakura T, Ohashi N, Kato A, et al. (2015). Prevalence of enhanced granular expression of thrombospondin type-1 domain-containing 7A in the glomeruli of Japanese patients with idiopathic membranous nephropathy. PLoS One. **10**: e0138841.

Jha V, Ganguli A, Saha TK, et al. (2007). A randomized, controlled trial of steroids and cyclophosphamide in adults with nephrotic syndrome caused by idiopathic membranous nephropathy. J Am Soc Nephrol. **18**: 1899–904.

Jiang X, Mei X, Feng D, et al. (2015). Prophylaxis and treatment of *Pneumocystis Jiroveci* pneumonia in lymphoma patients subjected to rituximab-contained therapy: A systematic review and meta-analysis. PloS One. **10**: e0122171.

Kalliakmani P, Koutroulia E, Sotsiou F, et al. (2010). Benefit and cost from the long-term use of cyclosporine-A in idiopathic membranous nephropathy. Nephrology (Carlton). **15**: 762–7.

Kanigicherla DAK, Hamilton P, Czapla K, et al. (2018). Intravenous pulse cyclophosphamide and steroids induce immunological and clinical remission in new-incident and relapsing membranous nephropathy. Nephrology (Carlton). **23**: 60–8.

Kanigicherla DAK, Short CD, Roberts S, et al. (2016). Long-term outcomes of persistent disease and relapse in primary membranous nephropathy. Nephrol Dial Transplant. **31**: 2108–14.

Kao L, Lam V, Waldman M, et al. (2015). Identification of the immunodominant epitope region in phospholipase A2 receptor-mediating autoantibody binding in idiopathic membranous nephropathy. J Am Soc Nephrol. **26**: 291–301.

Kattah A, Ayalon R, Beck LH Jr, et al. (2015). Anti-phospholipase A_2 receptor antibodies in recurrent membranous nephropathy. Am J Transplant. **15**: 1349–59.

KDIGO Clinical Practice Guideline for glomerulonephritis. (2012). Kidney Int. **2S**: 1–274.

Kearney N, Podolak J, Matsumura L, et al. (2011). Patterns of IgG subclass deposits in membranous glomerulonephritis in renal allografts. Transplant Proc. **43**: 3743–6.

Kim YG, Choi YW, Kim SY, et al. (2015). Anti-phospholipase A2 receptor antibody as prognostic indicator in idiopathic membranous nephropathy. Am J Nephrol. **42**: 250–7.

Kimura Y, Miura N, Debiec H, et al. (2017). Circulating antibodies to α-enolase and phospholipase A2 receptor and composition of glomerular deposits in Japanese patients with primary or secondary membranous nephropathy. Clin Exp Nephrol. **21**: 117–26.

Kobayashi M, Usui J, Sakai K, et al. (2015). Membranous nephropathy with solitary immunoglobulin A deposition. Intern Med. **54**: 1081–4.

Lai AS, Lai KN. (2006). Viral nephropathy. Nat Clin Pract Nephrol. **2**: 254–62.

Larsen CP, Ambuzs JM, Bonsib SM, et al. (2014). Membranous-like glomerulopathy with masked IgG kappa deposits. Kidney Int. **86**: 154–61.

Larsen CP, Cossey LN, Beck LH. (2016). THSD7A staining of membranous glomerulopathy in clinical practice reveals cases with dual autoantibody positivity. Mod Pathol. **29**: 421–6.

Larsen CP, Walker PD. (2013). Phospholipase A2 receptor (PLA2R) staining is useful in the determination of *de novo* versus recurrent membranous glomerulopathy. Transplantation. **95**: 1259–62.

Lawitz E, Poodard F, Gutierrez JA, et al. (2017). Short-duration treatment with elbasvir/grazoprevir and sofosbuvir for hepatitis C: A randomized trial. Hepatology. **65**: 439–50.

Le WB, Shi JS, Zhang T, et al. (2017). HLA-DRB1*15:01 and HLA-DRB3*02:02 in PLA2R-related membranous nephropathy. J Am Soc Nephrol. **28**: 1642–50.

Lee SM, Yang S, Cha RH, et al. (2014). Circulating TNF receptors are significant prognostic biomarkers for idiopathic membranous nephropathy. PLoS One. **9**: e104354.

Lee T, Biddle AK, Lionaki S, et al. (2014). Personalized prophylactic anticoagulation decision analysis in patients with membranous nephropathy. Kidney Int. **85**: 1412–20.

Lee T, Derebail VK, Abhijit V, et al. (2016). Patients with primary membranous nephropathy are at high risk of cardiovascular events. Kidney Int. **89**: 1111–18.

Leeaphorn N, Kue-A-Pai P, Thamcharoen N, et al. (2014). Prevalence of cancer in membranous nephropathy: a systematic review and meta-analysis of observational studies. Am J Nephrol. **40**: 29–35.

Lefaucheur C, Stengel B, Nochy D, et al. (2006). Membranous nephropathy and cancer: Epidemiologic evidence and determinants of high-risk cancer association. Kidney Int. **70**: 1510–17.

Li SJ, Guo JZ, Zuo K, et al. (2012). Thromboembolic complications in membranous nephropathy patients with nephrotic syndrome-a prospective study. Thromb Res. **130**: 501–5.

Lin KM, Lin JC, Tseng WY, et al. (2013). Rituximab-induced hepatitis C virus reactivation in rheumatoid arthritis. J Microbiol Immunol Infect. **46**: 65–7.

Lionaki S, Vimal K. Derebai VK, et al. (2012). Venous thromboembolism in patients with membranous nephropathy. Clin J Am Soc Nephrol. 7: 43–51.

van de Logt AE, Beerenhout CH, Brink HS, et al. (2015). Synthetic ACTH in high risk patients with idiopathic membranous nephropathy: A prospective, open label cohort study. PLoS One. 10: e0142033.

Lönnbro-Widgren J, Ebefors K, Mölne J, et al. (2015). Glomerular IgG subclasses in idiopathic and malignancy-associated membranous nephropathy. Clin Kidney J. 8: 433–9.

Lorusso P, Bottai A, Mangione E, et al. (2015). Low-dose synthetic adrenocorticotropic hormone-analog therapy for nephrotic patients: Results from a single-center pilot study. Int J Nephrol Renovasc Dis. 8: 7–12.

Luo W, Olaru F, Miner JH, et al. (2018). Alternative pathway is essential for glomerular complement activation and proteinuria in a mouse model of membranous nephropathy. Front Immunol. 9: 1433.

Ma H, Sandor DG, Beck LH Jr. (2013). The role of complement in membranous nephropathy. Semin Nephrol. 33: 531–42.

Madkova N, Kiryluk K. (2017). Genetic complexity of the HLA region and idiopathic membranous nephropathy. J Am Soc Nephrol. 28: 1331–34.

Malik GH, Al-Harbi AS, Al-Mohaya S. (2002). Repeated pregnancies in patients with primary membranous glomerulonephritis. Nephron. 91: 21–4.

Mathrani V, Alejmi A, Griffin S, et al. (2017). Intravenous cyclophosphamide and oral prednisolone is a safe and effective treatment option for idiopathic membranous nephropathy. Clin Kidney J. 10: 450–4.

Matsumoto Y, Shimada Y, Nojima Y, et al. (2013). Efficacy of mizoribine followed by low-dose prednisone in patients with idiopathic membranous nephropathy and nephrotic-range proteinuria. Ren Fail. 35: 936–41.

McGrogan A, Franssen CFM, de Vries CS. (2011). The incidence of primary glomerulonephritis worldwide: a systematic review of the literature. Nephrol Dial Transplant. 26: 414–43.

Meyrier A. (1992). Antiproteinuric and immunological effects of cyclosporin A in the treatment of glomerular diseases. Nephrol Dial Transplant. 7: 80–4.

Michel PA, Dahan K, Ancel PY, et al. (2011). Rituximab treatment for membranous nephropathy: A French clinical and serological retrospective study of 28 patients. Nephron Extra. 1: 251–61.

Morita M, Mii A, Shimizu A, et al. (2015). Glomerular endothelial cell injury and focal segmental glomerulosclerosis lesion in idiopathic membranous nephropathy. PLoS One. 10: e0116700.

Moroni G, Depetri F, Del Vecchio L, et al. (2017). Low-dose rituximab is poorly effective in patients with primary membranous nephropathy. Nephrol Dial Transplant. 32: 1691–6.

Moroni G, Gallelli B, Quaglini S, et al. (2010). Long-term outcome of renal transplantation in patients with idiopathic membranous glomerulonephritis (MN). Nephrol Dial Transplant 23: 208–16.

Mozessohn L, Chan KK, Feld JJ, et al. (2015). Hepatitis B reactivation in HBsAg-negative/HBcAb-positive patients receiving rituximab for lymphoma: A meta-analysis. J Viral Hepat. 22: 842–9.

Müller-Deile J, Schiffer L, Hiss M, et al. (2015). A new rescue regimen with plasma exchange and rituximab in high-risk membranous glomerulonephritis. Eur J Clin Invest. **45**: 1260–9.

Murtas C, Ghiggeri GM. (2016). Membranous glomerulonephritis: Histological and serological features to differentiate cancer-related and non-related forms. J Nephrol. **29**: 469–78.

Niel O, Dallocchio A, Thouret MC, et al. (2015). C3 nephritic factor can be associated with membranous glomerulonephritis. Pediatr Nephrol. **30**: 353–5.

Obana M, Nakanishi K, Sako M, et al. (2006). Segmental membranous glomerulonephritis in children: Comparison with global membranous glomerulonephritis. Clin J Am Soc Nephrol. **1**: 723–9.

Okyay GU, Inal S, Öneç K, et al. (2012). Remission of *de novo* membranous nephropathy in a kidney allograft recipient: A case report. Ren Fail. **34**: 1341–3.

Pippias M, Stel VS, Aresté-Fosalba N, et al. (2016). Long-term kidney transplant outcomes in primary glomerulonephritis: Analysis from the ERA-EDTA Registry. Transplantation. **100**: 1955–62.

Polanco N, Gutiérrez E, Covarsí A, et al. (2010). Spontaneous remission of nephrotic syndrome in idiopathic membranous nephropathy. J Am Soc Nephrol. **21**: 697–704.

Polanco N, Gutiérrez E, Rivera F, et al. (2012). Spontaneous remission of nephrotic syndrome in membranous nephropathy with chronic renal impairment. Nephrol Dial Transplant. **27**: 231–4.

Ponticelli C, Altieri P, Scolari F, et al. (1998). A randomized study comparing methylprednisolone plus chlorambucil versus methylprednisolone plus cyclophosphamide in idiopathic membranous nephropathy. J Am Soc Nephrol. **9**: 444–50.

Ponticelli C, Escoli R, Moroni G. (2018). Does cyclophosphamide still play a role in glomerular diseases? Autoimmun Rev. **17**: 1022–7.

Ponticelli C, Glassock RJ. (2010). Posttransplant recurrence of primary glomerulonephritis. Clin J Am Soc Nephrol. **5**: 2363–72.

Ponticelli C, Glassock RJ. (2012). *De novo* membranous nephropathy (MN) in kidney allografts. A peculiar form of alloimmune disease? Transpl Int. **25**: 1205–10.

Ponticelli C, Glassock RJ. (2013). Treatment of membranous nephropathy in patients with renal insufficiency: What regimen to choose? J Nephrol. **26**: 427–9.

Ponticelli C, Glassock RJ. (2014). Glomerular diseases: Membranous nephropathy--a modern view. Clin J Am Soc Nephrol. **9**: 609–16.

Ponticelli C, Passerini P. (2010). Can prognostic factors assist therapeutic decisions in idiopathic membranous nephropathy? J Nephrol. **23**: 156–63.

Ponticelli C, Passerini P, Salvadori M, et al. (2006). A randomized pilot trial comparing methylprednisolone plus a cytotoxic agent versus synthetic adrenocorticotropic hormone in idiopathic membranous nephropathy. Am J Kidney Dis. **47**: 233–40.

Ponticelli C, Sala G, Glassock RJ. (2015). Drug management in the elderly adult with chronic kidney disease: A review for the primary care physician. Mayo Clin Proc. **90**: 633–45.

Ponticelli C, Zucchelli P, Passerini P, et al. (1989). A randomized trial of methylprednisolone and chlorambucil in idiopathic membranous nephropathy. N Engl J Med. **320**: 8–13.

Ponticelli C, Zucchelli P, Passerini P, et al. (1992). Methylprednisolone plus chlorambucil as compared with methylprednisolone alone for the treatment of idiopathic membranous nephropathy. N Engl J Med. **327**: 599–603.

Ponticelli C, Zucchelli P, Passerini P, et al. (1995). A 10-year follow-up of a randomized study with methylprednisolone and Chlorambucil in membranous nephropathy. Kidney Int. **48**: 1600–4.

Praga M, Barrio V, Juárez GF, et al. (2007). Tacrolimus monotherapy in membranous nephropathy: a randomized controlled trial. Kidney Int. **71**: 924–30.

Prunotto M, Carnevali ML, Candiano G, et al. (2010). Autoimmunity in membranous nephropathy targets aldose reductase and SOD2. J Am Soc Nephrol. **21**: 507–19.

Qiao Y, Berg AL, Wang P, et al. (2016). MC1R is dispensable for the proteinuria reducing and glomerular protective effect of melanocortin therapy. Sci Rep. **6**: 27589.

Qin HZ, Liu L, Liang SS, et al. (2017). Evaluating tacrolimus treatment in idiopathic membranous nephropathy in a cohort of 408 patients. BMC Nephrol. **18**: 2.

Qin HZ, Zhang MC, Le WB, et al. (2016). Combined assessment of phospholipase A2 receptor autoantibodies and glomerular deposits in membranous nephropathy. J Am Soc Nephrol. **27**: 1137–43.

Qin W, Beck LH Jr, Zeng C, et al. (2011). Anti-phospholipase A2 receptor antibody in membranous nephropathy. J Am Soc Nephrol. **22**: 1137–43.

Quintana LF, Blasco M, Seras M, et al. (2015). Antiphospholipase A2 receptor antibody levels predict the risk of post-transplantation recurrence of membranous nephropathy. Transplantation. **99**: 1709–14.

Radhakrishnan J. (2012). Venous thromboembolism and membranous nephropathy: So what's new? Clin J Am Soc Nephrol. **7**: 3–4.

Radice A, Trezzi B, Maggiore U, et al. (2016). Clinical usefulness of autoantibodies to M-type phospholipase A2 receptor (PLA2R) for monitoring disease activity in idiopathic membranous nephropathy (IMN). Autoimmun Rev. **15**: 146–54.

Ramachandran R, Hn H, Kumar V, et al. (2016a). Tacrolimus combined with corticosteroids versus modified Ponticelli regimen in treatment of idiopathic membranous nephropathy: Randomized control trial. Nephrology (Carlton). **21**: 139–46.

Ramachandran R, Kumar V, Jha V. (2016c). Cyclical cyclophosphamide and steroids is effective in resistant or relapsing nephrotic syndrome due to M-type phospholipase A2 receptor-related membranous nephropathy after tacrolimus therapy. Kidney Int. **89**: 1401–2.

Ramachandran R, Kumar V, Kumar A, et al. (2016b). PLA2R antibodies, glomerular PLA2R deposits and variations in *PLA2R1* and *HLA-DQA1* genes in primary membranous nephropathy in South Asians. Nephrol Dial Transplant. **31**: 1486–93.

Reddy YN, Siedlecki AM, Francis JM. (2017). Breaking down the complement system: A review and update on novel therapies. Curr Opin Nephrol Hypertens. **26**: 123–8.

Remuzzi G, Chiurchiu C, Abbate M, et al. (2002). Rituximab for idiopathic membranous nephropathy. Lancet. **360**: 923–4.

Ren S, Wu C, Zhang Y, et al. (2018). An update on clinical significance of use of THSD7A in diagnosing idiopathic membranous nephropathy: A systematic review and meta-analysis of THSD7A in IMN. Ren Fail. **40**: 306–13.

Roccatello D, Sciascia S, Di Simone D, et al. (2016). New insights into immune mechanisms underlying response to Rituximab in patients with membranous nephropathy: A prospective study and a review of the literature. Autoimmun Rev. **15**: 529–38.

Rocha KB, Soares VA, Viero RM. (2004). The role of myofibroblasts and interstitial fibrosis in the progression of membranous nephropathy. Ren Fail. **26**: 445–51.

Rodriguez EF, Cosio FG, Nasr SH, et al. (2012). The pathology and clinical features of early recurrent membranous glomerulonephritis. Am J Transplant. **12**: 1029–38.

Rodriguez EF, Nasr SH, Larsen CP, et al. (2014). Membranous nephropathy with crescents: A series of 19 cases. Am J Kidney Dis. **64**: 66–73.

Ronco P, Debiec H. (2010). Antigen identification in membranous nephropathy moves toward targeted monitoring and new therapy. J Am Soc Nephrol. **21**: 564–9.

Rosenzwajg M, Languille E, Debiec H, et al. (2017). B- and T-cell subpopulations in patients with severe idiopathic membranous nephropathy may predict an early response to rituximab. Kidney Int. **92**: 227–37.

Rostoker G. Belghiti D, Ben Maadi A, et al (1993). Long-term cyclosporin A therapy for severe idiopathic membranous nephropathy.Nephron **63**:335-41

Ruggenenti P, Chiurchiu C, Abbate M, et al. (2006). Rituximab for idiopathic membranous nephropathy: Who can benefit? Clin J Am Soc Nephrol. **1**: 738–48.

Ruggenenti P, Cravedi P, Chianca A, et al. (2012). Rituximab in idiopathic membranous nephropathy. J Am Soc Nephrol. **23**: 1416–25.

Ruggenenti P, Debiec H, Ruggiero B, et al. (2015). Anti-phospholipaseA2 receptor antibody titer predicts post-rituximab outcome of membranous nephropathy. J Am Soc Nephrol. **10**: 2545–58.

Saeed M, Beggs ML, Walker PD, et al. (2014). DQA1 associated membranous glomerulopathy is modulated by common variants in PLA2R1 and HLA-DQA1 genes. Genes Immun. **15**: 556–561.

Saito T, Iwano M, Matsumoto K, et al. (2017). Mizoribine therapy combined with steroids and mizoribine blood concentration monitoring for idiopathic membranous nephropathy with steroid-resistant nephrotic syndrome. Clin Exp Nephrol. **21**: 961–70.

Sam R, Joshi A, James S, et al. (2015). Lupus-like membranous nephropathy: Is it lupus or not? Clin Exp Nephrol. **19**: 395–402.

Schwarz A, Krause PH, Offermann G, et al. (1994). Impact of *de novo* membranous glomerulonephritis on the clinical course after kidney transplantation. Transplantation. **58**: 650–4.

Segawa Y, Hisano S, Matsushita M, et al. (2010). IgG subclasses and complement pathway in segmental and global membranous nephropathy. Pediatr Nephrol. **25**: 1091–9.

Seitz-Polski B, Debiec H, Rousseau A, et al. (2018). Phospholipase A2 receptor 1 epitope spreading predicts reduced likelihood of remission in membranous nephropathy. J Am Soc Nephrol. **29**: 401–8.

Seitz-Polski B, Payre CD, Ambrosetti D, et al. (2014). Prediction of membranous nephropathy recurrence after transplantation by monitoring of anti-PLA2R1 (M-type phospholipase A2 receptor) autoantibodies: A case series of 15 patients. Nephrol Dial Transplant. **29**: 2334–42.

Senthyl Nayagam LS, Ganguli A, Rathi M, et al. (2008). Mycophenolate mofetil or standard therapy for membranous nephropathy and focal segmental glomerulosclerosis: A pilot study. Nephrol Dial Transplant. **23**: 1926–30.

Shiiki H, Saito T, Nishitani Y, et al. (2004). Prognosis and risk factors for idiopathic membranous nephropathy with nephrotic syndrome in Japan. Kidney Int. **65**: 1400–7.

Song EJ, Jeong KH, Yang YA, et al. (2018). Anti-phospholipase A2 receptor antibodies as a prognostic marker in patients with primary membranous nephropathy. Kidney Res Clin Pract. **37**: 248–56.

Souqiyyeh MZ, Shaheen FA, Alsuwaida A, et al. (2015). Rituximab as a rescue therapy in patients with glomerulonephritis. Saudi J Kidney Dis Transpl. **26**: 47–55.

Spinner ML, Bowman LJ, Horwedel TA, et al. (2015). Single-dose rituximab for recurrent glomerulonephritis post-renal transplant. Am J Nephrol. **41**: 37–47.

Sprangers B, Lefkowitz GI, Cohen SD, et al. (2010). Beneficial effect of rituximab in the treatment of recurrent idiopathic membranous nephropathy after kidney transplantation. Clin J Am Soc Nephrol. **5**: 790–7.

Stanescu HC, Arcos-Burgos M, Medlar A, et al. (2011). Risk HLA-DQA1 and PLA(2)R1 alleles in idiopathic membranous nephropathy. N Engl J Med. **364**: 616–26.

Stehlé T, Audard V, Ronco P, et al. (2015). Phospholipase A2 receptor and sarcoidosis-associated membranous nephropathy. Nephrol Dial Transplant. **30**: 1047–50.

Stylianou K, Maragkaki E, Tzanakakis M. (2014). Acute interstitial nephritis and membranous nephropathy in the context of IgG4-related disease. Case Rep Nephrol Dial. **5**: 44–8.

Tao JL, Liu LL, Wen YB, et al. (2011). Cyclosporine treatment in idiopathic membranous nephropathy nephrotic syndrome in adults: A retrospective study spanning 15 years. Chin Med J (Engl). **124**: 3490–4.

Thompson A, Cattran DC, Blank M, et al. (2015). Complete and partial remission as surrogate end points in membranous nephropathy. JASN. **26**: 2930–7.

Timmermans SA, Abdul Hamid MA, Cohen Tervaert JW, et al. (2015). Anti-PLA2R antibodies as a prognostic factor in PLA2R-related membranous nephropathy. Am J Nephrol. **42**: 70–7.

Timmermans SA, Ayalon R, van Paassen P, et al. (2013). Anti-phospholipase A2 receptor and malignancy in membranous nephropathy. Am J Kidney Dis. **62**: 1223–5.

Tomas NM, Beck LH Jr, Meyer-Schwesinger C, et al. (2014). Thrombospondin type-1 domain-containing 7A in idiopathic membranous nephropathy. N Engl J Med. **371**: 2277–87.

Tomas NM, Hoxha E, Reinicke AT, et al. (2016). Autoantibodies against thrombospondin type 1 domain-containing 7A induce membranous nephropathy. J Clin Invest. **126**: 2519–32.

Tran THJ, Hughes G, Greenfeld C, et al. (2015). Overview of current and alternative therapies for idiopathic membranous nephropathy. Pharmacotherapy. **35**: 396–411.

Trivin C, Tran A, Moulin B, et al. (2017). Infectious complications of a rituximab-based immunosuppressive regimen in patients with glomerular disease. Clin Kidney J. **10**: 461–9.

Troyanov S, Wall CA, Miller JA, et al. (2004). Idiopathic membranous nephropathy: definition and relevance of a partial remission. Kidney Int. **66**: 1199–205.

Truong L, Gelfand J, D'Agati V, et al. (1989). *De novo* membranous glomerulonephropathy in renal allografts: A report of ten cases and review of the literature. Am J Kidney Dis. **14**: 131–44.

Vivarelli M, Emma F, Pelle T, et al. (2015). Genetic homogeneity but IgG subclass–dependent clinical variability of alloimmune membranous nephropathy with anti-neutral endopeptidase antibodies. Kidney Int. **87**: 602–9.

Wang J, Cui Z, Lu J, et al. (2017). Circulating antibodies against thrombospondin type-I domain-containing 7A in Chinese patients with idiopathic membranous nephropathy. Clin J Am Soc Nephrol. **12**: 1642–51.

Wang L, Ye Z, Liang H, et al. (2016). The combination of tacrolimus and entecavir improves the remission of HBV-associated glomerulonephritis without enhancing viral replication. Am J Transl Res. **8**: 1593–600.

Wang X, Song X, Liu Y, et al. (2016). Treatment of membranous nephropathy with mizoribine: A control trial. Life Sci. **154**: 75–8.

Wei SY, Wang YX, Li JS, et al. (2016). Serum anti-PLA2R antibody predicts treatment outcome in idiopathic membranous nephropathy. Am J Nephrol. **43**: 129–40.

Wen J, Xie K, Zhang M, et al. (2016). HLA-DR, and not PLA2R, is expressed on the podocytes in kidney allografts in *de novo* membranous nephropathy. Medicine (Baltimore). **95**(37): e4809.

Wen M, Kuckle C, Sarkar O, et al. (2014). Plasmapheresis combined with rituximab for refractory idiopathic membranous nephropathy. J Urol Nephrol. **46**: 847–8.

Wu W, Shang J, Tao C, et al. (2018). The prognostic value of phospholipase A2 receptor autoantibodies on spontaneous remission for patients with idiopathic membranous nephropathy: A meta-analysis. Medicine (Baltimore). **97**: e11018.

Xie Q, Li Y, Xue J, et al. (2015). Renal phospholipase A2 receptor in hepatitis B virus-associated membranous nephropathy. Am J Nephrol. **41**: 345–53.

Xipell M, Rodas LM, Villareal J, et al. (2018). The utility of phospholipase A2 receptor autoantibody in membranous nephropathy after kidney transplantation. Clin Kidney J. **11**: 422–8.

Yamaguchi M, Ando M, Yamamoto R, et al. (2014). Patient age and the prognosis of idiopathic membranous nephropathy. PLoS One. **20**: 9.

Yang Y, Ma YP, Chen DP, et al. (2016). A meta-analysis of antiviral therapy for hepatitis B virus-associated membranous nephropathy. PLoS One. **6**: 11.

Yokoyama H, Goshima S, Wada T, et al. (1999). The short- and long-term outcomes of membranous nephropathy treated with intravenous immune globulin therapy. Kanazawa Study Group for Renal Diseases and Hypertension. Nephrol Dial Transplant. **14**: 2379–86.

Yu X, Cai J, Jiao X, et al. (2018). Response predictors to calcineurin inhibitors in patient with primary membranous nephropathy. Am J Nephrol. **47**: 266–74.

Zhang BO, Cheng M, Yang M, et al. (2016). Analysis of the prognostic risk factors of idiopathic membranous nephropathy using a new surrogate end-point. Biomed Rep. **4**: 147–52.

Zhang LJ, Zhang Z, Li SJ, et al. (2014). Pulmonary embolism and renal vein thrombosis in patients with nephrotic syndrome: prospective evaluation of prevalence and risk factors with CT. Pulmonary embolism and renal vein thrombosis in patients with nephrotic syndrome: prospective evaluation of prevalence and risk factors with CT. Radiology. **273:** 897–906.

Chapter 7

Immunoglobulin A nephropathy

Richard J Glassock, Claudio Ponticelli,
and Kar Neng Lai

Introduction and overview

The term *immunoglobulin A nephropathy* (IgA nephropathy or IgA N) refers to
a primary glomerular disease characterized by the dominant or co-dominant,
diffuse, and generalized mesangial deposition of IgA, typically of the IgA_1 subclass, often accompanied by deposition of IgG and the C3 and/or C4, but not
C1q, components of complement in a similar distribution (Glassock, 2009; Lai,
2009; Lai et al., 2016; Floege and Amann, 2016; Rodriguez et al., 2017). In the
past, it has also been referred to as Berger's disease, to signify the senior author
of the original publication describing the disorder that first appeared five decades ago in September of 1968 (Berger and Hinglais, 1968). IgA N is most likely
the commonest primary glomerular disease in the developed world (D'Amico,
1987). The disease is characterized principally by episodes of glomerular
haematuria often with persistent proteinuria of a variable degree. Spontaneous
remissions are uncommon, except in young children. It most often pursues an
indolent, slowly progressive course, but it can also produce rapidly progressive
disease and leads to end-stage renal disease (ESRD) in about 30–50 per cent of
cases after 25 years or more of follow-up. At present the disorder can only be
diagnosed by renal biopsy.

Pathology

The light microscopic appearance of IgA N varies widely, but the most common
findings are mesangial proliferation and expansion of the mesangial matrix
(Soares and Roberts, 2017). These lesions are commonly focal and segmental
(see Plate 9) but may also be diffuse and generalized in distribution. As the lesion progresses areas of segmental or global glomerulosclerosis often ensue.
The other lesions observed include diffuse crescentic glomerulonephritis (uncommon), membranoproliferative glomerulonephritis (rare), and the minimal
change lesion. It may co-exist with thin basement membrane nephropathy

(TBMN, see Chapter 11). Membranous nephropathy is very uncommon histo-logic pattern. A focal, necrotizing lesion ('capillaritis') may be seen and can sig-nify the presence of a 'low-grade' renal-limited angiitis (D'Amico et al., 2001). Crescentic lesions (cellular or fibrocellular) are seen in about one-third cases and contribute to a poor prognosis when extensive (Tumlin and Henniger, 2004; Haas et al., 2017).

The glomerular IgA deposits are typically confined to the mesangial area with occasional segmental extensions into the capillary sub-endothelium (see Plate 10). These deposits are often accompanied by IgG and/or IgM and C3 and or C4, but the C1q component of complement is seldom found. C3 deposits are seen in over 80 per cent of cases and C4d deposits are found in about 40–50 per cent of cases, indicating prominent involvement of the alternate or man-nose binding lectin pathways for complement activation (Oortwijn et al., 2008; Faria et al., 2015; Sethi et al., 2015; Coppo, 2017). The presence of C4d in glom-erular deposits can be associated with a worse prognosis (Espinosa et al., 2014; Rath et al., 2015; Heybeli et al., 2015), Mannose binding lectin deposits are seen in about 25 per cent of cases (Roos et al., 2006). The J-chain is often found in the glomerular deposits of IgA, particularly after partial elution, indicating the polymeric nature of the deposits. The secretory component of IgA may also be present, but this is not very common (about 30 per cent) (Oortwijn et al., 2008; Zhang et al., 2008).

The IgA deposits are principally composed of polymeric IgA_1 (Conley et al., 1980; Mestecky et al., 2008). The polymeric IgA_1 deposits very likely repre-sent the deposition of immune complexes from the circulation composed of an under-galactosylated and over-sialylated form of IgA_1 and an IgA or IgG auto-antibody to the glycan or peptide region of the abnormal IgA_1 (see 'Pathogenesis').

Predominant IgA deposits in the glomeruli are also seen in a wide variety of other underlying diseases (also known as 'secondary' IgA nephropathy—see Box 7.1), including cirrhosis of the liver, various malignancies (lung cancer, mycosis fungoides), acute infections (staphylococcus, toxoplasmosis, human immunodeficiency virus), psoriasis, celiac disease (non-tropical sprue) some-times accompanied dermatitis herpetiformis, and rheumatoid factor nega-tive (sero-negative) spondyloarthropathies (Pouria and Barratt, 2008; Helin et al., 1983).

Deposits very similar to that described in subjects with clinical findings com-patible with IgA N can also be found in otherwise normal individuals (revealed by autopsy following sudden accidental or suicidal death or by routine pre-implantation biopsies of donated kidneys in renal transplantation). The fre-quency of this finding varies from about 2–16 per cent, depending on the study

Box 7.1 A classification of disorders associated with glomerular IgA deposition (dominant or co-dominant)

Primary:

IgA nephropathy (historically known as Berger's disease)

Multisystem:

Henoch-Schönlein purpura (now known as IgA Vasculitis)

Secondary: (alphabetical)

Coeliac disease (with or without dermatitis herpetiformis)
Chronic liver disease (cirrhosis, of any kind; often asymptomatic)
Crohn's disease
Cytomegalovirus infection
Episcleritis
Familial immune thrombocytopenia
Galactosialidosis
Goodpasture's disease (anti-GBM antibody disease—rare)
Hepatitis B infection (may be coincidental, especially in endemic areas)
HIV infection
Leprosy
Mucin-secretin carcinoma
Multiple myeloma (and IgA monoclonal gammopathy)
Mycosis fungoides
Porto-systemic shunts
Staphylococcal-related acute nephritis with dominant IgA deposition
Psoriasis
Pulmonary haemosiderosis
Recurrent mastitis
Sero-negative spondyloarthropathies
Sézary syndrome
Sicca syndrome
Small cell cancer of the lung
Thromboangiitis obliterans (Buerger's disease)
Toxoplasmosis
Vogt–Koyanagi–Harada syndrome

(Sinniah, 1983; Waldherr et al., 1989; Rosenberg et al., 1989, 1990; Curschellas et al., 1991; Varis et al., 1993; Suzuki et al., 2003; Glassock, 2008). These so called 'lanthanic' deposits of IgA are frequently not accompanied by C3 deposition suggesting the complement activation is somehow involved in promoting the clinical expression of disease.

IgA N is also closely related to a multi-system small vessel vasculitic disease known as Henoch–Schönlein purpura (HSP, now also called IgA vasculitis; Pillebolut et al., 2002). IgA N may be considered to be a *mono-symptomatic* or *renal-limited form* of HSP, and conversely HSP may be regarded as a multisystem form of IgA N. As IgA vasculitis is a multisystem disorder, not a *primary* glomerular disease, it will not be discussed here. Intermediate forms having the renal-limited character of IgA N and the small vessel vasculitic features of HSP have been described (see 'Pathology'; D'Amico et al., 2001). A uniform approach to the classification of the glomerular and tubulo-interstitial pathology of IgA N has been agreed upon (The OXFORD-MEST system; Working Group of the International IgA Nephropathy Network and the Renal Pathology Society et al., 2009, 2010; Trimarchi et al., 2017) and its utility as a prognostic tool in untreated patients has been validated in numerous studies in adults and children (Barbour et al., 2015; Coppo et al., 2014). This classification system scores lesions of the mesangium (MO and M1), endothelium (E0 and E1), glomerulosclerosis (S0 and S1), and tubular atrophy and interstitial fibrosis (T0, T1, or T2). Recently a C classification (MEST-C) has been added to signify the involvement of glomeruli with crescents (Soares and Roberts, 2017; no crescents = C0; any crescents less than 25 per cent involvement = C1, and 25 per cent or greater crescents = C2). These T and C lesions have significant effects on prognosis (see 'Renal biopsy morphology').

Pathogenesis

The 'multi-hit' pathogenesis of primary IgA N is now reasonably well understood (Mestecky et al., 2008; Novak et al., 2008; Novak et al., 2013; Robert et al., 2015; Floege and Feehally, 2016; Yeo et al., 2017). A subset of B-cells, including those in the palatine tonsils, bone marrow, and peripheral lymphoid tissue manufacture a form of IgA_1 that is deficient in galactose residues ($gdIgA_1$) and has a surfeit of N-acetyl glucosamine (sialic acid) at several O-linked glycan side chains located in the 'hinge-region' of the molecule (Mestecky et al., 2008; Novak et al., 2008; Suzuki et al., 2008). This abnormality is the 'first hit'. The cellular and molecular mechanisms underlying this glycosylation abnormality is not yet completely understood. It may be due to an acquired imbalance of glycosylation/sialylation in a subset of B cells, perhaps driven by a perturbed local cytokine milieu (Mestecky et al., 2008; Suzuki et al., 2008). It might also be due to somatic or germ-line gene abnormalities of the main enzymes responsible for adding galactose or sialic acid to the glycan side chains (core β 1,3 galactosyltransferase or 1,6-sialyltrasferase or the molecular chaperone for these enzymes (COSM; Beerman et al., 2007; Buck et al., 2008; Mestecky et al., 2008; Magistroni et al., 2015; Kiryluk et al., 2017). The circulating IgA_1 of patients with IgA N has an increased concentration of these abnormally glycosylated molecules (which can be detected by abnormal binding to *Helix aspersa* agglutinin; Moldoveanu et al., 2007; Novak et al., 2008). This abnormality may provide a useful non-invasive diagnostic test for IgA N (Moldoveanu et al., 2007). An auto-antibody response (IgA or IgG class) to these abnormally glycosylated IgA_1 molecules, the 'second hit', results in the formation of immune complexes in the circulation, which can bind and localize to mesangial structures (predominantly via binding to the mesangial transferrin receptor; Moura et al., 2008; Novak et al., 2008; Novak et al., 2013) and accumulate in the mesangium. The immune complexes also appear to be inefficiently cleared by the hepatic Kupfer cell mechanism. The deposition of aberrantly glycosylated IgA containing immune complexes provokes elaboration of various cytokines and growth factors and induces local activation of complement, via the alternative and mannose-binding lectin (MBL) pathways. The 'third hit' of complement activation via the alternative or lectin pathways of complement activation plays a crucial role in the development and progression of IgA N (Malliard et al., 2015; Floege and Daha, 2018). IgA deposition alone may be insufficient to evoke a recognizable disease, as demonstrated by the high frequency (4–16 per cent) of glomerular mesangial IgA deposits in otherwise normal healthy individuals (such as kidney transplant donors, and suicide/accident victims). Some additional events are required to bring the disease to its full clinical (and recognizable) form, e.g. that a quantitative threshold for $gdIgA_1$ deposition be exceeded; that anti-gdIgA antibodies rise to a sufficient titre to active mediator pathways; that characteristics of the IgA deposits (or the co-deposition of IgG) result in activation of mediators (such as the alternate or lectin complement pathways). Clearly something more than mere IgA deposition in the glomerular mesangium must be involved in determining the clinical expression of the disease.

Mesangial IgA deposits are predominantly polymeric in nature with more lambda- than kappa-light chain (Lai, Chui et al., 1988). These deposits consist mostly of underglycosylated polymeric IgA_1 with the absence of the secretory component and the presence of the J chain. Polymeric lambda-light chain IgA_1 from patients with IgA N exhibits enhanced affinity to mesangial cells and granulocytes (Lai et al., 2002). The migration and/or sequestration of leukocytes with high affinity to lambda light chain-IgA in the mononuclear phagocytic system or inflammatory tissues may bear important pathologic significance in

IgA N. Prominent infiltration of mononuclear cells is frequently detected in renal biopsies from patients with IgA N and the glomerular and interstitial infiltration by neutrophils increases with the histopathologic severity (Li et al., 1990; Pei et al., 2014). Intriguingly, this unusual glycosylation and sialylation pattern of the lambda-light chain IgA_1 may have important implications for the pathogenesis of IgA N, as both the masking effect of sialic acid on galactose and the reduced galactosylation will hinder the clearance of macromolecular lambda-light chain IgA_1 by asialoglycoprotein receptor of hepatocytes (Lai et al., 1996). The negative charge from sialic acid may also favour mesangial deposition of polymeric lambda-light chain IgA_1 in IgA N (Leung et al., 2001).

The study of subjects who undergo renal biopsy for the diagnosis of IgA N may underestimate the true nature of the disease, as expressed by glomerular mesangial deposits, both covert and overt. Although the pathogenesis of primary IgA N is reasonably well understood, it remains possible that the lesion is a phenotype and that several pathogenic mechanisms, acting alone or in concert, are responsible for the development of the full spectrum of the disease.

Aetiology and genetic predisposition

The precise aetiology of the primary form of IgA N is unknown and may well be heterogeneous. It has been suggested that repeated exposure to a variety of environmental agents (bacterial, viruses) generates an over-stimulated B-cell population (in tonsils and bone marrow), which, in turn, secretes the abnormal IgA_1. It is also possible that environmental agents (e.g. *Staphylococcus aureus*) create a cytokine milieu within lymphoid tissue (including the tonsils) that favours the production of abnormal IgA_1. The mucosal immune system of patients with IgA N appears to be deficient in its protective response to ubiquitous neo-antigens in the environment, perhaps due to a fundamental defect in dendritic cells (antigen recognizing cells; Eijgenraam et al., 2005, 2008). A condition closely resembling primary IgA N can be associated with staphylococcal infection (skin, viscera, or wounds). This entity is called *IgA-dominant staphylococcal-related acute nephritis* (Nasr et al., 2003, 2007; Haas et al., 2008). There is little evidence to incriminate such staphylococcal infections in the overwhelming majority of patients with primary IgA N. From time to time, reports have appeared identifying various antigens related to environmental agents (viruses, bacteria) in the glomerular mesangium of patients with otherwise typical IgA N (Hung et al., 1996; Ogura et al., 2000). These observations have been difficult to replicate (Park et al., 1994). Rarely, cytomegalovirus has been strongly implicated in the development of IgA N (Ortmanns et al., 1998), but this appears to be a rare event. Currently, the abnormally glycosylated *endogenous* IgA_1 is believed to provide the dominant pathogenetic antigen in the primary form of IgA N. Thus, IgA N must be regarded is an auto-immune disease involving pathogenic immune complex formation with an endogenous antigen (aberrantly glycosylated IgA_1 and a polyclonal auto-antibody (IgA or IgG class), but the precise trigger for auto-antibody production remains uncertain.

A clear genetic influence is present in many cases of IgA N (Beerman et al., 2007; Gharavi et al., 2008; Magistroni et al., 2015; Feehally and Barratt, 2015). Specific somatic mutations seem to modulate the development of autoantibodies to $gdIgA_1$ (Huang et al., 2016). Familial clustering of cases of IgA N is seen, particularly in Europe (Italy) and the Southern US (Kentucky, Tennessee, Alabama, Mississippi, and Louisiana; Beerman et al., 2007). A familial tendency is seen in 10–50 per cent of cases, depending on the geographic region and case ascertainment. A genetic 'founder' effect has been suggested by genetic haplomapping. Several gene loci have been identified, particularly 6q22 (the IgA N1 locus; Beerman et al., 2007). Multiple rare genetic variants co-segregating with familial IgA N seem to act within a common immune network (Cox et al., 2017; Zhai et al., 2016). Significantly susceptibility to sporadic IgA N is linked strongly to the HLA sites on chromosome 6 (HLADQB1- DQBw7 allele; (Feehally et al., 2010; Kiryluk et al., 2014). Genome-wide association studies (GWAS) have also identified new genetic loci (ITGAM, ITGSAX, VAV3, CARD9, DEFA) associated with IgA N that also link to inflammatory bowel disease and the barrier to intestinal pathogens, including helminths (Kiryluk et al., 2014). Critical genetic determinants for the development of abnormal levels of gdIgA due to enzyme alteration affecting O-glycosylation pathways have been identified by GWAS (Kiryluk et al., 2017). Genetic variation is the complement Factor H gene on Chromosome 1 may impact the expression of IgA N and deletions of Complement Factor H related genes may afford protection from IgA N, at least in Han Chinese (Xie et al., 2016). The precise relationship of these genetic loci to pathogenesis of sporadic IgA N remains unknown, but is of intense interest.

Genetic polymorphisms may also influence susceptibility and /or progression of IgA N, but this has not been well worked out and some associations are hard to reproduce in all geographic sites and ancestry, perhaps because of the effect of population stratification. At the present time, it is not possible to *diagnose* IgA nephropathy by genetic testing alone nor does such testing offer much in the way of prognostication. However, as methods improve, particularly whole genome scanning for single nucleotide polymorphisms (SNP) this may change dramatically.

It seems very clear at present that the IgA galactosylation abnormality underlying idiopathic (primary) IgA N is inherited (Gharavi et al., 2008). As many as 25 per cent of the (apparently healthy) blood relatives of subjects with proven IgA N and about 50 per cent of the at-risk blood relatives of subjects with familial IgA N (assuming autosomal dominant inheritance) have abnormally elevated serum levels of the aberrantly glycosylated IgA (Gharavi et al., 2008). Elevated serum levels of aberrantly glycosylated IgA appear not to be an acquired abnormality. Renal biopsies of the apparently normal subjects with elevated serum levels of aberrantly glycosylated IgA_1 have not yet been systematically performed but they might be presumed to contain IgA mesangial deposits.

Clinical presentation and diagnosis

Primary IgA nephropathy typically presents in older children and young or middle-aged adults (Lau et al., 2007; Lai et al., 2016). but the average age at diagnosis seems to be increasing over time. IgA N is seldom seen in infancy or after the age of 80 years, at least in the idiopathic (primary) form. However, this observation may be due to the infrequency in which such patients at the extremes of age are subjected to renal biopsy. The peak age at diagnosis is somewhat older in males than in females (Briganti et al., 2001; Nair and Walker, 2006). Males are more commonly affected than females, in a ratio of about 2 to 1, in most populations (Briganti et al., 2001). IgA N is much less often observed in African-American blacks but is particularly common in Caucasians, Asians, American Indians, Eskimos, and Hispanics. IgA N remains as the most common primary glomerular disease in young adult Caucasians in the US (Nair and Walker, 2006).

Recurrent self-limited episodes of visible (macroscopic or gross) *dysmorphic (glomerular)* haematuria with or without proteinuria, often in association with upper respiratory infection (with or without tonsillitis), is a hallmark of the disorder, and the most common reason for its discovery. However, a substantial number of patients with IgA N do not have any history of recurrent bouts of macroscopic haematuria. Commonly about 50 per cent of the erythrocytes in the urinary sediment are dysmorphic. In addition, asymptomatic non-visible (microscopic) haematuria with or without proteinuria can also be a presenting feature in those individuals whose disease is discovered upon screening testing of urine or when a urinalysis is performed for another indication. *Persistent non-visible (microscopic) haematuria*, without any episodes of visible haematuria at all, is more suggestive of TBMN or variants of Alport syndrome (see also Chapter 11). Loin pain—either unilateral or bilateral—and low-grade fever may also be present during these episodes. This may give rise to initial confusion with urinary tract infection or urolithiasis and prompt an erroneous referral to a urologist. Patients may (often unnecessarily) then undergo repeated urological investigations before the true diagnosis is established, because the presence of more than trivial proteinuria (1–2 + proteinuria on dipstick or >100 mg/dl) or other urinary casts and dysmorphic erythrocytes (especially acanthocytes) are either not sought or their presence ignored. A frank nephrotic syndrome (NS) at presentation is relatively uncommon (<5–10 per cent). Episodes of reversible acute renal failure in association with acute bacterial or viral upper respiratory infections and severe gross haematuria are not infrequent (Delclaux et al., 1993) but true rapidly progressive renal failure (with underlying extensive crescentic glomerulonephritis; see also Chapter 10) is an uncommon event (<5 per cent). This latter phenomenon is likely a manifestation of a severe form of renal-limited vasculitis. The Cure Glomerulonephropathy Network reported that, in comparison with IgA N, those with IgA vasculitis were younger, more frequently white, and had a higher eGFR and a lower serum albumin (Selewski et al., 2018). Severe hypertension, even resembling malignant essential hypertension may occasionally be observed present (Clarkson et al., 1977; Sevilliano et al., 2015). Rarely, patients may present with features identical to atypical haemolytic uremic syndrome (Isnard et al., 2014).

The diversity of clinical presentation of IgA nephropathy has recently been emphasized by Philibert and co-workers (Philibert et al., 2008), and others. The major differential diagnostic considerations are: TBMN (Chapter 11), membranoproliferative glomerulonephritis (C3 glomerulonephritis or Dense Deposit Disease; Chapter 8), fibrillary glomerulonephritis, resolving post-infectious glomerulonephritis (Chapter 9), crescentic glomerulonephritis (Chapter 10) and in familial cases both Alport syndrome (hereditary nephritis and deafness) and Fabry's disease need to be considered as well. Henoch–Schönlein purpura (IgA vasculitis) can develop in a patient previously diagnosed as having primary IgA N.

Laboratory evaluation is of little help in establishing the diagnosis, but several abnormalities may provide clues. Serum IgA and IgA secretory-piece levels are elevated in about 50 per cent of patients (Zhang et al., 2008). Serum IgA/C3 concentration ratios are elevated (>4.0–4.5) but this has poor sensitivity despite reasonable specificity (Ishiguro et al., 2002; Shen et al., 2007; Nakayama et al., 2008). Elevated IgA levels, presence of moderate albuminuria (also known as micro-albuminuria) or overt proteinuria, elevated blood pressure, and increased IgA/C3 ratio ≥3.0 has a reasonable ability to separate IgA N from other diseases causing haematuria, with a correct diagnosis rate of over 75 per cent (Nakayama et al., 2008). Micro-albuminuria in association with haematuria is a useful clue to underlying IgA N, at least in children (Assadi, 2005). This would likely be of less utility in adults and in obese or diabetic subjects.

The most promising new tools for non-invasive diagnosis of IgA N are urinary proteomics measurement of the serum levels of abnormally glycosylated IgA$_1$ (by the *Helix aspersa* assay) (Haubitz et al., 2005; Lai et al., 2007) or antibodies to the gdIgA$_1$ (Renfrow and Novak, 2017; Yanagawa et al., 2014). IgA rheuma-toid factor may be found in 80–85 per cent of patients, and a variety of auto-antibodies to mesangial structural proteins may also be present, but of little diagnostic utility. These latter antibodies are very likely epiphenomena. Serum complement levels are usually normal, but complement degradation products may be elevated in the serum, particularly during episodes of macroscopic haematuria (Janssen et al., 2000). A decrease in serum C4 concentration can be seen in up to 20 per cent of cases and might be associated with a worse prognosis, but this has not yet been confirmed (Zhu et al., 2015). Low C3 levels are more common in IgA vasculitis but may also reflect activity of disease in primary IgA N (Suzuki et al., 2013). CH50, C4, factor B, properdin, and factor H and I levels can be abnormal in IgA N (Onda et al., 2007). Interestingly, C-reactive protein (CRP) levels, even with high-sensitivity methods, are not usually increased in IgA N (Baek et al., 2008). ANCA titres may be elevated in IgA N but tests using purified antigens (MPO and PR3) are often negative; thus, a positive ANCA in IgA N might be a 'false positive' (Sinico et al., 1994). However, ANCA-positive patients with systemic symptoms have lower cumu-lative renal survival rate compared with both ANCA-positive patients without systemic symptoms and ANCA-negative patients (Xie et al., 2018). Biopsies of apparently normal skin on the volar surface of the forearm will show de-posits of IgA in the dermal vessels in 30–70 per cent of patients (Hasbargen and Copley, 1985).

Despite the advances in laboratory testing, at the present time a renal biopsy is still required for the definitive diagnosis of IgA N. Importantly, TBMN (see Chapter 11) cannot reliably be distinguished from IgA N on a clinical basis (Packham, 2007). However, patients presenting with persistent isolated visible (glomerular) haematuria and a positive family history of glomerular haema-turia (autosomal dominant pattern) will more likely have TBMN than IgA N (Packham, 2007; see also Chapter 11). Patients with isolated non-visible haema-turia and a positive family history of haematuria (X-linked pattern) will more likely have Alport syndrome than IgA N. Persistent hypocomplementaemia (low C3, normal C4) is a feature of C3 glomerulonephritis or Dense Deposit Disease (Chapter 8) or transiently in post-streptococcal GN (Chapter 9), not typically in IgA N.

Epidemiology

As mentioned, asymptomatic, unrecognized (covert or 'lanthanic') depos-ition of IgA in the glomeruli (without any clinical abnormalities) is relatively common (averaging about 10 per cent) in the general population. Thus, it is not surprising that the frequency (incidence and prevalence) of IgA N in any given population is very intimately related to the indications for and the performance of renal biopsy. If the usual policy is to perform a renal biopsy in individuals with isolated non-visible haematuria (in the absence of any overt proteinuria) then the frequency of recognized IgA N in the population will be high, whereas if a more restrictive policy of renal biopsy is employed, then the frequency of IgA N in the population will be lower. Due to the ancestral influences on the frequency of IgA N, populations with a high fraction of African-Americans will have a low frequency of IgA N (Kohout and Waldo, 1989). In Victoria, Australia, which has a relatively liberal renal biopsy policy (about 260 renal biopsies per million population per year in adults), the *incidence* of newly diagnosed IgA N is approximately 57 per million population per year in males and 30 per million population per year in females (Briganti et al., 2001). Lower values would be expected in the US and Europe, where the frequency of performing renal biopsies for a diagnosis of isolated haematuria tend to be lower. Thus, the *prevalence* of IgA N among adults undergoing renal biopsies of native kidneys for presumed primary glomerular disease is high, 25–50 per cent, depending upon age and geographic region. IgA N remains as the most common primary renal disease encountered in *young* adults, at least in the *developed* world (Nair and Walker, 2006). A rise in the frequency of IgA N over time and a decline in the prevalence of membranoproliferative glomerulonephritis (see Chapter 8) has been suggested to be due to better hygiene and control of endemic infections (Johnson et al., 2003).

Differential diagnosis

The main conditions which need to be considered in a patient presenting with non-visible or visible dysmorphic haematuria, with or without proteinuria, in the *absence* of a systemic disease are IgA N, TBMN, and variants of Alport syndrome (the type IV collagen disorders), membranoproliferative glomerulonephritis (MPGN due to C3GN or DDD), non-IgA mesangial proliferative glomerulonephritis, resolving acute post-infectious glomerulonephritis (AGN), fibrillary glomerulonephritis, and rarely crescentic glomerulonephritis (see relevant chapters for details). Persistence of low-grade non-visible dysmorphic haematuria in the absence of hypertension or proteinuria (including microalbuminuria), and normal renal function suggests TBMN, especially if there is a family history of haematuria with an autosomal dominant form of transmission. However, it should be pointed out that the association of TBMN with IgA nephropathy is frequent (Żurawski et al., 2016). A persistently low C3 level is a clue for the presence of C3GN or DDD. A history of a streptococcal or staphylococcal infection or a high anti-streptolysin O or anti-DNAase titre may suggest resolving AGN. Fibrillary glomerulonephritis is almost always associated with a NS; whereas, in IgA N NS as a presenting feature in uncommon. A renal biopsy may be needed in most cases for accurate differentiation.

Natural history

Primary IgA N pursues a highly variable (and often unpredictable) course (D'Amico et al., 1993; Coppo and D'Amico, 2005; Berthoux, Mohey et al., 2008). Most patients will experience multiple episodes of self-limited macroscopic haematuria, often occurring shortly (within one to two days) after an acute symptomatic viral or bacterial upper respiratory infection (synpharyngitic nephritis; Clarkson et al., 1977; Kincaid-Smith et al., 1983; Praga et al., 1985). The majority of these patients will also display some degree of abnormal microscopic haematuria between episodes of gross haematuria. A minority will have only persistent microscopic haematuria, without any overt episodes of gross haematuria. The haematuria is dysmorphic in character (see Chapter 1), but not uncommonly only about 50 per cent of the erythrocytes in the urine specimen have the characteristic dysmorphism of glomerular haematuria. Proteinuria may be absent initially and slowly develop over many years. The presence of micro-albuminuria (excretion of albumin in the urine below the level usually detectable by qualitative testing [dipstick] but above normal) in conjunction with persistence of low-grade haematuria may predict the future evolution to a progressive disease (Nakayama et al., 2008). Persisting high-grade haematuria and overt proteinuria is a marker of a poor prognosis in IgA N (Sevillano et al., 2017). Haematuria with mild or absent proteinuria may not necessarily confer a poor prognosis, albeit over short follow-up periods (Tanaka et al., 2015). Occasionally, frank NS is present initially and may undergo partial or complete remission in response to glucocorticoid therapy (see 'Glucocorticoids'). Spontaneous complete remissions and permanent disappearance of all abnormal findings are distinctly uncommon in adults (about 6 per cent) but may be much more common in children (about 25–30 per cent; see Schena et al., 1990).

Progressive renal failure occurs in a substantial number of patients. Over 25 years of follow-up, about 30–50 per cent of patients with IgA nephropathy will develop end-stage renal disease (ESRD; Coppo and D'Amico, 2005; Berthoux, Mohey et al., 2008). The average rate of development of ESRD is about 1.5 per cent per year of follow-up. Some patients will experience a reduction in renal function and then stabilize at an abnormal level for many years (Fellin et al., 1988; D'Amico et al., 1993). Episodes of acute renal failure developing in association with macroscopic haematuria and upper respiratory infections is most often spontaneously reversible unless renal biopsy shows ESRD or very extensive (greater than 25 per cent) diffuse crescentic involvement (Delclaux et al., 1993). A very prolonged course of macroscopic haematuria (>10 days) in association with acute renal failure in an older subject with IgA N may confer an adverse prognosis for compete recovery of renal function (Gutierrez et al., 2007). A rapidly progressive course to ESRD is distinctly unusual. The magnitude of proteinuria at follow–up or time-averaged proteinuria is the main determinant of the rate of progression to ESRD (Barbour et al., 2015; Coppo et al., 2017). The OXFORD-MEST score also provides additional prognostic information, at least in untreated patients (Barbour et al., 2015). Extensive crescents (>25 per cent) also imply a poor outcome (Haas et al., 2017).

In those patients who develop progressive renal insufficiency, the course to ESRD is usually slow but relentless in the absence of therapy. Arterial hypertension is very common and may precede the development of progressive renal impairment by many years giving rise to a 'mis-diagnosis' of essential 'primary' hypertension. This seems to be particularly true in Caucasians and is much less true in African-Americans. Elevated blood pressure is a significant contributor to the rate of progression towards ESRD (see Chapter 1).

Once impaired renal function is well established (e.g. an eGFR of about 30 ml/min/1.73 m^2 or less or a serum creatinine level above 2.0–3.0 mg/dl, (depending on age, ancestry, and gender) with chronic fibrotic and irreversible changes in the renal biopsy it becomes increasingly unlikely that any specific intervention will slow the rate of subsequent progression (other than control of blood pressure and the use of inhibitors of renin-angiotensin system (RAS inhibitors). This stage of IgA N is often referred to as the *point of no return* (D'Amico et al., 1993; Scholl et al., 1999; Komatsu et al., 2005). The mortality risk (mostly from cardiovascular disease) is also increased in patients with IgA N, usually after ESRD has developed (Knoop et al., 2013).

Prognostic factors

Also see Table 7.1.

Age

As stated previously, children have a higher likelihood of spontaneous clinical remission, providing they do not have established and persistent proteinuria or impaired renal function at the time of diagnosis. There is some unconfirmed clinical evidence that older age at presentation is associated with a worse prognosis (Cameron, 1993). However, in a comprehensive review, the incidence of ESRD in the older IgA N patients was 1.95 times higher than that in the

Table 7.1 Factors possibly indicating a poorer prognosis of IgA nephropathy.

Clinical	Morphologic

◆ Impaired renal function at discovery (serum creatinine >1.4 mg/dl)
◆ *Hypertension (uncontrolled or poorly controlled; >130/80 mmHg)
◆ *Magnitude, persistence and quality of proteinuria (>500 mg/day total protein excretion; increased fractional excretion of IgG)
◆ Older age at diagnosis
◆ Character of haematuria (macroscopic vs. microscopic)
  • *Persistence of non-visible haematuria
◆ HLA specificities (some studies)
◆ *Low urinary EGF/MCP-1 ratio
◆ Elevated IgA/C3 ratio (>3–4:1)
◆ Increased serum C4bp levels; Low serum C4 levels
◆ Increased secretory IgA levels (?)
◆ Angiotensin converting enzyme gene polymorphisms (DD genotype)
◆ *Lack of use of inhibitors of the renin–angiotensin system
◆ Co-existent metabolic syndrome (obesity/hyperuricemia/hypertriglyceridaemia)
◆ Markers of inflammation (increased, low albumin, increased leukocytes)
◆ Increased excretion of podocytes in urine
◆ Exposure to volatile hydrocarbons (?)
  • Low birth weight and nephron endowment
	◆ *Chronic tubulo-interstitial infiltrates/fibrosis OXFORD-MEST-T-Score 1 or 2)
	◆ *Extensive crescents (OXFORD MEST C score 1 or 2)
	◆ *Advanced glomerulosclerosis (OXFORD-MEST Score- G-1
	◆ Arteriosclerosis and arteriolosclerosis (hypertension related)
	◆ Extensive mesangial proliferation (some studies)
	◆ 'Capillaritis' (IgA Vasculitis)
	◆ Extensive peripheral capillary deposits of IgA
	◆ *Fibroblast specific protein-1 in interstitium
	◆ *'Tubulitis' (with GMP+ T-lymphocytes in tubules)
	◆ *C3c/C4d deposits in mesangium
	◆ Reduced podocyte density

(* Most important)

non-older IgA N patients (Duan et al., 2013), and a large observational study from Japan (n = 31; representing about 5 per cent of all cases of IgA N studied; Oshima et al., 2015) suggested that subjects over age 60 years had lower renal survival, higher levels of proteinuria, more histological damage, and a poorer prognosis (>70 per cent reaching ESRD within 20 years) compared to younger subjects.

Gender

Gender-related differences in long-term outcome of IgA N have been inconsistently noted. Some studies have suggested a worse prognosis in males by univariate analysis (Cameron, 1993; Hogg, 1995; Deng et al., 2018).

Ancestry

Black children appear to have a worse prognosis than Caucasian children (Hogg, 1995). However, ascertainment (lead-time) bias, may contribute to the differences observed.

Geographic site

Differences in long-term outcome have been reported according to the geographic site of diagnosis. Most, but not all, of these differences are probably due to differences in renal biopsy policy and the effects of an ascertainment (lead-time) bias (Geddes et al., 2003; McGrogan et al., 2011).

Renal function

In general, impaired renal function at discovery (e.g. an abnormally elevated serum creatinine concentration) is a poor prognostic sign unless it develops acutely in conjunction with macroscopic haematuria and acute upper respiratory infection (Delclaux et al., 1993). However, even mildly impaired renal function at the time of diagnosis does not guarantee a future progressive course (Fellin et al., 1988). An initial eGFR of <90 ml/min/1.73 m^2 associated with proteinuria of ≥0.4 g/day/1.73 m^2 was determined to be a risk factor for renal disease progression in patients with IgA N (Coppo et al., 2017).

Hypertension

Established hypertension (blood pressure >140/90 mmHg) generally reflects relatively advanced underlying disease and is often associated with a progressive course if untreated (Coppo and D'Amico, 2005). Management of hypertension is an important element in retardation of progression (see also Chapter 2). In the presence of proteinuria, the level at which *hypertension* is diagnosed and treated in a subject with IgA N should be lowered from ≥140/90 mmHg to ≥130/80 mmHg in adults, or perhaps even lower.

Proteinuria

The presence of *persistent proteinuria* over 500 mg/day has been repeatedly demonstrated to be associated with an adverse long-term prognosis, unless the renal biopsy shows only minimal change disease by light microscopy (Coppo and D'Amico, 2005; Lv et al., 2008; Cattran et al., 2008; Barbour et al., 2015; Coppo et al., 2017). Persistence of >3.0 g/day of proteinuria at presentation is an ominous finding (see 'Persistent proteinuria and haematuria (with or without reduced renal function'; see also Coppo and D'Amico, 2005; Coppo et al., 2017), except when accompanied by minimal changes on light microscopy. The quality of proteinuria (e.g. increased fractional excretion of

IgG) may indicate a worse prognosis, even at equivalent degrees of total daily urinary protein exertion (Bazzi and D'Amico, 2005). It is very clear from well-done retrospective studies in large cohorts of patients with IgA N that a partial remission of proteinuria to levels less than 0.75–1.0 g/day after treatment with RAS inhibition (see 'Angiotensin-converting enzyme inhibitors (ACEi) and angiotensin receptor blockers (ARB)') are associated with a dramatically better prognosis (Reich et al., 2007; Rauen et al., 2015). However, even patients with mild disease (normal GFR and mild proteinuria) may have a long-term adverse outcome. Almost 20 per cent of subjects with assumed 'benign' IgA N at discovery (as judged clinically and pathologically) had progressive disease after a follow-up of more than 20 years (Knoop et al., 2017). Accurate prediction of this course at the time of diagnosis of IgA N was not possible.

Haematuria

It has been reported that the *persistence of non-visible (microscopic) haematuria* carries a less favourable poor prognosis (Rauta et al., 2002; Yuste et al., 2015; Sevillano et al., 2017), even in mild-to-moderate disease, but particularly when this is accompanied by overt proteinuria. Increasingly, studies show a deleterious effect for the combination of persistent microhaematuria and albuminuria on prognosis in IgA N (Shen et al., 2007; Sevillano et al., 2017). Persistent microhaematuria may be a sign of underlying *capillaritis* (see 'Pathogenesis'). On occasion, the authors have associated episodes of *macrohaematuria* with progression to ESRD and a higher frequency of crescentic lesions. (Nicholls et al., 1984; Hogg et al., 1995), but others have shown the reverse (Ibels and Gyory, 1994; Rauta et al., 2002).

HLA antigens

Some, but not all, investigators have found an association between a poor prognosis and certain HLA specificities, most notably HLA Bw35 (Berthoux et al., 1988; Almartine et al., 1991). At least 20 susceptibility loci of IgA nephropathy have been identified by genome-wide association studies to date (Feehally et al., 2010; Gharavi et al., 2011; Yu et al., 2011; Kiryluk et al., 2014). Most loci are either directly associated with risk of inflammatory bowel disease or maintenance of the intestinal epithelial barrier and response to mucosal pathogens. The geospatial distribution of risk alleles is highly suggestive of multi-locus adaptation and the genetic risk correlates strongly with variation in local pathogens, particularly helminth diversity, suggesting a possible role for host–intestinal pathogen interactions in shaping the genetic landscape of IgA N (Kiryluk et al., 2014).

Genetically-based polymorphisms

Polymorphisms of the angiotensin-converting enzyme (ACE) gene have been associated with prognosis in IgA N. A deletion polymorphism in the ACE gene, the DD genotype, may be a risk factor for progression and predict therapeutic efficacy of ACE inhibitors in IgA nephropathy (Yoshida et al., 1995; Hunley et al., 1996), but this is not consistent across all populations (Woo et al., 2004). The angiotensinogen-M235T polymorphism may predispose to progressive disease (Bantis et al., 2004). In epidemiologic cross-sectional studies, many other single nucleotide polymorphisms (SNP) have been associated with susceptibility and/or prognosis of IgA N. These findings have been difficult to replicate and may have been due to systematic errors introduced by population stratification. At the present time, assessment of SNP in IgA N does not have any established role in determining prognosis. However, as methods improve for rapid and inexpensive genome-wide scanning for SNP, it remains possible, or even likely, that markers of susceptibility and/or progression may emerge that will have great value in both epidemiologic studies as well as in individual patients.

Familial disease

At one time, patients with a family history of IgA N were thought to have a worse prognosis; however, follow-on studies have failed to replicate this effect (Izzi et al., 2006). The genetic loci currently identified as having an association with IgA N (such as the Chromosome 6;22 locus, *IGAN1*) do not appear to have any prognostic significance.

Serum IgA and complement levels

Although commonly ($\approx$50 per cent) elevated in patients with IgA N, the actual serum total or polymeric IgA levels have no prognostic utility (D'Amico, 1992). The C3 level is almost always normal or slightly reduced. Some authors have suggested that an elevated IgA/C3 concentration ratio (>3–4:1) is a sign predicting a progressive disease, but this has not yet been confirmed in multiple populations (Ishiguro et al., 2002; Maeda et al., 2003; Komatsu et al., 2004; Nakayama et al., 2008). Elevated levels of Complement 4 binding protein (C4bp) may influence prognosis (Nakayama et al., 2008) and low C4 levels can be associated with a worse, perhaps due to activation of the mannose-binding lectin pathway of complement (Zhu et al., 2015).

Urinary epidermal growth factor (EGF) to monocyte chemotactic peptide-1 (MCP-1) ratio (EGF/MCP1)

Torres and colleagues (2008) have described the utility of measuring the urinary EGF/MCP-1 ratio at the time of renal biopsy in the determination of the prognosis of IgA N. A *low* value for the EGF/MCP1 ratio (lowest tertile) was strongly associated with a progressive course. Over 60 per cent of patients with the lowest tertile of the EGF/MCP-1 ratio developed progressive renal disease after 84 months of follow-up. None of the patients in the highest tertile had any manifestation of progressive disease. At a cut-off value of 23.2 (using concentrations of ECP and MCP-1 in ng/mg urinary creatinine) the sensitivity and specificity of the EGF/MCP1 ratio for the prediction for progression was 89 per cent and 86 per cent, respectively. The actual levels of urinary protein excretion or blood pressure control *following* the diagnostic renal biopsy were not included in the multivariate model. There was also no adjustment for the red-cell excretion and the predictive power of the assay was not tested independently in another unselected cohort.

Obesity, hyperuricaemia, and hypertriglyceridaemia

Obesity, elevated blood levels of uric acid and elevated triglyceride levels have been independently associated with a worse prognosis for IgA N (Syrjanen et al., 2000; Bonnet et al., 2001; Myllymaki et al., 2005; Ruan et al., 2018). These are all components of the metabolic syndrome.

Inflammatory markers

Increased CRP, low serum albumin, and increased leukocyte count may be markers of a poor prognosis; however, these may simply reflect the state of underlying renal function (Kaartinen et al., 2008), but serum CRP levels are often normal in primary IgA N. Markedly increased CRP levels might be an indication that IgA vasculitis is present.

Exposure to volatile hydrocarbons (solvents)

Exposure to volatile hydrocarbons does not appear to be involved in the induction of IgA N. However, some studies have suggested that heavy and prolonged exposure to these substances may have a deleterious effect on prognosis and enhance progression to ESRD in patients with established IgA N (Yaqoob et al., 1994; Jacob et al., 2007). These findings are based on case-control and cohort studies. It may be prudent to advise individuals with established IgA N to avoid such exposures whenever possible.

Auto-antibodies to gdIgA$_1$ and/or serum levels of gdIgA$_1$

Measuring serum levels of gdIgA$_1$ or assessing the serum levels of IgG auto-antibodies to gdIgA$_1$ may have clinical utility in predicting outcome (Berthoux et al., 2012), but such assays are not yet broadly available nor are they well standardized, so they may not be quite ready for routine clinical application beyond research studies or clinical trials.

Low birth weight

Low birth weight (<2.5 kg) or small for gestational age is a moderate predictor of a propensity for progression to ESRD in IgA N patients (Hazard Ratio 2.9 [95 per cent–CI = 1.1–3.7]) compared to normal birth weight) based on registry data in Norway (Ruggajo et al., 2016). This effect is likely mediated by low nephron number.

Other laboratory tests

Increased urinary excretion of podocytes may indicate a poor prognosis (Hara et al., 2007).

Renal biopsy morphology

Several morphologic findings in renal biopsy have been related to a poor prognosis, including the extent of *glomerulosclerosis, chronic tubulo-interstitial fibrosis, arteriosclerosis* and *arteriolosclerosis,* and *glomerular crescents* (Coppo and D'Amico, 2005). Podocyte injury and glomerular podocytopenia has also been noted as a feature of severe and progressive injury to the glomerulus in IgA N (Lemley et al., 2002).

Several classifications and scoring systems for evaluating the character and the severity of these lesions have been developed and related to outcome in population studies (Radford et al., 1997; Cook, 2007). All these show predictive power of the classification and scoring systems in determining the course of the disease to renal failure or ESRD, especially in untreated. The OXFORD-MEST system is the best studied and validated (Working Group of the International IgA Nephropathy Network and the Renal Pathology Society, 2009, 2010; Coppo et al., 2014; see 'Pathology'). However, the prognostic power of this classification system is significantly blunted in treated patients and the improvement of prognostic accuracy by adding pathology to clinical estimation of prognosis (by hypertension, proteinuria and renal function) can be somewhat marginal (Cook, 2007). However, the OXFORD-MEST score provides an earlier risk prediction than does clinical information (Barbour et al., 2016). Subclassification of the podocytopathic features associated with FSGS lesions can add prognostic value to the classification system (Bellur et al., 2017; see also Chapter 5). The addition of crescentic lesions to the OXFORD-MEST system improves its overall utility. C1 and C2 lesions (crescents present but involving less than 25 per cent of glomeruli) and C2 lesions (crescents involving over 25 per cent of glomeruli) are associated with poorer outcomes, even with treatment (Haas et al., 2017; Trimarchi et al., 2017). Other than defining the presence of IgA N, the details of immunofluorescence microscopy are not included in the OXFORD-MEST classifications. The extent and degree of IgA deposits as assessed by immunofluorescence microscopy do not uniformly predict the outcome, although some investigators have noted that very extensive peripheral capillary wall deposits of IgA are associated with a poorer outcome (D'Amico, 1992). The presence of capillaritis and associated focal and segmental crescentic lesions likely imply an active vasculitic disease process and a poorer long-term prognosis (Ferrario et al., 1995; D'Amico et al., 2001; Haas et al., 2017).

The coexistence of thin-basement membrane nephropathy is seen more commonly in females with a family history of renal disease, but is not accompanied by an improved prognosis (Berthoux et al., 1995). Superimposition of a lesion compatible with Minimal Change Disease and the presence of NS is associated with a favourable prognosis, so long as the patient is 'steroid-responsive (see 'Nephrotic syndrome associated with minimal glomerular lesions'). The presence of extensive lesions of FSGS confers a worse prognosis, but identification of FGGS lesions appropriate for age does not (see Chapter 5).

The application of newer techniques to the study of renal biopsy specimens, such as in situ hybridization, immuno-staining for specific molecules (such as fibroblast specific protein-1, cell surface markers for T-cells infiltrating the interstitium and/or tubules (tubulitis), and quantitative polymerase chain reaction assays on microdissected glomeruli) may yet prove to add great value to the more conventional approaches to estimating prognosis from renal biopsy (Nishitani et al., 2005; van Es et al., 2008). Extensive mesangial deposits of C4d (Espinosa et al., 2009; Rath et al., 2015) or peri-tubular deposits of C3d (Gherghiceanu et al., 2005) may also be a sign of progressive disease. Morphometric analysis of podocyte density may also be of value in prognostication (Lemley et al., 2002). Glomerular hypertrophy may be a sign of low birth weight and compensatory change (Ruggajo et al., 2016).

However, it must be remembered that renal biopsy is only a 'snapshot' of a disease at a single moment in time. Thus, the findings in a single biopsy sample will reflect the cumulative and lasting effects of past events and only by inference be viewed as a 'window' to the future, absent any intervention on the natural course of disease. Whether the OXFORD–MEST-C classification system will aid decision making concerning treatment choices is not yet full known, and deserves greater study (Palumuthusingam et al., 2018; Cambier et al., 2018). However, some studies (uncontrolled) have shown improvement with combined immunosuppression in the presence of glomerular inflammation and proliferation, even in advanced disease—including crescents in some cases (Tan et al., 2018). Extensive podocyte lesions may be predictive of a poor outcome (Cambier et al., 2018). A study of the role of renal histologic findings in treatment of IgA N is in progress in France (TIGER, NCT#003188887). In addition, because IgA N is relatively common disease, it is possible for other diseases (e.g. LECT2 amyloidosis, collagen IV membranopathies, infection-related glomerulopathies, monoclonal immunoglobulin deposition disease) to be superimposed on IgA N (overt or latent) and alter its prognosis.

Formulas or indices to predict prognosis in an individual patient

Several multi-variate analyses have been carried out in an attempt to refine the ability to reliably determine the prognosis in individual patients (Beukhof et al., 1986; D'Amico, 1992; Bartosik et al., 2001; Rauta et al., 2002; Magistroni et al., 2006; Wakai et al., 2006; Manno et al., 2007; Ballardie and Cowley, 2008; Lemley et al., 2008; Mackinnon et al., 2008; Berthoux et al., 2011). These studies have attempted to deduce 'scores', 'indices', or formulae that will allow prognosis to be determined from simple assessment of the additive effect of a variety of clinical and/or histological features present at the time of diagnosis or after a relatively short period of follow-up. While these analyses have been helpful in the determination of the factors that independently contribute to prognosis, the associations have been derived in *populations* of patients, usually examined retrospectively, and thus they have severe limitations when applied to *individual* patients. Because the course of IgA N can be very indolent with long periods of stable renal function punctuated by episodes of transient renal functional impairment, one should be cautious about prognosticating in individual patients using these methods, especially since they often give conflicting results when applied at the individual patient level. Nevertheless, groupings of prognostic indicators such as proteinuria (magnitude, persistence and quality), renal function, and renal histologic classifications (OXFORD–MEST-C) have been quite useful for the selection of patients for studies of the influence of therapy on the course of disease and for the calculation of the expected frequency of selected end points in a placebo population—a critical part of determining sample size and power of a study (Ballardie and Cowley, 2008). Some, but not all, of these formulas have been validated across populations and samples (MacKinnon et al., 2008; Berthoux et al., 2011).

It should also be re-emphasized that these systems for prognostication generally account for only about 50 per cent of the variability in long-term outcome in IgA N, and some formulas *do not* include renal histologic abnormalities as such factors have not been *consistently* demonstrated to have a totally *independent* effect on prognosis, over and above simple clinical assessment, e.g. renal function, blood pressure, proteinuria, red cell excretion (Bartosik et al., 2001). Importantly, the application of several different formulas, scoring systems, or indices to individual patients with similar or identical clinical characteristics do not always provide consistent and comparable results. Much improvement is needed in prognostic tools before they can be routinely applied to individual patients, beyond dividing patients into 'good', 'moderate', and 'poor' prognostic categories. In the future, a scoring system may be produced that is valid for all patients with IgA N, even at early stages of presentation, long before any impairment in renal function is evident (Lemley et al., 2008; Nakayama et al., 2008). At this moment the Absolute Renal Risk prediction algorithm seems to work well, even in treated patients (Berthoux et al., 2011). Modification of this schema with the addition of crescentic lesion score (OXFORD-MEST-C) may be even better.

Specific treatment

No universal, evidence-based consensus recommendations have yet emerged on the specific treatment of IgA N (Barratt and Feehally, 2006). In the 2012 KDIGO clinical practice guidelines (KDIGO, 2012), evaluation for secondary causes, assessing the risk of progression by clinical and/or pathological means before commencing any treatment was advised. The only strong recommendation (Based on grade-B evidence) was to use long- term RAS inhibition (with an ACEi or an ARB) when the proteinuria persists (duration not defined) at >1.0 g/day. Less strenuous suggestions (Based on grade-C/D evidence) were that the RAS inhibition be considered when proteinuria persists at 0.5–1.0g/ day (0.5–1.0 g/day per 1.73 m² in children) and that the doses of these agents be titrated upwards (as tolerated) to achieve a proteinuria of <1.0 g/day and a blood pressure of 130/80 mmHg when proteinuria is <1.0 g/day or <125/ 75 mmHg when proteinuria is >1.0 g/day. No recommendations were made regarding combined use of ACEi and ARB or concomitant use of salt restriction, diuretics, or aldosterone receptor antagonists to achieve the desired goals of blood pressure or proteinuria. A minimum of a three-to-six-month course of such optimized supportive care was suggested (on grade-C evidence) before considering the patient a candidate for additional specific treatment and only if the GFR was >50 ml/min/1.73 m² (at the conclusion of the course of supportive therapy). The suggested next step was a six-month course or corticosteroid therapy, without any suggestions as to the optimal regimen of steroid treatment. The addition of immunosuppressive agents (such as cyclophosphamide, azathioprine, MMF [or MPA], calcineurin inhibitors) was not suggested unless crescentic disease with rapidly deteriorating renal function was present, and anti-platelet agents or tonsillectomy were also not suggested. Oral fish oils (omega-3 fatty acids) could be used, largely based on weak evidence of efficacy and a very low risk of serious side effects. Any specific treatment of IgA N and a chronic slowly progressive decline to <30 ml/min/1.73 m² was to be avoided. Exception to these general suggestions were made for IgA N and minimal change disease, AKI with visible haematuria, and crescentic disease (defined as >50 per cent crescents and a rapidly progressive course (see 'With extensive crescentic glomerulonephritis').

This was the evidence-based, state-of-the-art treatment of IgA nephropathy in about 2012, when the KDIGO guidelines were published and it was clear that much further research on treatment was needed to better define efficacy and safety of existing regimens and to establish a role for novel approaches. As the clinical course of IgA N is protracted and indolent, a large sample size and prolonged follow-up is necessary in order to yield meaningful results of randomized trials, using clinically relevant event-based, 'hard' end-points such as doubling of serum creatinine, dialysis, or transplantation or death, rather than surrogate end-points, such as declining proteinuria, haematuria, or slowing of the pace of GFR change.

Based on our current understanding of IgA N as an 'auto-immune', immune-complex mediated disease, many of the therapeutic interventions have been directed at altering the abnormal immune response and its consequences including cellular proliferation, inflammation, glomerulosclerosis and interstitial fibrosis (Table 7.2). The use of these therapeutic options in the following four clinical settings will be discussed:

- Isolated haematuria.
- Haematuria with abnormal but non-nephrotic range proteinuria (normal or impaired renal function).
- NS or nephrotic- range proteinuria.
- Acute renal failure or rapidly progressive glomerulonephritis.

Isolated haematuria

Isolated haematuria (haematuria in the absence of abnormal proteinuria) is a relatively common mode of presentation for IgA N, especially when the disease is discovered a part of a 'screening' program or incidentally when a urinalysis is performed for some other indication. Various studies suggest that the outcome of IgA N is generally favourable (at least over the short-term range of five to ten years) in patients presenting with isolated episodes of gross or microscopic haematuria without any abnormal proteinuria or histological signs of indicating an active or severe disease process. Longer-term outcome is less certain in such patients (Knoop et al., 2017) when mild proteinuria (or albuminuria) is present. Hence, aggressive therapy is not usually recommended in this group of patients and there are no prospective randomized clinical trials in this area. Nevertheless, long-term studies have indicated that ESRD can develop after 15 or 20 years in such cases, usually with the new development of

Table 7.2 Specific agents/regimens that have been used to treat IgA N.

Prevention or reduction of exogenous antigen entry:	◆ Reduction of dietary antigens (gluten-free diets; low-antigen diets) ◆ Removal of infective antigens (tonsillectomy, antimicrobials) ◆ Alteration of mucosal permeability (sodium cromoglycate, 5-amino salicylic acid, avoidance of alcohol, budesonide
Alteration of abnormal immune response or inflammations:	◆ Reduction of serum IgA levels (phenytoin) ◆ Immunosuppression/immunomodulation (prednisone, prednisolone, MP, Budesonide, cyclophosphamide, calcineurin inhibitors, azathioprine, MMF or MPA, mizoribine, RTX, leflunomide, high-dose IVIg, plasma exchange) ◆ Dissolution of immune complexes (danazol) ◆ Anti-inflammation (glucocorticoids, fish oils, angiotensin inhibition, ACTH), hydroxychloroquine, complement inhibition (eculizumab and others)
Alteration of coagulation/ thrombosis:	Inhibition of platelet aggregation (aspirin, dipyridamole, dilazep) Anti-coagulation (heparin, warfarin)
Other:	Anti-proteinuric agents (angiotensin-converting enzyme inhibitors, angiotensin receptor blockers, calcineurin inhibitors, ACTH, statins)

proteinuria (Vivante et al., 2011). Additionally, studies have also suggested that the prognosis may not be so benign in subjects with a biopsy- proven lesion of IgA N who have in addition to haematuria, an increase in albumin exertion above the normal range but below that usually detected by qualitative tests (moderate albuminuria, also known as micro-albuminuria; Sevillano et al., 2017) and those in whom the renal biopsy show early changes associated with future progression, including tubulo-interstitial inflammation (tubulitis), deposition of fibroblast specific protein-1 (FSP-1), T-cell markers. or glomerular capillaritis (see 'Pathology').

Scoring of the renal pathology by OXFORD-MEST-C criteria can also aid in the early identification of potential progression in such patients (Barbour et al., 2015). Perhaps, some of the patients with 'so-called' isolated haematuria demonstrating these 'poor prognosis' features early in the course of disease may become candidates for more aggressive specific therapy. However, it will be difficult to perform randomized controlled therapeutic trials with 'hard' end points (such as a decline renal function or ESRD) because of the slow and indolent progression in these patients. If an '*early*' therapeutic intervention in patients presenting with isolated haematuria were found to be safe and effective, then there would be a radical change in the indications for performing renal biopsy in patients presenting with isolated haematuria. If blood pressure is elevated in subjects with IgA N and isolated haematuria it should be aggressively treated, preferably with angiotensin inhibition (see Chapter 11); however, at this juncture no specific therapeutic intervention is recommended in such patients. But careful and regular follow-up with periodic examination of the urine sediment, blood pressure recordings, and evaluation of proteinuria (albuminuria) is indicated.

Haematuria with non-nephrotic range proteinuria (normal or impaired renal function)

This is a quite common mode of presentation for patients ultimately diagnosed as having IgA N, accounting for as many as 50–75 per cent of such patients in some series. Most of the therapeutic trials of IgA N have been conducted in this group of patients (see Table 7.3). Although it would be ideal to discuss treatment of patients with normal renal function separate from those with abnormal renal function, this is not possible as many of the clinical trials have included both categories of patients in the same trial. The level of proteinuria which was required for eligibility into a trial has varied, but most demanded persistent protein excretion above about 0.75–1.0 g/day, in order to enrich the trial for the expectation of events of distinctly impaired renal function and in order to assess the *surrogate* end point of a reduction in proteinuria consequent to treatment. Unfortunately, many early trials did not require that all patients receive baseline treatment with RAS inhibitors (ACEi or ARB, or both), as a condition of entry into the trial (see Chapter 1). Any imbalance in the arms of the study concerning treatment with these agents or in the degree of blood pressure control during follow-up could introduce a bias into the results.

Angiotensin-converting enzyme inhibitors (ACEi) and angiotensin receptor blockers (ARB)

Inhibition of the renin-angiotensin system with ACEi or ARB (RAS inhibition), alone or in combination, have shown beneficial effects on proteinuria and renal function in many experimental models of renal disease (reviewed in Chapter 2; GISEN, 1997; Ruggenenti et al., 1999). Apart from their ability to reduce glomerular capillary hypertension and thus provide protection against glomerular injury there is additional evidence that ACEi/ARB also have a direct effect on mesangial cell growth and proliferation, upon podocyte integrity and on inflammation and fibrosis. RAS-inhibition has pleiotropic effects, including haemodynamic, anti-inflammatory, anti-fibrotic, anti-proliferative, and anti-oxidant

Table 7.3 Effects of various therapies in patients with IgA nephropathy with haematuria and proteinuria.

	IgA levels	IgAIC	Urine RBC	Urine protein	Histology	Renal function
Gluten-free diet	↓	↓	0	↓	↓	↓
Low-antigen diet	↓	↔	0	↓	↑	↔
Tonsillectomy	↓	↓	↓	sl ↓	0	↔
Tetracycline	0	0	↓	↔	0	↔
Sodium cromoglycate	↓	↔	0	↓	0	↔
Phenytoin	↓	↓	↓	↔	↓	↓
Danazol	↔	0	↔	↓	0	↔
Corticosteroids	0	0	↓c	↓	↑*	↔**
Azathioprine	0	0	↔	↔	↑	↑
Cyclosporin A	↓	0	0	↓	0	↓
IV immunoglobulin	↔	0	↓	↓	↑	↔
Antiplatelet agents	0	0	↔	↓	↔	↔
Urokinase	0	0	↓	↓	0	↑
Fish oil	0	0	↔	↔	0	↔, ↑
ACE inhibitors	0	0	0	↓	0	↔, ↑
Mycophenolate mofetil	0	0	↔	↓→	↓→	↔
Cyclophosphamide	0	0	↓	↓	↓→	↑

0 = not done; ↔ = not changed; ↑ = improved; ↓ = decreased; * = improved in children; ** = only in patients with preserved renal function; c = in children. See text for references.

effects. Maximum effects on proteinuria are dose-related and are augmented by dietary sodium chloride restriction and/or diuretic-induced volume depletion (see also Chapter 2). The beneficial effects of these agents on the course of renal disease appear to be independent of the degree of blood pressure lowering, although some of the reported effects do appear to be directly due to lowering of systemic arterial (systolic) blood pressure (Reid et al., 2011).

RAS inhibition significantly reduces proteinuria by 30–60 per cent in patients with IgA N, although the effect is variable and those that respond appear to have higher pre-treatment proteinuria and are more likely to maintain stable renal function. In a landmark retrospective analysis of 115 patients with IgA N, Cattran and colleagues (1994) showed better preservation of renal function among hypertensive patients receiving ACEi compared with other anti-hypertensive agents.

In one of the first controlled trials in patients with IgA N, Rekola and colleagues (1991) studied the effects of enalapril (an ACEi) in patients with IgA N and a GFR above 40mL/min/1.73 m^2 and hypertension. Patients treated with β-blockers served as controls. Other medications were used when hypertension could not be controlled with monotherapy. After a mean follow-up of 1.7 years there was no deterioration in the GFR in the enalapril-treated group compared to the control group. There was also a decrease in proteinuria and increase in urine protein selectivity which did not reach statistical significance. Mean arterial blood pressures were not different between the two groups. However, no change in proteinuria was observed. Yoshida and colleagues (Yoshida et al., 1995) found that the DD genotype of the ACE gene is found in 43 per cent of Japanese patients with 'progressive' IgA nephropathy compared with only 7 per cent of those with 'non-progressive' disease. Furthermore, proteinuria declined significantly only in patients with DD and not in ID or II genotypes when ACE inhibitors were employed. Similar findings have also been described in Caucasian populations (Hunley et al., 1996). Therefore, the analysis of effectiveness of ACE inhibitors in IgA N probably should take into account ACE gene polymorphisms (Woo et al., 2004).

The combination of an ACE1 with an ARB, both at maximal recommended dosage may be more effective than either drug given alone, in terms of reducing proteinuria, slowing the progression of renal disease and offering protection from ESRD. This finding was demonstrated in the COOPERATE study, which included a large number of subjects with IgA N (Nakao et al., 2003). Unfortunately, concerns surfaced regarding the validity of the COOPERATE trial (Kunz, Friedrich et al., 2008), and the report was retracted. Nevertheless, a recent meta-analysis (excluding the COOPERATE trial results) supported the view that combinations of ACE inhibitors and ARB are more effective in reducing proteinuria than either drug used alone (Kunz, Wolbers et al., 2008), and recent trials have allowed such therapy to be employed in supportive regimens determining eligibility for randomization to specified treatment regimens (Rauen et al., 2015). More trials of dual ACEi and ARB (in maximal tolerated dosage) for retarding progression of IgA N to ESRD are needed (Fernandez-Juarez et al., 2006). Short-term studies have also shown that dual therapy (losartan and enalapril) exerts additive anti-proteinuric effects in IgA N (Russo et al., 2001). The effect of adding direct renin inhibitors (e.g. aliskerin; see Szeto et al., 2013) or mineralocorticoid receptor antagonists (e.g. spironolactone) have not been adequately explored in IgA N (see Chapter 2).

Although relatively few controlled trials of monotherapy using an ACEi or an ARB have been carried out exclusively in those with IgA N and proteinuria (Praga et al., 2003; Coppo et al., 2007), the bulk of evidence strongly indicates a substantial number (25–35 per cent) of IgA N patients with proteinuria, above at least 1 g/day and perhaps lower, benefit from therapies designed to inhibit the systemic and intra-renal effects of angiotensin II both in terms of reduction of proteinuria and slowing of the progression of renal disease. Therapy of proteinuric subjects (>500–1000 mg/day) with an ACEi or ARB (or perhaps both if either one alone fails to reduce proteinuria to goal levels) is now considered the initial treatment of choice. A period of three to six months is desirable in order to fully assess the benefits of such a regimen (Rauen et al., 2015). Some studies have suggested that ARB are the preferred initial RAS-inhibiting agents in IgA N (Woo et al., 2008).

As mentioned in the KDIGO 2012 guideline, other therapies (discussed further on in the chapter) should be reserved for those patients who exhibit unresponsiveness to ACEi or ARB, given in maximum tolerated doses or in combination of the two drugs, in terms of a decline in proteinuria of at least 30–40 per cent from baseline to a value of <0.75–1.0 g/day or who show progressive loss of renal function despite this therapy. Even a 'partial remission', a reduction of protein excretion to values of 1–2 g/day is beneficial as measured by a delay in the progression of disease to ESRD (Reich et al., 2007). The goals of RAS-inhibition therapy should be to lower the protein excretion to the lowest possible value (preferably <500–750 mg/day) without disabling or dangerous side effects. Sitting blood pressure levels should be maintained at between 120–130 mmHg systolic and 70–80 mmHg diastolic. Whether RAS-inhibition will also be effective in retarding progression of IgA N in milder cases is not well understood. The addition of steroids to RAS-inhibition as the *initial* approach needs to be confirmed in a large trial (Lv et al., 2009). The added value of aldosterone receptor antagonism upon optimal RAS inhibition is uncertain, but may be accompanied by more episodes of hyperkalaemia (see Chapter 2). Such an approach has a sound experimental rationale (Leung et al., 2011) and deserves testing in future prospective trials. The use of a direct renin inhibitor (aliskiren) has shown promising effects on proteinuria when added to ACE inhibitor or ARB treatment in IgA N (Szeto et al., 2013). Although there may be a risk of hyperkalaemia, this agent might be considered as add on therapy for RAS inhibitor-resistant patients (Simeon et al., 2018). The recent discovery that renin cleaves a C3 convertase may reawaken interest in use of this agent in IgA N and other complement dependent diseases (Békássy et al., 2018).

Fish oils

Fish oil (menhaden oil, mackerel oil) is rich in omega-3 fatty acids (eicosa-pentaenoic and docosahexaenoic acid) and appears to exert its effects through limiting the production or action of inflammatory lipids and cytokines released during the inflammatory response (Donadio and Grande, 2004; van Ypersele de Strihou et al., 1994; Dillon, 1997). One uncontrolled trial (Cheng et al., 1990) and six controlled trials of varying size and duration (Hamazaki et al., 1984; Bennett et al., 1989; Donadio et al., 1994; Petterson et al., 1994; Alexopoulos et al., 2004; Hogg, Fitzgibbons et al., 2006: Hogg, Lee et al., 2006) have been published using fish oil in IgA N.

The largest trial to date was reported from the Mayo Clinic (Donadio et al., 1994) where 55 patients and 51 controls, who were stratified by serum creatinine levels, proteinuria, and blood pressure, received fish oil (Omacor®) for two years at doses similar to the studies of Hamazaki and colleagues (1984) and Bennett and colleagues (1989). The primary end point of a doubling of serum creatinine was observed in 6 per cent of patients in the fish-oil group and 33 per cent of patients in the control group. These findings were independent of the presence of renal impairment, degree of proteinuria, or presence of hypertension at base-line. There were no changes in bleeding times or lipid levels and no sustained effect on the magnitude of proteinuria. These encouraging results have to be tempered by the fact that the control group experienced a greater deterioration in renal function (7.1 ml/min/year) than the controls in the study by Petterson (1.3 ml/min/year) (Petterson et al., 1994) and another study by Rekola and co-workers (1991a) who examined the deterioration of renal function in IgA N using Cr^{51} EDTA clearance (3.6 ml/min/year). The patients enrolled in the original Donadio et al. trial continued to show favourable results with more extended follow-up, so long as the patients continued to receive fish oil (Donadio and Grande, 2004). An additional study of fish oils in IgA N was underpowered, but showed no beneficial effects on progression (Hogg, Fitzgibbons et al., 2006). Alexopoulos and colleagues in a small study (2004) also suggested that very low dose fish oils (0.85g of EPA and 0.57g of DHA daily) also slowed the rate of progression of IgA N. If the latter study is correct, then there is no established 'dose-response' relationship for fish oils. Some studies have suggested that dosage of fish oil should be on a weight basis (40 mg/kg/day optimally; Hogg, Fitzgibbons et al., 2006) but this has not been consistently observed (Donadio et al., 2006).

A meta-analysis of all reported trials through 1996 suggested that the overall effects of fish oil were modest at best (Dillon, 1997). In addition, fish oils may act synergistically with steroids or ACEi and/or ARB. The source of the fish oil (prescription grade versus over-the-counter diet supplements) might also be a factor in the effects. Side-effects are minimal, except for mild gastrointestinal distress, excess flatulence, and an unpleasant 'fishy' odour to the breath and perspiration. Easy bruising has been very minor and not of serious concern. Fish oil therapy seems to have little effect on the magnitude of proteinuria in IgA N but its putative reno-protective effect may be more evident in those with nephrotic-range proteinuria and those with more severe disease, as manifested by renal biopsy changes or impaired renal function (Donadio and Grande, 2004). Despite the caveats regarding overall effectiveness, fish oil therapy was suggested by the KDIGO guidelines (2012), largely based on its track record of safety rather than consistent efficacy.

Glucocorticoids

As with other forms of glomerulonephritis, glucocorticoids (oral prednisone or prednisolone, intravenous (IV) methyl-prednisolone) have been used in the treatment of IgA N, in both uncontrolled and in randomized controlled trials (RCTs). Despite this, considerable uncertainty still exists concerti the overall efficacy and safety of steroids in treatment of IgA N (Glassock, 2016) and the KDIGO guidelines in 2012 judged the evidence for a benefit of steroids added to maximum supportive therapy to be of low-quality and only justifying a suggestion for their use (KDIGO, 2012).

Among the early trials of the use of steroids in IgA N was a small uncontrolled observational study of patients with IgA N and proteinuria of 2.0g/day or more by Kobayashi and co-workers (Kobayashi et al., 1988). They used an initial dose of prednisolone of 40 mg/day and subsequently tapered the dosage to a maintenance level of 15mg/day given for a period of one to three years. Patients who had initially well-preserved renal function (creatinine clearances of 70 ml/min or above) appeared to have stabilization of renal function with only one out of 15 patients developing renal failure after a follow-up of 74 months. Renal function, as measured by the serum creatinine level and creatinine clearance, continued to deteriorate at the same rate as before treatment in the group with creatinine clearances of <70 ml/min. The complications from steroid therapy included one patient with avascular necrosis of the femoral head and another with a duodenal ulcer, but no serious adverse infectious events were noted.

In another somewhat larger 'quasi-controlled' trial Kobayashi and co-workers (Kobayashi et al., 1989) studied 60 patients with IgA N and moderate proteinuria of 1–2 g/day, of which 18 were placed on a similar regimen of prednisolone for a period of two years and who were compared to 42 'controls' treated with either indomethacin or dipyridamole. As with the previous study, patients with renal impairment (creatinine clearances <70 ml/min) did poorly regardless of therapy. In patients with preserved renal function (creatinine clearance 70 ml/min or above) and those with histological scores of 6 or less according to the Pirani and Salinas-Madrigal (1968) scoring method remained stable in both the treatment and control groups. However, in patients with well-preserved renal function and histological scores of 7 or more, steroid therapy appeared to reduce proteinuria and slow the rapid deterioration of creatinine clearance. At the end of a follow-up of 79 months, six of ten (60 per cent) patients in the steroid group were stable compared to only one out of 20 (5 per cent) in the control group. Another small controlled trial (Lai et al., 1986) failed to demonstrate any benefit of glucocorticoids in smaller doses overall, but such treatment may be beneficial in NS with minimal glomerular lesions.

In order to reduce the potential problem of steroid toxicity, Waldo and colleagues (1993) used an alternate-day prednisolone therapy given at a dose of 60 mg/m^2 for a period of two to four years in an uncontrolled trial in children with IgA N and proteinuria of more than 1 g/day (using historical controls). This study revealed that therapy normalized the urinalysis, preserved glomerular filtration rate, and resulted in a fall in the glomerular activity score in repeat renal biopsies. No steroid toxicity was observed in that there was no increase in the incidence of hypertension, cataracts, growth retardation, infections or bone disease. Alternate-day steroid treatment might be a useful alternative to daily steroids in IgA N (Julian and Barker, 1993).

In a pivotal open-label randomized and controlled study of adult patients with IgA N and well preserved renal function (serum creatinine levels ≤1.5 mg/dl; 132 μmol/l; n = 86) but with established proteinuria of 1–3 g/day (average = 1.9gms/d), Pozzi and colleagues (Pozzi et al., 1999, 2004) demonstrated a long-term benefit (>10 years) of a six-month course of glucocorticoid therapy, in terms of a significant reduction in the end-point of doubling of the serum creatinine concentration over time, using a regimen of steroid treatment compared to conservative treatment (Box 7.2A shows details of the protocol). After ten years of follow-up, renal survival was 97 per cent in the patients assigned to steroids and 53 per cent of those assigned to conservative management (Pozzi et al., 2004). Renoprotection was seen mainly in those subjects who experienced a reduced protein excretion; from 1.9 g/day at baseline to 0.6 g/day at seven years (Pozzi et al., 2004; Sarcina et al., 2016). The withdrawal rate was 14 per cent and was equal in both groups. Very few of the patients randomized in this trial had received treatment with ACEi or ARB (about 16 per cent in each group), so the relevance of this approach to subjects with IgA N who fail to reduce proteinuria after aggressive treatment with ACEi or ARB is unknown. Nevertheless, the benefit persisted over a long-term follow-up and adverse effects were mild (Pozzi et al., 1999, 2004). The lasting effect of a short

---

Box 7.2A A suggested regimen for glucocorticoid therapy in IgA nephropathy: The 'Pozzi' protocol

- Beginning of months 1, 3, and 5: 1.0g IV MP for three consecutive days.
- Months 1–6: oral prednisone in doses of 0.5mg/kg every other day (at 8–9 am).
- Angiotensin-converting enzyme inhibitors or angiotensin receptor blocker to maintain blood pressure <125/70 mmHg.

Data sourced from Pozzi C, et al. (2004). Corticosteroid effectiveness in IgA nephropathy: long term results of a controlled randomized clinical trial. J Am Soc Nephrol 15:157–62.

*Note: only a fraction of patients also received continued RAS-inhibition, and there was no uniform mandatory pre-randomization supportive care regimen employed. Patients were allocated to steroid treatment + 'conventional' care or 'conventional' care only on an open-label basis).

---

course of treatment with steroids has suggested a 'legacy effect' of such therapy (Coppo, 2013).

Subsequently, additional studies have appeared adding to the controversy concerning the role of steroids in treatment of IgA N. In 2009, Manno and colleagues (2009) reported on a European randomized, open-label trial of steroids plus an ACEi inhibitor (ramipril) compared to an ACEi inhibitors alone (n = 97; see Box 7.2B for details of the treatment protocol). The baseline serum creatinine level was <1.5 mg/dl in most patients (average eGFR = 99ml/min/1.73 m^2) and urine protein was about 1.7 g/day. After a follow-up of eight years, renal survival was 96 per cent in the steroid + ACEi group, compared to 73 per cent in the ACEi monotherapy group. Side effects were mild in both groups. No lead-in period of intensive RAS-inhibition was performed and there was no steroid monotherapy arm of the study; all enrolled subjects received RAS inhibition.

A similar study carried out in China and employing open label trial design (n = 63) was reported by Lv and colleagues (2009), using cilazapril as the ACEi and somewhat higher baseline proteinuria, averaging about 2.3 g/day. Most patients had an eGFR >60 ml/min/1.73 m^2 and none had an eGFR <30 ml/min/1.73 m^2 at baseline. The steroid dosage was very similar to the Manno (2009) study. The trial was stopped prematurely at two years as interim analysis showed efficacy in the steroid + ACEi groups. After a follow-up of four years renal survival was 97 per cent in the steroid + ACEi group and 75 per cent in the ACEi only group. About 32 per cent of the enrolled subjects had received

---

Box 7.2B A suggested regimen for glucocorticoid therapy in IgA nephropathy: The 'Manno' protocol

- Months 1–2: oral prednisone in doses of 1 mg/kg/day (maximum 75 mg/day).
- Months 3–6: prednisone dosage tapered by 0.2 mg/kg/day each month.

Data sourced from Manno C, Torres DD, Rossini M, et al. (2009). Randomized controlled clinical trial of corticosteroids plus ACE-inhibitors with long-term follow-up in proteinuric IgA nephropathy. Nephrol Dial Transplant. 24: 3694–701.

*Note: 100 per cent of the patients receiving steroids also received ramipril in doses of 2.5 mg/day sufficient to achieve a blood pressure of 120/80 mmHg or less and urine protein less than 1.0 g/day). No protocol-defined period of supportive care was employed prior to randomization into ramipril only, or ramipril + steroid groups on an open-label basis).

RAS-inhibitor therapy prior to enrolment, but there was no mandatory aggressive RAS-inhibition regimen required before randomization. Side effects were generally mild.

Between 2012 and 2015 several meta-analyses and systematic reviews of steroid therapy of IgA N appeared (Lv et al., 2012; Vecchio et al., 2015); Lv and colleagues, who conducted nine RCTs involving 536 patients all with proteinuria >1.0 g/day at baseline, noted that the dose of steroids was important, in that high-dose therapy (>30 mg/day) afforded renoprotection but low-dose therapy did not, but an effective dosage threshold could not be clearly identified. Steroid therapy was associated with a lower risk of kidney failure (relative risk of 0.32; CI = 0.15–0.67), but there was a 55 per cent higher risk for adverse events (mostly non-serious). Overall the quality of the trials was low, rendering concerns about reliability and generalizability. Vecchio and colleagues (2015) came to similar conclusions but gave the trials a better rating for quality. Importantly, the studies could not consistently identify patient characteristics that might predict a better (or worse) response to treatment, such as renal pathology and OXFORD-MEST scores, or serum or urinary biomarkers.

This historical background is necessary to better understand the events of 2015–2017 that had a marked impact on our understanding of the potential benefits and hazards of steroids in IgA N. Two of the largest studies of steroids in IgA N appeared over this interval. The first of these was the STOP-IgA N trial (Rauen et al., 2015). This trial was a multicentre (European), open-label randomized trial with a unique two group, parallel, group sequential design and two hierarchal primary end-points. One of the two groups the comparison was between comprehensive supportive care vs. steroid therapy administered according to the Pozzi protocol (see Box 7.2A) combined with supportive care in patients with an eGFR of >60 ml/min/1.73 m^2 at baseline. The other group consisted of comprehensive supportive care vs. steroids (40 mg/day in tapering dosage + low-dose cyclophosphamide (three months) followed by azathioprine 1.5 mg/day for the subsequent 33 months (see 'Combined immunosuppressive therapy'). A common hierarchical primary end-point was used for both groups and consisted of a full clinical remission (UPCR <0.2 gm/gm and stable renal function) or a decrease of at least 15ml/min/1.73 m^2 from baseline level of eGFR over 36 months. A unique aspect of this trial compared to all prior trials was that 98 per cent of patients randomized had completed a six-month 'run-in' phase of comprehensive dose-titrated RAS inhibition (42 per cent ACEi alone, 23 per cent ARB only, and 24 per cent ACEi + ARB). Patients randomized to the supportive care group (n = 80) had a baseline 24-hour urine protein excretion of 1.6 g/day, while those receiving steroids + supportive care (n = 55) also had a baseline 24-hour urine protein of 1.6 g/day. The baseline UPCR of both groups was comparable at about 0.9–1.1 gm/gm. At 36 months post-randomization, the UPCR was 0.57 gm/gm, complete clinical remissions had occurred in 31 per cent, and complete disappearance of haematuria occurred in 48 per cent of the patients receiving steroids + supportive care. At 36 months, the UPCR remained unchanged at about 0.9 gm/gm in the supportive care only group, 6 per cent had developed a complete clinical remission, and 16 per cent had complete disappearance of haematuria.

Thus, steroid therapy added to continued supportive therapy induced a significantly higher rate of remission than with continued supportive care. However, no benefits could be ascertained in the change of renal function over the 36 months of the study. In the supportive care only group, 9 per cent had a decrease of eGFR >30 ml/min/1.73 m^2; similar declines were seen in the steroid + supportive care groups, but the duration of follow-up may have been too short to ascertain if such a difference might have occurred with longer follow-up (Pozzi, 2016). Observational data from VALIGA and other studies suggest that with partial (or complete) remission of proteinuria and disappearance of haematuria the long-term prognosis would have been improved (Tesar et al., 2015; Coppo, 2017; Sevillano et al., 2017). Important aspects of this study were that patients with proteinuria >3.5 g/day were not enrolled and no patient had a pre-randomization eGFR of <30 ml/min. Marked nephrotic range proteinuria is expected to be associated with a more rapid decline in eGFR than observed in this study (Tesar et al., 2015; Coppo et al., 2017). Furthermore, the OXFORD-MEST classification of patients was not used to stratify the subjects at randomization. Additionally, this study shows very clearly that a 'run in' period of intensive supportive care for six months with optimum dosing of RAS inhibitors (alone or in combination) can safely and effectively diminish proteinuria in a substantial number (about 50 per cent) of patients with IgA N and proteinuria >0.75–1.0 g/day. Serious adverse events related to therapy were relatively uncommon (<10 per cent) in the steroid + supportive care group. But severe infections, weight gain, and impaired glucose tolerance were observed in the steroid treated groups. There were no deaths reported in this group. Mild hyperkalaemia was rare.

Finally, in 2017 the results of the TESTING study of steroids in IgA N was published (Lv et al., 2017). This trial was a double-blind, placebo controlled randomized trial of steroids in IgA N with persisting proteinuria >1.0gms/d after 3 or more months of blood pressure control with RAS-inhibitors. Entry criteria included an eGFR of between 20 and 120 ml/min/1.73 m². Patients were stratified according to proteinuria < or > 3 g/day; eGFR < or > 50 ml/min/ 1.73 m² and by OXFORD-MEST scores in a renal biopsy for endocapillary pro- liferation (E0 or E1). Steroid treatment consisted of 0.6–0.8 mg/kg/day (oral methylprednisolone (MP) or a matching placebo—maximum dose 48 mg/day) for two months, then tapered by 8 mg/day each month for a total treatment time of six to eight months. This regimen is quite comparable to that employed by Manno and colleagues (2009; see also Box 7.2B). Prophylactic administra- tion of trimethoprim-sulfamethoxazole (TMP-SMX) was not required, con- sistent with other trials of a similar nature. The primary composite end-point was the first occurrence of a 50 per cent decrease in eGFR (modified later to a 40 per cent decline in eGFR), development of ESRD, or death due to kidney dis- ease. Adverse events were very carefully monitored. The study was conducted mainly in China.

The trial was well powered and it was anticipated that 750 patients would be randomized in a 1:1 fashion to the two groups and that three years should be sufficient to accumulate enough primary end-points for analysis. However, the trial was stopped early (after 262 subjects had been randomized) due to an increase incidence of serious adverse events (including death), primarily, infection-related issues occurring in 14.7 per cent of the steroid- treated group (n = 136) and 3.3 per cent of the placebo group (n = 126). An analysis of the results was conducted after the trial was stopped.

The two groups were well balanced for clinical characteristics at randomiza- tion. The urine protein excretion was 2.6 g/day in the steroid group and 2.2 g/ day in the placebo group (both values considerably higher than at baseline in the STOP-IgA N trial cited previously). The average eGFR was 60 ml/min/1.73 m² in the steroid group and 59 ml/min/1.73 m² min the placebo group. About

39 per cent of the subjects in the steroid group had an eGFR ≤50 ml/min/1.73 m² and 44 per cent of the placebo group had an eGFR <50 ml/min/1.73 m² at baseline.

After a mean follow-up of 1.5 years the primary efficacy outcome had developed in 5.9 per cent of the steroid group and 15.9 per cent of the placebo group (p = 0.019). A complete or partial remission of proteinuria occurred by 24 months in 48 per cent of the steroid group and 22 per cent in the placebo group (p = 0.05). The annual rate of decline of eGFR was -1.7 ml/min/1.73 m² in the steroid group and -6.8 ml/min/1.73 m² in the placebo group (p = 0.03). A remission of haematuria occurred in 62 per cent of the steroid group and 40 per cent of the placebo group (p = 0.005). Due to the early termination of the trial these impressive results can only be viewed as suggestive evidence of efficacy for steroid therapy and further investigation is needed to find safer and effective steroid regimens. Generalization of these finding to non-Chinese cannot be made with confidence. The benefits seen are likely the results of randomization of subjects with higher levels of residual proteinuria after RAS inhibition (e.g. > 2.0 g/day) and thus a more unfavourable short-term prognosis (Pozzi, 2016; Glassock, 2016). The adverse event profile of daily high-dose steroids was not entirely unexpected, but its severity was a surprise. This points out that there remains considerable uncertainty over the optimum dose, regimen and duration of steroid therapy that best balances efficacy and safety. A study addressing these issues involving lower doses of steroids is currently underway (TESTING-II- Low Dose Trial; NCT#01560052). In this trial daily oral MP 0.4 mg/kg/day initially (32 mg/day maximum, 24 mg/day minimum) with slow tapering over six to nine months will be studied in comparison to a matching placebo.

Taken collectively these studies on use of steroids in IgA N carried out over the last three decades strongly indicates that patients with relatively well-preserved renal function (eGFR >50 ml/min/1.73 m²), moderate proteinuria (usually well over 1.0 g/day) that persists after a three- to six-month course of vigorous RAS-inhibition, and poor histological (OXFORD- MEST) M and E scores will benefit from steroid therapy, but at a possible cost of adverse events that can be serious (Schena et al., 1990; Glassock, 2016; Coppo, 2017; Pozzi, 2016). Optimum dosing regimens are still uncertain.

Very recently, a new twist on steroid therapy of IgA N has surfaced. It has long been presumed that the putative benefits of steroids were produced via a systemic effect on pathogenesis, but the lymphoid system of the gut has also been invoked as major participant in IgA N. Thus, the rationale for a therapy that would target the mucosal system of the intestines is very reasonable. The NEFIGAN trial explored the effects of a form of potent glucocorticoid (budesonide) as a modified formulation (TRF budesonide) designed to deliver the agent to the distal ileum (and beyond) such that it would be effective locally and be metabolized after a first pass thru the liver, theoretically avoiding major systemic effects (Fellstrom et al., 2017). The trial was designed as a randomized, double-blind, placebo-controlled proof of concept (Phase 2B) study. Two doses of TRF budesonide (8 mg/day and 15 mg/day) were compared to a matching placebo with continuation of RAS-inhibition in both groups. A total of 149 patients (analysis set) were randomized after a six-month run-in of optimized RAS-inhibition. All randomized subjects had a UPCR of ≥0.5 gm/gm (or a 24-hour urine protein of ≥0.75 g/day) and an eGFR of ≥45 ml/min/1.73 m^2 at entry. They were followed for 12 months (nine-month treatment and three-month follow-up off therapy). The primary outcome was the mean change of UPCR from baseline. Patients who received active drug (8 or 16 mg/day) experienced a 24 per cent declined UPCR at nine months ($p = 0.007$), while in the placebo group UPCR increased by 2.6 per cent ($p = NS$). Side effects were common in all groups, but glucocorticoid related adverse events were particularly common in the TRF-Budesonide groups (and were more frequent in the 16 mg/day than in the 8 mg/day groups), implying a systemic effect of the TRF-Budesonide. While these are encouraging results and fully justify an extension into a pivotal Phase 3 trial, the lack of a low-dose oral absorbable steroid group for comparison and absence of plasma cortisol and ACTH levels to assess the magnitude of the systemic effects of TRF-Budesonide are weaknesses of the study and raise questions as to whether the observed changes in proteinuria are due to a localized intestinal effect (as postulated) or a systemic effect of an absorbed very potent glucocorticoid. Since the minimally effective dose of potent glucocorticoid on IgA N is largely unknown, these issues will be relevant for the further evaluation of this promising new agent (Glassock, 2017).

The role of steroids or combined immunosuppressive therapy in patients with more advanced degrees of renal insufficiency (Serum creatinine levels 1.5–2.5 mg/dl; eGFR <50 ml/min/1.73 m^2 is highly uncertain, as to date, few RCT have been performed in this group (Pozzi et al., 2002; Locatelli et al., 2003; Pozzi, 2017; see 'Special circumstances in management of IgA N').

Calcineurin inhibitors

The calcineurin inhibitors (cyclosporin A [CsA] and tacrolimus [TAC]) inhibit activation of both T and B lymphocytes and theoretically could have a beneficial therapeutic effect in IgA N. The cumulative experience with these drugs in IgA N is very limited and the results inconclusive, at best. Nephrotoxicity over prolonged use is a major concern. Lai and co-workers (Lai, Lai et al., 1988) conducted a small controlled trial comparing CsA (5 mg/kg body weight/day for

12 weeks) to untreated placebo controls. All subjects had proteinuria of at least 1.5 g/day and a creatinine clearance of >50 ml/min. There was a significant reduction in proteinuria and increase in serum albumin as early as one week after the start of therapy. These effects were present even 12 months after discontinuation of treatment. There was also a significant *rise* in serum creatinine which returned to baseline level in all but one patient after cessation of treatment (presumably a manifestation of calcineurin toxicity). This study suggests a short course of CsA may be beneficial in patients with hypo-albuminaemia and heavy proteinuria (largely because of the pronounced direct anti-proteinuric effects of CsA rather than via any systemic 'immunosuppressive' actions). However, nephrotoxicity severely limits the utility of this agent in the long-term management of the disorder unless it can be shown that CsA is effective at even lower doses (1–2 mg/kg/day). Similar short-term results have been described for tacrolimus (Zhang et al., 2012), but nephrotoxicity remains a concern and these studies did not make any comparisons to patients treated with ACEi or ARB alone.

Song and colleagues (2017) conducted a comprehensive meta-analysis of seven randomized and controlled trials involving 374 patients using calcineurin inhibiting agents in IgA N. As expected, evidence of an anti-proteinuric effect of these agents was demonstrated, but no beneficial and sometimes an adverse effect on eGFR was observed. It seems likely that the effects of calcineurin inhibitors are no better than and perhaps inferior to RAS inhibition therapy, and this class of agents is not recommended for treatment of IgA N, especially in the presence of impaired renal function (e.g. an eGFR <50 ml/min/1.73 m^2). Additional meta-analyses have suggested efficacy and safety for use of Tacrolimus plus low-dose steroids in IgA N (Zhang et al., 2018). Successful therapy with Tacrolimus has also been reported in IgA N with monoclonal Ig deposition (Sato et al., 2018).

Mizoribine

Mizoribine is a purine synthesis inhibitor with similar effects to mycophenolate mofetil. Preliminary trials of mizoribine (carried out exclusively in Japan where the agent is approved for use) has shown efficacy, but only with short term-follow-up (Nagaoka et al., 2002; Kawasaki et al., 2004; Ikezumi et al., 2008). This agent may be of value in the treatment of patients who fail to benefit from steroids, but further RCTs are needed to establish a role for this agent in IgA N (Ikezumi et al., 2008). In a small trial, 40 patients with moderate-to-severe glomerular injuries were randomly administered either pulse MP followed by a 25-month course of oral prednisolone or in combination with mizoribine.

Both therapeutic regimens significantly reduced the levels of proteinuria, but no additional effect of mizoribine was seen (Masutani et al., 2016).

Mycophenolate mofetil and mycophenolate sodium

Salts of mycophenolic acid (mycophenolate mofetil [MMF] and mycophenolate sodium [MPS]) have been used to treat IgA N. Only the former has been subjected to prospective randomized clinical trials and meta-analysis (Navaneethan et al., 2008; Chen et al., 2014; Liu et al., 2016). The results of the trials of MMF in IgA N have thus far been inconsistent or inconclusive. Two trials from China showed beneficial effects on proteinuria in short-term follow-up (Tang et al., 2005; Chen et al., 2002). Two trials in the US showed no clear benefit for MMF, but both had low power to demonstrate efficacy and one enrolled only patients with far-advanced disease (Hogg et al., 2004; Hogg et al., 2015; Frisch et al., 2005). One well-conducted randomized trial in Europe showed no benefit (Maes et al., 2004), despite a design that was very similar to the Chinese studies. It is possible that the divergent effects observed in these trials are consequent to some confounding variable, such a pharmacokinetics or pharmacodynamics of MMF which differ among the enrolled subjects (Yau et al., 2007). A fixed dose regimen may not be appropriate for all subjects (Yau et al., 2007). A meta-analysis of eight RCTs did not find significant difference between therapeutic regimens with and without MMF for renal remission and ESRD. A subgroup analysis showed that MMF was significantly more effective compared with the placebo. This data demonstrated that MMF is more effective than placebo, had similar efficacy to other immunosuppressants in inducing renal remission, and did not increase the risk of adverse events (Zheng et al., 2018). Therapeutic monitoring of plasma MPA levels might provide better results.

Histological improvement (reduced endocapillary hypercellularity and crescents) has been observed following treatment with MMF, often combined with IV pulses of MP. This approach to therapy might have some beneficial effect in the more severe proliferative and crescentic forms of the disease (OXFORD-MEST-C1 or C2) and impaired renal function with marked proteinuria (Beckwith et al., 2017; Roccatello et al., 2012). Poor results from MMF therapy can be expected in those cases with advanced interstitial fibrosis (OXFORD-MEST-T1/T2; Kang et al., 2015). MMF may exhibit some degree of a steroid-sparing effect (Hou et al., 2017). Further trials will be necessary to establish a role for MMF in the therapy of IgA N as the evidence for efficacy is presently contradictory and of low quality (Chen et al., 2014). This agent is not recommended for use in IgA N except perhaps in individuals of Asian ancestry or those with florid proliferative/crescentic disease and impaired renal function (Roccatello et al., 2012).

Sequential cyclophosphamide–azathioprine

A small RCT of low-dose (1.5mg/kg/day) oral daily cyclophosphamide for three months followed by long-term low dose azathioprine (also at 1.5 mg/kg/day) (plus low-dose steroids) has been carried out by Ballardie and Roberts (2002). The patients were selected for randomization on the basis of progressive decline in renal function during a period of observation (in the absence of crescentic disease on renal biopsy). All patients had a significant decline in renal function prior to randomization and the rate of decline would have predicted the early onset of ESRD. The use of the sequential cyclophosphamide/azathioprine regimen was associated with a marked protection from further decline in renal function and from ESRD, but the control group fared particularly poorly. Not all of the patients randomized were treated with ACEi or ARB.

The STOP-IgA N trial (see 'Glucocorticoids') also randomized 27 patients with IgA N and a baseline eGFR between 30 and 60ml/min/1.73 m^2 to receive a Ballardie–Roberts regimen (Rauen et al., 2016). No benefits were observed compared to continued supportive care with RAS inhibition. Similar regimens have been reported to be successful in the treatment of severe crescentic glomerulonephritis associated with IgA N in case reports or small series, but no controlled trials have been done (McIntyre et al., 2001). This regimen is currently not recommended for patients with progressive IgA N, except in the presence of severe (OXFORD-MEST-C1/2) crescentic disease a rapidly progressive course.

Leflunomide

Small trials with short-term follow-up have suggested beneficial effects of this agent in IgA N (Lou et al., 2006). Lou and colleagues (2006) ran a controlled comparative trial involving 60 patients with IgA N, where 30 were treated with leflunomide and 30 were treated with fosinopril, an ACEi. The composite complete remission rate (both groups combined) was 62 per cent and there was no overall difference in the efficacy of leflunomide compared to fosinopril. Side effects were mild and equal in both groups. In a small short-term comparison trial from China, Liu and colleagues (2010) showed equal efficacy to MMF in patients with IgA N presenting with NS. Leflunomide, like MMF, may have steroid sparing effects in patients with progressive disease (Min et al., 2017). Leflunomide combined with telmisartan might also have beneficial effects but this has not yet been independently confirmed (Wu et al., 2016). The long-term safety and benefits of this drug (approved for use in rheumatoid arthritis in the US), including protection from the development of ESRD, are not yet known and further trials are needed in order to establish a role for this drug in the treatment of IgA N. Leflunomide is not recommended for treatment of IgA N, except as part of an ongoing trial, or as 'rescue' therapy for treatment resistant cases with progressive disease.

Azathioprine

Azathioprine has been regarded as a weak and largely ineffective immunosuppressive agent for IgA N, despite its low risk for side effects and good long-term record of safety in renal allografts. However, the results of an extensive retrospective observational study conducted by Goumenos and colleagues (1995) at Sheffield Kidney Institute (UK) stimulated a re-evaluation of this position. They studied 114 patients (adults and children) with IgA N; 66 were treated with long-term azathioprine (2 mg/kg/day) plus low-dose prednisolone and were compared with 48 patients not receiving either azathioprine or steroids. Both received vigorous conservative measures, including blood-pressure control, usually with agents other than ACEi or ARB. The clinical course in the treated patients was different from that in the 'untreated' patients only for those who presented with initial renal impairment (serum creatinine >110 μmol/l, >1.25 mg/dl). A 'non-progressive' course was seen in 80 per cent of the treated group and in only 36 per cent of the untreated group. No consistent effect on proteinuria was noted. Side effects occurred in 15 per cent of treated patients, which were serious in 3 per cent. Repeat renal biopsies showed stable lesions in patients with a 'non-progressive' course and deterioration in those with a 'progressive' course. Pre-treatment biopsies showing mesangial proliferation, interstitial inflammation, and C3 and fibrin deposition (possibly indicative of a capillaritis) predicted a beneficial response to therapy. Although this is an observational and retrospective study, the treated group had more factors indicating an unfavourable prognosis.

However, RCTs comparing the Pozzi regimen of steroid therapy (see Box 7.2A) with and without added azathioprine have not confirmed a beneficial effect of azathioprine, and have also pointed out the potential for harm (Pozzi, 2007; Pozzi et al., 2010; Pozzi et al., 2016). No additional benefits of adding azathioprine were observed, and an increase in side effects were noted in those subjects assigned to the azathioprine arm of the study. Thus, azathioprine, at least when given with steroids, is not considered to be effective and safe therapy for IgA N, and it is not recommended.

Rituximab (RTX) and other B-cell depleting agents

Rituximab (RTX) is a chimeric anti-CD20 monoclonal antibody that was originally used to eradicate CD20⁺ B-cell lymphomas. More recently, the drug has been applied with success in minimal change disease (Ravani et al., 2016), primary membranous nephropathy (Ruggenenti et al., 2012), lupus nephritis (Rovin et al., 2012), and vasculitis (Jones et al., 2015).

No clear evidence exists that RTX is effective in IgA N (Barbour and Feehally, 2017). A small open-label, randomized trial in patients with IgA N (serum creatinine 0.9–2.4 mg/dl) showed no benefits of RTX compared to conventional therapy (Lafayette et al., 2017), despite adequate depletion of circulating B-cells. Interestingly RTX therapy also failed to decrease the serum level of anti-gdIgA$_1$ antibodies, perhaps explaining the absence of benefit. Anecdotal cases of patients with IgA N or IgA vasculitis (including those with crescentic disease) treated with RTX or other B-cell depleting agents have been more encouraging (Lundberg et al., 2017). The efficacy of RTX in IgA vasculitis has been reported in a few cases (Fenoglio et al., 2017). Larger studies with adequate follow-up are needed to assess the value of RTX in patients with ANCA-associated crescentic glomerulonephritis and IgA N.

Very limited trials of proteasome inhibiting agents (e.g. bortezomib) to affect B-cell elaboration of antibodies in IgA N have been reported so far (Hartono et al., 2018), but preliminary findings indicate a potential anti-proteinuric effect. Toxicity of these compounds may limit their usefulness for long treatment term treatment, but development of less toxic analogues may change this pessimistic outlook.

Adrenocorticotrophic hormone (ACTH)

Very few cases of IgA N treated with ACTH (intact natural ACTH in an intramuscular long-acting gel formulation; ACTHAR gel®, Mallinckrodt) have been reported (Bomback et al., 2012). Reductions of proteinuria by 50 per cent or more have been seen in about one-third of cases of IgA N refractory to other therapies (Prasad et al., 2018). Based on current evidence it is not possible to determine whether this treatment is efficacious or safe, or able to prevent progression to ESRD. The preparation is approved by the US Food and Drug Administration (USFDA) for use in primary IgA N accompanied by NS (in the absence of 'uraemia'). A trial of ACTHAR gel® in IgA N is underway (NCT#02282930). A small pilot uncontrolled study of ACTHAR gel in IgA N was presented in Abstract form at the American Society of Nephrlogy meeting in 2018, with promising short term results (Zand L, et al- ASN Abstracts, 2018). A full publication is eagerly awaited.

Other combinations of immunosuppressive agents

Yoshikawa and colleagues (1999, 2006) conducted a series of controlled trials of a combination therapy approach, using prednisolone, azathioprine, heparin–warfarin, and dipyridamole, in children with 'severe' forms of IgA N associated with diffuse mesangial proliferation, including crescents in 16–21 per cent of glomeruli. No studies of this combination approach have been carried out in adults. The comparison has been with the four-drug combination of prednisolone, azathioprine, heparin–warfarin, and dipyridamole to the two-drug combination of heparin–warfarin and dipyridamole (Yoshikawa et al., 1999), or the four-drug combination to prednisolone alone (Yoshikawa et al., 2006). In the study involving the four-drug comparison to the two-drug regimen of heparin and dipyridamole, the four-drug combination was superior in terms of reducing 'immune injury', proteinuria and haematuria, and glomerulosclerosis. No differences in renal function could be shown at two years of follow-up; most of the subjects had normal renal function at entry. In the study comparing the four-drug regimen to prednisolone alone, the primary end-point of a complete remission of proteinuria (<0.1 $g/m^2/day$) the group receiving the four-drug combination was 92 per cent of patients randomized; while those assigned to the prednisolone-only arm of the study reached the primary end-point in 74 per cent of instances (p = 0.0007 by log rank statistics). Glomerulosclerosis progressed only in the prednisolone-only treated subjects. Adverse events were similar. These encouraging results have not yet been duplicated in adults with IgA N, so no recommendations can be made. A more recent RCT has suggested that with addition of warfarin/dipyridamole to a regimen of mizoribine and prednisolone offers little in the way of additional efficacy and adds concerns of safety (Shima et al., 2018).

Small observational trials have suggested that sequential therapy of progressive IgA N with oral cyclophosphamide and Mycophenolic acid (Rasche et al., 2016) or IV MP pulses followed by oral prednisone and MMF (Roccatello et al., 2012) might be beneficial. Such suggestions have not yet been examined by RCTs.

High-dose intravenous immunoglobulins

High-dose IV immunoglobulin (IVIg) therapy (see Chapter 3) have been effective in some forms of immune-mediated diseases (Hammarstromm et al., 1992) as there appears to be a deficiency in the IgG_1 subclass in proteinuric patients with IgA N and Henoch–Schönlein purpura (Rostoker et al., 1994). Rostoker and colleagues (1995) studied the effects of high-dose IVIg in a small uncontrolled study of patients with IgA N or Henoch-Schönlein purpura disease who had moderate to severe histological changes, proteinuria of >2 g/day, and a glomerular filtration rate >35 ml/min. IVIg were given at a dose of 1g/kg/body weight/day on two successive days each month for three months, followed by intramuscular immunoglobulins at a dose of 0.35ml/kg/body weight twice each month for another six months. At the end of the study period there was a decrease in proteinuria, haematuria, and leukocyturia. The rate of decline in the GFR was reduced and repeat renal biopsies following therapy revealed a reduction in histological index of activity and a decrease in the staining intensity of glomerular IgA and C3 deposits. This may be a promising approach, especially in patients with a relatively rapid course of declining renal function, but randomized trials are necessary to fully evaluate the benefits and risks of this approach to treatment. Additional uncontrolled trials have in general supported these findings (Rasche et al., 2006). The discovery that an extremely potent anti-inflammatory fraction of heavily sialyted IgG can be isolated from polyclonal Ig preparations, may change the way we view this form of treatment (Kaveri et al., 2008; see also Chapter 2), but at this moment such therapy cannot be recommended for treatment of IgA N until further trials confirm its efficacy and safety.

Tonsillectomy

Surgical removal of the palatine tonsils has long-been advocated as a therapy for IgA N (particularly in some prefectures in Japan and in parts of France), usually combined with oral or pulse glucocorticoids (Bene et al., 1993; Rasche et al., 1999; Hotta et al., 2001; Miyazaki et al., 2007; Suwabe et al., 2007; Komatsu et al., 2008; Moriyama et al., 2014; Hoshino et al., 2016; Liu et al., 2015; Duan et al., 2017). All of the observational, cohort, and 'quasi-controlled' studies reported so far are biased by possible confounding or patient selection and most have used historical rather than concurrent case-controls. Komatsu and colleagues (2008) reported on a trial where steroid 'pulse' therapy alone was compared to tonsillectomy plus 'pulse' steroids. This was not an RCT. Nevertheless, patients who had their tonsils removed (all of whom had had 'chronic tonsillitis') did demonstrate a higher clinical remission rate at 24 months and had fewer proliferative lesions on re-renal biopsy. It could not be demonstrated that the treatment altered the progression to ESRD due to the short-term follow-up. In a non-randomized, long-term cohort study Hoshino and colleagues (2016) suggested a better outcome with tonsillectomy + pulse corticosteroids in those patients with proteinuria over 1 g/day. Two meta-analyses of observational studies focusing on long-term outcomes, suggested that this therapy might produce some protection form ESRD (Lie et al., 2015; Duan et al., 2017). Also, tonsillectomy may be more beneficial in those with marked mesangial hypercellularity of diffuse C1q deposition (Hirano et al., 2016; Nishiwaki et al., 2015). The size of the tonsils has no bearing on the 'success' of the therapy (Sato et al., 2017). The mechanisms underlying the putative benefits of tonsillectomy are unclear but might be due to removal of pathogen sources and a reduction in the mucosal production of gdIgA$_1$ (Vergano et al., 2015; Nakata et al., 2014).

Unfortunately, until recently this treatment strategy has not been subjected to a randomized clinical trial. In 2014, Kawamura and co-workers reported on a multicentre RCT of tonsillectomy combined with steroid pulse therapy compared to steroid pulse therapy alone in patients with IgA N. The results were disappointing, showing no clear benefits of the tonsillectomy + pulse steroid treatment compared to steroid pulses alone for clinical remission or reduction of haematuria. The trial was too short to ascertain any effect on ESRD incidence. A modest anti-proteinuric effect of the combined treatment was shown, but the long-term significance of this effect is uncertain. In a post hoc, subanalysis of this trial, it was suggested that the presence of crescents (active cellular or fibrous) might predict a better response to tonsillectomy + steroid pulse therapy (Katafuchi et al., 2016). This hypothesis has not yet been tested in a prospective trial. Studies if this therapy in Europe have been largely negative and not supportive of the findings reported by Japanese investigators (Feriozzi and Polci, 2016; Feehally et al., 2016).

Despite its lack of proven long-term benefits, this form of therapy remains popular in certain prefectures in Japan, but is seldom used for treatment of IgA N in the US or in many other geographic areas. In a large survey of over 1000 patients with IgA N treated at a single centre in Japan, 12 per cent of subjects were treated with this therapy (Moriyama et al., 2014). Rarely, tonsillectomy may be associated with the development of macroscopic haematuria and acute renal failure. Tonsillectomy apparently does not prevent the recurrence of IgA N in the transplanted kidney (Sato et al., 2014). Therefore, at the present time, tonsillectomy (with pulse steroids) is not regarded as an established form of therapy for IgA N (Zand and Fervenza, 2014). This treatment is not recommended for therapy of IgA N.

Anti-platelet, anti-coagulant, and thrombolytic agents

The rationale for the use of anti-platelet, anti-coagulant, or fibrinolytic therapy in IgA N has been based on the findings that platelets and coagulation play a role in the pathogenesis of glomerular disease, and also that microthrombotic lesions within the glomerulus may contribute to the progression of renal disease (Cameron, 1984). This subject area was extensively reviewed in the last edition of this book (Glassock and Lee, 2009) and very few new studies have been reported. A meta-analysis of anti-thrombotic therapy of IgA N concluded that such agents might have an effect on proteinuria, but have no reno-protective effects on progression to ESRD (Liu et al., 2011). A small, randomized study of combinations of steroids, azathioprine, heparin-warfarin and dipyridamole compared to heparin-warfarin and dipyridamole alone suggested benefits on long term outcome for the combination regimen of in childhood IgA N (Kamei et al., 2011). At the present time, none of these agents have a role in therapy of primary IgA N.

The overall long-term benefits (and risks) of anti-platelet and anti-coagulant therapy in IgA N remain very unclear at present, although the therapy generally reduces proteinuria modestly over the short term. Warfarin may induce episodes of AKI and be harmful (Brodsky et al., 2012). Therapy of IgA N with anti-thrombotic agents is not recommended. A recent RCT also emphasizes the potential hazards of anticoagulants in IgA N (Shima et al., 2018).

Anti-microbials

There is only one brief report of a controlled trial using *tetracycline* for one year in patients with IgA N (Kincaid-Smith and Nicholls, 1983). This small trial showed that although there was a significant reduction in the magnitude of haematuria, the serum creatinine and proteinuria remained unchanged. There have also been numerous anecdotal reports of the use of antibiotics in children with IgA N where they were found not to change the rate of gross haematuria. Anti-microbial may be of clinical value in treatment of IgA-dominant infection-related glomerulonephritis (see Chapter 9).

Sodium cromoglycate, 5-aminosalicylic acid, danazol, and phenytoin

Both sodium cromoglycate, an anti-allergic agent, and 5-aminosalicylic acid alter mucosal permeability to food antigens. However, as reviewed by Glassock and Lee in the last edition of this book (2009), there are no clear benefits in IgA N and no new information has been published subsequently. Phenytoin sodium, an anticonvulsant agent with pleotropic properties, has been shown to consistently reduce serum total IgA levels (Seager et al., 1975) thus justifying the trial of its use in patients with IgA N. But no evidence of efficacy in IgA N has been forthcoming (Glassock and Lee, 2009). Danazol, a heterocyclic anabolic steroid, increases serum complement levels in patients with complement deficiency such as hereditary angioneurotic oedema (Pappalardo et al., 2003) and may thus assist in solubilizing IgA glomerular deposits. But no clear evidence of efficacy in IgA N has been reported to date (Glassock and Lee, 2009). These therapies are not currently recommended for treatment of primary IgA N.

Restricted diets and weight reduction

Increased levels of IgA antibodies to a variety of alimentary antigens, most frequently anti-gliadin IgA (Fornasieri et al., 1987; Fornasieri et al., 1998; Rodriguez-Soriano et al., 1988; Rostoker et al., 1988) have been described in patients with IgA N and a few studies have also demonstrated that food antigens participate in the formation of IgA immune complexes (Fornasieri et al., 1988;

Sancho et al., 1988). Coeliac disease and dermatitis herpetiformis, both linked to gluten sensitivity, can be associated with IgA N (Cheung and Barratt, 2015). The gut microbial and diet might interact with a genetic predisposition to promote IgA N (Coppo, 2017). Very few trials of dietary treatment of IgA N have been conducted. To study the effects of a reduction in dietary antigens, Coppo and co-workers (Coppo et al., 1990) used a *gluten-free* diet in adults with serum creatinine ranging from 0.5–2.7 mg/dl, for a period of six months to four years. There was a reduction in proteinuria and microscopic haematuria after six months on the gluten-free diet. However, serum creatinine levels continued to rise suggesting that although some immunological abnormalities were corrected, the diet did not favourably alter the clinical course. A short anecdotal report by Ferri and colleagues (1992) showed that an *oligo-antigenic diet* could reduce proteinuria, but there were no changes in renal function. Follow-up of patients upon return to 'normal' diet was lacking. It appears from these limited trials that dietary restrictions (gluten) do not offer much benefit apart from a reduction in proteinuria, but larger-scale trials and longer follow-up are probably warranted. It is noteworthy that patients with proven gluten-sensitive enteropathy (with anti-gliadin antibody positivity and an abnormal small intestinal biopsy) do have an increased incidence of IgA glomerular deposits and in such patients a gluten-free diet may be beneficial.

In obese subjects with IgA N, caloric restriction will result in a diminution of proteinuria if weight loss occurs, but the long-term benefits are unknown (Kittiskulnam et al., 2014).

Oral calcitriol

A small trial reported beneficial effects on proteinuria of oral calcitriol (0.5 µg twice weekly) in IgA nephropathy (Szeto et al., 2008). A small open label, non-placebo RCT comparing oral calcitriol (0.5 µg twice a week) for 48 weeks to not treatment in patients with IgA N and proteinuria >0.8 g/day found a short-term decline in proteinuria but no effect on eGFR (Liu et al., 2012). Both groups received RAS inhibition. A meta-analysis of seven trials and 310 (mainly Chinese) subjects conclude that calcitriol will lower proteinuria in IgA N with few adverse events, but no effects are seen on GFR over short-term observations (Deng et al., 2017). Calcitriol is not yet recommended for treatment of IgA N.

Complement inhibition

No major clinical trials of complement inhibition in IgA have yet been reported, although there is interest in the subject as activation of the lectin and alternative pathways of complement are involved in the pathogenesis of IgA N (Maillard et al., 2015). Trials of a MASP inhibitor (Lectin Pathway;

OMS-721l NCT#03060833) and a C3 inhibitor (Alternative Pathway; APL-2; NCT#03453619) are currently in progress. Very rarely a clinically expressed atypical haemolytic uremic syndrome and a thrombotic micro-angiopathy may occur in IgA N. It is possible that eculizumab—a C5 convertase inhibitor (see Chapter 3)—therapy might be useful in such patients. In addition, anecdotal cases suggest short-term benefits of eculizumab in severe crescentic forms of IgA N unresponsive to conventional therapy (Ring et al., 2015).

Statins

Only one small observational trial of the effect statin therapy for IgA N has been reported (Moriyama et al., 2014). While proteinuria did not decline the eGFR stabilized. The evidence is insufficient to recommend statin therapy or IgA N except when it is indicated to manage abnormal levels of LDL-cholesterol.

Hydroxychloroquine

Two studies, one an RCT, have suggested that hydroxychloroquine has potent anti-proteinuric action in IgA N, when added to RAS inhibition (Gao et al., 2017; Yang et al., 2018). These have been short-term studies so it is not known if hydroxychloroquine has reno-protective properties. However, the agent is reasonably safe (serial retinal examinations are required to evaluate retinal toxicity) so it might be a candidate for treatment of patients with low-grade proteinuria or those who fail to achieve a target level of proteinuria after aggressive RAS inhibition.

Other investigational agents

The use of microRNAs for treatment of IgA N remains in the sphere of investigation, but their potential is great and might be a paradigm-shifting advance in treatment if efficacy and safety can be shown in an RCT (Selvaskandan et al., 2018). Trials are also underway to examine the effects of a CTLAIg fusion protein (abatacept; NCT#02808429) and a Nrf-2 agonist (bardoxolone; NCT# 03366337) I in IgA N. An inhibitor of spleen tyrosine kinase (fostamanitib; NCT#02112838) is in progress (McAdoo and Tam, 2018).

Special circumstances in IgA N management

IgA N and moderately reduced renal function

Often, patients with IgA N present with moderately advanced CKD (eGFR 20–50 ml/min/1.73 m^2) after a relatively silent but slowly progressive course. Such patients represent a conundrum in therapeutics as little if any data from randomized clinical trials is available and applicable to these subjects (Locatelli et al., 2003). Observational studies have suggested that steroid therapy might be beneficial even at levels of eGFR less than 50 ml/min/1.73 m², especially in the presence of high-grade proteinuria, but the threshold of eGFR where treatment efficacy is lost is not well understood (Tesar et al., 2015). A consensus has developed that an eGFR of 25–30 ml/min/1.73 m² or less in the presence of advanced chronic changes on renal biopsy (glomerulosclerosis and interstitial fibrosis) are signs of futility of immunosuppressive therapy—the 'point-of-no-return'. In a small randomized study Pozzi and colleagues (2013) compared the effects of a Pozzi steroid regimen + azathioprine to a Pozzi regimen alone (see Box 7.2A) in 46 patients with IgA N and an initial serum creatinine of >2.0 mg/dl (eGFR 20–31 ml/min/1.73 m²). Proteinuria fell in both groups and the six-year renal survival (defined as freedom from a 50 per cent increase in serum creatinine from baseline) was 50 per cent in the steroid + azathioprine group and 57 per cent in the steroid only group (p = ns). Adverse events were twice as common in the steroid + azathioprine group (30 per cent) compared to the steroid only group (15 per cent). There was no untreated control group for comparison. Additionally, Frisch and co-workers found no benefit (or even harm) for MMF therapy of a similar group of IgA N patients with moderately reduced renal function (mean serum creatinine = 2.4 mg/dl; Frisch et al., 2005) and a sequential cyclophosphamide-azathioprine + low dose steroids was ineffective in a subset of IgA N with eGFR 30–60 ml/min/1.73 m² in the STOP-IgA N study discussed previously (Rauen et al., 2015).

Management of IgA N in pregnancy

There is virtually no data on treatment of IgA N during pregnancy but pregnancy seems to have little or no impact on the long-term outcome of IgA N, as long as the serum creatinine is <1.2 mg/dl at the time of diagnosis (Limardo et al., 2010). However, pregnancy in women with IgA N have a higher risk of infant loss, preterm delivery, low birth weight, and toxaemia of pregnancy (Liu et al., 2016). RAS inhibition, MMF and MPA, and cyclophosphamide, but not steroids, CNI, or azathioprine, are contraindicated during pregnancy. Glucocorticoids, azathioprine, and CNI may be considered to be relatively safe.

Atypical forms of IgA N

Nephrotic syndrome (NS) associated with minimal glomerular lesions

The NS is a rather uncommon presentation of IgA N with a frequency ranging from 0–13 per cent (average about 5 per cent). Although nephrotic-range proteinuria has been associated with a poor prognosis. Virtually all the reported cases of *steroid-responsive NS* in adults and children with IgA

N have only minimal glomerular changes on renal biopsy. In such cases, the NS runs a course similar to *idiopathic* minimal change nephropathy (see also Chapter 4) with relapses that usually remain steroid responsive. It is uncertain, at present, if this entity is a variant of IgA N, or whether it is actually minimal change disease with incidental IgA deposits (Southwest Pediatric Nephrology Study Group, 1985). Two studies (Cheng et al., 1989; Fukushi et al., 1989) report the disappearance of the IgA deposits in four patients following steroid therapy, with one concluding that this was more likely the result of a variant of minimal change nephropathy (Fukushi et al., 1989) and the other suggesting that it is a distinct clinical syndrome (Cheng et al., 1989).

Despite the confusion in classifying this entity, there is general agreement that this group of patients should be treated with steroids as they have a favourable prognosis (Lai et al., 1986). Lai and colleagues (1986) conducted a small open-label controlled trial in nephrotic patients with IgA N, with varying severity of histology on renal biopsy, using prednisolone or prednisone at a dose of 40–60 mg/day with subsequent tapering of the dose after eight weeks and a total treatment period of four months compared to no treatment in the controls. After a mean follow-up of 38 months there was no significant difference in the serum creatinine levels and creatinine clearances between the two groups. Moreover, 40 per cent of patients on steroid therapy developed complications. However, despite the *overall* lack of benefit of steroid therapy in IgA N with NS, there was excellent remission rate of 80 per cent of patients with mild histological changes only. This study confirms the observation that patients with IgA N, mild renal histology and the NS clearly benefit from steroid therapy. Relapses in these patients usually respond again to steroids although cyclophosphamide at a dose of 1.5–2.0 mg/kg/body weight for about 8–12 weeks (Southwest Pediatric Nephrology Study Group, 1985) may be required in the frequent relapsing patient. Patients with IgA N and minimal glomerular lesions with NS should be treated as described in Chapter 4 on minimal change disease. Newer therapies, such as MMF or RTX have not been studied in this group of patients.

In a more recent study, 33 patients with biopsy-proven IgA N and NS were followed for 62 ± 45 months. Complete remission occurred in ten steroid users and two steroid non-users. Partial remission occurred in seven steroid users, and eight steroid non-users. During follow-up, six patients showed progressive deterioration of renal function. Among the IgA N patients with NS, 36 per cent and 45 per cent of patients had complete and partial remission, respectively. Steroid treatment may effectively reduce proteinuria. However, spontaneous remission occurs in some case (Jeong et al., 2017).

Acute and/or rapidly progressive renal failure

Acute or rapidly progressive renal failure are uncommon presentations in IgA N, occurring in about 10 per cent or less of patients of which 20–25 per cent might require temporary dialysis. Acute renal failure occurs: (i) in association with the development of *diffuse and extensive crescentic glomerulonephritis;* or (ii) following an episode of *gross haematuria* in which the renal biopsy reveals minor glomerular changes (including occasional segmental crescents most often involving <10–20 per cent of glomeruli) but marked *acute tubular necrosis, interstitial nephritis,* and marked red cell casts in the tubule lumina (Kincaid-Smith et al., 1993; Delclaux et al., 1993; Fogazzi et al., 1995). A separate discussion of these two clinical forms are needed. IgA dominant infection-related glomerulonephritis is discussed in Chapter 9.

With extensive crescentic glomerulonephritis

Any crescents are seen in about 36 per cent of renal biopsies in IgA N (Haas et al., 2017) but only 14 per cent have over 10 per cent, and 3 per cent have crescents involving over 25 per cent of glomeruli. As discussed earlier, crescents have now been added to the OXFORD-MEST-C classification of renal pathology in IgA N. Any crescentic involvement (C1 or C2) increases the risk of a poor outcome (without immunosuppression), but a precise threshold of percentage involvement above which an aggressive immunosuppressive approach to therapy should be pursued has been difficult to establish but values between 16 and 25 per cent or more of glomerular involvement (with an adequate sample of at least glomeruli in the biopsy specimen), especially in the presence of a rapidly progressive clinical course. Segmental crescents involving less than 10 per cent of glomeruli seem to have only a minor and inconsistent effect on prognosis (Shi et al., 2011). Anti-neutrophil cytoplasmic antibody (ANCA)-positive crescentic glomerulonephritis is uncommon in IgA N (about 1–2 per cent), but it may indicate a better prognosis (with therapy) than ANCA-negative crescentic glomerulonephritis (Yang et al., 2015).

Not surprisingly, there have been no controlled therapeutic studies as the condition of rapidly progressive glomerulonephritis with extensive crescents is uncommon in IgA N (around 5 per cent of cases have this presentation). Anecdotal reports have described the use of various therapeutic regimens which include steroids, cytotoxic agents, anticoagulants, and plasmapheresis. Most of the regimens use a combination of glucocorticoid—either oral prednisolone or IV MP pulses—and cytotoxic agents such as cyclophosphamide (see also Chapter 10). The combination of prednisolone and cytotoxic agents does not appear to be universally effective in controlling progression of the disease (Lai et al., 1987; Itami et al., 1989), but several reports of success have been claimed (Yang et al., 2015) and treatment with combined immunosuppression is often advocated.

Plasmapheresis added to a regular dose of steroids and cytotoxic agents has been shown to stabilize renal function during treatment (Hene et al., 1982) but a variable course was observed following cessation of therapy with some reporting a deterioration of function several months later (Coppo et al., 1985). Lai and others have reported a more sustained effect (Lai et al., 1987; Boobes et al., 1990; Roccatello et al., 1995; Xie et al., 2016). IV MP pulse therapy has been thought to be beneficial according to the observational study of Habib and colleagues (1994) who reported that in a group of 38 patients who had crescent formation in 50 per cent or more of glomeruli, NS, or both, all nine (100 per cent) who remained untreated progressed to ESRD, whereas seven out of 17 (41 per cent) who were treated with combination therapies including oral steroids immunosuppressive agents, anticoagulants, and non-steroidal anti-inflammatory agents progressed to end-stage renal failure, while none of the 12 (0 per cent) who were given MP alone were in ESRD. However, this observation has not always been reproducible as others have found no benefit with the use of MP pulse therapy alone (Coppo et al., 1985; Itami et al., 1989). Alveolar haemorrhage can occasionally complicate the course of IgA N, especially in the presence of progressive loss of renal function (Rajagopala et al., 2017). Treatment of such alveolar haemorrhage with plasmapheresis, high-doses of steroids, and combined immunosuppression may be life-saving.

Without extensive crescentic glomerulonephritis

Some patients with IgA N accompanied by with acute kidney injury (AKI) have been noted to exhibit minor glomerular abnormalities and/or scattered segmental glomerular crescents (<10 per cent of glomeruli involved) accompanied by acute tubulo-interstitial lesions on renal biopsy (Kincaid-Smith et al., 1983; Delclaux et al., 1993; Fogazzi et al., 1995). These patients typically present with an episode of macrohaematuria, sometimes associated with flank pain, shortly following an acute upper respiratory illness. The episodes of acute renal failure may be recurrent in individual patients. Rarely, these episodes may follow surgical tonsillectomy, especially in the face of an active or chronic tonsillitis. The episodes of AKI are thought to occur as a result of extensive glomerular bleeding, leading to tubular damage due to the local production of toxic haemoglobin degradation products and/or toxic oxygen radicals (Fogazzi et al., 1995) within the tubular lumina. Temporary dialysis therapy is required in some patients during the period of AKI, but nearly all patients eventually recover renal function. Warfarin-induced nephropathy can also occur in patients with IgA N who are receiving this anticoagulant for thrombosis/emboli prophylaxes or therapy (deep venous thrombosis or atrial fibrillation; Brodsky et al., 2012).

Practical recommendations

Isolated haematuria

Because of an intrinsically favourable intermediate-term prognosis (five to ten years) prognosis, in the absence of progression to overt proteinuria, this group of patients requires no specific therapy. Observation with RAS inhibition for hypertension is indicated.

Persistent proteinuria and haematuria (with or without reduced renal function)

The treatment of patients with IgA nephropathy who present with haematuria and significant (but often non-nephrotic) proteinuria (e.g., >0.5–3.0 g/day) with or without mild renal impairment has received a great deal of attention in the past few years. Table 7.3 provides a summary of the effects of various therapies in this group of patients and Figure 7.1 provides a suggested algorithm for *initial* management. A three-to-six-month trial of RAS inhibition (with an ACEi and/or ARB) is recommended in all patients. The doses of ACEi or ARB should be gradually increased to maximum recommended dosage using proteinuria and blood pressure as the guidepost of an effect, with a goal of reducing proteinuria to < 0.75–1.0 g/day (or lower, if RAS-inhibitor treatment is well tolerated). The addition of a low-salt diet and/or diuretics potentiates the anti-proteinuric actions of these agents. Blood pressure should be maintained at 120–130 mmHg systolic and 70–80 mmHg diastolic. If goal proteinuria cannot be met with the use of one agent alone, then treatment with both agents (an ACEi and an ARB) should be considered. Even a partial reduction of proteinuria to levels between 1–2 g/day can be of benefit in slowing the pace of progression of renal disease.

If a substantial reduction in proteinuria cannot be achieved by monotherapy with ACEi or ARB therapy in maximum tolerated dosage or by a combination of an ACEi and an ARB (or if disabling side-effects ensue limiting this treatment approach), then adjunctive therapy can be considered. There is no reason not to use fish oils (preferably prescription forms) in doses of 40 mg/kg/day usually in two divided doses, concomitantly with the ACEi/ARB regimens, but the true added value of this treatment approach is not well understood. Treatment with fish-oils alone is not advisable. Side effects are usually mild. Monotherapy with anti-platelet agents, alone or in combination with anti-coagulants, cannot be recommended.

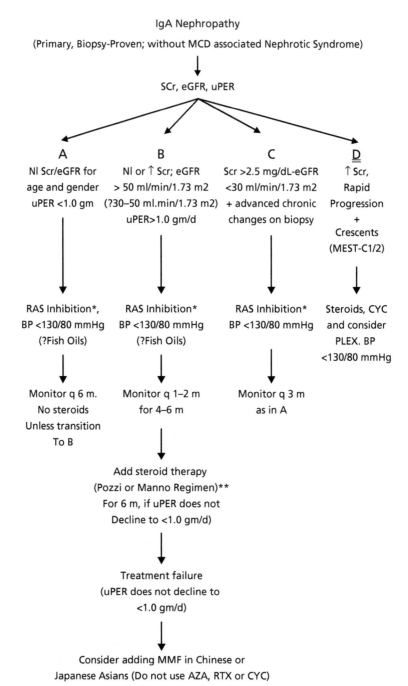

Figure 7.1 A suggested algorithm for initial treatment of IgA nephropathy based on urine protein excretion and serum creatinine (without minimal change lesions, extensive crescents, or advanced glomerulosclerosis/interstitial fibrosis on renal biopsy).
See text for additional details.

The choice of adjunctive therapy for patients who do not respond to these suggested regimens and continue to excrete protein at rates above 0.75–1.0 g/day (particularly above 2.0 g/day) should be individualized. Evidence from controlled trials suggests that a six-month course of steroids using the Pozzi or Manno regimens will reduce proteinuria and haematuria and likely slow the rate of progression of renal disease. However, the potential for side effects (especially opportunistic infections) at higher doses of steroids needs to be taken into account. Prophylaxis with TMP-SMX should be considered. The level of renal function at the time such treatment is started may influence the response, and patients with serum creatinine concentrations ≤1.5 mg/dl (132 μmol/l, eGFR >50 ml/min/1.73 m²) without moderate-to-marked tubulo-interstitial fibrosis on renal biopsy appear to respond better than those with more advanced chronic disease, but exception to this general rule do exist (Mitsuiki et al., 2007). Thus, the decision to use steroids for therapy of IgA N should be made before significant progression of disease has occurred. The addition of oral azathioprine to the steroid regimen is of no proven benefit and may even be harmful. If the serum creatinine concentration is >2.5 mg/dl (220 μmol/l; eGFR <30 ml/min/1.73 m²) and advanced tubulo-interstitial chronic lesions are present in the renal biopsy—'the point-of-no-return'—further treatment is generally futile, except that RAS inhibition should be continued with intensified monitoring of serum potassium concentration in order to retard the rate of progression to ESRD.

Adult patients who exhibit features of progression with a loss of estimated GFR >5–7 ml/min/year and an eGFR of 30–50 ml/min/1.73 m² (in the absence of rapidly progressive glomerulonephritis with extensive glomerular crescent involvement) should be considered candidates for a steroid therapy as well but the value of treatment and its side effects are less well understood The therapeutic roles of other adjunctive agents, such as MMF (or MPA), cyclophosphamide, sirolimus, cyclosporin, tacrolimus, IVIg, leflunomide, RTX, or anti-thrombotic agents are not well established and cannot be generally recommended. While MMF (or MPA) as therapeutic option for IgA N has been studied in randomized and controlled trials (conducted in China, Europe, and the US), the results are inconsistent and contradictory. The effects of MMF (or MPA) appear to be better in Japanese and Chinese patients than in Caucasians, but this has not been formally evaluated in a prospective fashion. High-dose IVIg has been claimed to have a benefit in IgA N, but this is based on small uncontrolled trials only. There is no consistent body of evidence that calcineurin inhibitors on sirolimus may be indicated for long-term use in IgA N.

Tonsillectomy, usually performed in conjunction with short-term oral or 'pulse' steroids, might to have an effect to promote 'clinical remission', particularly in children. However, a single randomized, controlled long-term trial has not confirmed this effect and the available observational studies do not strongly support the view that this therapy has any material and consistent effect on long-term outcome, even though episodes of haematuria may decrease in frequency and urinary protein excretion may modestly diminish contemporaneously with this treatment. Thus, at the present time, tonsillectomy (with pulse steroid therapy) cannot be generally recommended for the treatment of IgA N (Zand and Fervenza, 2014). Other therapies, such as danazol, phenytoin, urokinase, sodium cromoglycate, or chronic broad-spectrum antimicrobials have no significant lasting effect on the course of IgA N and are also not recommended.

Nephrotic syndrome (NS) with minimal glomerular changes

Treatment of the NS associated with minimal glomerular histological changes in IgA N should follow the lines of treatment in patients with idiopathic NS and MCN as pointed out in Chapter 4. Patients can be given a course of prednisone at an initial dose of 40–60 mg/day (60 mg/m^2 in children) for a total treatment period of three to four months. Relapses usually respond to steroids although cyclophosphamide at a dose of 1.5–2.0 mg/kg/body weight for 8–12 weeks may be required in the frequent relapse. Treatment of patients with the NS *and* IgA N who have more severe changes on renal histology is more difficult to define as there has only been one controlled study (Lai et al., 1986), which showed that a short course of prednisolone did not confer any overall benefits on this group of patients. As discussed, other controlled trials have shown benefits when steroids are given to patients with IgA N exhibiting lower levels of proteinuria. Consistent with other recommendation in other settings, patients with the NS and IgA deposits in glomeruli, should be offered RAS inhibition therapy, although the benefit of this approach in those with underlying minimal change disease who are also very steroid-sensitive is not well understood.

Acute or rapidly progressive glomerulonephritis

With extensive crescents

Because of the conflicting findings in small uncontrolled trials using different regimens, it is difficult to provide any 'evidence-based' recommended therapy in patients with rapidly progressive IgA N associated with extensive glomerular crescents (>25–50 per cent glomerular crescents), but aggressive therapy, including IV MP pulses and even plasma exchange might be justified because of the uniformly dismal outcome in untreated patients. Thus, until more definitive data are available, patients with rapidly progressive IgA N associated with very extensive glomerular crescents should be treated in the standard fashion, as other forms of crescentic glomerulonephritis (see Chapter 10), with prednisolone at an initial dose of 1 mg/kg/body weight/day and oral cyclophosphamide at a dose of 2 mg/kg/body weight/day. A methylprednisolone pulse of 500mg to 1 g/day for three days can be given prior to initiation of the oral prednisolone. There is no standard regimen for plasma exchange and, if required, the plasma exchanges can be tailored according to the clinical progress of the patient.

Without extensive crescents

No definitive treatment, apart from supportive therapy (including dialysis), is recommended for this group of patients, who often have a picture like acute tubular necrosis with mild crescentic involvement (<25 per cent of glomeruli affected by segmental crescents), because of the marked tendency for 'spontaneous' recovery. It should be emphasized that a renal biopsy is often needed to separate these two differing forms if IgA N with rapid loss of renal function, even though the patient may already carry a diagnosis of IgA N from a prior diagnostic renal biopsy.

Advanced chronic kidney disease

Patients with IgA N who present with or who advance to chronic kidney disease (Stage 4) with eGFR of <30 ml/min/1.73 m^2 and serum creatinine concentrations >2.0–3.0 mg/dl and who show very chronic tubulo-interstitial changes and advanced glomerulosclerosis are not very likely to benefit from any of the 'specific' treatment modalities discussed earlier. This stage is often called the *point-of-no-return* (D'Amico et al., 1993; Lai et al., 2002; Coppo and D'Amico, 2005). At this period, management of hypertension should be aggressive with a goal for systolic blood pressures of 120/70–130/80 mmHg, using inhibitors of angiotensin II action as preferred agents.

Transplantation

Glomerular IgA deposition occurs in between 10 and 60 per cent of renal allografts in patients who have undergone renal transplantation for progressive IgA N (Floege et al., 2004; Kim et al., 2017). According to Ponticelli and colleagues (Ponticelli et al., 2001, 2004; Moroni et al., 2013; Ponticelli and Glassock, 2010), a recurrence of IgA deposits was found in about 20 per cent of patients at a median of four years post-transplantation, but this may not be a true reflection of the 'recurrence rate' since only patients with microhaematuria and/or proteinuria underwent a transplant kidney biopsy. The combination of dysmorphic haematuria and low-grade proteinuria may signify recurrent disease.

Rarely, crescentic glomerulonephritis with rapidly progressive renal failure may be a manifestation of recurrent disease. This is seen more often in patients who present with IgA vasculitis, than with IgA N. Serial serum gdIgA levels can be useful in detecting recurrences- elevated levels are commonly found in recurrent IgA N compared to IgA transplant recipients without recurrence (Temurhan et al., 2017).

A recurrence of IgA deposition can develop in both living related, living unrelated, and deceased (cadaveric) donor organ recipients. Some studies have shown a slightly increased risk for recurrence in living related donors are used (Wang et al., 2001; Kennard et al., 2017). In the Australia and New Zealand Dialysis and Transplant Registry, the ten-year recurrence rate for IgA N was 16.7 per cent for living related donors compared to only 7.1 per cent for living unrelated donors and 9.2 per cent for deceased, but this is not a consistent finding. Very likely these IgA deposits represent recurrence of the original disease, rather than *de novo* IgA N, however, the risk of finding such deposits in subsequent renal biopsies of the transplanted kidney might be enhanced if the donor had (clinically unrecognizable) glomerular deposits of IgA *prior* to implantation of the kidney (Moriyama et al., 2005; Sanfillipo et al., 1986); however, a deleterious effect of this type of IgA deposition on outcomes of transplantation has not been confirmed (Sofue et al., 2013). Early rejection episodes may also be increased when patients receive kidneys from donors with mesangial IgA deposits (Ji et al., 2004). The prevalence of *recurrent* deposits of IgA in recipients with IgA N as their original disease depends on the duration of the post-transplant period, but by five to ten years post-transplant, about 20–40 per cent or more of renal allograft biopsies reveal IgA deposits (Hartung et al., 1995).

The eventual risk of recurrences of IgA deposition may approach 50 per cent or more for very long post-transplant graft survival (≥20 years). Such recurrences of IgA deposition very likely have an unfavourable impact on kidney survival. In an analysis of US registry data (in 4,589 patients with IgA N and 107,747 patients without IgA N receiving kidney transplants between 1999 and 2008, the hazard ratio for death censored graft survival was no different between IgA N and all non-IgA N recipients, but patient survival was better for IgA N, perhaps because of younger age in the IgA N group (Kadiyala et al., 2015). However, compared to subjects with polycystic kidney disease, patients with IgA N have a 1.6 (1.3–2.0) times greater hazard of graft failure (Pruthi et al., 2016). In Italian single-centre studies, renal transplantation in patients with IgA N compared to non-diabetic controls had a slightly (non-significant) better patient survival but significantly inferior death- censored graft survival at 15 years (Moroni et al., 2013). Re-transplantation in patients with IgA N suffering graft loss is overall accompanied by good results, at least over mid-term follow-up (Kim et al., 2017).

Therefore, a recurrence of IgA N in a renal allograft (or isograft) carries with it a risk of eventual graft failure. In the experience of Moroni and colleagues, IgA N recurred in 42 or 190 kidney grafts (22.1 per cent). Among them recurrence directly caused or contributed to kidney graft loss in 18 cases (43 per cent; Moroni et al., 2013). Similar findings have been reported by other, but not all, investigators (Nijim et al., 2016; Kawabe et al., 2015). Without any recurrence the graft survival is similar to that of controls (Moroni et al., 2013). A recurrence of IgA N in the renal allograft 'is not a benign condition' (Floege and Grone, 2013). An early recurrence of NS is a particularly ominous finding (Otsuka et al., 2014).

The deleterious effect of recurrent IgA deposition may be offset by a somewhat greater freedom from acute or chronic allograft rejection in recipients with IgA N, particularly when the donor and recipient are well-matched (zero mismatches; (McDonald and Russ, 2006). These adverse consequences of using zero-mismatched kidneys in patients with IgA N has not yet been thoroughly studied and have not been universally confirmed. Graft loss due to recurrence was as low as 3 per cent in a series of 101 patients from Malaysia (Ng et al., 2007). Also, in a very large series of patients from Hong Kong, only three of 75 patients (4 per cent) had graft loss due to recurrence after a mean follow-up of about eight years (Choy et al., 2003). However, longer term follow-up (>12 years) shows a suggestion of greater graft loss due to recurrence compared to non-IgA N recipients (Choy et al., 2003; Moroni et al., 2013). Some studies have shown 'blocking' IgA antibodies in the sera of patients with IgA N, which might contribute to better graft survival (in the absence of a recurrence of IgA N (Lim et al., 1991).

The following factors seem to be consistently associated with an increased risk of recurrent IgA N:

i. younger age at presentation;

ii. a rapid course to ESRD;

iii. the existence of aggressive crescentic disease in the recipient (including IgA vasculitis; see Moriyama et al., 2005; Mousson et al., 2007; Ponticelli and Glassock, 2010);

iv. use of a living related donor.

Selected biomarkers may also be useful in predicting risk of recurrences. Serum levels of gdIgA$_1$ are poor and rather inconsistent predictor of recurrence (Coppo et al., 2007; Berthelot et al., 2015; Berthoux et al., 2017; Temurhan et al., 2017). Normalized values for circulating levels of IgG antibodies to gdIgA$_1$ may predict recurrences (Berthoux et al., 2017). Polymorphisms of IL-10 and/or TNF alpha may be associated with protection from recurrence of IgA N (Coppo et al., 2007). A recurrence of IgA N is predicted by the presence of elevated IgA-IgG immune complexes in serum and by elevated IgA-sCD89 complexes in serum pre-transplant (Berthelot et al., 2015).

In addition, Berthoux, El Deeb, and colleagues (2008) have suggested that renal allograft recipients who receive anti-thymocyte globulin (ATG) therapy for prevention of allograft rejection have a lower risk of recurrence of IgA N. Patients receiving MMF for post-transplant maintenance immunosuppression do not apparently have a lower risk of recurrence (Chandrakantan et al., 2005), but this was not confirmed in a later study (Von Visger et al., 2014). In this later study, MMF use was associated with a lower risk of recurrence. CsA use did not affect recurrence rates but sirolimus use was associated with a higher risk of recurrence as did the absence of ALG induction (Von Visger et al., 2014), confirming the findings of Berthoux, El Deeb, and colleagues (2008).

Very importantly, steroid-free post-transplant immunosuppressive regimens are associated with a greatly increased risk of IgA recurrence (Hazard Ratio of 8.59; 3.03–24.38 CI) compared to steroid-based regimens (Von Visger et al., 2014). *In summary*, IgA N should not be regarded as a contraindication for renal transplantation, but prospective recipients should be informed regarding the likelihood of a recurrence and efforts should be made to predict risk based on the available demographic and biological parameters discussed earlier. Other than the avoidance of a steroid-free post-transplant immunosuppressive protocol and sirolimus, along with ALG induction, the standard post-transplant regimen for rejection prophylaxis or prevention of recurrence does not have to be modified. An intra-operative, pre-implantation renal biopsy is suggested to determine if the donor has clinically unrecognized IgA deposits.

The management of an identified post-transplant recurrence of IgA N (usually following a transplant renal biopsy, either for clinical indications or according to protocol), remains rather poorly defined (Lionaki et al., 2017). Ordinarily, no specific therapy is needed for mild-moderate recurrent disease, without evidence of NS or a progressive decline in eGFR. No data are available on the safety or efficacy of fish oil, low-antigen diets, IVIg, or cytotoxic agents for recurrent disease. Small case reports have suggested benefits for RTX or tonsillectomy as treatments for recurrent IgA N (Chancharoenthana et al., 2017; Hoshino et al., 2014; Koshino et al., 2013). Whether these are chance observations or real effects cannot be determined. RAS inhibitors should be prescribed if hypertension and/or proteinuria >500 mg–1.0 g are present, taking into account that these agents may reduce haemoglobin levels and favour hyperkalaemia and a reversible increase in serum creatinine concentrations (Ponticelli and

Cucchiari, 2017). Recurrent crescentic glomerulonephritis, which is quite uncommon, should be treated as the *de novo* disease is treated with steroids, cytotoxic agents, and possibly plasma exchange (see Chapter 10). Eculizumab has recently also been reported to be effective in post-transplant crescentic GN due to IgA N recurrence (Herzog et al., 2017).

References

Alexopoulos E, Stangou M, Pantzaki A, et al. (2004). Treatment of severe IgA nephropathy with omega-3 fatty acids: the effect of a 'very-low-dose' regimen. Ren Fail. **26**: 453–9.

Almartine E, Sabatier J, Guerin C, et al. (1991). Prognostic factors in mesangial IgA glomerulonephritis: an extensive study with invariable and multivariable analysis. Am J Kidney Dis. **18**: 1–19.

Assadi FJ. (2005). Value of urinary excretion of microalbumin in predicting glomerular lesions in children with isolated microscopic hematuria. Pediatr Nephrol. **20**: 1131–5.

Baek JE, Chang JW, Min WK, et al. (2008). Serum high-sensitivity C-reactive protein is not increased in patients with IgA nephropathy. Nephron Clin Pract. **108**: c35–c40.

Ballardie F, Roberts TS. (2002). Controlled prospective trial of prednisolone and cytotoxics in progressive IgA nephropathy. J Am Soc Nephrol. **13**: 142–8.

Ballardie FW, Cowley RD. (2008). Prognostic indices and therapy in IgA nephropathy: Toward a solution. Kidney Int. **73**: 249–51.

Bantis C, Ivens K, Kreusser W, et al. (2004). Influence of genetic polymorphisms of the renin–angiotensin system on IgA nephropathy. Am J Nephrol. **24**: 258–67.

Barbour SJ, Cattran DC, Espino-Hernandez G, et al. (2015). Identifying the ideal metric of proteinuria as a predictor of renal outcome in idiopathic glomerulonephritis Kidney Int. **88**: 1392–401.

Barbour SJ, Espino-Hernandez G, Reich HN, et al. (2016). The MEST score provides earlier risk prediction in IgA nephropathy. Kidney Int. **89**: 167–75.

Barbour S, Feehally J. (2017). An update on the treatment of IgA nephropathy. Curr Opin Nephrol Hypertens. **26**: 319–26.

Barratt J, Feehally J. (2006). Treatment of IgA nephropathy. Kidney Int. **69**: 1934–8.

Bartosik LP, Lajoie G, Sugar L, et al. (2001). Predicting progression in IgA nephropathy. Am J Kidney Dis. **38**. 728–35.

Bazzi G, D'Amico G. (2005). Qualitative aspects of proteinuria predict progression and response to therapy better than its quantity. NephSAP. **4**: 111–16.

Beckwith H, Medjeral-Thomas N, Galliford J, et al. (2017). Mycophenolate mofetil therapy in immunoglobulin A nephropathy: Histological changes after treatment. Nephrol Dial Transplant. **32**: i123–8.

Beerman L, Novak J, Wyatt RJ, et al. (2007). The genetics of IgA nephropathy. Nat Clin Pract Nephrol. **3**: 325–38.

Békássy ZD, Kristoffersson AC, Rebetz J, et al. (2018). Aliskiren inhibits renin-mediated complement activation. Kidney Int. **94**: 689–700.

Bellur SS, Lepeytre F, Vorobyeva O, et al. (2017). Evidence from the Oxford Classification cohort supports the clinical value of subclassification of focal segmental glomerulosclerosis in IgA nephropathy. Kidney Int. **91**: 235–43.

Bene MG, Hurault de Ligny B, Kessler M, et al. (1993). Tonsils in IgA nephropathy. In MC Bene, GC Faure, M Kessler (eds), *International Symposium on IgA Nephropathy: the 25th Year. Proceedings. Nancy, France, August 31-September 2, 1992*. Vol. **104**, pp. 153–61. Karger, Basel.

Bennett WM, Walker RG, and Kincaid-Smith P. (1989). Treatment of IgA nephropathy with eicosapentaenoic acid (EPA): A two-year prospective trial. Clin Nephrol. **31**: 128–31.

Berger J, Hinglais N. (1968). Les depots intercapillaries d'IgA–IgG. J Urol Nephrol (Paris). **74**: 694–700.

Berthelot L, Robert T, Vuiblet V, et al. (2015). Recurrent IgA nephropathy is predicted by altered glycosylated IgA, autoantibodies and soluble CD89 complexes. Kidney Int. **88**: 815–22.

Berthoux F, Alamartine F, Pommier G, et al. (1988). HLA and IgA-nephritis revisited 10 years later. HLA-B35 antigen as a prognostic factor. New Eng J Med. **319**: 1609–10.

Berthoux F, El Deeb S, Mariat C, et al. (2008). Antithymocyte globulin (ATG) induction therapy and disease recurrence in renal transplant recipients with primary IgA nephropathy. Transplantation. **85**: 1505–7.

Berthoux F, Laurent B, Koller J-M, et al. (1995). Primary IgA glomerulonephritis with thin glomerular basement membrane: A peculiar pathological marker versus thin membrane nephropathy association. In A Clarkson, A Woodroffe (eds), *IgA Nephropathy: Pathogenesis and Treatment*, vol. III, pp. 1–7. Karger, Basel.

Berthoux FC, Mohey H, Afiani A. (2008). Natural history of primary IgA nephropathy. Semin Nephrol. **28**: 4–9.

Berthoux F, Mohey H, Laurent B, et al. (2011). Predicting the risk for dialysis or death in IgA nephropathy. J Am Soc Nephrol. **22**: 752–61.

Berthoux F, Suzuki H, Mohey H, et al. (2017). Prognostic value of serum biomarkers of autoimmunity for recurrence of IgA nephropathy after kidney transplantation. J Am Soc Nephrol. **28**: 1943–50.

Berthoux F, Suzuki H, Thibaudin L, et al. (2012). Autoantibodies targeting galactose-deficient IgA1 associate with progression of IgA nephropathy. J Am Soc Nephrol. **23**: 1579–87.

Beukhof J, Kardaun O, Schaafsma W, et al. (1986). Towards individual prognosis of IgA nephropathy. Kidney Int. **29**: 549–56.

Bomback AS, Canetta PA, Beck LH Jr, et al. (2012). Treatment of resistant glomerular diseases with adrenocorticotropic hormone gel: A prospective trial. Am J Nephrol. **36**: 58–67.

Bonnet F, Deprele C, Sassolas A, et al. (2001). Excessive body weight as a new independent risk factor for clinical and pathological progression in primary IgA nephritis. Am J Kidney Dis. **37**: 720–27.

Boobes Y, Baz M, Durand C, et al. (1990). Early start of intensive therapy in malignant form of IgA nephropathy. Nephron. **54**: 351–3.

Briganti EM, Dowling J, Finlay M, et al. (2001). The incidence of biopsy-proven glomerulonephritis in Australia. Nephrol Dial Transplant. **16**: 1364–7.

Brodsky SV, Rovin BH, Hebert LA. (2012). Benefit of cyclophosphamide therapy in IgA nephritis may have been obscured by warfarin-related nephropathy in the randomized trials in which warfarin and dipyridamole were used in combination with cyclophosphamide. Nephrol Dial Transplant. **27**: 475–7.

Buck KS, Smith AC, Molyneux K, et al. (2008). B-cell O-galactosyltransferase activity and expression of O-glycosylation genes in bone marrow in IgA nephropathy. Kidney Int. **73**: 1128–36.

Cambier A, Rabant M, Peuchmaur M, et al. (2018). Immunosuppressive treatment in children with IgA nephropathy and the clinical value of podocytopathic features. Kidney Int Rep. **3**: 916–25.

Cameron JS. (1984). Platelets in glomerular disease. Ann Rev Med. **35**: 175–80.

Cameron JS. (1993). The long-term outcome of glomerular disease. In R Schrier, G Gottskalk (eds), *Disease of the Kidney*. 5th Edition. pp. 1914–16. Little Brown, Boston.

Cattran D, Greenwood G, Ritchie S. (1994). Long-term benefit of angiotensin converting enzyme inhibitor therapy in patients with severe immunoglobulin A nephropathy: A comparison to patients receiving treatment with other antihypertensive agents and to patients receiving no therapy. Am J Kidney Dis. **23**: 247–54.

Cattran D, Reich HN, Beanlands HJ, et al. (2008). The impact of sex in primary glomerulonephritis. Nephrol Dial Transplant. **23**: 2247–53.

Chancharoenthana W, Townamchai N, Leelahavanichkul A, et al. (2017). Rituximab for recurrent IgA nephropathy in kidney transplantation: A report of three cases and proposed mechanisms. Nephrology (Carlton). **22**: 65–71.

Chandrakantan A, Ratanapanichkich P, Said M, et al. (2005). Recurrent IgA nephropathy after renal transplantation despite immunosuppressive regimens with mycophenolate mofetil. Nephrol Dial Transplant. **20**: 1214–31.

Chen X, Chen P, Cai G, et al. (2002). A randomized trial of mycophenolate mofetil treatment in severe IgA nephropathy. Zhonghua Yi Xue Za Zhi. **82**: 796–801.

Chen Y, Li Y, Yang S, et al. (2014). Efficacy and safety of mycophenolate mofetil treatment in IgA nephropathy: A systematic review. BMC Nephrol. **15**: 193–9.

Cheng IKP, Chan KW, Chan MK. (1989). Mesangial IgA nephropathy with steroid-responsive nephrotic syndrome: Disappearance of mesangial IgA deposits following steroid-induced remission. Am J Kidney Dis. **14**: 361–4.

Cheng, IKP, Chan PG K, Chan MK. (1990). The effects of fish-oil dietary supplement on the progression of mesangial IgA glomerulonephritis. Nephrol Dial Transplant. **5**: 241–6.

Cheung CK, Barratt J. (2015). Gluten and IgA nephropathy: You are what you eat? Kidney Int. **88**: 215–18.

Choy BY, Chan TM, Lo SK, et al. (2003). Renal transplantation in patients with primary immunoglobulin A nephropathy. Nephrol Dial Transplant. **18**: 2399–404.

Clarkson AR, Seymour AE, Thompson AJ, et al. (1977). IgA nephropathy: A syndrome of uniform morphology, diverse clinical features and uncertain prognosis. Clin Nephrol. **8**: 458–71.

Conley ME, Cooper MD, Michael AF. (1980). Selective deposition of immunoglobulin A1, in immunoglobulin A nephropathy, anaphylactoid purpura nephritis, and septuric lupus erythematosus. J Clin Invest. **66**: 1342–9.

Cook HT. (2007). Interpretation of renal biopsies in IgA nephropathy. Contr Nephrol. **157**: 44–9.

Coppo R. (2013). Is a legacy effect possible in IgA nephropathy? Nephrol Dial Transplant. **28**: 1657–62.

Coppo R. (2015). The intestine-renal connection in IgA nephropathy. Nephrol Dial Transplant. **30**: 360–6.

Coppo R. (2017). Corticosteroids in IgA nephropathy: Lessons from recent studies. J Am Soc Nephrol. **28**: 25–33.

Coppo R. (2017). The gut-kidney axis in IgA nephropathy: Role of microbiota and diet on genetic predisposition. Pediatr Nephrol. **33**: 53–61.

Coppo R. (2017). C4d deposits in IgA nephropathy: Where does complement activation come from? Pediatr Nephrol. **32**: 1097–101.

Coppo R, Amore A, Chiesa M, et al. (2007). Serological and genetic factors in early recurrence of IgA nephropathy after renal transplantation. Clin Transplant. **21**: 728–37.

Coppo R, Basolo B, Giachino O, et al. (1985). Plasmapheresis in a patient with rapidly progressive idiopathic IgA nephropathy: Removal of IgA-containing circulating immune complexes and clinical recovery. Nephron. **40**: 488–90.

Coppo R, D'Amico G. (2005). Factors predicting progression of IgA nephropathy. J Nephrol. **18**: 503–12.

Coppo R, Rocatello D, Amore A, et al. (1990). Effects of a gluten-free diet on primary IgA nephropathy. Clin Nephrol. **33**: 72–86.

Coppo R, Lofaro D, Camilla RR, et al. (2017). Risk factors for progression in children and young adults with IgA nephropathy: An analysis of 261 cases from the VALIGA European cohort. Pediatr Nephrol. **32**: 139–50.

Coppo R, Peruzzi L, Amore A, et al. (2007). IgACE: A placebo-controlled, randomized trial of angiotensin-converting enzyme inhibition in children and young adults with IgA nephropathy and moderate proteinuria. J Am Soc Nephrol. **18**: 1880–8.

Coppo R, Troyanov S, Bellur S, et al. (2014). VALIGA study of the ERA-EDTA Immunonephrology Working Group. Validation of the Oxford classification of IgA nephropathy in cohorts with different presentations and treatments. Kidney Int. **86**: 828–36.

Cox SN, Pesce F, El-Sayed Moustafa JS, et al. (2017). European IgAN Consortium Multiple rare genetic variants co-segregating with familial IgA nephropathy all act within a single immune-related network. J Intern Med. **281**: 189–205.

Curschellas E, Landmann J, Dürig M, et al. (1991). Morphologic findings in 'zero-hour' biopsies of renal transplants. Clin Nephrol. **36**: 215–22.

D'Amico G. (1987). The commonest glomerulonephritis in the world: IgA nephropathy. Quart J Med. **245**: 709–27.

D'Amico G. (1992). Influence of clinical and histologic features on actuarial renal survival in adult patients with idiopathic IgA nephropathy, membranous nephropathy, and membranoproliferative glomerulonephritis. Survey of the recent literature. Am J Kidney Dis. **20**: 315–23.

D'Amico G, Ragni A, Gandini E, et al. (1993). Typical and atypical natural history of IgA nephropathy in adult patients. Contr Nephrol. **104**: 6–13.

D'Amico G, Napodano P, Ferrario F, et al. (2001). Idiopathic IgA nephropathy with segmental necrotizing lesions of the capillary wall. Kidney Int. **59**: 682–92.

Delclaux C, Jacquot C, Callard P, et al. (1993). Acute reversible renal failure with macroscopic hematuria in IgA nephropathy. Nephrol Dial Transplant. **8**: 195–9.

Deng W, Tan X, Zhou Q et al. (2018). Gender-related differences in clinicopathological characteristics and renal outcomes of Chinese patients with IgA nephropathy. BMC Nephrol. **19**: 31.

Deng J, Zheng X, Xie H, et al. (2017). Calcitriol in the treatment of IgA nephropathy with non-nephrotic range proteinuria: A meta-analysis of randomized controlled trials. Clin Nephrol. **87**: 21–7.

Dillon JJ. (1997). Fish oil therapy for IgA nephropathy: Efficacy and interstudy variability. J Am Soc Nephrol. **8**: 1739–44.

Donadio JV, Bergstrahl EJ, Offord KP, et al. (1994). A controlled trial of fish oil in IgA nephropathy. New Eng J Med. **331**: 1194–9.

Donadio JV, Bergstrahl EJ, Bibus DM, et al. (2006). Is body size a biomarker for optimizing dosing of omega-3 polyunsaturated fatty acids in the treatment of patients with IgA nephropathy? Clin J Am Soc Nephrol. **1**: 933–99.

Donadio JV, Grande JP. (2004). The role of fish oil/omega-3 fatty acids in the treatment of IgA nephropathy. Semin Nephrol. **24**: 225–43.

Duan Z, Cai GY, Chen YZ, et al. (2013). Aging promotes progression of IgA nephropathy: A systematic review and meta-analysis. Am J Nephrol. **38**: 241–52.

Duan J, Liu D, Duan G, Liu Z. (2017). Long-term efficacy of tonsillectomy as a treatment in patients with IgA nephropathy: A meta-analysis. Int Urol Nephrol. **49**: 103–12.

Eijgenraam JW, Woltman AM, Kamerling SW, et al. (2005). Dendritic cells of IgA nephropathy patients have an impaired capacity to induce IgA production in naive B cells. Kidney Int. **68**: 1604–12.

Eijgenraam JW, Reinartz SM, Kamerling SW, et al. (2008). Immuno-histological analysis of dendritic cells in nasal biopsies of IgA nephropathy patients. Nephrol Dial Transplant. **23**: 612–20.

van Es LA, et al. (2008). GMP-17-positive T-lymphocytes in renal tubules predict progression in the early stages of IgA nephropathy. Kidney Int. **73**: 1426–38.

Espinosa M, Ortega R, Gomez-Carrasco JM, et al. (2009). Mesangial cell C4d deposition: A new prognostic factor in IgA nephropathy. Nephrol Dial Transplant. **24**: 886–91.

Espinosa M, Ortega R, Sánchez M, et al. (2014). Association of C4d deposition with clinical outcomes in IgA nephropathy. Clin J Am Soc Nephrol. **9**: 897–904.

Faria B, Henriques C, Matos AC, et al. (2015). Combined C4d and CD3 immunostaining predicts immunoglobulin (Ig)A nephropathy progression. Clin Exp Immunol. **179**: 354–61.

Feehally J, Barratt J. (2015). The genetics of IgA nephropathy: An overview from Western countries. Kidney Dis (Basel). **1**: 33–41.

Feehally J, Coppo R, Troyanov S, et al. (2016). Tonsillectomy in a European cohort of 1,147 patients with IgA nephropathy. Nephron. **32**: 15–24.

Feehally J, Farrall M, Boland A, et al. (2010). HLA has strongest association with IgA nephropathy in genome-wide analysis. J Am Soc Nephrol. **21**: 1791–7.

Fellin G, Gentile MG, Duca G, et al. (1988). Renal function in IgA nephropathy with established renal failure. Nephrol Dial Transplant. **3**: 17–23.

Fellström BC, Barratt J, Cook H, et al. (2017). Targeted-release budesonide versus placebo in patients with IgA nephropathy (NEFIGAN): A double-blind, randomised, placebo-controlled phase 2b trial. Lancet. **389**: 2117–27.

Fenoglio H, Naretto C, Basolo B, et al. (2017). Rituximab therapy for IgA vasculitis with nephritis: A case series and review of the literature. Immunol Res. **65**: 186–92.

Feriozzi S, Polci R. (2016). The role of tonsillectomy in IgA nephropathy. J Nephrol. **29**: 13–19.

Fernandez-Juarez G, Barrio V, de Vinuesa SG, et al. (2006). Dual blockade of the renin-angiotensin system in the progression of renal disease: The need for more clinical trials. J Am Soc Nephrol. **17**: s250–4.

Ferrario F, Napodano P, Rastaldi MP, et al. (1995). Capillaritis in IgA nephropathy. Contrib Nephrol. **111**: 8–12.

Ferri C, Puccini R, Paleologo G, et al. (1992). IgA nephropathy: Preliminary results of low-antigen-content diet treatment. Arch Int Med. **152**: 249.

Floege J. (2004). Recurrent IgA nephropathy after renal transplantation. Semin Nephrol. **24**: 287–91.

Floege J, Amann K. (2016). Primary glomerulonephritides. Lancet. **387**: 2036–48.

Floege J, Daha MR. (2018). IgA nephropathy: New insights into the role of complement. Kidney Int. **94**: 16–18.

Floege J, Gröne HJ. (2013). Recurrent IgA nephropathy in the renal allograft: Not a benign condition. Nephrol Dial Transplant. **28**: 1070–3.

Floege J, Feehally J. (2016). The mucosa-kidney axis in IgA nephropathy. Nat Rev Nephrol. **12**: 147–56.

Fogazzi G, Imbasciati E, Moroni G, et al. (1995). Reversible acute renal failure from gross hematuria due to glomerulonephritis, not only in IgA nephropathy and not associated with intratubular obstruction. Nephrol Dial Transplant. **10**: 624–9.

Fornasieri A, Sinico RA, Maldifassi P, et al. (1987). IgA-antigliadin antibodies in mesangial IgA nephropathy (Berger's disease). BMJ. **295**: 78–80.

Fornasieri A, Sinico RA, Maldifassi P, et al. (1988). Food antigens, IgA immune complexes and IgA mesangial nephropathy. Nephrol Dial Transplant. **3**: 738–43.

Frisch G, Lin J, Rosenstock J, et al. (2005). Mycophenolate mofetil (MMF) vs. placebo in patients with moderately advanced IgA nephropathy: A double blind randomized controlled trial. Nephrol Dial Transplant. **21**: 39–45.

Fukushi K, Yamabe H, Ozawa K, et al. (1989). Disappearance of glomerular IgA deposits in steroid-responsive nephrotic syndrome. Nephron. **51**: 553–4.

Gao R, Wu W, Wen Y, et al. (2017). Hydroxychloroquine alleviates persistent proteinuria in IgA nephropathy. Int Urol Nephrol. **49**: 1233–41.

Geddes CC, Rauta V, Gronhagen-Riska C, et al. (2003). A tricontinental view of IgA nephropathy. Nephrol Dial Transplant. **18**: 1541–8.

Gharavi AG, Kiryluk K, Choi M, et al. (2011). Genome wide association study identifies susceptibility loci for IgA nephropathy. Nat Genet. **43**: 321–7.

Gharavi AG, Moldoveanu Z, Wyatt RJ, et al. (2008). Aberrant IgA1 glycosylation is inherited in familial and sporadic IgA nephropathy. J Am Soc Nephrol. **19**: 1008–14.

Gherghiceanu M, Penescu M, Mandache E. (2005). The predictive value of peritubular C3d deposition in IgA glomerulonephritis. J Cell Mol Med. **9**: 143–52.

GISEN (Gruppo Italiano di Studi Epidemiolgici in Nefrologia. (1997). Randomized placebo-controlled trial of the effect of ramipril on decline in glomerular filtration rate and risk of terminal renal failure in proteinuric, non-diabetic nephropathy. Lancet. **349**: 1857–63.

Glassock RJ. (2009). Future prospects for IgA nephropathy. In **KN Lai** (ed), *Recent Advances in IgA Nephropathy*. World Scientific, London.

Glassock RJ. (2016). Moderator's view: Treatment of IgA nephropathy-getting comfortable with uncertainty. Nephrol Dial Transplant. **31**: 1776–80.

Glassock RJ. (2017). Glomerular disease: Targeted steroid therapy for IgA nephropathy. Nat Rev Nephrol. **13**: 390–2.

Glassock RJ, Lee G. (2009). Immunoglobulin A Nephropathy. In **C Ponticelli, RJ Glassock** (eds), *Treatment of Primary Glomerulonephritis*. 2nd Edition, pp. 313–74. OUP, Oxford.

Goumenos D, Ahuja M, Shortland J, et al. (1995). Can immuno-suppressive drugs slow the progression of IgA nephropathy? Nephrol Dial Transplant. **10**: 1173–81.

Gutierrez E, González E, Hernández E, et al. (2007). Factors that determine an incomplete recovery of renal function in macrohematuria-induced acute renal failure in IgA nephropathy. Clin J Am Soc Nephrol. **2**: 51–7.

Haas M, Racusen LC, Bagnasco SM. (2008). IgA-dominant postinfectious glomerulonephritis: A report of 13 cases with common ultrastructural features. Hum Pathol. **39**: 1309–16.

Haas M, Verhave JC, Liu ZH, et al. (2017). A multicenter study of the predictive value of crescents in IgA nephropathy. J Am Soc Nephrol. **28**: 691–701.

Habib R, Niaudet P, Levy M. (1994). Schönlein-Henoch purpura nephritis and IgA nephropathy. In **C Tisher, BM Bremner** (eds), *Renal pathology: With Clinical and Pathological Correlations*. 2nd Edition. pp. 472–523. Lippincott, Philadelphia.

Hamazaki T, Tateno S, Shishido S. (1984). Eicosapentaenoic acid and IgA nephropathy. Lancet. **1**: 1017–18.

Hammarstromm L, Lundkvist I, Petterson A, et al. (1992). The use of IVIG in immunological disorders other than cytopenias. In **PL Yap** (ed), *Clinical Applications of Intravenous Immunoglobulin Therapy*, pp. 117–37. Churchill Livingstone, Edinburgh.

Hara M, Yanagihara T, Kihara I. (2007). Cumulative excretion of urinary podocytes reflects disease progression in IgA nephropathy and Schönlein–Henoch purpura. Clin J Am Soc Nephrol. **2**: 231–8.

Hartono C, Chung M, Perlman AS, et al. (2018). Bortezomib for reduction of proteinuria in IgA nephropathy. Kidney Int Rep. **3**: 861–6.

Hartung R, Livingston B, Excell L, et al. (1995). Recurrence of IgA deposits/disease in grafts. In **A Clarkson, A Woodroffe** (eds), IgA nephropathy: Pathogenesis and Treatment, Vol. **III**. pp. 13–17. Karger, Basel.

Hasbargen J, Copley J. (1985). Utility of skin biopsy in the diagnosis of IgA nephropathy. Am J Kidney Dis. **6**: 100–6.

Haubitz M, Wittke S, Weissinger EM, et al. (2005). Urine protein patterns can serve as diagnostic tools in patients with IgA nephropathy. Kidney Int. **67**: 2313–20.

Helin H, Mustonen J, Reunala T, et al. (1983). IgA nephropathy associated with celiac disease and dermatitis herpetiformis. Arch Pathol Lab Med. **107**: 324–7.

Hene RJ, Valentijin RM, Kater L. (1982). Plasmapheresis in nephropathy of Henoch–Schönlein purpura and primary IgA nephropathy. Kidney Int. **22**: 409 (Abstract).

Herzog AL, Wanner C, Amann K, et al. (2017). First treatment of relapsing rapidly progressive IgA nephropathy with eculizumab after living kidney donation: A case report. Transplant Proc. **49**: 1574–7.

Heybeli C, Unlu M, Yildiz S, et al. (2015). IgA nephropathy: Association of C4d with clinical and histopathological findings and possible role of IgM. Ren Fail. **37**: 1464–9.

Hirano K, Amano H, Kawamura T, et al. (2016). Tonsillectomy reduces recurrence of IgA nephropathy in mesangial hypercellularity type categorized by the Oxford classification. Clin Exp Nephrol. **20**: 425–32.

Hogg RJ. (1995). Prognostic indicators and treatment of childhood IgA nephropathy. Contrib Nephrol. **111**: 194–9.

Hogg RJ, Bay RC, Jennette JC, et al. (2015). Randomized controlled trial of mycophenolate mofetil in children, adolescents, and adults with IgA nephropathy. Am J Kidney Dis. **66**: 783–91.

Hogg RJ, Fitzgibbons L, Atkins C, et al. (2006). Efficacy of omega-3 fatty acid in children and adults with IgA nephropathy is dosage and size-dependent. Clin J Am Soc Nephrol. **1**: 1167–72.

Hogg RJ, Lee J, Nardelli N, et al. (2006). Clinical trial to evaluate omega-3 fatty acids and alternate day prednisone in patients with IgA nephropathy: Report from the Southwest Pediatric Nephrology Study Group. Clin J Am Soc Nephrol. **1**: 467–74.

Hogg RJ, Wyatt RJ; Scientific Planning Committee of the North American IgA Nephropathy Study. (2004). A randomized controlled trial of mycophenolate mofetil in patients with IgA nephropathy [ISRCTN62574616]. BMC Nephrology. **5**: 3.

Hoshino J, Fujii T, Usui J, et al. (2016). Renal outcome after tonsillectomy plus corticosteroid pulse therapy in patients with immunoglobulin A nephropathy: Results of a multicenter cohort study. Clin Exp Nephrol. **20**: 618–27.

Hoshino Y, Abe Y, Endo M, et al. (2014). Five cases of tonsillectomy and steroid pulse therapy for recurrent immunoglobulin A nephropathy after kidney transplantation. CEN Case Rep. **3**: 118–22.

Hotta O, Miyazaki M, Furuta T, et al. (2001). Tonsillectomy and steroid pulse therapy significantly impact on clinical remission in patients with IgA nephropathy. Am J Kidney Dis. **38**: 736–43.

Hou JH, Le WB, Chen N, et al. (2017). Mycophenolate mofetil combined with prednisone versus full-dose prednisone in IgA nephropathy with active proliferative lesions: A randomized controlled trial. Am J Kidney Dis. **69**: 788–95.

Huang ZQ, Raska M, Stewart TJ, et al. (2016). Somatic mutations modulate autoantibodies against galactose-deficient IgA1 in IgA nephropathy. J Am Soc Nephrol. **27**: 3278–84.

Hung KY, Chen WY, Yen TS, et al. (1996). Adult primary IgA nephropathy and common viral infections. J Infect. **32**: 227–30.

Hunley TE, Julian BA, Phillips JA 3rd, et al. (1996). Angiotensin converting enzyme gene polymorphism: Potential silencer motif and impact on progression in IgA nephropathy. Kidney Int. **49**: 571–7.

Ibels LS, Gyory AZ. (1994). IgA nephropathy: Analysis of the natural history, important factors in the progression of renal disease, and a review of the literature. Medicine (Baltimore). **73**: 79–102.

Ikezumi Y, Suzuki T, Karasawa T, et al. (2008). Use of mizoribine as a rescue drug for steroid-resistant pediatric IgA nephropathy. Pediatr Nephrol. **23**: 645–50.

Ishiguro C, Yaguchi Y, Funabiki K, et al. (2002). Serum IgA/C3 ratio may predict diagnosis and prognosis grading in patients with IgA nephropathy. Nephron. **91**: 755–8.

Isnard P, Labaye J, Bourgault M, et al. (2014). TTP or HUS? About a case revealing an IgA nephropathy. Nephrol Ther. **10**: 532–6.

Itami N, Akutsu V, Kusonoki Y, et al. (1989). Does methylprednisolone pulse therapy deteriorate the course of rapidly progressive IgA nephropathy? Am J Dis Child. **143**: 441–2 (Letter).

Izzi C, Ravani P, Torres D, et al. (2006). IgA nephropathy: The presence of familial disease does not confer an increased risk for progression. Am J Kidney Dis. **47**: 761–69.

Jacob S, Héry M, Protois JC, et al. (2007). Effect of organic solvent exposure on chronic kidney disease progression: The GN-PROGRESS Cohort study. J Am Soc Nephrol. **18**: 274–81.

Janssen U, Bahlmann F, Köhl J, et al. (2000). Activation of the acute phase response and complement C3 in patients with IgA nephropathy. Am J Kidney Dis. **35**: 21–8.

Jeong EG, Hyoun S, Lee SM, et al. (2017). Clinical outcomes of nephrotic syndrome in immunoglobulin A nephropathy. Saudi J Kidney Dis Transplant. **28**: 1314–20.

Ji S, Liu M, Chen J, et al. (2004). The fate of glomerular mesangial deposition in the donated kidney after allograft transplantation. Clin Transplant. **18**: 536–40.

Johnson RJ, Hurtado A, Merszei J, et al. (2003). Hypothesis: Dysregulation of immunologic balance resulting from hygiene and socioeconomic factors may influence the epidemiology and causes of glomerulonephritis worldwide. Am J Kidney Dis. **42**: 575–81.

Jones RB, Furuta S, Tervaert JW, et al. (2015). Rituximab versus cyclophosphamide in ANCA-associated vasculitis: 2-year results of a randomized trial. Ann Rheum Dis. **74**: 1178–82.

Julian BA, Barker C. (1993). Alternate-day prednisone therapy in IgA nephropathy. Control Nephrol. **104**: 198–206.

Kaartinen K, Syrjänen J, Pörsti I, et al. (2008). Inflammatory markers and the progression of IgA glomerulonephritis. Nephrol Dial Transplant. **23**: 1285–90.

Kadiyala A, Mathew AT, Sachdeva M, et al. (2015). Outcomes following kidney transplantation in IgA nephropathy: A UNOS/OPTN analysis. Clin Transplant. **29**: 911–19.

Kamei K, Nakanishi K, Ito S, et al. (2011). Long-term results of a randomized controlled trial in childhood IgA nephropathy. Clin J Am Soc Nephrol. **6**: 1301–7.

Kang Z, Li Z, Duan C, et al. (2015). Mycophenolate mofetil therapy for steroid-resistant IgA nephropathy with the nephrotic syndrome in children. Pediatr Nephrol. **30**: 1121–9.

Katafuchi R, Kawamura T, Joh K, et al. (2016). Pathological sub-analysis of a multicenter randomized controlled trial of tonsillectomy combined with steroid pulse therapy versus steroid pulse monotherapy in patients with immunoglobulin A nephropathy. Clin Exp Nephrol. **20**: 244–52.

Kaveri SV, Lacroix-Desmazes S, Bayry J. (2008). The anti-inflammatory IgG. N Engl J Med. **17**: 307–9.

Kawabe M, Yamamoto I, Komatsuzaki Y, et al. (2017). Recurrence and graft loss after renal transplantation in adults with IgA vasculitis. Clin Exp Nephrol. **21**: 714–20.

Kawamura T, Yoshimura M, Miyazaki Y, et al. (2014). A multicenter randomized controlled trial of tonsillectomy combined with steroid pulse therapy in patients with immunoglobulin A nephropathy. Nephrol Dial Transplant. **29**: 1546–53.

Kawasaki Y, Hosoya M, Suzuki J, et al. (2004). Efficacy of multidrug therapy combined with mizoribine in children with diffuse IgA nephropathy in comparison with multidrug therapy without mizoribine and methylprednisolone pulse therapy. Am J Nephrol. **24**: 576–81.

KDIGO Clinical Practice Guidelines for Glomerulonephritis. (2012). Kidney Int Suppl. **2**: 209–17.

Kennard AL, Jiang SH2, Walters GD. (2017). Increased glomerulonephritis recurrence after living related donation. BMC Nephrol. **18**: 25–31.

Kim Y, Yeo SM, Kang SS, et al. (2017). Long-term clinical outcomes of first and second kidney transplantation in patients with biopsy-proven IgA nephropathy. Transplant Proc. **49**: 992–6.

Kincaid-Smith P, Bennett WM, Dowling JP, et al. (1983). Acute renal failure and tubular necrosis associated with hematuria due to glomerulonephritis. Clin Nephrol. **19**: 206–10.

Kincaid-Smith P, Nicholls K. (1983). Mesangial IgA nephropathy. Am J Kidney Dis. **3**: 90–102.

Kiryluk K, Li Y, Moldoveanu Z, Suzuki H, et al. (2017). GWAS for serum galactose-deficient IgA1 implicates critical genes of the O-glycosylation pathway. PLoS Genet. **13**: e1006609.

Kiryluk K, Li Y, Scolari F, et al. (2014). Discovery of new risk loci for IgA nephropathy implicates genes involved in immunity against intestinal pathogens. Nat Genet. **46**: 1187–9.

Kittiskulnam P, Kanjanabuch T, Tangmanjitjaroen K, et al. (2014). The beneficial effects of weight reduction in overweight patients with chronic proteinuric immunoglobulin a nephropathy: A randomized controlled trial. J Ren Nutr. **24**: 200–7.

Knoop T, Vikse BE, Mwakimonga A, et al. (2017). Long-term outcome in 145 patients with assumed benign immunoglobulin A nephropathy. Nephrol Dial Transplant. **32**: 1841–50.

Knoop T, Vikse BE, Svarstad E, et al. (2013). Mortality in patients with IgA nephropathy. Am J Kidney Dis. **62**: 883–90.

Kobayashi Y, Fujii K, Hiki Y, et al. (1988). Steroid therapy in IgA nephropathy: A retrospective study in heavy proteinuric cases. Nephron. **48**: 12–17.

Kobayashi Y, Hiki Y, Fujii K, et al. (1989). Moderately proteinuric IgA nephropathy: Prognostic prediction of individual clinical courses and steroid therapy in progressive cases. Nephron. **53**: 250–6.

Kohaut E, Waldo F. (1989). IgA nephropathy in black children. Pediatr Nephrol. **3**: C135.

Komatsu H, Fujimoto S, Hara S, et al. (2004). Relationship between serum IgA/C3 ratio and the progression of IgA nephropathy. Intern Med. **43**: 1023–8.

Komatsu H, Fujimoto S, Hara S, et al. (2008). Effect of tonsillectomy plus steroid pulse therapy on clinical remission of IgA nephropathy: A controlled study. Clin J Am Soc Nephrol. **3**: 1301–7.

Komatsu H, Fujimoto S, Sato Y, et al. (2005). 'Point of no return (PNR)' in progressive IgA nephropathy: Significance of blood pressure and proteinuria management up to PNR. J Nephrol. **18**: 690–5.

Koshino K, Ushigome H, Sakai K, et al. (2013). Outcome of tonsillectomy for recurrent IgA nephropathy after kidney transplantation. Clin Transplant. **26**: 22–8.

Kunz R, Friedrich C, Wolbers M, et al. (2008). Meta-analysis: Effect of monotherapy and combination therapy with inhibitors of the renin-angiotensin system on proteinuria in renal disease. Ann Intern Med. **148**: 30–48.

Kunz R, Wolbers M, Glass T, et al. (2008). The COOPERATE trial. A letter of concern. Lancet. **371**: 1575–6.

Lafayette RA, Canetta PA, Rovin BH, et al. (2017). A randomized, controlled trial of rituximab in IgA nephropathy with proteinuria and renal dysfunction. J Am Soc Nephrol. **28**: 1306–13.

Lai FM, Szeto CC, Choi PC, et al. (2002). Primary IgA nephropathy with low histologic grade and disease progression: Is there a 'point of no return'? Am J Kidney Dis. **39**: 401–6.

Lai KN, Chan LY, Tang SC, et al. (2002). Characteristics of polymeric lambda-IgA binding to leukocytes in IgA nephropathy. J Am Soc Nephrol. **13**: 2309–13.

Lai KN, Chui SH, Lai FM, et al. (1988). Predominant synthesis of IgA with lambda light chain in IgA nephropathy. Kidney Int. **33**: 584–9.

Lai KN, Lai FM, Ho CP, et al. (1986). Corticosteroid therapy in IgA nephropathy with nephrotic syndrome: A long-term controlled trial. Clin Nephrol. **26**: 174–80.

Lai KN, Lai FM, Leung ACT, et al. (1987). Plasma exchange in patients with rapidly progressive idiopathic IgA nephropathy: A report of two cases and review of literature. Am J Kidney Dis. **10**: 66–70.

Lai KN, Lai FM, Vallance-Owen J. (1988). A short-term controlled trial of cyclosporin A in IgA nephropathy. Trans Proceedings. **20**: 297–303.

Lai KN, Tang SC, Schena FP, et al. (2016). IgA nephropathy. Nat Rev Dis Primers. **2**: 16001.

Lai KN, To WY, Li PK, et al. (1996). Increased binding of polymeric lambda-IgA to cultured human mesangial cells in IgA nephropathy. Kidney Int. **49**: 839–45.

Lau KK, Wyatt RJ, Moldoveanu Z, et al. (2007). Serum levels of galactose deficient IgA in children with IgA nephropathy and Henoch-Schönlein purpura. Pediatr Nephrol. **22**: 2067–72.

Lemley KV, Lafayette RA, Derby G, et al. (2008). Prediction of early progression in recently diagnosed IgA nephropathy. Nephrol Dial Transplant. **23**: 213–22.

Lemley KV, Lafayette RA, Safai M, et al. (2002). Podocytopenia and disease severity in IgA nephropathy. Kidney Int. **61**: 1475–85.

Leung JC, Chan LY, Tang SC, et al. (2011). Oxidative damages in tubular epithelial cells in IgA nephropathy: Role of crosstalk between angiotensin II and aldosterone. J Transl Med. **9**: 169.

Leung JC, Tang SC, Lam MF, et al. (2001). Charge-dependent binding of polymeric IgA1 to human mesangial cells in IgA nephropathy. Kidney Int. **59**: 277–85.

Li HL, Hancock WW, Hooke DH, et al. (1990). Mononuclear cell activation and decreased renal function in IgA nephropathy with crescents. Kidney Int. **37**: 1552–6.

Lim E, Chia D, Terasaki P. (1991). Studies of sera from IgA nephropathy patients to explain high kidney graft survival. Hum Immunol. **32**: 81–6.

Limardo M, Imbasciati E, Ravani P, et al. (2010). Pregnancy and progression of IgA nephropathy: Results of an Italian multicenter study. Am J Kidney Dis. **56**: 506–12.

Lionaki S, Panagiotellis K, Melexopoulou C, et al. (2017). The clinical course of IgA nephropathy after kidney transplantation and its management. Transplant Rev (Orlando). **31**: 106–14.

Liu LJ, Lv JC, Shi SF, et al. (2012). Oral calcitriol for reduction of proteinuria in patients with IgA nephropathy: A randomized controlled trial. Am J Kidney Dis. **59**: 67–74.

Liu LL, Wang LN, Jiang Y, et al. (2015). Tonsillectomy for IgA nephropathy: A meta-analysis. Am J Kidney Dis. **65**: 80–7.

Liu XJ, Geng YQ, Xin SN, et al. (2011). Antithrombotic drug therapy for IgA nephropathy: A meta-analysis of randomized controlled trials. Intern Med. **50**: 2503–10.

Liu XW, Li DM, Xu GS, et al. (2010). Comparison of the therapeutic effects of leflunomide and mycophenolate mofetil in the treatment of immunoglobulin A nephropathy manifesting with nephrotic syndrome. Int J Clin Pharmacol Ther. **48**: 509–13.

Liu Y, Ma X, Zheng J, et al. (2016). A systematic review and meta-analysis of kidney and pregnancy outcomes in IgA nephropathy. Am J Nephrol. **44**: 187–93.

Liu Y, Xiao J, Shi X, et al. (2016). Immunosuppressive agents versus steroids in the treatment of IgA nephropathy-induced proteinuria: A meta-analysis. Exp Ther Med. **11**: 49–56.

Locatelli F, Pozzi M, Del Vecchio L, et al. (2003). Advanced IgA nephropathy: To treat or not to treat? Nephron Clin Pract. **93**: c119–21.

Lou T, Wang C, Chen Z, et al. (2006). Randomized controlled trial of leflunomide in the treatment of Immunoglobulin A nephropathy. Nephrology (Carlton). **11**: 113–16.

Lundberg S, Westergren E, Smolander J, et al. (2017). B cell-depleting therapy with rituximab or ofatumumab in immunoglobulin A nephropathy or vasculitis with nephritis. Clin Kidney J. **10**: 20–6.

Lv J, Xu D, Perkovic V, et al. (2012). Corticosteroid therapy in IgA nephropathy. J Am Soc Nephrol. **23**: 1108–16.

Lv J, Zhang H, Chen Y, et al. (2009). Combination therapy of prednisone and ACE inhibitor versus ACE inhibitor therapy alone in patients with IgA nephropathy: A randomized controlled trial. Am J Kidney Dis. **53**: 26–32.

Lv J, Zhang H, Wong MG, et al. (2017). Effect of methylprednisolone on clinical outcomes in patients with IgA nephropathy. The TESTING randomized clinical trial. JAMA. **318**: 432–42.

Lv J, Zhang H, Zhou Y, et al. (2008). Natural history of immunoglobulin A nephropathy and predictive factors of prognosis: A long-term follow-up of 204 cases in China. Nephrology (Carlton). **13**: 242–6.

MacKinnon B, Fraser EP, Cattran DC, et al. (2008). Validation of the Toronto formula to predict progression of IgA nephropathy. Nephron Clin Pract. **109**: c148–53.

McAdoo S, Tam FWK. (2018). Role of the spleen tyrosine kinase pathway in driving inflammation in IgA nephropathy. Semin Nephrol. **38**: 496–503.

McDonald SP, Russ GR. (2006). Recurrence of IgA nephropathy among renal allograft recipients from living donors is greater among those with zero HLA mismatches. Transplantation. **27**: 759–62.

McGrogan A, Franssen CSM, De Vries CS. (2011). The incidence of primary glomerulonephritis worldwide: A systematic review of the literature. Nephrol Dial Transplant. **26**: 414–43.

McIntyre CW, Fluck RJ, Lambie SH. et al. (2001). Steroid and cyclophosphamide therapy for IgA nephropathy associated with crescentic change: An effective treatment. Clin Nephrol. **56**: 193–8.

Maeda A, Gohda T, Funabiki K, et al. (2003). Significance of serum IgA levels and serum IgA/C3 ratio in diagnostic analysis of patients with IgA nephropathy. J Clin Lab Anal. **17**: 73–6.

Maes BD, Oyen R, Claes K, et al. (2004). Mycophenolate mofetil in IgA nephropathy: Results of a 3-year prospective placebo-controlled randomized study. Kidney Int. **65**: 1842–9.

Magistroni R, D'Agati VD, Appel GB, et al. (2015). New developments in the genetics, pathogenesis, and therapy of IgA nephropathy. Kidney Int. **88**: 974–89.

Magistroni R, Furci L, Leonelli M, et al. (2006). A validated model of disease progression in IgA nephropathy. J Nephrol. **19**: 32–40.

Maillard N, Wyatt RJ, Julian BA, et al. (2015). Current understanding of the role of complement in IgA nephropathy. J Am Soc Nephrol. **26**: 1503–12.

Manno C, Strippoli GF, D'Altri C, et al. (2007). A novel simple histological classification for renal survival in IgA nephropathy: A retrospective study. Am J Kidney Dis. **49**: 763–5.

Manno C, Torres DD, Rossini M, et al. (2009). Randomized controlled clinical trial of corticosteroids plus ACE-inhibitors with long-term follow-up in proteinuric IgA nephropathy. Nephrol Dial Transplant. **24**: 3694–701.

Masutani K, Tsuchimoto A, Yamada T, et al. (2016). Comparison of steroid-pulse therapy and combined with mizoribine in IgA nephropathy: A randomized controlled trial. Clin Exp Nephrol. **20**: 896–903.

Mestecky J, Tomana M, Moldoveanu Z, et al. (2008). Role of aberrant glycosylation of IgA1 in the pathogenesis of IgA nephropathy. Kidney Blood Pres Res. **31**: 29–37.

Min L, Wang Q, Cao L, et al. (2017). Comparison of combined leflunomide and low-dose corticosteroid therapy with full-dose corticosteroid monotherapy for progressive IgA nephropathy. Oncotarget. **8**: 48375–84.

Mitsuiki K, Harada A, Okura T, et al. (2007). Histologically advanced IgA nephropathy treated successfully with prednisolone and cyclophosphamide. Clin Exp Nephrol. **11**: 297–303.

Miyazaki M, Hotta O, Komatsuda A, et al. (2007). A multicenter prospective cohort study of tonsillectomy and steroid therapy in Japanese patients with IgA nephropathy: A 5-year report. Control Nephrol. **157**: 94–8.

Moldoveanu Z, Wyatt RJ, Lee JY, et al. (2007). Patients with IgA nephropathy have increased serum galactose-deficient IgA1 levels. Kidney Int. **71**: 1148–54.

Moriyama T, Nitta K, Suzuki K, et al. (2005). Latent IgA deposition from donor kidney is the major risk factor for recurrent IgA nephropathy in renal transplantation. Clin Transplant. **19**: 41–8.

Moriyama T, Oshima Y, Tanaka K, et al. (2014). Statins stabilize the renal function of IgA nephropathy. Ren Fail. **36**: 356–60.

Moriyama T, Tanaka K, Iwasaki C, et al. (2014). Prognosis in IgA nephropathy: 30-year analysis of 1,012 patients at a single center in Japan. PLoS One. **9**: e91756.

Moroni G, Longhi S, Quaglini S, et al. (2013). The long-term outcome of renal transplantation of IgA nephropathy and the impact of recurrence on graft survival. Nephrol Dial Transplant. **28**: 1305–14.

Moura IC, Benhamou M, Launay P, et al. (2008). The glomerular response to IgA deposition in IgA nephropathy. Semin Nephrol. **28**: 88–95.

Mousson C, Charon-Barra C, Funes de la Vega M, et al. (2007). Recurrence of IgA nephropathy with crescents in kidney transplants. Transplant Proc. **39**: 2595–6.

Myllymaki J, Honkanen T, Syrjänen J, et al. (2005). Uric acid correlates with the severity of histopathological findings in IgA nephropathy. Nephrol Dial Transplant. **20**: 89–95.

Nagaoka R, Kaneko K, Ohtomo Y, et al. (2002). Mizoribine treatment for IgA nephropathy. Pediatr Int. **44**: 217–23.

Nair R, Walker PD. (2006). Is IgA nephropathy the commonest primary glomerulopathy among young adults in the USA? Kidney Int. **69**: 1455–8.

Nakao M, Yoshimura A, Morita H, et al. (2003). Combination treatment of angiotensin II receptor blocker and angiotensin converting enzyme inhibitor in non-diabetic renal disease (COOPERATE): A randomized controlled trial. Lancet. **361**: 117–24.

Nakata J, Suzuki Y, Suzuki H, et al. (2014). Changes in nephritogenic serum galactose-deficient IgA1 in IgA nephropathy following tonsillectomy and steroid therapy. PLoS One. **9**: e89707.

Nakayama K, Ohsawa I, Maeda-Ohtani A, et al. (2008). Prediction of diagnosis of immunoglobulin A nephropathy prior to renal biopsy and correlation with urinary sediment findings and prognostic grading. J Clin Lab Anal. **22**: 114–19.

Nasr SH, Markowitz GS, Whelan JD, et al. (2003). IgA-dominant acute post-staphylococcal glomerulonephritis complicating diabetic nephropathy. Hum Pathol. **34**: 1235–41.

Nasr SH, Share DS, Vargas MT, et al. (2007). Acute post-staphylococcal glomerulonephritis superimposed on diabetic glomerulosclerosis. Kidney Int. **71**: 1317–21.

Navaneethan SD, Viswanathan G, Strippoli GF. (2008). Meta-analysis of mycophenolate mofetil in IgA nephropathy. Nephrology (Carlton). **13**: 90.

Ng YS, Vathsala A, Chew ST, et al. (2007). Long-term outcome of renal allografts in patients with immunoglobulin A nephropathy. Med J Malaysia. **62**: 109–13.

Nicholls K, Fairley KF, Dowling JP, et al. (1984). The clinical course of mesangial IgA associated nephropathy in adults. Quart J Med. **210**: 227–36.

Nijim S, Vujjini V, Alasfar S, et al. (2016). Recurrent IgA nephropathy after kidney transplantation. Transplant Proc. **48**: 2689–94.

Nishitani Y, Iwano M, Yamaguchi Y, et al. (2005). Fibroblast specific protein-1 is a specific prognostic marker for renal survival in patients with IgAN. Kidney Int. **68**: 1078–85.

Nishiwaki H, Hasegawa T, Nagayama Y, et al. (2015). Absence of mesangial C1q deposition is associated with resolution of proteinuria and hematuria after tonsillectomy plus steroid pulse therapy for immunoglobulin a nephropathy. Nephron. **130**: 1–7.

Novak J, Julian BA, Tomana M, et al. (2008). IgA glycosylation and IgA immune complexes in the pathogenesis of IgA nephropathy. Semin Nephrol. **28**: 78–87.

Novak J, Renfrow MB, Gharavi AG, et al. (2013). Pathogenesis of immunoglobulin A nephropathy. Curr Opin Nephrol Hypertens. **22**: 287–94.

Ogura Y, Suzuki S, Shirakawa T, et al. (2000). Hemophilus influenza antigen and antibody in children with IgA nephropathy and Henoch–Schönlein purpura. Am J Kidney Dis. **36**: 47–52.

Onda K, Ohi H, Tamano M, et al. (2007). Hypercomplementemia in adult patients with IgA nephropathy. J Clin Lab Anal. **211**: 77–84.

Oortwijn BD, Eijgenraam JW, Rastaldi MP, et al. (2008). The role of secretory IgA and complement in IgA nephropathy. Semin Nephrol. **28**: 58–65.

Ortmanns A, Ittel TH, Schnitzler N, et al. (1998). Remission of IgA nephropathy following treatment of cytomegalovirus with ganciclovir. Clin Nephrol. **49**: 379–84.

Oshima Y, Moriyama T, Itabashi M, et al. (2015). Characteristics of IgA nephropathy in advanced-age patients. Int Urol Nephrol. **47**: 137–45.

Otsuka Y, Takeda A, Horike K, et al. (2014). Early recurrence of active IgA nephropathy after kidney transplantation. Nephrology (Carlton). **3**: 45–8.

Packham DK. (2007). Thin basement membrane nephropathy and IgA glomerulonephritis: Can they be distinguished without a renal biopsy? Nephrology (Carlton). **12**: 481–6.

Palamuthusingam D, Castledine C, Lawman S. (2018). Outcomes of immunosuppression in IgA nephropathy based on the oxford classification. Saudi J Kidney Dis Transpl. **29**: 341–50.

Pappalardo E, Zingale LC, Cicardi M. (2003). Increased expression of C1-inhibitor mRNA in patients with hereditary angioedema treated with Danazol. Immunol Lett. **86**: 271–6.

Park JS, Song JH, Yang WS, et al. (1994). Cytomegalovirus is not specifically associated with immunoglobulin A nephropathy. J Am Soc Nephrol. **4**: 1623–6.

Pei G, Zeng R, Han M, et al. (2014). Renal interstitial infiltration and tertiary lymphoid organ neogenesis in IgA nephropathy. Clin J Am Soc Nephrol. **9**: 255–64.

Petterson EE, Rekola S, Berglund L, et al. (1994). Treatment of IgA nephropathy with omega-3-polyunsaturated fatty acids: A prospective, double-blind, randomised study. Clin Nephrol. **41**: 183–90.

Philibert D, Cattran D, Cook T. (2008). Clinicopathologic correlations in IgA nephropathy. Semin Nephrol. **28**: 10–17.

Pillebout E, Thervet E, Hill G, et al. (2002). Henoch-Schönlein purpura in adults: Outcome and prognostic factors. J Am Soc Nephrol. **13**: 1271–8.

Pirani CL, Salinas-Madrigal L. (1968). Evaluation of percutaneous renal biopsy. Pathol Ann. **3**: 249–96.

Ponticelli C, Cucchiari D. (2017). Reninn-angiotensin system inhibitors in kidney transplantation: A benefit risk assessment. J Nephrol. **30**: 155–7.

Ponticelli C, Glassock R. (Eds). (2009). *Treatment of Primary Glomerulonephritis*. 2nd Edition. OUP, Oxford.

Ponticelli C, Glassock RJ. (2010). Posttransplant recurrence of primary glomerulonephritis. Clin J Am Soc Nephrol. **5**: 2363–72.

Ponticelli C, Traversi L, Banfi G. (2004). Renal transplantation in patients with IgA mesangial glomerulonephritis. Pediatr Transplant. **8**: 334–8.

Ponticelli C, Traversi L, Feliciani A, et al. (2001). Kidney transplantation in patients with IgA mesangial glomerulonephritis. Kidney Int. **60**: 1948–54.

Pouria S, Barratt J. (2008). Secondary IgA nephropathy. Semin Nephrol. **28**: 27–37.

Pozzi C. (2007). Treatment of IgA nephropathy with chronic renal failure. G Ital Nefrol. **25**: 83–7.

Pozzi C. (2016). Pro: STOP immunosuppression in IgA nephropathy? Nephrol Dial Transplant. **31**: 1766–70.

Pozzi C, Andrulli S, Del Vecchio L, et al. (2004). Corticosteroid effectiveness in IgA nephropathy: Long-term results of a controlled randomized clinical trial. J Am Soc Nephrol. **15**: 157–62.

Pozzi C, Andrulli S, Pani A, et al. (2010). Addition of azathioprine to corticosteroids does not benefit patients with IgA nephropathy. J Am Soc Nephrol. **21**: 1783–90.

Pozzi C, Andrulli S, Pani A, et al. (2013). IgA nephropathy with severe chronic renal failure: a randomized controlled trial of corticosteroids and azathioprine. J Nephrol. **26**: 86–93.

Pozzi C, Bolasco PG, Fogazzi GB, et al. (1999). Corticosteroids in IgA nephropathy: A randomised controlled trial. Lancet. **353**: 883–7.

Pozzi C, Del Vecchio L, Locatelli F. (2002). Can immunosuppression therapy be useful in IgA nephropathy when the 'point of no return' has already been exceeded? Nephron. **92**: 699–701.

Pozzi C, Sarcina C, Ferrario F. (2016). Treatment of IgA nephropathy with renal insufficiency. J Nephrol. **29**: 551–8.

Praga M, Gutiérrez E, González E, et al. (2003). Treatment of IgA nephropathy with ACE inhibitors: A randomized and controlled trial. J Am Soc Nephrol. **14**: 1578–83.

Praga M, Gutierrez-Millet V, Navas JJ, et al. (1985). Acute worsening of renal function during episodes of macroscopic hematuria in IgA nephropathy. Kidney Int. **28**: 69–74.

Prasad B, Giebel S, McCarron MCE, et al. (2018). Use of synthetic adrenocorticotropic hormone in patients with IgA nephropathy. BMC Nephrol. **19**: 118.

Pruthi R, McClure M, Casula A, et al. (2016). Long-term graft outcomes and patient survival are lower posttransplant in patients with a primary renal diagnosis of glomerulonephritis. Kidney Int. **89**: 918–26.

Radford MG, Donadio JV Jr, Bergstrahl EJ, et al. (1997). Predicting renal outcome in IgA nephropathy. J Am Soc Nephrol. **8**: 199–207.

Rajagopala S, Parameswaran S, Ajmera JS, et al. (2017). Diffuse alveolar hemorrhage in IgA nephropathy: Case series and systematic review of the literature. Int J Rheum Dis. **20**: 109–21.

Rasche FM, Keller F, Lepper PM, et al. (2006). High-dose intravenous immunoglobulin pulse therapy in patients with progressive immunoglobulin A nephropathy: A long-term follow-up. Clin Exp Immunol. **146**: 47–53.

Rasche FM, Keller F, Rasche WG, et al. (2016). Sequential therapy with cyclophosphamide and mycophenolic acid in patients with progressive immunoglobulin A nephropathy: A long-term follow-up. Clin Exp Immunol. **183**: 307–16.

Rasche FM, Schwarz A, Keller F. (1999). Tonsillectomy does not prevent a progressive course in IgA nephropathy. Clin Nephrol. **51**: 147–52.

Rath A, Tewari R, Mendonca S, et al. (2015). Oxford classification of IgA nephropathy and C4d deposition; correlation and its implication. J Nephropharmacol. **5**: 75–9.

Rauen T, Eitner F, Fitzner C, et al. (2015). Intensive supportive care plus immunosuppression in IgA nephropathy. N Engl J Med. **373**: 2225–36.

Rauen T, Eitner F, Fitzner C, et al. (2016). Con: STOP immunosuppression in IgA nephropathy. Nephrol Dial Transplant. **31**: 1771–4.

Rauta V, Finne P, Fagerudd J, et al. (2002). Factors associated with progression of IgA nephropathy are related to renal function: A model for estimating risk of progression in mild disease. Clin Nephrol. **58**: 85–94.

Ravani P, Bonanni A, Rossi R, et al. (2016). Anti-CD20 antibodies for idiopathic nephrotic syndrome in children. Clin J Am Soc Nephrol. **11**: 710–20.

Reich HN, Troyanov S, Scholey JW, et al. (2007). Remission of proteinuria improves prognosis in IgA nephropathy. J Am Soc Nephrol. **18**: 3177–83.

Reid S, Cawthon PM, Craig JC, et al. (2011). Non-immunosuppressive treatment for IgA nephropathy. Cochrane Database Syst Rev. **1**: CD003962.

Rekola S, Bergstrand A, Bucht H. (1991a). Deterioration in GFR in IgA nephropathy as measured by 51Cr-EDTA clearance. Kidney Int. **40**: 1050–4.

Rekola S, Bergstrand, A, Bucht H. (1991b). Deterioration rate in hypertensive IgA nephropathy: Comparison of a converting enzyme inhibitor and β-blocking agents. Nephron. **59**: 57–60.

Renfrow MB, Novak J. (2017). What insights can proteomics give us into IgA nephropathy (Berger's disease)? Expert Rev Proteomics. **29**: 1–3.

Ring T, Pedersen BB, Salkus G, et al. (2015). Use of eculizumab in crescentic IgA nephropathy: proof of principle and conundrum? Clin Kidney J. **8**: 489–91.

Robert T, Berthelot L, Cambier A, et al. (2015). Molecular insights into the pathogenesis of IgA nephropathy. Trends Mol Med. **21**: 762–75.

Rocatello D, Ferro M, Coppo R, et al. (1995). Treatment of rapidly progressive IgA nephropathy. In **A Clarkson, A Woodroffe** (eds), *IgA Nephropathy: Pathogenesis and Treatment*, vol. **3**, pp. 177–83. Karger, Basel.

Roccatello D, Rossi D, Marletto F, et al. (2012). Long-term effects of methylprednisolone pulses and mycophenolate mofetil in IgA nephropathy patients at risk of progression. J Nephrol. **25**: 198–203.

Rodrigues JC, Haas M, Reich HN. (2017). IgA nephropathy. Clin J Am Soc Nephrol. **12**: 677–86.

Rodriguez-Soriano J, Arrieta A, Vallo A, et al. (1988). IgA antigliadin antibodies in children with IgA mesangial glomerulonephritis. Lancet. **1**: 1109–10 (Letter).

Roos A, Rastaldi MP, Calvaresi N, et al. (2006). Glomerular activation of the lectin pathway of complement in IgA nephropathy is associated with more severe renal disease. J Am Soc Nephrol. **17**: 1724–34.

Rosenberg H, Martínez P, Vaccarezza A, et al. (1989). A morphologic study of 103 kidneys donated for renal transplantation. Rev Med Chil. **117**:1344–50.

Rosenberg H, Martínez P, Vaccarezza A, et al. (1990). Morphological findings in 70 kidneys of living donors for renal transplants. Pathol Res Pract. **186**: 619–24.

Rostoker G, Desvaux-Belghiti D, Pilatte Y, et al. (1994). High-dose immunoglobulin therapy for severe IgA nephropathy and Henoch–Schönlein purpura. Ann Intern Med. 120: 476–84.

Rostoker G, Desvaux-Belghiti D, Pilatte Y, et al. (1995). Immunomodulation with low-dose immunoglobulins for moderate IgA nephropathy and Henoch-Schönlein purpura. Preliminary results of a prospective uncontrolled trial. Nephron. 69: 327–34.

Rostoker G, Laurent J, Andre C, et al. (1988). High levels of IgA antigliadin antibodies in patients who have IgA mesangial glomerulonephritis but no coeliac disease. Lancet. 1: 356–7.

Rovin BH, Furie R, Latinis K, et al. (2012). Efficacy and safety of rituximab in patients with active proliferative lupus nephritis: The Lupus Assessment with Rituximab study. Arthritis Rheum. 64: 1215–26.

Ruan Y, Hong F, Wu J, et al. (2018). Clinicopathological characteristics, role of immunosuppressive therapy and progression in IgA nephropathy with hyperuricemia. Kidney Blood Press Res. 43: 1131–40.

Ruggajo P, Svarstad E, Leh S, et al. (2016). Low birth weight and risk of progression to end stage renal disease in IgA nephropathy: A retrospective registry-based cohort study. PLoS One. 11: e0153819.

Ruggenenti P, Cravedie P, Chianca A, et al. (2012). Rituximab in idiopathic membranous nephropathy. J Am Soc Nephrol. 23: 1416–25.

Ruggenenti P, Perna A, Benini R, et al. (1999). In chronic nephropathies prolonged ACE inhibition can induce remission: Dynamics of time-dependent change in GFR. Investigations of the GISEN Group. Gruppo Italiano Studi Epidemiologici in Nefrologia. J Am Soc Nephrol. 10: 997–1006.

Russo D, Minutolo R, Pisani A, et al. (2001). Coadministration of losartan and enalapril exerts additive antiproteinuric effect in IgA nephropathy. Am J Kidney Dis. 38: 18–25.

Sancho J, Egido J, Rivera F, et al. (1988). Immune complexes in IgA nephropathy: Presence of antibodies against diet antigens and delayed clearance of specific polymeric IgA immune complexes. Clin Exp Immunol. 73: 295–301.

Sanfilippo F, Crocker P, Bollinger R. (1986). Fate of four cadaveric donor allografts with mesangial IgA deposits. Transplantation. 42: 511–15.

Sarcina C, Tinelli C, Ferrario F, et al. (2016). Changes in proteinuria and side effects of corticosteroids alone or in combination with azathioprine at different stages of IgA nephropathy. Clin J Am Soc Nephrol. 11: 973–81.

Sarcina C, Tinelli C, Ferrario F, et al. (2016). Corticosteroid treatment influences ta-proteinuria and renal survival in IgA nephropathy. PLoS One. 11: e0158584.

Sato M, Adachi M, Kosukegawa H, et al. (2017). The size of palatine tonsils cannot be used to decide the indication of tonsillectomy for IgA nephropathy. Clin Kidney J. 10: 221–8.

Sato Y, Ishida H, Shimizu T, et al. (2014). Evaluation of tonsillectomy before kidney transplantation in patients with IgA nephropathy. Transpl Immunol. 30: 12–17.

Sato K, Makabe S, Iwabuchi Y, et al. (2018). Successful treatment with steroid and cyclosporine A in a patient with immunoglobulin A-proliferative glomerulonephritis with monoclonal immunoglobulin deposits. Nephrology (Carlton). doi: 10.1111/nep.13261.

Schena FR, Montenegro M, Scivittaro V. (1990). Meta-analysis of randomised controlled trials in patients with IgA nephropathy (Berger's disease). Nephrol Dial Transplant. **5**: 47–52.

Scholl U, Wastl U, Risler T, et al. (1999). The 'point of no return' and the rate of progression in the natural history of IgA nephritis. Clin Nephrol. **52**: 285–92.

Seager J, Wilson J, Jamieson DL, et al. (1975). IgA deficiency, epilepsy and phenytoin treatment. Lancet. **306**: 632–5.

Selewski DT, Ambruzs JM, Appel GB, et al. (2018). Clinical characteristics and treatment patterns of children and adults with IgA nephropathy or IgA vasculitis: findings fom the CureGn study. Kidney Int Rep. **3**: 373–84.

Selvaskandan H, Pawluczyk I, Barratt J. (2018). MicroRNAs: A new avenue to understand, investigate and treat immunoglobulin A nephropathy? Clin Kidney J. **11**: 29–37.

Sethi S, Nasr SH, De Vriese AS, et al. (2015). C4d as a diagnostic tool in proliferative GN. J Am Soc Nephrol. **26**: 2852–9.

Sevilliano AM, Cabrera J, Gutierrez E, et al. (2015). Malignant hypertension: A type of IgA nephropathy manifestation with poor prognosis. Nefrologia. **35**: 42–9.

Sevillano AM, Gutiérrez E, Yuste C, et al. (2017). Remission of hematuria improves renal survival in IgA nephropathy. J Am Soc Nephrol. **28**: 3089–99.

Shen P, He L, Jiang Y, et al. (2007). Useful indicators for performing a renal biopsy in adult patients with isolated microscopic hematuria. Int J Clin Pract. **61**: 789–94.

Shi SF, Wang SX, Jiang L, et al. (2011). Pathologic predictors of renal outcome and therapeutic efficacy in IgA nephropathy: Validation of the Oxford classification. Clin J Am Soc Nephrol. **6**: 2175–84.

Shima Y, Nakanishi K, Kaku Y, et al. (2018). Combination therapy with or without warfarin and dipyridamole for severe childhood IgA nephropathy: An RCT. Pediatr Nephrol. doi: 10.1007/s00467-018-4011-6

Simeoni M, Nicotera R, Pelagi E, et al. (2018). Successful use of Aliskiren in a case of IgA-mesangial glomerulonephritis unresponsive to conventional therapies. Rev Recent Clin Trials. doi: 10.2174/1574887113666180726103648

Sinico RA, Tadros M, Radice A, et al. (1994). Lack of IgA neutrophil cytoplasmic antibodies in Henoch–Schönlein purpura and IgA nephropathy. Clin Immunol Immunopathol. **73**: 19–26.

Sinniah R. (1983). Occurrence of mesangial IgA and IgM deposition in a control necropsy population. J Clin Pathol. **36**: 276–9.

Soares MF, Roberts IS. (2017). IgA nephropathy: An update. Curr Opin Nephrol Hypertens. **26**: 165–71.

Sofue T, Inui M, Hara T, et al. (2013). Latent IgA deposition from donor kidneys does not affect transplant prognosis, irrespective of mesangial expansion. Clin Transplant. **27**: 14–21.

Song YH, Cai GY, Xiao YF, et al. (2017). Efficacy and safety of calcineurin inhibitor treatment for IgA nephropathy: A meta-analysis. BMC Nephrol. **18**: 61–9.

Southwest Pediatric Nephrology Study Group. (1985). Association of IgA nephropathy with steroid-responsive nephrotic syndrome. Am J Kidney Dis. **5**: 157–64.

Suwabe T, Ubara Y, Sogawa Y, et al. (2007). Tonsillectomy and corticosteroid therapy with concomitant methylprednisolone pulse therapy for IgA nephropathy. Control Nephrol. **157**: 99–103.

Suzuki H, Moldoveanu Z, Hall S, et al. (2008). IgA1-secreting cells lines from patients with IgA nephropathy produce aberrantly glycosylated IgA1. J Clin Invest. **118**: 629–39.

Suzuki H, Ohsawa I, Kodama F, et al. (2013). Fluctuation of serum C3 levels reflects disease activity and metabolic background in patients with IgA nephropathy. J Nephrol. **26**: 708–15.

Suzuki K, Honda K, Tanabe K, et al. (2003). Incidence of latent mesangial IgA deposition in renal allograft donors in Japan. Kidney Int. **63**: 2286–94.

Syrjanen J, Mustonen J, Pasternack A. (2000). Hypertriglyceridemia and hyperuricemia are the risk factors for progression of IgA nephropathy. Nephrol Dial Transplant. **15**: 34–42.

Szeto CC, Chow KM, Kwan BC, et al. (2008). Oral calcitriol for the treatment of persistent proteinuria in immunoglobulin A nephropathy: An uncontrolled trial. Am J Kidney Dis. **51**: 724–31.

Szeto CC, Kwan BC, Chow KM, et al. (2013). The safety and short-term efficacy of aliskiren in the treatment of immunoglobulin a nephropathy: A randomized cross-over study. PLoS One. **8**: e62736.

Tan L, Tang Y, Peng W, et al. (2018). Combined immunosuppressive treatment may improve short-term renal outcomes in Chinese patients with advanced IgA nephropathy. Kidney Blood Press Res. **43**: 1333–43.

Tanaka K, Moriyama T, Iwasaki C, et al. (2015). Effect of hematuria on the outcome of IgA nephropathy with mild proteinuria. Clin Exp Nephrol. **19**: 815–21.

Tang S, Leung JC, Chan LY, et al. (2005). Mycophenolate mofetil alleviates proteinuria in IgA nephropathy. Kidney Int. **68**: 802–12.

Temurhan S, Akgul SU, Caliskan Y. (2017). A novel biomarker for post-transplant recurrent IgA nephropathy. Transplant Proc. **49**: 541–5.

Tesar V, Troyanov S, Bellur S, et al. (2015). Corticosteroids in IgA nephropathy: A retrospective analysis from the VALIGA Study. J Am Soc Nephrol. **26**: 2248–58.

Torres DD, Rossini M, Manno C, et al. (2008). The ratio of epidermal growth factor to monocyte chemotactic peptide-1 in the urine predicts renal prognosis in IgA nephropathy. Kidney Int. **73**: 327–33.

Trimarchi H, Barratt J, Cattran DC, et al. (2017). Oxford Classification of IgA nephropathy 2016: An update from the IgA Nephropathy Classification Working Group. Kidney Int. **91**: 1014–21.

Tumlin JA, Henniger RA. (2004). Clinical presentation, natural history and treatment of crescentic proliferative IgA nephropathy. Semin Nephrol. **24**: 256–68.

Varis J, Rantala I, Pasternack A, et al. (1993). Immunoglobulin and complement deposition in glomeruli of 776 subjects who had committed suicide or met with a violent death. J Clin Pathol. **46**: 215–22.

Vecchio M, Bonerba B, Palmer SC, et al. (2015). Immunosuppressive agents for treating IgA nephropathy. Cochrane Database Syst Rev. **8**: CD003965.

Vergano L, Loiacono E, Albera R, et al. (2015). Can tonsillectomy modify the innate and adaptive immunity pathways involved in IgA nephropathy? J Nephrol. **28**: 51–8.

Vivante A, Afek A, Frenkel-Nir Y, et al. (2011). Persistent asymptomatic isolated microscopic hematuria in Israeli adolescents and young adults and risk for end-stage renal disease. JAMA. **306**: 729–36.

Von Visger JR, Gunay Y, Andreoni KA. (2014). The risk of recurrent IgA nephropathy in a steroid-free protocol and other modifying immunosuppression. Clin Transplant. **28**: 845–54.

Wakai K, Kawamura T, Endoh M, et al. (2006). A scoring system to predict renal outcomes in IgA nephropathy: From a nationwide prospective study. Nephrol Dial Transplant. **21**: 2800–8.

Waldherr R, Rambausek M, Duncker WD, et al. (1989). Frequency of mesangial IgA deposits in a non-selected autopsy series. Nephrol Dial Transplant. **4**: 943–46.

Waldo B, Wyatt RJ, Kelly DR, et al. (1993). Treatment of IgA nephropathy in children: Efficacy of alternate-day prednisolone. Pediat Nephrol. **7**: 529–32.

Wang AY, Lai FM, Yu AW, et al. (2001). Recurrent IgA nephropathy in renal transplant allografts. Am J Kidney Dis. **38**: 588–96.

Woo KT, Lau YK, Chan CM, et al. (2008). Angiotensin-converting enzyme inhibitor versus angiotensin 2 receptor antagonist therapy and the influence of angiotensin-converting enzyme gene polymorphism in IgA nephritis. Ann Acad Med Singapore. **37**: 372–6.

Woo KT, Lau YK, Choong LH, et al. (2004). Polymorphisms of renin–angiotensin system genes in IgA nephropathy. Nephrology (Carlton). **9**: 304–9.

Working Group of the International IgA Nephropathy Network and the Renal Pathology Society, et al. (2009). The Oxford classification of IgA nephropathy: Pathology definitions, correlations, and reproducibility. Kidney Int. **76**: 546–56.

Working Group of the International IgA Nephropathy Network and the Renal Pathology Society, et al. (2009). The Oxford classification of IgA nephropathy: Rationale, clinicopathological correlations, and classification. Kidney Int. **76**: 534–45.

Working Group of the International IgA Nephropathy Network and the Renal Pathology Society, et al. (2010). The Oxford IgA nephropathy clinicopathological classification is valid for children as well as adults. Kidney Int. **77**: 921–7.

Wu J, Duan SW, Sun XF, et al. (2016). Efficacy of leflunomide, telmisartan, and clopidogrel for immunoglobulin a nephropathy: A randomized controlled trial. Chin Med J (Engl). **129**: 1894–903.

Xie J, Kiryluk K, Li Y, et al. (2016). Fine mapping implicates a deletion of CFHR1 and CFHR3 in protection from IgA nephropathy in Han Chinese. J Am Soc Nephrol. **27**: 3187–94.

Xie L, He J, Liu X, et al. (2018). Clinical value of systemic symptoms in IgA nephropathy with ANCA positivity. Clin Rheumatol. **37**: 1953–61.

Xie X, Lv J, Shi S, Zhu L, et al. (2016). Plasma exchange as an adjunctive therapy for crescentic IgA nephropathy. Am J Nephrol. **44**: 141–9.

Yanagawa H, Suzuki H, Suzuki Y, et al. (2014). A panel of serum biomarkers differentiates IgA nephropathy from other renal diseases. PLoS One. **9**: e98081.

Yang YZ, Liu LJ, Shi SF, et al. (2018). Effects of hydroxychloroquine on proteinuria in immunoglobulin A nephropathy. Am J Nephrol. **47**: 145–52.

Yang YZ, Shi SF, Chen YQ, et al. (2015). Clinical features of IgA nephropathy with serum ANCA positivity: A retrospective case-control study. Clin Kidney J. **8**: 482–8.

Yaqoob M, King A, McClelland P, et al. (1994). Relationship between hydrocarbon exposure and nephropathology in primary glomerulonephritis. Nephrol Dial Transplant. **9**: 1575–9.

Yau WP, Vathsala A, Lou HX, et al. (2007). Is a standard fixed dose of mycophenolate mofetil ideal for all patients? Nephrol Dial Transplant. **22**: 3638–45.

Yeo SC, Cheung CK, Barratt J. (2017). New insights into the pathogenesis of IgA nephropathy. Pediatr Nephrol. **33**:763–77.

Yoshida H, Mitarai T, Kawamura T, et al. (1995). Role of deletion polymorphisms of the angiotensin converting enzyme gene in the progression and therapeutic responsiveness of IgA nephropathy. J Clin Invest. **86**: 2162–9.

Yoshikawa N, Honda M, Iijima K, et al. (2006). Steroid treatment for severe childhood IgA nephropathy: A randomized, controlled trial. Clin J Am Soc Nephrol. **1**: 511–17.

Yoshikawa N, Ito H, Sakai T, et al. (1999). A controlled trial of combined therapy for newly diagnosed severe childhood IgA nephropathy. J Am Soc Nephrol. **10**: 101–9.

van Ypersele de Strihou C. (1994). Fish oil for IgA nephropathy? New Eng J Med. **331**: 1227–9.

Yu XQ, Li M, Zhang H, et al. (2011). A genome-wide association study in Han Chinese identifies multiple susceptibility loci for IgA nephropathy. Nat Genet. **44**: 178–82.

Yuste C, Rubio-Navarro A, Barraca D, et al. (2015). Haematuria increases progression of advanced proteinuric kidney disease. PLoS One. **10**: e0128575.

Zand L, Fervenza FC. (2014). Does tonsillectomy have a role in the treatment of patients with immunoglobulin A nephropathy? Nephrol Dial Transplant. **29**: 1456–9.

Zhai YL, Meng SJ, Zhu L, et al. (2016). Rare variants in the complement factor H-related protein 5 gene contribute to genetic susceptibility to IgA nephropathy. J Am Soc Nephrol. **27**: 2894–905.

Zhang JJ, Xu LX, Liu G, et al. (2008). The level of serum secretory IgA of patients with IgA nephropathy is elevated and associated with pathological phenotypes. Nephrol Dial Transplant. **23**: 207–12.

Zhang Q, Shi SF, Zhu L, et al. (2012). Tacrolimus improves the proteinuria remission in patients with refractory IgA nephropathy. Am J Nephrol. **35**: 312–20.

Zhang Y, Luo J, Hu B, et al. (2018). Efficacy and safety of tacrolimus combined with glucocorticoid treatment for IgA nephropathy: A meta-analysis. J Int Med Res. **46**: 3236–50.

Zheng JN, Bi TD, Zhu LB, et al. (2018). Efficacy and safety of mycophenolate mofetil in IgA nephropathy: An updated meta-analysis of randomized controlled trials. Exp Ther Med. **16**: 1882–90.

Zhu B, Zhu CF, Lin Y, et al. (2015). Clinical characteristics of IgA nephropathy associated with low complement 4 levels. Ren Fail. **37**: 424–32.

Żurawski J, Burchardt P, Moczko J, et al. (2016). The presence of thin glomerular basement membranes in various glomerulopathies. Ultrastruct Pathol. **40**: 77–82.

Chapter 8

C3 glomerulopathies and 'idiopathic' immune complex membranoproliferative glomerulonephritis (MPGN)

Richard J Glassock and Fernando C Fervenza

Introduction and overview

Definitions

In the previous edition of this book (Ponticelli and Glassock, 2009) this chapter was titled membranoproliferative glomerulonephritis (MPGN; also known as mesangiocapillary glomerulonephritis). The term MPGN is a designation given to a 'pattern of injury' consequent to an extremely heterogeneous collection of disorders that manifest by *light microscopy* both mesangial hypercellularity and proliferation accompanied by broadening of the peripheral capillary loops (Glassock, 2009) due to reduplication of the glomerular capillary basement membrane (known as 'double-contour'). As such, MPGN is not a disease diagnosis per se, but a descriptive term covering a patterned (stereotypic) response seen on light microscopy to a variety of injurious pathogenetic processes affecting the glomerular capillaries.

In the past, MPGN has been classified by the location and appearance of electron dense deposits (EDD) within in or closely associated with the basement membrane (BM) of the capillary wall. In this schema MPGN was divided into type I (subendothelial EDD, see Plate 11 and Plate 12); type II (intramembranous EDD; Dense Deposit Disease (DDD), Plate 13); or other types (type III, type IV with various locations of EDD (subendothelial, subepithelial) accompanied by lesion of the glomerular BM itself (e.g. fragmentation) (Levy et al., 1978; Burkholder et al., 1970; Strife et al., 1975; Anders et al., 1977; Donadio and Holley, 1982).

This long-standing *ultrastructural* approach to categorization of MPGN has now been largely replaced by a more *pathogenetic-based* system using the pattern of immunoglobulin (Ig) and complement (C) deposits seen on immunofluorescence (IF) (Sethi and Fervenza, 2011, 2012; Sethi et al., 2012; (Plate 14). Based on this new classification system, the 'pattern of injury' lesion of MPGN can be divided as either immune complex-mediated (Ig + C) or complement-mediated (C) or neither. Immune complex-mediated MPGN shows deposition of immunoglobulin and/or complement factors in glomeruli on IF studies. Complement-mediated MPGN shows complement factors and lack of significant (but often not totally absent) immunoglobulin deposition on IF studies. Immune complex-mediated MPGN results from chronic infections (e.g. hepatitis C viral infection), autoimmune diseases (systemic lupus erythematosus), and monoclonal gammopathies. Complement-mediated MPGN (C3 glomerulopathy; C3G) is caused by genetic or acquired dysregulation of the alternative pathway of complement and can be further classified into C3 glomerulonephritis (C3GN) and DDD (formerly type II MPGN) based on electron microscopy (EM).

In a small group of patients, the light microscopic lesion of MPGN appears to have an immune complex basis, although no known cause for immune complex-mediated MPGN can be identified. These cases have been called 'idiopathic' immune complex MPGN.

A MPGN 'pattern of injury' can also result from damage to the endothelial cells in cases associated with a chronic thrombotic microangiopathy and a few other causes. In these cases, however, immunoglobulin and complement are typically absent on IF, and EM does not show electron dense deposits along the capillary walls (see Box 8.1).

This chapter discusses the primary C3 glomerulopathies (C3GN and DDD) and the 'idiopathic' immune complex forms of MPGN as together they constitute a distinct category of primary glomerulonephritis (GN; Floege and Amann, 2016).

For the purposes of this chapter, the secondary forms of MPGN are not discussed or are only mentioned tangentially (see Box 8.1). IF and EM are particularly useful in separating the various underlying causes of MPGN (Rennke and Renounce, 1995; Glassock, 2009; Sethi and Fervenza, 2012).

C3 glomerulopathy

The term C3 glomerulopathy (C3G) is utilized to describe two distinct lesions identified by ultrastructural analysis—C3GN, often revealing the type I or type III lesions by EM and DDD, formerly known as type II MPGN (Appel et al., 2005; Servais et al., 2007; Nasr et al., 2009; Servais et al., 2013; Pickering et al., 2013; Medjeral-Thomas et al., 2014; Barbour et al., 2016; Master Sankar Raj et al., 2016). While these two lesions are usually quite separable according to

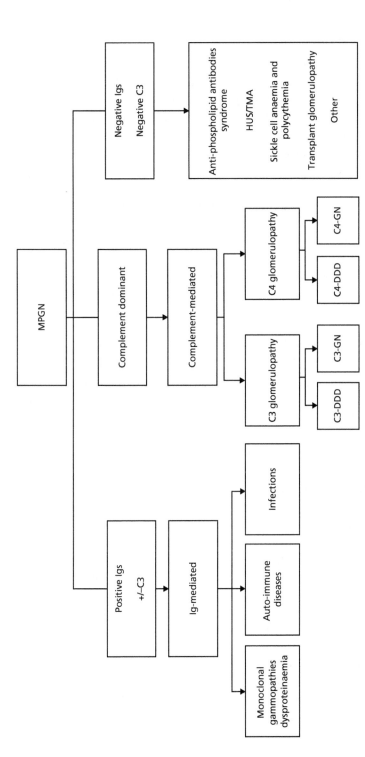

Figure 8.1 An immunopathogenetic classification of the MPGN lesion.

Source: data from Sethi S, Fervenza FC. (20′ 2) Membranoproliferative glomerulonephritis : A new look at an old entity. *N Engl J Med.* 366: 1119–31.

EM morphology, overlaps occasionally can be seen (Sethi et al., 2015). The clinical and laboratory features of these two sub-categories of C3G are quite similar, so they will be discussed together with the dissimilar features highlighted as needed. C3GN occurs in familial and sporadic forms. It should be stressed that C3G, both C3GN and DDD, do not uniformly produce lesions of MPGN by light microscopy—other lesions, e.g. pure mesangial proliferative GN, acute proliferative and exudative or crescentic GN, can also be seen (Walker et al., 2007; Cook and Pickering, 2015). Indeed, Walker and colleagues (2017) have suggested that DDD should not be categorized as a lesion with uniform MPGN features. Familial and sporadic cases of C3GN or DDD are often linked to mutations in the complement factor H related genes (*CFH or CFHR1-5*), C3, factor I, complement receptor 1, thrombomodulin (Gale et al., 2010; Servais et al., 2011; Servais et al., 2012; Medjeral-Thomas et al., 2014; Chauvet et al., 2016; Iatropoulos et al., 2016; Gale and Maxwell, 2013; Bu et al., 2016) and the existence of such mutations can have a pronounced impact on natural history of disease progression and management.

Pathology and pathogenesis

C3GN and DDD may display a variety of findings by light microscopy; including mesangial proliferative GN, acute proliferative and exudative GN, crescentic GN, and MPGN (Sethi and Fervenza, 2014). In DDD, the most common lesion by light microscopy is mesangial proliferative GN (40 per cent), while typical MPGN lesions only account for about 20 per cent of cases (Walker et al., 2007). Crescentic GN is more common in DDD than in C3GN, while mesangial proliferative GN and MPGN patterns of injury are quite common in C3GN. By immunofluorescence, both subcategories of C3G show dominant C3 deposition (in reality C3c or C3dg), with no or much less intense deposition of IgG and IgM (Houi et al., 2014). The C3GN consensus report defines that 'glomerulonephritis with dominant C3' should be used as a morphological term for those cases with dominant staining for C3c. Dominant is defined as C3c intensity ≥2 orders of magnitude more than any other immune reactant on a scale of 0 to 3 (including 0, trace, 1+, 2+, 3+; Pickering et al., 2013).

In C3GN, the deposits are mainly mesangial and in DDD deposits can also involve the peripheral capillaries with nodules of deposition in the mesangium. In both C3GN and DDD the predominating form of C3 in the deposits is C3dg, with lesser amounts of C3a, C3b, and C5–C9 (Sethi et al., 2016). C1q and C4d are typically absent or weakly deposited (Sethi et al., 2012) C4 deposition is more commonly seen in immune complex-mediated C3GN (auto-immune disease and infections) (Sethi et al., 2015; Cook, 2015). Prominent C4d deposition without C3dg deposition can be seen in the rare form of C4 glomerulopathy

Box 8.1 Causes of a membranoproliferative pattern of injury by light microscopy

Immune complex-mediated:

Deposition of antigen-antibody immune complexes as a result of an infection

◆ Viral: hepatitis C, hepatitis B with or without cryoglobulinemia

◆ Bacterial: endocarditis, infected ventriculo-atrial shunt, visceral abscesses, leprosy, meningococcaemia

◆ Protozoal/other infections: malaria, schistosomiasis, leishmaniasis. filariasis, histoplasmosis, mycoplasma

Deposition of immune complexes as a result of an auto-immune disease

◆ Lupus nephritis (Class IV)

◆ Sjögren's syndrome

◆ Rheumatoid arthritis

◆ Mixed connective tissue disease

Deposition of monoclonal Ig (in an immune complex pattern) a result of a monoclonal gammopathy from to a plasma cell or B-cell neoplastic disorder

◆ Light- or heavy-chain disease

◆ Proliferative GN and monoclonal Ig deposition disease

◆ Immunotactoid GN

◆ Fibrillary GN

◆ Mixed (essential) IgG/IgM cryoglobulinemia

◆ Other

Complement-mediated (C3/4 GN and DDD):

◆ Mutations in complement regulating proteins: CFH, CFI, CFHR5

◆ Polyclonal or monoclonal antibodies to or inhibitors of complement regulating proteins: C3 nephritic factor, CFH, CFI, CFB

◆ Mutations in complement factors: C3

◆ C4 GN and C4 DDD

Non-immunoglobulin/complement mediated:

◆ Healing phase of HUS/TTP

◆ Anti-phospholipid (anti-cardiolipin) antibodies syndrome

Box 8.1 Causes of a membranoproliferative pattern of injury by light microscopy (*continued*)

- POEMS syndrome and thrombotic microangiopathy
- Radiation nephritis
- Nephropathy associated with bone marrow transplantation
- Drug-associated thrombotic angiopathies
- Sickle cell anaemia and polycythaemia
- Dysfibrinogenemia, cryofibrinogenemia, and other pro-thrombotic states
- Transplant glomerulopathy
- Anti-trypsin deficiency

'Idiopathic' forms of MPGN

- None of the conditions above are present

Modified from Fervenza FC, Sethi S, Glassock RJ. (2012). Nephrol Dial Transplant. 27(12): 4288–94 with permission from Oxford University Press.

(Sethi et al., 2014; Sethi et al., 2016). C3 deposits can also be seen in Bowman's Capsule and tubular basement membrane in DDD. One needs to be cognizant of the fact that monoclonal Ig proteins can be masked in renal biopsies, leading to an appearance of C3N (Larsen et al., 2015; Messias et al., 2015). This is especially true in patients with a circulating monoclonal gammopathy. Special treatment of paraffin embedded renal biopsy material with Pronase® can unmask these deposits and lead to a correct diagnosis of a proliferative GN with monoclonal immunoglobulin deposits (PGNMID; Messias et al., 2015; Larsen et al., 2015). Laser dissection and mass spectrometry can also uncover such monoclonal gammopathy mediated lesions of MPGN (Jain et al., 2014). The C5b-C9 membrane attack complex can also be detected in the glomerular deposits in C3GN and DDD.

Importantly, the ultrastructural findings usually separate C3GN from DDD, although overlap features may sometimes be found (Sethi et al., 2015). In C3GN the deposits are of varying electron density and predominantly localize in the subendothelial and mesangial areas (formerly known as type I MPGN) or in both subendothelial, intramembranous or subepithelial locations accompanied by 'fraying' or fragmentation of the GBM (formerly known as the Strife or Anders variant, or type III MPGN) (Strife et al., 1977; Anders et al., 1977). In DDD the deposits are very electron- dense and typically localize in the glomerular basal lamina) as sausage-shaped structures. Subepithelial deposits, even resembling 'humps', can occasionally be seen in both subcategories of C3G.

Recent advances in the understanding of the pathogenesis of the C3G show that both genetic anomalies and acquired auto-antibody responses appear to be involved (Servais et al., 2012; Xiao et al., 2014; Sethi et al., 2012; Bu et al., 2016). Mutations (or pathogenetic polymorphisms) of the regulatory complement factor H (CfH, which down-regulates the C3b component of the C3 convertase) leading to deficient CfH action and unregulated C3 activation via the alternate pathway are found in DDD and, to a lesser extent, in C3GN. Mutations or polymorphisms in the complement factor H-related genes (CFHR 1-5) that regulate the function of CfH can also be associated with familial forms of C3GN (Chauvet et al., 2016; Gale and Maxwell, 2013). Inhibitory auto-antibodies to CfH or gain of function auto-antibodies to factor B can also be found, more so in C3GN than in DDD (Józsi et al., 2014). Auto-antibodies to C3 convertase of the alternate pathway (also termed C3-nephritic factor, C3Nef) leading to stabilization of the C3 convertase are found in both subcategories of C3N, but more frequently in DDD (Jokiranta et al., 1999; Zhang et al., 2014; Nicolas et al., 2014). Very rarely, monoclonal light chains capable of interfering with the action of CfH on C3b can be observed in both C3GN and DDD (Zand et al., 2013; Bridoux et al., 2011).

Taken together, these findings strongly suggest that both C3GN and DDD are due to activation and dysregulation of the alternative pathway of C activation (Servais et al., 2012; Zipfel et al., 2015). The precise ways that these abnormalities (genetic and acquired) contribute to the different disease phenotypes are largely unknown, but likely reflect differential glomerular accumulation of complement proteins (e.g. C3b, C3dg) in subendothelial and intramembranous sites along with the generation of inflammatory and cytolytic by-products (such as C3a, C5a, and the C5b-C9 membrane attack complex) from the complement cascade activation, are likely involved. C4d is seldom found in the lesion of C3GN or DDD, but can be prominent in the rare cases of C4 DDD (Sethi et al., 2015).

An intriguing and novel approach to analysing the complexities of C3G (and immune complex-mediated GN, ICGN) has been presented by Iatropoulos and colleagues (2018). Using an unbiased, hierarchical cluster analysis involving histologic, genetic, clinical, and C abnormality phenotypes, they arranged C3G and ICGN into four different pathogenetic patterns (clusters). Patterns 1, 2, and 3 exhibited fluid phase C activation, low C3 levels, and a high prevalence of genetic and acquired alternate pathway abnormalities. Pattern 4 had solid phase C activations and usually normal C3 levels. Pattern 2 had

Table 8.1 The correspondence of 'conventional' and 'cluster' analysis of 173 cases of C3 glomerulopathy and immune complex glomerulonephritis.

Conventional histologic	Pattern (cluster) diagnosis			
Diagnosis	1	2	3	4
C3 GN	42	2	4	20
DDD	4	0	21	0
Immune complex MPGN	16	30	8	26

Source: data from Iatropoulos P., Daina E., Curreri M. et. al. (2018). Cluster analysis identifies distinct pathogenetic patterns in c3 glomerulopathies/immune complex-mediated membranoproliferative GN. *Journal of the American Society of Nephrology*, 29(1), 283–94.

evidence of concomitant classical pathway activation. Pattern 3 was associated with prominent activation of C3 convertase and features of DD by EM. This type of analysis can be applied in an algorithmic fashion to improve risk assessment and clarify disease pathogenesis. Overlap between conventional C3G and ICGN categorization is extensive when a cluster-type analysis is employed, perhaps due to histologic interpretations of renal biopsy findings in the latter (see Table 8.1) The role of cluster analysis in making treatment decisions requires further experience and validation.

Clinical presentation

The clinical expression of C3G, in both of its forms (C3GN and DDD), are quite varied (Medjeral-Thomas et al., 2014) but share many common features. Persistent hypocomplementaemia (low C3, normal C4) is common, but by no means universal (West et al., 1965; Varade et al., 1990). Patients with DDD tend to be more likely to have a low C3, are usually younger (children or young adults), but C3 complement levels are common in both diseases (Ravindran et al., 2018a). Low C3 levels can also be found in immune complex-mediated forms of MPGN (Servais et al., 2012). Patients with C3GN tend to be older and have less renal impairment at presentation. Older adults with a C3 glomerulopathy (C3GN or DDD) should always be suspected of having a monoclonal gammopathy that functions to inhibit the action of CfH on the C3b component of the C3 convertase (Zand et al., 2013; Bridoux et al., 2011). Males and females are approximately equally affected and no racial predilections are evident.

The development of macroscopic or microscopic haematuria and marked proteinuria (including nephrotic syndrome) is common in both DDD and C3GN (Ravindran et al., 2018a). Hypertension, which is sometimes severe, is also a common finding. The serological findings in C3N, e.g. the presence or absence of C3Nef (an auto-antibody to C3 convertase) or the extent of lowering of C3, do not often differ systematically with the clinical findings at presentation. The genetic forms of C3N, such as a factor H mutation or a CFHR polymorphism, may show familial aggregation or affect specific geographic populations (such as Cypriots in the case of a CFHR polymorphism). C3GN associated with a CFHR polymorphism tends to be associated with haematuria and non-nephrotic proteinuria (Athanasiou et al., 2011). Some patients with DDD or C3GN can present in fashion closely resembling acute post-infectious GN (PIGN; Khalighi et al., 2016), often in the absence of a prior infection (so-called 'atypical' APIGN; Alexander et al., 2016; Sethi et al., 2013); however, in classical PIGN the low C3 levels return to normal within eight weeks, whereas they may persist in C3N and atypical PIGN associated with persistence of C3 activation (Sethi et al., 2013). Similarly, haematuria and proteinuria persist and kidney function may progressively decrease, which would be atypical in classical PIGN (see also Chapter 9). Cases of PSGN that evolve into DDD have been described (Prasto et al., 2014; see also Chapter 9).

Partial lipodystrophy with insulin resistance (Dunnigan–Köbberling syndrome) and macular drusen (sometimes with vision impairment) associate with DDD but not typically with C3GN (Gullín-Amarelle et al., 2016; Savige et al., 2016; Owen et al., 2004). A subset of patients with otherwise typical C3GN (about 10 per cent) may have an array of auto-immune phenomena, including positive antinuclear antibody and anti-dsDNA auto-antibody (Alexander et al., 2016). These patients are typically young females and they appear to have an excellent short-term prognosis. DDD can also mimic a small-vessel vasculitis (Singh et al., 2016) and both C3GN and DDD can sometime be associated with severe crescentic GN and rapidly progressive renal failure (Mao et al., 2015).

Laboratory values

A complete laboratory evaluation of the alternative pathway of complement, including genetic testing, is crucial in defining the pathogenesis of C3G and may be important in prognosis and therapeutic decision making (Angioi et al., 2016).

Genetic testing involves searching for loss of function mutations or pathogenetic polymorphisms of *CFH*, complement factor I (*CFI*)and membrane co-factor protein (*MCP*) (CD46) genes, as well as other gain of function mutations in factor B or C3. Familial C3N has been associated with genomic re-arrangements in the complement factor H-related (*CFHR*) genes (*CFHR1, CFHR2, CFHR3, CFHR4, and CFHR5*). The *CFHR5* mutation, termed familial CFHR5 nephropathy (Athanasiou et al., 2011; Medjeral-Thomas et al., 2014; Gale and Maxwell, 2013), is common in Cyprus is associated with C3GN, but other gene re-arrangements can be found in familial DDD (Chen et al., 2014). Mutations in the C3 gene can also be associated with DDD (Martínez-Barricarte et al., 2010).

In Servais and colleagues (2012) landmark study, mutations in *CFH* gene were found in 17.5 per cent of DDD and 12.5 per cent of C3GN. *CFI* and *MCP* mutations were found only in C3GN (7.1 per cent). Rare polymorphisms of *CFH, CFI, or MCP* were found about equally in DDD (6.9 per cent) and C3GN (7.2 per cent). Overall, a *CFH* gene mutation or polymorphism was found in 27.1 per cent of DDD and 15.1 per cent of C3GN. Thus, screening for a *CFH* mutation or polymorphism is more likely to be revealing in DDD than in C3GN. It is noteworthy that identification of a genetic origin of DDD or C3GN may have important therapeutic significance. High throughput genetic analysis of the complement is a promising new development (Bu et al., 2016).

Complement serology is vital to the recognition and diagnosis of DDD and C3GN. As mentioned, both disorders tend to manifest persistent hypocomplementaemia, typically with low levels of C3 and normal levels of C4. In the aforementioned Servais and colleagues' study (2012), 60 per cent of subjects with DDD had low levels of C3 and only 4.5 per cent had low levels of C4. In C3GN, the corresponding values for low C3 and C4 are 40 per cent and 0 per cent, respectively.

Thus, C3 and C4 levels alone do not distinguish DDD or C3GN, and they may be commonly found in immune complex GN with MPGN histological features. C3Nef (the auto-antibody to C3bB of the C3 convertase) is found in roughly 45 per cent of C3GN and 85 per cent of DDD and C3Nef + patients tend to have much lower levels of C3. Low CfH levels are found in 18 per cent of DDD, 4 per cent of C3GN. Antibodies to factor B and factor H are uncommon, but have been described.

Older subjects with DDD or C3GN may have a monoclonal gammopathy, so screening for free light chain (FLC) and serum protein electrophoresis and/or immunofixation is essential (Zand et al., 2013). Patients with PIGN may have clinical, serological, and morphological features quite similar to C3N (Al-Ghaithi et al., 2016; Sethi et al., 2015); however, the prognosis for recovery is much better in acute PIGN.

Measurement of serum factor B, serum C5, assessment of activation of the AP (soluble serum C5b-C9 or soluble membrane attack complex, sMAC), anti-factor-B or factor-H auto-antibodies can be helpful in individual cases in pinpointing the pathogenetic processes involved in disease production. For example, normal plasma levels of sMAC would not be expected to be observed in C3GN, unless the disease is inactive (Bomback A, personal communication). These sophisticated studies can only be done in a few laboratories and require very careful collection and storage procedures to avoid in vitro artefacts, but from time to time can be very helpful in assessing disease activity, deciding treatment or following the effect of treatment on the course of the disease. Finally, it should be stressed that, in many cases of DDD and C3GN, the precise nature of the underlying complement dysregulation cannot be determined by contemporary methods.

Epidemiology

Overall, the 'pattern of injury' lesion of MPGN by light microscopy appears to be decreasing in frequency in developed countries, but remains as a relatively common finding in patients presenting with the NS in the developing countries of Asia and Africa (Barbiano di Belgiojoso et al., 1985; Simon et al., 2004; Asinobi et al., 1999). This phenomenon is likely due to better control of infectious diseases. However, the epidemiology of C3G (both C3GN and DDD) has been little studied so far, and there may be no corresponding secular decrease in the incidence of these lesions. We do know that certain types of C3GN due to CFHR5 mutations/polymorphisms are more common in certain geographic regions (especially in Cyprus).

Overall, C3G is an uncommon disorder, accounting for 1 to 3 per cent of renal biopsies done for evaluation of apparently primary GN. The incidence of MPGN in most developed countries is on the order of <1–2 cases per million population per year (McGrogan et al., 2011); only about 4 to 5 per cent of renal biopsies showing a MPGN pattern are due to C3N (Xu et al., 2016), so it is a very uncommon disorder. The distribution of DDD and C3GN among biopsies categorized as C3N will vary according to age, with DDD tending to be seen in younger subjects.

Natural history

The long-term prognosis for C3G varies widely and is not well understood. Progression to ESRD seems to be more common in the DDD subcategory, probably because of the association with extensive crescentic disease. The overall prognosis for adults and children with C3N is similar (Servais et al., 2012). Older studies that did not differentiate the underlying causes of MPGN are rather useless for estimating prognosis of C3N in contemporary terms. Nevertheless, older studies in children with a MPGN pattern of injury on light microscopy, undergoing various therapies, suggested a ten-year actuarial renal survival of about 50–60 per cent (Habib et al., 1973; Cameron et al., 1983; Glassock, 2009), quite similar to studies in adults. In the comprehensive study of Servais and colleagues (2012), the ten-year renal survival of C3GN and

Table 8.2 Factors indicating a poor prognosis in C3 glomerulonephropathy.

Clinical:	Older age at presentation (not consistently observed)
	Persistent nephrotic-range proteinuria (>3.5g/d)
	Impaired renal function at diagnosis
	Persistent poorly controlled hypertension (systolic>diastolic)
	Lack of treatment with inhibitors of the renin angiotensin system
Pathological:	Extensive crescents (>50% glomerular involvement)
	Superimposed segmental glomerulosclerosis
	Advanced tubulointerstitial fibrosis
	Arteriolo-nephrosclerosis (hypertension-related)

DDD overall (adults + children) was similar, at about 64 per cent. However, the long-term prognosis for DDD is much worse in adults (0 per cent renal survival at ten years) and C3GN has a better prognosis (83 per cent at ten years), although adult cases of DDD with preserved renal function are well recognized. Spontaneous complete remissions of C3G (showing a lesion of MPGN by light microscopy) are quite rare. Several clinical and morphological features affect the likelihood of developing end-stage renal failure (see also Table 8.2).

Prognostic factors

Age/sex

Neither the age at presentation nor gender seems to have has any consistent or unique effect on long-term prognosis, other than that conveyed by clinical features at presentation or underlying pathology.

Proteinuria

The magnitude of proteinuria and its persistence has a significant effect on prognosis as is true for all primary glomerular diseases. It is generally agreed that the greater the proteinuria the worse the long-term prognosis. In subjects with the 'full-blown' NS the 50 per cent actuarial survival will be reached somewhere between five and nine years after diagnosis, depending on how well the blood pressure is controlled.

Impaired renal function at presentation

An elevated serum creatinine and/or reduced creatinine clearance (or estimated GFR) at diagnosis is often, but not invariably, associated with a poor long-term outcome both in adults and in children. Fluctuations in the level of renal function, representing exacerbations of disease due to superimposed infection or other triggering factors (e.g. drugs), may punctuate the course of the disease.

The pattern of complement levels (C3, C4) has little impact on prognosis in either DDD or C3GN (Servais et al., 2012). The levels may fluctuate and show no clear-cut relationship to the clinical activity of the disease. Persistently low C3 levels are more commonly observed in DDD than in C3GN.

Hypertension

As is commonly noted in many glomerular diseases, the presence of hypertension (usually now defined for proteinuric subjects as >130/80 mm/Hg) is usually a feature indicating a worse prognosis. Use of inhibitors of the renin-angiotensin system (RAS) are associated with a better prognosis in observational studies (Servais et al., 2012) but there are no prospective, randomized interventional trials proving a long-term benefit of such therapy on patient-centred outcomes (see also Chapter 2). However, such treatment may lower proteinuria somewhat, especially in hypertensive patients.

Morphologic features

The presence of superimposed extensive crescents and/or chronic tubulo-interstitial lesions have consistently been shown to affect prognosis adversely. The severity of mesangial cellular interposition and/or hypercellularity are not particularly helpful in prognostication. Arteriolar damage, perhaps reflecting the severity of hypertension, can indicate a poor outcome. The worse prognosis of DDD seen in adults could be explained by a greater tendency for superimposition of crescents in this subcategory. Superimposed focal and segmental glomerulosclerosis might also have an adverse effect on renal survival. Overall, C3GN lesions have a much better prognosis in adults (Servais et al., 2012). A large review of 114 cases of C3G from the Mayo Clinic concluded that the response to treatment is highly variable, with an overall risk of developing ESRD of about 9 per cent after approximately two years of follow-up (Ravindran et al., 2018). In this study, only the extent of global glomerulosclerosis, but not the pattern of injury (mesangial proliferative, membranoproliferative, and crescentic glomerulonephritis), was predictive of ESRD (Ravindran et al., 2018).

Specific treatment

At present there is no proven effective treatment for C3G, either in the DDD or C3GN subcategories). In its evidence-based clinical practice guideline, KDIGO (2012) made no specific recommendations or suggestions for treatment of C3G (in its MPGN form), other than suggesting that combined immunosuppression be used when extensive crescents and rapidly progressive deterioration of renal function were encountered. This is largely due to the absence of randomized controlled trials (RCTs) of therapy for these uncommon disorders. The pre-2010 literature undoubtedly included such patients in trials using a light microscopic pattern of injury of MPGN for entry. Evidence-based guidelines for therapy of MPGN published before 2010 have little relevance today (Levin, 1999). However, the inability to separate out the cases of C3N in these trials renders them rather unsatisfactory as evidence for therapeutic efficacy specifically in C3G; nevertheless, many of these studies did separately identify DDD, but not C3GN. In nearly all the therapeutic trials of 'generic' MPGN reported to date, the analysis of the effect of treatment is confounded by the pathogenetic heterogeneity of the subjects with MPGN enrolled in the treatment trials (since patients with immune complex-mediated and complement-mediated MPGN were grouped together as part of a general diagnosis of MPGN) and by the use of short-term surrogate end-points, such as a change in proteinuria. Additionally, many trials have used historical controls as the basis for comparison. Such analyses are biased since treatment groups must survive from clinical onset to the initiation of treatment, whereas control patients have no such constraints. By intention-to-treat analysis from the onset or discovery of disease, many of the claims of efficacy cannot be supported (Donadio and Offord, 1989).

Glucocorticoids

Long-term but uncontrolled studies of children with predominantly type I MPGN by EM (some of whom had C3GN) conducted at the University of Cincinnati Children's Hospital in the 1970s–1990s suggested that *high-dose, alternate-day prednisone therapy* preserves renal function, reduces glomerular inflammation, and increases renal survival (McAdams et al., 1975; McEnery et al., 1985). Alternate-day prednisone at 2–2.5 mg/kg or 60 mg/m^2 (maximum dose 80 mg) every other day subsequently slowly reduced to 1–1.5 mg/kg every other day at two years and 0.2–1.0 mg/kg every other day at four years was the protocol used. Repeat biopsies in patients so treated showed resolution of hypercellularity and 'improved' glomerular architecture. In the absence of an untreated cohort of patients with similar characteristics at onset, it was not possible to definitively conclude that glucocorticoid therapy itself is responsible for the observed changes, and whether this therapy had beneficial effects in C3GN or DDD is impossible to state with certainty.

In 1990, McEnery updated the cumulative University of Cincinnati Children's Hospital uncontrolled experience with a high-dose, alternate-day prednisone regimen in MPGN (McEnery, 1990). Seventy-one paediatric patients with presumed primary MPGN seen at this centre have been treated *exclusively* with the alternate-day prednisone regimen described. Of the patients treated with this regimen since 1957, 43 per cent have been type I MPGN (including some with C3GN, some immune complex MPGN as well as others with 'idiopathic' immune complex MPGN), 22 per cent type II MPGN (DDD), and 34 per cent other types of MPGN. The average duration of disease prior to treatment was 1.5 years and the average total duration of treatment was 7.7 years. Overall, nineteen of 71 treated patients (27 per cent) developed ESRD and the actuarial renal survival in this group at ten and 20 years from the *start of therapy* was 75 per cent and 59 per cent, respectively. Survival at ten and 20 years from the *time of diagnosis* was 82 per cent and 56 per cent, respectively. The development of ESRD was not greater in patients treated for one or more years (averaging 3.5 years) after the diagnosis compared to patients treated early in the course of disease (average 0.3 years following discovery). While an 82 per cent ten-year renal survival rate from disease diagnosis is substantially greater than the expected 50–60 per cent ten-year renal survival rate mentioned earlier, the absence of contemporaneous controls makes it difficult to ascribe the better outcome to glucocorticoid therapy alone (Glassock, 2009). Other improvements in management, particularly better control of hypertension or the use of angiotensin II inhibiting agents (Guo et al., 2008), could have also affected the outcome in comparison to historical controls. Nevertheless, repeat renal biopsies in treated patients showed improvement in inflammation (McAdams et al., 1975), and patients with normal or near-normal renal function 15 or more years after the onset (more accurately, discovery) of disease continued to enjoy stable renal function, although with discontinuation of glucocorticoid therapy exacerbations and relapses have been observed. Only one prospective, randomized, placebo-controlled trial of alternate-day glucocorticoids in apparently primary MPGN has been reported. The full-length report of the International Study of Kidney Disease in Children trial appeared in 1992 (Tarshish et al., 1992), approximately 12 years following the closure of the study to entry of new patients and ten years after the initial abstract appeared recording the preliminary results of the trial. All patients admitted to the trial were children with MPGN, subtyped according to EM but not by immunopathogenesis. Eligibility included a creatinine clearance ≥ 70 ml/min/1.73 m^2 and persistent proteinuria >40 mg/ h/m^2. A total of 80 patients were randomized to receive either prednisone 40 mg/m^2 every other day, or a placebo (lactose). The average duration of treatment was 41 months, with the onset of renal failure the most common reason for termination of treatment. Forty-two patients (52 per cent) had MPGN type I (including an unspecified number with C3GN), 14 (18 per cent) had MPGN type II (DDD), and 24 (30 per cent) had other ultrastructural or unclassified types of MPGN (not likely to include C3GN). Treatment failure was defined as a 30 per cent *increase* in serum creatinine from baseline and this event occurred in 33 per cent of patients with non-type II (DDD) allocated to prednisone treatment compared with 58 per cent in the placebo group (p = 0.05). No clear benefits were observed in type II MPGN (DDD). Kaplan–Meier analysis indicated that 61 per cent of treated patients and 12 per cent of placebo patients had stable renal function over the first ten years of follow-up (p = 0.07). Repeat renal biopsy showed no important differences between treated and placebo patients. There was no difference in outcome relative to whether treatment was instituted early (<1 year) after diagnosis or discovery compared with late treatment (>1 year). It is noteworthy that the duration of disease prior to entry was only 8.9 ± 1.3 months in the prednisone-treated group, and 18.1 ± 3.9 months in the placebo group (p <0.05). A stable course was noted more often in patients whose red cell excretion rate fell and whose urinary protein excretion decreased during the observation periods. Side effects were encountered, particularly worsening of hypertension. Aggravation of hypertension led to discontinuance of prednisone in five of 47 treated patients, and in two of 33 placebo patients. The conclusion offered by the authors was that long-term treatment with prednisone appears to improve the outcome of children with MPGN. The differences in outcome were of marginal statistical significance and the power to detect substantial differences was small (0.35). In terms of stability of renal function, the differences between treated and placebo patients were not observed until after 90 months of observation when only eleven prednisone and seven placebo patients were still under observation. Thus, the strength of the data supporting the conclusions is weak and, when interpreted strictly, the study is at best inconclusive and not applicable to the contemporary subdivision of MPGN, except for strongly suggesting lack of efficacy of steroid treatment in DDD.

Most of the older studies of steroids in MPGN have indicated that all non-type IMPGN, including DDD, are resistant to steroid therapy (Braun et al., 1999). Data on the use of oral alternate-day prednisone in adults in non-type I MPGN (mainly DDD) is scarce and largely anecdotal—no controlled trials of alternate-day steroids have yet been reported in adults.

Ford and colleagues (1992) carried out a small uncontrolled trial of oral and/or intravenous (IV) glucocorticoids in nineteen children with type I MPGN (not sub-divided according to C3 deposition) utilizing regimens that were 'tailored to the severity of disease based on creatinine clearance and proteinuria' (treatment was generally instituted within one year of the diagnosis of disease. The most intensive regimens included IV methylprednisone (30 mg/kg/day for three doses) and oral prednisolone (2 mg/kg/day, up to 60 mg/day). This regimen was utilized for patients with creatinine clearance of <50 ml/min and any level of proteinuria. The least intensive regimen was 20 mg of prednisone every other day. This regimen was used for patients with a creatinine clearance >80 ml/min and proteinuria <40 mg/h/m². Those with disease severity between these two extremes received oral glucocorticoids either daily or every other day in doses of 2 mg/kg. Therapy was subsequently tapered slowly according to clinical course. Other immunosuppressive agents were not used. Hypertension was controlled medically and 90 per cent of patients received an angiotensin-converting enzyme (ACE) inhibitor. Follow-up averaged 6.5 years with total duration of therapy of 38 ± 3 months. Repeat renal biopsies were performed after about three years of treatment and showed reduced inflammatory activity in the great majority of patients. Interestingly, progressive glomerulosclerosis was seen only in those patients treated with *daily* as opposed to *every other day* glucocorticoid regimens. Eight of nineteen (42 per cent) treated patients entered a complete remission with normal urinalyses. The average creatinine clearance for the entire group rose from 78 ± 7 to 126 ± 5 ml/min over the course of treatment and follow-up. No patient developed ESRD. Significant side effects were observed in the treated patients, which included seizures, hypertension, growth retardation, osteoporosis, and obesity. It is possible that the good outcomes observed in this trial were also a function of better control of hypertension and the use of ACE inhibitors. It is also worth re-emphasizing that progressive glomerulosclerosis was associated with the use of *daily* glucocorticoid regimens. Other limited studies of prednisone therapy conducted in children have suggested that the initiation of therapy early in the course of disease, before the establishment of chronic irreversible lesions, may be important in determining the final outcome of treatment (Warady et al., 1985; Yanagihara et al., 2005; Bahat et al., 2007; Glassock, 2009; Holle et al., 2018).

Very limited trials of glucocorticoids have been conducted (none controlled) in adults with MPGN (unclassified as immune complex-mediated or complement-mediated), but they have generally reached conclusions similar to those in children. In extensive reviews of data from several trials using an intention-to-treat analysis, Donadio and Offord (1989) at the Mayo Clinic and a meta-analysis by Schena (1999) have concluded that the available information does not support a beneficial effect of glucocorticoids in adults with MPGN (unspecified as to pathogenesis, since in many studies treatment was started years after onset of disease). A role for very intensive therapies with high-dose IV pulses of glucocorticoids (with or without concomitant cytotoxic agents) in adults has been suggested by small observational trials with limited follow-up (Emre et al., 1995; Bahat et al., 2007).

In sum, due to deficiencies inherent to older (pre-2000) trials, it is not possible to conclude that steroid monotherapy has any beneficial effect in either C3GN or DDD. These studies were not adequately powered to be able to detect steroid-responsiveness in a small subset of C3GN (such as those with an auto-antibody to CfH or factor B) but they do generally suggest lack of efficacy for steroids in DDD and they also demonstrate the propensity for adverse events, particularly worsening of hypertension. It is evident that steroid monotherapy is not effective in DDD, but a definitive answer regarding efficacy of steroid treatment of C3GN is still elusive.

Alkylating agents

Prior to 1980, numerous anecdotes had appeared regarding the use of adjunctive cytotoxic (alkylating) immunosuppressive agents in MPGN (see Kincaid-Smith, 1972; Chapman et al., 1980; Glassock, 2009). These reports were generally unimpressive and mostly demonstrated unfavourable results. As a consequence, the use of these agents in any form of MPGN has, until recently, not been recommended and no prospective trials of this category of therapeutic modalities have been conducted, except in combination with warfarin or heparin and dipyridamole (see 'Anticoagulants and anti-thrombotics'). These latter trials also concluded that cytotoxic therapy was ineffective in MPGN (Chapman et al., 1980; Tiller et al., 1981; Cattran et al., 1985).

A few studies, largely of an uncontrolled nature, have suggested that more aggressive regimens combining IV 'pulse' methylprednisolone with oral cyclophosphamide initially followed by short-term maintenance therapy with alternate-day prednisone and oral cyclophosphamide may be beneficial. Faedda and colleagues (1994) studied nineteen patients, ages nine to 65 years, with a variety of types of MPGN. Fifteen of nineteen (79 per cent) patients treated with this aggressive glucocorticoid and cytotoxic regimen experienced complete remission while three additional patients (15 per cent) experienced partial remissions. Relapses occurred in six of the eighteen responders and overall, four patients progressed to ESRD. After an average follow-up of 7.4 ± 0.8 years, the renal survival rate was 79 per cent. Because of the lack of contemporaneous controls, it is not possible to conclude that the favourable outcome was a result of treatment, although a complete remission rate of 79 per cent is higher than would have been predicted from historical controls. However, it worth noting that a renal survival rate of approximately 80 per cent following 7.5 years of follow-up is not greatly different from that found in other trials that utilized glucocorticoids alone in children. Taken in aggregate, these data give us no information on the effects of alkylating agents in the treatment of C3GN or DDD, at least in the absence of extensive crescent formation.

Inhibitors of purine synthesis

Azathioprine and mycophenolate mofetil

No controlled trials of azathioprine (AZA), mycophenolate mofetil (MMF), or MMF's parent compound mycophenolate sodium have been reported to date in

C3GN or DDD. Numerous anecdotes and small short-term observational trials have been reported, usually in combination with steroids (Choi et al., 2002; Bayazit et al., 2004; Jones et al., 2004; Glassock, 2009; Holle et al., 2018). Short-term results have included a reduction in proteinuria and stabilization of renal function. The long-term benefits and risks of azathioprine and/or MMF in C3GN or DDD are largely unknown. However, Rabasco and colleagues (2015) has reported on the results of an uncontrolled, observational study of immune-suppressive therapy (IST), including use of MMF, in 60 patients with C3GN. Conservative non-IST therapy (mainly blood pressure control with RAS inhibition) was associated with clinical remission in 20 per cent of such cases, but 35 per cent went on to develop ESRD after an average of 39 months of follow-up, mostly without any clinical remission. Interestingly, of those who received MMF-based IST, remissions developed in 86 per cent (mostly partial remissions) and no patient developed ESRD after a follow-up averaging 44 months. Non-MMF based IST (steroid monotherapy or cyclophosphamide-based therapy) was associated with a 50 per cent rate of remissions, but almost 40 per cent developed a doubling of serum creatinine and 17 per cent developed ESRD after a follow up averaging 54 months. Patients who were C3Nef positive fared better with IST (80 per cent clinical remissions in C3Nef + IST vs. only 37 per cent clinical remission's in C3Nef patients). While uncontrolled and hypothesis generating, this study provides some encouragement for use of IST in C3GN (particularly the C3Nef + IST subgroup), with MMF + steroids as the preferred regimen. #

Also, in a retrospective study, Avasare and colleagues (2018) reported on 30 patients treated with MMF for at least three months and follow-up for at least one year. Patients were categorized as 'responders' if they had either CR (stable or improved eGFR with decline in proteinuria to <0.5 g/g creatinine determined by the urine protein-to-creatinine ratio) or PR (stable or improved eGFR with >50 per cent decline in proteinuria between (urine protein-to-creatinine ratio 0.5 and 3.5 g/g) while on MMF treatment. Stable eGFR was defined as eGFR within 15 per cent of the baseline value. 'Nonresponders' were defined as those who did not achieve remission on MMF. Twenty patients (67 per cent) were classified as responders. 'Responders' had lower proteinuria (median = 2,468 mg/g creatinine) than nonresponders (median = 5,000 mg/g creatinine). Patients in the Avasare and colleagues' study were younger (median age = 25 years) and had lower proteinuria (median UPCR = 3.2 g/g of creatinine) than patients treated with MMF in the Rabasco and colleagues' (2015) study (median age = 35 years; median proteinuria value = 6,500 mg/24 hours), and more patients progressed to ESRD (10 per cent) when compared to Rabasco and colleagues (0 per cent; 2015).

In the largest study to date by investigators at the Mayo Clinic, featuring a series of patients with C3G ESRD or doubling of serum creatinine level was worse in patients managed conservatively vs. those treated with immunosuppressive therapy (Ravindran et al., 2018a). However, when patients treated with MMF were analysed separately, the results were less impressive than that reported in the two studies discussed here. This difference may be related to the greater degree of kidney failure at baseline in the Mayo cohort (median creatinine level = 1.4 mg/dl) than those in Avasare and colleagues' study (median creatinine level = 1.0 mg/dl). However, this does not explain the discrepancy between this study and the Rabasco and colleagues' study, which included patients of similar age (median age = 35 years) and kidney function (median serum creatinine level = 1.3 mg/dl). Both the Rabasco (2015) and Ravindran (2018a) studies had similar numbers of patients with biopsies showing moderate to severe interstitial fibrosis and tubular atrophy (25 per cent vs. 21 per cent). However, in the Ravindran study (2018a), patients with C3G without a circulating monoclonal gammopathy had a significantly higher number of patients with genetic forms (58.5 per cent) than did the Rabasco (2015) study population (13 per cent). In addition, the Ravindran study (2018a) had a lower number of patients with C3Nef (37.8 per cent) than did the Rabasco study (48 per cent; 2015). This raises the possibility that the lower response rate to MMF observed by Ravindran and colleagues (2018a) may be due to the enrichment of genetic forms of C3G in this study. Taken together, these studies suggest that genetic forms of C3G are less likely to respond to immunosuppressive therapy. An RCT is sorely needed to confirm these preliminary observations.

Calcineurin inhibitors

Cyclosporine A and tacrolimus

Limited uncontrolled trials and case-reports of cyclosporine A (CsA), usually in doses of 4–6 mg/kg/day and tacrolimus (0.1–0.15 mg/kg/day) accompanied by low doses of oral prednisolone have demonstrated a modest and non-specific decline in proteinuria in not otherwise characterized MPGN (Erbay et al., 1988; Cattran, 1991; Glassock, 1994; Matsumoto et al., 1995; Kiyomasu et al., 2002; Glassock, 2009) or more rarely complete remission (Haddad et al., 2007). However, because of the potential for nephrotoxicity with a drug- and dose-related decline in GFR and aggravation of hypertension, these agents are not currently widely used or recommended (Radhakrishnan and Halevy, 2000; Glassock, 2009), for treatment of C3GN.

Plasma exchange (PLEX)/infusion

The rationale for plasma exchange (PLEX) is based on the following:

i. it replaces deficient or defective regulatory proteins,

ii. it removes autoantibodies and/or mutant proteins that may compete with the functional proteins, and

iii. it enables the administration of higher volumes of plasma.

Intensive PLEX with immunosuppression may be of benefit for the occasional patient with superimposed extensive crescentic GN and the syndrome of rapidly progressive GN (D'Apice and Kincaid-Smith, 1979; Montoliu et al., 1982; McGinley et al., 1985; Morton and Bannister, 1993; Kurtz and Schlueter, 2002; Häffner, et al., 2015). However, the results of the recently completed PEXIVAS trial in ANCA-associated vasculitis trial raises question about the overall efficacy of PLEX in these disorders (see Chapter 9). The effect of PLEX on C3Nef levels appears not to be involved in its putative beneficial effects (Häffner et al., 2015).

In a patient with DDD due to a CFHR2/CFHR5 deregulating hybrid protein, PLEX substantially reduced the levels of the mutant protein, but the response was short lived, and within one to two days, complement activation rebounded (Chen et al., 2014).

Plasma infusion might conceivably be of benefit in DDD associated with factor H deficiency (Licht et al., 2005; Habbig et al., 2009), but only anecdotes exist in the literature, so the efficacy and safety of this approach cannot be evaluated. In these patients, however, persistent disease control requires life-long substitution therapy.

In patients with gain-of-function mutations in complement activation proteins, plasma infusion may not only be ineffective but may be counterproductive, as it provides additional complement substrate for the hyperfunctioning mutant protein. In a patient with DDD associated with a mutant C3 convertase resistant to CFH control, replacement therapies providing CFH was futile (Martínez-Barricarte et al., 2010). In a case of DDD caused by a hybrid CFHR2/CFHR5 protein that rendered the C3 convertase refractory to inhibition and decay by CFH, plasma infusion proved detrimental (Chen et al., 2014).

Anticoagulants and anti-thrombotics

As mentioned, early uncontrolled trials suggested that anticoagulants (heparin or warfarin), frequently combined with glucocorticoids and cytotoxic agents, had beneficial effects in MPGN, but prospective trials generally failed to support this view and this therapeutic approach fell out of favour (Tiller et al., 1981; Cattran et al., 1985; Glassock, 2009). Additionally, while several studies showed some effects of platelet inhibitors on MPGN, they were short-term, rather inconsistent, and unconvincing. Thus, at the present time, there are no compelling reasons to use anti-thrombotics or anticoagulants in C3GN or DDD. They are not likely to be of benefit and may be harmful.

Monoclonal antibodies

Rituximab (RTX)

Rituximab (RTX; Rituxan®, Genetech/Roche) has been used very infrequently to treat DDD or C3GN, so its efficacy and safety are unknown, but so far, the results are rather unimpressive and anecdotal (Reviewed in Smith et al., 2007; Nester and Smith, 2013, 2016; Rousset-Rouvière et al., 2014; Giaime et al., 2015). A small pilot study (n = 6) of RTX therapy in patients with type I MPGN (idiopathic or associated with cryoglobulinaemia showed only a reduction in urinary protein excretion but no change in renal function (Dillon et al., 2012). It would not be expected to be effective in genetic forms of DDD or C3GN. In the author's unpublished observations, RTX is ineffective in DDD. Whether RTX would be effective in cases where auto-antibody inhibition of complement regulatory proteins (e.g. anti-CfH or CeNef) be effective has not yet been adequately tested.

Eculizumab and other complement inhibitors

Eculizumab (Soliris®, Alexion Pharmaceuticals) is a chimeric, IgG2/4 κ-humanized monoclonal antibody against the C5 component of complement (see also Chapter 3), and inhibits ability of C5 convertase to cleave C5 to C5a (a potent pro-inflammatory, pro-thrombotic anaphylatoxin/chemotactin) and C5b, thus also preventing the formation of the membrane attack complex (MAC; C5b-C9; Nester and Smith, 2016). It is approved by the US Food and Drug Administration (FDA) for treatment of paroxysmal nocturnal haemoglobinuria and aHUS, but not C3G (either DDD or C3GN). The rationale for use of an agent that interferes with the production of C5a and C5b upon dysregulated activation of the alternative pathway complement is very reasonable. However, at present the available data on use of eculizumab for treatment of C3GN or DDD are mostly anecdotes or very small trials with short-term follow-up only (Zuber et al., 2012; Bomback, 2014; Bomback et al., 2012). No RCTs have yet been conducted. A consensus group recommended that a formal trial be undertaken (Pickering et al., 2013). The response of C3G to eculizumab is heterogeneous (Welte et al., 2018; Ravindran et al., 2018), and appears to be most effective when rapidly progressive disease is present (Le Quintrec et al., 2018). Two open-label, non-randomized clinical trials are in progress (Clintrials.gov, NCT02093533 and NCT01221181). The doses used and duration of treatment have varied. The usual dosing regimen has been 900 mg IV once weekly for four weeks, then 1200 mg every other week for up to one year (Bomback et al., 2012). It is noteworthy that the half-life of the agent can be affected by proteinuria, so dosage adjustments may be required in patients with severe NS. The minimum dose and duration of treatment necessary for optimum effectiveness and long-term safety is not established.

Most cases treated with eculizumab have had DDD (native or recurrent in allografts, see 'Recurrence in renal transplants'), some with underlying *CFH* or *MCP* mutations and some without such mutations (Oosterveld et al., 2015). Fewer patients with C3GN have been treated with eculizumab (Bomback, 2014). In general, the short-term responses have been impressive with improvements in serum creatinine levels, reduction of proteinuria, and a decrease in signs of glomerular inflammation (Bomback et al., 2012; Herlitz et al., 2012). Circulating soluble C5b-C9 levels have also declined with treatment. However, not unexpectedly, the C3c/dg deposition in glomeruli continues unabated and eventually the chimeric monoclonal antibody can itself be detected in glomerular deposits, possibly along with host antibody to the deposited foreign protein (Herlitz et al., 2012; Bomback et al., 2012). After discontinuation of therapy these deposits tend to resolve (Bomback, 2014). The long-term significance of these findings is uncertain but worrisome. It is also unknown how long treatment with eculizumab must be continued for optimal effects.

Some, but not all, patients may have long-term partial remissions despite stopping treatment, but others have immediate relapses as soon as treatment is stopped (Bomback, 2014). In patients with C3G, treatment benefit may be short lived. The authors have two patients who initially responded well to eculizumab but who later 'escaped' control and both progressed to ESRD despite continue eculizumab therapy. This is not surprising as C3 convertase activity persists or may even increase with blockade of C5 and illustrates the perils of making strong conclusions based on short-term follow-up.

The challenge is to determine which patients with C3G are most likely to respond to eculizumab and how long treatment is necessary. This is an important issue as eculizumab is a very expensive agent that can interfere with resistance to common, sometimes lethal, infections like *N. meningococcus*. Patients receiving eculizumab must be immunized with meningococcal vaccines concomitantly or prophylactically (see Chapter 3). So far, with limited experience, eculizumab appears to be a reasonably safe agent. It would be expected that patients displaying predominant dysregulation of C5 convertase (C3bBbC3B) rather than C3 convertase (C3bBb) would be more responsive to eculizumab. Patients with C3N show heterogeneity in regards to the degree of C3 convertase or C5 convertase dysregulation (Bomback, 2014). Increased levels of soluble

C5b-C9 may indicate strong activation of C5 convertase. So far, it seems that eculizumab can have pronounced effect in those patients with rapidly progressive C3N, unresponsive to immunosuppression, PLEX, or RTX (Le Quintrec et al., 2015). Eculizumab has even rescued a patient with C3GN from dialysis-dependent ESRD (Inman et al., 2015).

Additional complement inhibiting agents, such as soluble complement receptor 1, a recombinant fusion protein of complement receptor 2 and CfH, an engineered complement factor H construct, inhibitors of factors B, D, or C3, or an inhibitor of the C5a receptor, are all in the development pipeline, but still require formal evaluation for efficacy and safety in C3GN and DDD (Ruseva et al., 2016; Zhang et al., 2013; Bekker et al., 2016; Yang et al., 2018).

C3G associated with a monoclonal gammopathy

Two recent studies have evaluated patients with C3G and monoclonal gammopathy. Chauvet and colleagues (2017) reported on 50 adult patients with C3G associated with a monoclonal gammopathy extracted from the C3G French national database. At diagnosis, patients presented with nephrotic-range proteinuria in 20/46 (43 per cent) and CKD Stage 3 or above was present in 42/49 (86 per cent) patients. Monoclonal gammopathy was of IgG type in 47 (94 per cent) patients. Haematological diagnosis was monoclonal gammopathy of renal significance in 30 (60 per cent), multiple myeloma in 17 (34 per cent), and chronic lymphocytic leukaemia in three (6 per cent) patients. Complement studies showed low C3 level in 22/50 (43 per cent) and elevated soluble C5b-9 level in 27/34 (79 per cent) patients. Twenty-nine patients received monoclonal gammopathy targeted therapy, whereas eight and 13 patients, respectively, received various immunosuppressive drugs or symptomatic measures alone. Patients who achieved haematological response after targeted therapy had higher renal response rates and median renal survival than those receiving conservative/immunosuppressive therapy.

More recently, Ravindran and colleagues (2018b) reported on 36 patients with C3G and monoclonal gammopathy. Mean age at diagnosis was 60 years, and serum creatinine and proteinuria were 1.9 mg/dl and 3.0 g/24 hours respectively. Haematuria was present in 32 (88.9 per cent) patients. Twelve (34.3 per cent) patients had low C3 levels. C3 nephritic factor was detected in 45.8 per cent of patients, while pathogenic variants in complement protein genes were rare. Haematologic evaluation revealed monoclonal gammopathy of renal significance in 26 patients, multiple myeloma in five, smouldering multiple myeloma in two, and chronic lymphocytic leukaemia, lymphoma, or type I cryoglobulin each in one patient. After a median follow-up of 43.6 months, the median serum creatinine and proteinuria were 1.4 mg/dl and 0.8 g/24 hours. Nine patients developed ESRD. Sixteen patients received monoclonal gammopathy-targeted therapy, 17 patients received non-targeted treatment, and three patients were managed conservatively. Of the 16 patients who received targeted therapy, ten achieved complete/very good/partial haematologic response. Of these, seven achieved a complete/partial/stable renal response. Of the five patients receiving targeted therapy that did not achieve haematologic response, none had a renal response. Patients receiving non-targeted treatment were more likely to have monoclonal gammopathy of renal significance.

Thus, evaluating for the presence of a monoclonal protein in patients with C3G, especially in older patients, is *mandatory*. These studies suggest that targeted therapy aimed to induce haematological remission may result in remission and stabilization of kidney function in a subset of these patients, as rapid achievement of haematological response appears to result in improved renal survival.

Idiopathic immune complex-mediated MPGN

The category of 'idiopathic' immune complex-mediated MPGN is a difficult one to precisely characterize, as it is a 'diagnosis of exclusion' based on biopsy findings of an immune complex-mediated MPGN that is not due to infection, auto-immune disease, or monoclonal gammopathy. The extent to which it is 'idiopathic' depends on the vigour and comprehensiveness of the search for well-defined causes of the immune complex MPGN 'pattern-of-injury' (see also Table 8.1). In addition, the dividing lines between C3GN and immune complex-mediated MPGN may be hazy and based on comparative intensity of Ig deposition by IF microscopy. Criteria have been established that aid in this separation (Hou et al., 2014). In order to classify a biopsy as showing C3GN, the C3 intensity should be two orders of magnitude greater than the intensity of the deposits of IgG, IgM, or IgA. However small amounts of Ig are commonly found in biopsies with predominant C3 staining and immune deposits on EM. Indeed, some patients initially characterized as having 'idiopathic' immune complex MPGN may, in fact, have C3GN (Nargund et al., 2015) The pattern of Ig deposition in C3GN can also change over time (Hou et al., 2014; Kerns et al., 2013). Intense deposition of C4b is much more common in immune complex MPGN (Sethi et al., 2016), suggesting activation of the classical or lectin pathways of complement.

As such, 'idiopathic' MPGN is a diagnosis of exclusion and should only be applied after extensive laboratory evaluation has ruled out known causes of MPGN. Furthermore, these cases are rare (Sethi et al., 2012).

Based on the rigour with which we now have defined 'idiopathic' MPGN, it is impossible to discuss prognosis as these cases are rare and there is no literature upon which to base any firm conclusions.

Similarly, the treatment of 'idiopathic' immune complex MPGN is highly uncertain due to the lack of RCTs. However, some patients may 'respond' to combined immunosuppression (such as MMF + steroids) with a diminution of proteinuria and a stabilization of renal function. The roles of calcineurin inhibitors RTX or eculizumab are unknown. Patients with extensive crescentic disease and rapidly progressive GN should be empirically treated with combined immunosuppression (Cyclophosphamide + steroids) and possibly with PLEX as well (KDIGO, 2012).

Practical recommendations

Providing practical recommendations for treatment of C3G (DDD or C3GN) or 'idiopathic' MPGN is difficult because of the lack of RCTs and the anecdotal nature of the data base, increasing the possibility of publication bias. Furthermore, the intrinsic heterogeneity of the phenotypes and underlying pathogenic mechanisms provides an additional source of confounding. One must always carry out a thorough investigation of possible secondary causes before attempting to render a specific diagnosis and initiating any therapy for patients revealing a light microscopic MPGN 'pattern of injury'. One should never forget that MPGN is not a disease diagnosis. Finding such a lesion in a renal biopsy must always instigate a thorough search for secondary causes. This would include a careful search for chronic infections (particularly endocarditis, visceral abscesses, and viral hepatitis C or B), cryoglobulinaemia, auto-immune disease (particularly SLE), thrombotic microangiopathies, and various forms of plasma cell dyscrasia or immunoglobulin-deposition diseases (see also Box 8.1). Specific therapy of these disorders with antimicrobials, antivirals, PLEX/ plasma infusion, RTX, or chemotherapy will depend on the aetiology of MPGN.

When C3G is identified by light and IF microscopy, further classification into DDD or C3GN by EM is the next step, followed by characterization of the genetic, auto-immune or other pathomechanisms underlying the disorders by appropriate genetic screening studies and complement serological investigation, especially for *CFH* and *CFHR* mutations and testing for C3Nef, CfH function levels, and auto-antibodies to CfH or factor B.

The therapy for DDD is very problematic. Immunosuppressive therapy, of any kind, is not likely to be of benefit, in most cases, and may be harmful; therefore, it cannot be generally recommended. According to the Hixton Retreat on Dense Deposit Disease (Smith et al., 2007), if C3Nef is present then a trial of

PLEX/infusion therapy may be considered. If a factor H deficiency is present due to a factor H gene mutation, then plasma infusion therapy may be indicated. Patients with anti-factor H antibodies could be considered for treatment with immunosuppressants including RTX and/or PLEX. The use of eculizumab is a very promising approach, but long-term results are largely unknown, and treatment regimens may be prohibitively expensive.

Treatment of C3GN with immunosuppressive agents (such as steroid mono-therapy or MMF combined with steroids) may be more successful, especially in the presence of C3Nef, and a trial of this treatment may be indicated in cases that are not due to a genetic mutation. Eculizumab seems also to be effective and may be indicated in patients with progressive disease who fail to respond to other therapies, providing that activation of the AP and C5 convertase is well documented.

When C3G (either C3GN or DDD) is complicated by extensive crescentic disease, aggressive therapy with oral cyclophosphamide, high-dose steroids and possibly PLEX is indicated; however, if no response is evident after about two weeks, this treatment should be stopped and eculizumab initiated, if a renal biopsy has suggested the possibility of reversible disease.

Treatment of 'idiopathic' immune complex-mediated MPGN is highly uncertain. Although, retrospective analysis of older reports would suggest that immunosuppression (alternate day steroids or combined immunosuppression) may be useful in some cases, but modern day RCTs, excluding cases of C3N (DDD or C3GN), are lacking.

Recurrence in renal transplants

When classified according to 'pattern-of injury' rather than specific diseases all forms of MPGN have been noted to recur in renal allografts (Glassock, 2009; Ivanyi, 2008; reviewed in Ponticelli and Glassock, 2010). The recurrence rate is about 67–100 per cent in DDD, whereas only 20 33 per cent of patients with MPGN type I (which includes both C3N and 'idiopathic' immune complex MPGN) will manifest a clinical recurrence (Curtis et al., 1979; Briganti et al., 2002; Braun et al., 2005; Ivanyi, 2008).

Lorenz and colleagues (2010) reported on 29 patients who had recurrent MPGN. Excluded from this analysis were patients who had MPGN type II/ DDD, those with clear evidence of secondary MPGN, and those without a post-transplant biopsy. During an average of 53 months of follow-up using protocol biopsies, 12 patients had recurrent MPGN diagnosed one week to 14 months post-transplant. In four of the 12 patients, the MPGN presented clinically, whereas the remaining had subclinical disease. The risk of recurrence was significantly increased in patients with low complement levels. A serum monoclonal gammopathy was found in six patients. The presence of a monoclonal gammopathy was associated with earlier and more aggressive disease, and was more common in recurrent than non-recurrent disease. Some patients developed characteristic lesions within two months post-transplant, whereas others presented with minimal, atypical histological changes that progressed to MPGN. Of 29 patients, five lost their allograft and two patients were on chronic plasmapheresis. Other studies which antedate the current understanding of C3G as a cause of the MPGN 'pattern of injury' suggested that the recurrence rate of DDD was higher possibly due to the higher frequency of extensive crescentic disease (Little et al., 2006; Ivanyi, 2008).

The only study to evaluate clinical findings, pathology, and outcomes of recurrence in patients with C3GN was reported by Zand and colleagues (2014) in an extensive study at the Mayo Clinic (n = 21 cases). A recurrence of the disease was seen in 67 per cent of case after a period of follow-up of up to about 13 years. The recurrence rate at one year of follow-up was 30 per cent. The median time to recurrence was 32 months. Graft failure was about 50 per cent at ten years in the 14 patients with a recurrence—all but three of which had received living donor transplants. Proteinuria at the time of recurrence ranged widely (22–4288 mg/day). Recurrence rate was particularly high in those patients who were found to have an underlying monoclonal gammopathy (20 per cent of the entire group). Pathology of recurrence varied showing mesangial proliferative GN or MPGN. Treatment varied and its efficacy could not be evaluated. RTX or stem cell transplantation seemed to be of benefit in those with an underlying monoclonal gammopathy. No patient received eculizumab in this series, but there are anecdotal reports of successful treatment of recurrent C3GN (and DDD) with this agent (McCaughan et al., 2012; Sanchez-Moreno et al., 2014: Moog et al., 2018; Sahin et al., 2018). Recurrence of disease in renal allografts has also been reported for CFHR-5 nephropathy (Vernon et al., 2011).

Treatment of recurrent MPGN and/or C3G is generally unsatisfactory, but a few anecdotal reports have claimed success for aggressive treatment with oral cyclophosphamide, PLEX, and/or high-dose MMF and IV steroids; the true benefits of these approaches have not yet been tested in a controlled trial (Lien and Scott, 2000; Kurtz and Schlueter, 2002; Wu et al., 2004; Glassock, 2009). If a factor-H deficiency is the cause of DDD, PLEX/plasma infusion may be used in the pre- and post-transplant management to try to avoid a recurrence. A genetic deficiency of CfH causing recurrent MPGN and graft loss might conceivably be managed by combined liver and kidney transplantation, as has been done for CfH deficiency related aHUS (Jalanko et al., 2008). Patients with recurrent disease associated with a monoclonal gammopathy should be considered for targeted chemotherapy aimed to eliminate the monoclonal protein.

References

Al-Ghaithi B, Chanchlani R, Riedl M, et al. (2016). C3 Glomerulopathy and post-infectious glomerulonephritis define a disease spectrum. Pediatr Nephrol. 31: 2079–86.

Alexander MP, Fervenza FC, De Vriese AS, et al. (2016). C3 glomerulonephritis and autoimmune disease: More than a fortuitous association? J Nephrol. 29: 203–9.

Anders D, Agricola B, Sippel M, et al. (1977). Basement membrane changes in membranoproliferative glomerulonephritis II: Characterization of a third type by silver impregnation of ultra-thin sections. Virchows Arch A Pathol Anat Histol. 376: 1–19.

Angioi A, Fervenza FC, Sethi S, et al. (2016). Diagnosis of complement alternative pathway disorders. Kidney Int. 89: 278–88.

Appel GB, Cook HT, Hageman G, et al. (2005). Membranoproliferative glomerulonephritis type II (dense deposit disease): An update. J Am Soc Nephrol. 16: 1392–403.

Asinobi AO, Gbadegesin RA, Adeyemo AA, et al. (1999). The predominance of membranoproliferative glomerulonephritis in childhood nephrotic syndrome in Ibadan, Nigeria. West Afr J Med. 18: 203–6.

Athanasiou Y, Voskarides K, Gale DP, et al. (2011). Familial C3 glomerulopathy associated with CFHR5 mutations: Clinical characteristics of 91 patients in 16 pedigrees. Clin J Am Soc Nephrol. 6: 1436–46.

Avasare RS, Canetta PA, Bomback AS, et al. (2018). Mycophenolate mofetil in combination with steroids for treatment of C3 glomerulopathy: A case series. Clin J Am Soc Nephrol. 13: 406–13.

Bahat E, Akkaya BK, Akman S, et al. (2007). Comparison of pulse and oral steroid in childhood membranoproliferative glomerulonephritis. J Nephrol. 20: 234–45.

Barbiano di Belgiojoso G, Baroni M, Pagliari B, et al. (1985). Is membranoproliferative glomerulonephritis really decreasing? Nephrol. 40: 380–4.

Barbour TD, Ruseva MM, Pickering MC. (2016). Update on C3 glomerulopathy. Nephrol Dial Transplant. 31: 717–25.

Bayazit AK, Noyan A, Cengiz N, et al. (2004). Mycophenolate mofetil in children with multi-drug resistant nephrotic syndrome. Clin Nephrol. 61: 25–9.

Bekker P, Dairaghi D, Seitz L, et al. (2016). Characterization of pharmacologic and pharmacokinetic properties of CCX168, a potent and selective orally administered complement 5a receptor inhibitor, based on preclinical evaluation and randomized phase 1 clinical study. PLoS One. 11: e0164646.

Bomback AS. (2014). Eculizumab in the treatment of membranoproliferative glomerulonephritis. Nephron Clin Pract. 128: 270–6.

Bomback AS, Smith RJ, Barile GR, et al. (2012). Eculizumab for dense deposit disease and C3 glomerulonephritis. Clin J Am Soc Nephrol. 7:748–56.

Briganti EM, Russ GR, McNeil JJ, et al. (2002). Risk of renal allograft loss from recurrent glomerulonephritis. N Engl J Med. 347: 103–9.

Braun MC, Stablein DM, Hamiwka LA, et al. (2005). Recurrence of membranoproliferative glomerulonephritis type II in renal allografts: The North American Pediatric Renal Transplant Cooperative Study experience. J Am Soc Nephrol. 16: 2225–33.

Braun MC, West CD, Strife CF. (1999). Difference between membranoproliferative glomerulonephritis type I and III in long-term response to an alternate-day prednisone regimen. Am J Kidney Dis. **34**: 1022–32.

Bridoux F, Desport E, Frémeaux-Bacchi V, et al. (2011). Glomerulonephritis with isolated C3 deposits and monoclonal gammopathy: A fortuitous association? Clin J Am Soc Nephrol. **6**: 2165–74.

Bu F, Borsa NG, Jones MB, et al. (2016). High-throughput genetic testing for thrombotic microangiopathies and C3 glomerulopathies. J Am Soc Nephrol. **27**: 1245–53.

Burkholder P, Marchand H, Krueger R. (1970). Mixed membranous and proliferative glomerulonephritis: A correlative light, immunofluorescence and electron microscopic study. Lab Invest. **23**: 450–7.

Cameron J, Turner D, Heaton J, et al. (1983). Idiopathic mesangiocapillary glomerulonephritis: Comparison of type I and II in children and adults and long-term prognosis. Am J Med. **74**: 175–92.

Cattran D. (1991). Current status of cyclosporin A in the treatment of membranous, IgA and membranoproliferative glomerulonephritis. Clin Nephrol. **35**: 543–7.

Cattran DC, Cardella C, Roscoe J, et al. (1985). Results of a controlled drug trial in membranoproliferative glomerulonephritis. Kidney Int. **27**: 436–41.

Chapman S, Cameron J, Chantler C, et al. (1980). Treatment of mesangiocapillary glomerulonephritis in children with combined immunosuppression and anticoagulation. Arch Dis Child. **55**: 446–57.

Chauvet S, Frémeaux-Bacchi V, Petitprez F, et al. (2017). Treatment of B-cell disorder improves renal outcome of patients with monoclonal gammopathy-associated C3 glomerulopathy. Blood. **129**: 1437–47.

Chauvet S, Roumenina LT, Bruneau S, et al. (2016). Familial C3GN secondary to defective C3 regulation by complement receptor 1 and complement factor H. J Am Soc Nephrol. **27**: 1665–77.

Chen Q, Wiesener M, Eberhardt HU, et al. (2014). Complement factor H-related hybrid protein deregulates complement in dense deposit disease. J Clin Invest. **124**: 145–55.

Choi MJ, Eustace JA, Giminez LF, et al. (2002). Mycophenolate mofetil treatment for primary glomerular diseases. Kidney Int. **61**: 10981114.

Cook HT. (2015). C4d staining in the diagnosis of C3 glomerulopathy. J Am Soc Nephrol. **26**: 2601–11.

Cook HT, Pickering MC. (2015). Histopathology of MPGN and C3 glomerulopathies. Nat Rev Nephrol. **11**: 14–22.

Curtis J, Wyatt R, Bhathena D, et al. (1979). Renal transplantation for patients with type I and type II membranoproliferative glomerulonephritis: Serial complement and nephritic factor measurement and the problem of recurrence of disease. Am J Med. **66**: 216–23.

D'Apice AJF, Kincaid-Smith G. (1979). Plasma exchange in the treatment of glomerulonephritis. In P Kincaid-Smith, AJF D'Apice, R Atkins (eds), *Progress in Glomerulonephritis*, pp. 371–84. John Wiley, New York.

Dillon JJ, Hladunewich M, Haley WE, et al. (2012). Rituximab therapy for Type I membranoproliferative glomerulonephritis. Clin Nephrol. **77**: 290–5.

Donadio JV, Holley KE. (1982). Membranoproliferative glomerulonephritis. Semin Nephrol. **2**: 214–19.

Donadio J, Offord K. (1989). Reassessment of treatment results in membranoproliferative glomerulonephritis, with emphasis on life-table analysis. Am J Kidney Dis. **6**: 445–51.

Emre S, Sirin A, Alpay H, et al. (1995). Pulse methylprednisolone therapy in children with membranoproliferative glomerulonephritis. Acta Paediatr Jpn. **37**: 626–9.

Erbay B, Karatan O, Duman N, et al. (1988). The effect of cyclosporine in idiopathic nephrotic syndrome resistant to immunosuppressive therapy. Transplant Proc. **20**: 292.

Faedda R, Satta A, Tanda F, et al. (1994). Immunosuppressive treatment of membranoproliferative glomerulonephritis. Nephron. **67**: 59–65.

Fervenza FC, Sethi S, Glassock RJ. (2012). Idiopathic membranoproliferative glomerulonephritis: Does it exist? Nephrol Dial Transplant. **27**: 4288–94.

Floege J, Amann K. (2016). Primary glomerulonephritides. Lancet. **387**: 2036–48.

Ford P, Briscoe D, Shanley P, et al. (1992). Childhood membranoproliferative glomerulonephritis type I: Limited steroid therapy. Kidney Int. **41**: 1606–12.

Gale DP, de Jorge EG, Cook HT, et al. (2010). Identification of a mutation in complement factor H-related protein 5 in patients of Cypriot origin with glomerulonephritis. Lancet. **376**: 794–801.

Gale DP, Maxwell PH. (2013). C3 glomerulonephritis and CVFHR5 nephropathy. Nephrol Dial Transplant. **28**: 282–8.

Giaime P, Daniel L, Burtey S. (2015). Remission of C3 glomerulopathy with rituximab as only immunosuppressive therapy. Clin Nephrol. **83**: 57–60.

Glassock R. (1994). The role of cyclosporine in glomerular disease. Cleveland Clin J Med. **61**: 363–9.

Glassock RJ. (2009). Membranoproliferative glomerulonephritis. In D Molony and J Craig (eds), *Evidence-based Nephrology*, pp. 183–97. Wiley-Blackwell, Oxford.

Guillín-Amarelle C, Sánchez-Iglesias S, Castro-Pais A, et al. (2016). Type 1 familial partial lipodystrophy: Understanding the Köbberling syndrome. Endocrine. **54**: 411–21.

Guo S, Kowalewska J, Wietecha TA, et al. (2008). Renin-angiotensin system blockade is renoprotective in immune complex-mediated glomerulonephritis. J Am Soc Nephrol. **19**: 1168–76.

Habib R, Kleinknecht C, Gubler M-C, et al. (1973). Idiopathic membranoproliferative glomerulonephritis in children: Report of 105 cases. Clin Nephrol. **1**: 194–214.

Habbig S, Mihatsch MJ, Heinen S, et al. (2009). C3 deposition glomerulopathy due to a functional factor H defect. Kidney Int. **75**: 1230–4.

Haddad M, Lau K, Butani L. (2007). Remission of membranoproliferative glomerulonephritis type I with the use of tacrolimus. Pediatr Nephrol. **22**: 1787–91.

Häffner K, Michelfelder S, Pohl M. (2015). Successful therapy of C3Nef-positive C3 glomerulopathy with plasma therapy and immunosuppression. Pediatr Nephrol. **30**: 1951–9.

Herlitz LC, Bomback AS, Markowitz GS, et al. (2012). Pathology after eculizumab in dense deposit disease and C3 GN. J Am Soc Nephrol. **23**: 1229–37.

Holle J, Berenberg-Goßler L, Wu K, et al. (2018). Outcome of membranoproliferative glomerulonephritis and C3 glomerulopathy in children and adolescents. Pediatr Nephrol. **33**: 2389–98.

Hou J, Markowitz GS, Bomback AS, et al. (2014). Toward a working definition of C3 glomerulopathy by immunofluorescence. Kidney Int. **85**: 450–6.

Iatropoulos P, Daina E, Curreri M, et al. (2018). Cluster analysis identifies distinct pathogenetic patterns in C3 glomerulopathies/immune complex-mediated membranoproliferative GN. J Am Soc Nephrol. **29**: 283–94.

Iatropoulos P, Noris M, Mele C, et al. (2016). Complement gene variants determine the risk of immunoglobulin-associated MPGN and C3 glomerulopathy and predict long-term renal outcome. Mol Immunol. **71**: 131–42.

Imamura H, Konomoto T, Tanaka E, et al. (2015). Familial C3 glomerulonephritis associated with mutations in the gene for complement factor B. Nephrol Dial Transplant. **30**: 862–4.

Inman M, Prater G, Fatima H, Wallace E. (2015). Eculizumab-induced reversal of dialysis-dependent kidney failure from C3 glomerulonephritis. Clin Kidney J. **8**: 445–8.

Ivanyi B. (2008). A primer on recurrent and de-novo glomerulonephritis in renal allografts. Nat Clin Pract Nephrol. **4**: 446–57.

Jain D, Green JA, Bastacky S, et al. (2014). Membranoproliferative glomerulonephritis: The role for laser microdissection and mass spectrometry. Am J Kidney Dis. **63**: 324–8.

Jalanko H, Peltonen S, Koskinen A, et al. (2008). Successful liver-kidney transplantation in two children with aHUS caused by a mutation in complement factor H. Am J Transplant. **8**: 216–21.

Jokiranta TS, Solomon A, Pangburn MK, et al. (1999). Nephritogenic lambda light chain dimer: A unique human mini auto-antibody against complement factor H. J Immunol. **163**: 4590–6.

Józsi M, Reuter S, Nozal P, et al. (2014). Autoantibodies to complement components in C3 glomerulopathy and atypical hemolytic uremic syndrome. Immunol Lett. **160**: 163–71.

Jones G, Juszczak M, Kingdon E, et al. (2004). Treatment of idiopathic membranoproliferative glomerulonephritis with mycophenolate mofetil and steroids. Nephrol Dial Transplant. **19**: 3160–4.

KDIGO. (2012). KDIGO Practice Guidelines for Glomerulonephritis. Kidney Int. **2**: 198–9.

Kerns E, Rozansky D, Troxell ML. (2013). Evolution of immunoglobulin deposition in C3-dominant membranoproliferative glomerulopathy. Pediatr Nephrol. **28**: 2227–31.

Khalighi MA, Wang S, Henriksen KJ, et al. (2016). Revisiting post-infectious glomerulonephritis in the emerging era of C3 glomerulopathy. Clin Kidney J. **9**: 397–402.

Kincaid-Smith P. (1972). The treatment of chronic mesangiocapillary glomerulonephritis with impaired renal function. Med J Aust. **2**: 587–92.

Kiyomasu T, Shibata M, Kurosu H, et al. (2002). Cyclosporin A treatment for membranoproliferative glomerulonephritis type II. Nephron. **91**: 509–11.

Kurtz KA, Schlueter AJ. (2002). Management of membranoproliferative glomerulonephritis type II with plasmapheresis. J Cin Apher. **17**: 135–7.

Larsen CP, Messias NC, Walker PD, et al. (2015). Membranoproliferative glomerulonephritis with masked monotypic immunoglobulin deposits. Kidney Int. **88**: 867–73.

Le Quintrec M, Lapeyraque AL, Lionet A, et al. (2018). Patterns of clinical response to eculizumab in patients with C3 glomerulopathy. Am J Kidney Dis. **72**: 84–92.

Le Quintrec M, Lionet A, Kandel C, et al. (2015). Eculizumab for treatment of rapidly progressive C3 glomerulopathy Am J Kidney Dis. **65**: 484–9.

Levin A. (1999). Management of membranoproliferative glomerulonephritis: Evidence-based recommendations. Kidney Int. **55**: s41–6.

Levy M, Gubler MC, Sich M, et al. (1978). Immunopathology of membranoproliferative glomerulonephritis with subendothelial deposits (Type I MPGN). Clin Immunol Immunopathol. **10**: 477–92.

Licht C, Weyersberg A, Heinen S, et al. (2005). Successful plasma therapy for atypical hemolytic uremia syndrome caused by Factor H deficiency owing to a novel mutation in the complement cofactor protein domain 15. Am J Kidney Dis. **45**: 415–21.

Lien YH, Scott K. (2000). Long-term cyclophosphamide treatment for recurrent type I membranoproliferative glomerulonephritis after transplantation. Am J Kidney Dis. **35**: 539–43.

Little MA, Dupont P, Campbell E, et al. (2006). Severity of primary MPGN, rather than MPGN type determines renal survival and post-transplantation recurrence risk. Kidney Int. **69**: 504–11.

Lorenz EC, Sethi S, Leung N, et al. (2010). Recurrent membranoproliferative glomerulonephritis after kidney transplantation. Kidney Int. **77**: 721–8.

Mao S, Xuan X, Sha Y, et al. (2015). Crescentic acute glomerulonephritis with isolated C3 deposition: A case report and review of literature. Int J Clin Exp Pathol. **8**: 1826–9.

Martínez-Barricarte R, Heurich M, Valdes-Cañedo F, et al. (2010). Human C3 mutation reveals a mechanism of dense deposit disease pathogenesis and provides insights into complement activation and regulation. J Clin Invest. **120**: 3702–12.

Master Sankar Raj V, Gordillo R, Chand DH. (2016). Overview of C3 Glomerulopathy. Front Pediatr. **4**: 45.

Matsumoto H, Shibasaki T, Ohno I, et al. (1995). Effect of cyclosporin monotherapy on proteinuria in patients with membranoproliferative glomerulonephritis. Nippon Jinzo Gakkai Shi. **37**: 258–62.

McAdams A, McEnery P, West C. (1975). Mesangiocapillary glomerulonephritis: Changes in glomerular morphology with long-term alternate-day prednisone therapy. J Pediatr. **86**: 23–30.

McEnery P. (1990). Membranoproliferative glomerulonephritis: The Cincinnati experience—cumulative renal survival 1957–1989. J Pediatr. **116**: S109–14.

McEnery P, McAdams A, West C. (1985). The effect of prednisone in a high-dose, alternate-day regimen on the natural history of idiopathic membranoproliferative glomerulonephritis. Medicine (Baltimore). **6**: 401–18.

McGinley E, Watkins R, McLay A, et al. (1985). Plasma exchange in the treatment of mesangiocapillary glomerulonephritis. Nephron. **40**: 385–90.

McCaughan JA, O'Rourke DM, Courtney AE. (2012). Recurrent dense deposit disease after renal transplantation: An emerging role for complementary therapies. Am J Transplant. **12**: 1046–51.

McGrogan A, Franssen CF, de Vries CS. (2011). The incidence of primary glomerulonephritis worldwide: A systematic review of the literature. Nephrol Dial Transplant. **26**: 414–30.

Medjeral-Thomas N, Malik TH, Patel MP, et al. (2014). A novel CFHR5 fusion protein causes C3 glomerulopathy in a family without Cypriot ancestry. Kidney Int. **85**: 933–7.

Medjeral-Thomas NR, O'Shaughnessy MM, O'Regan JA, et al. (2014). C3 glomerulopathy: Clinicopathologic features and predictors of outcome. Clin J Am Soc Nephrol. **9**: 46–53.

Messias NC, Walker PD, Larsen CP. (2015). Paraffin immunofluorescence in the renal pathology laboratory: More than a salvage technique. Mod Pathol. **28**: 854–60.

Montoliu J, Bergada E, Arrizabalaga P, et al. (1982). Acute renal failure in dense-deposit disease: Recovery after plasmapheresis. BMJ. **384**: 940–3.

Moog P, Jost PJ, Büttner-Herold M. (2018). Eculizumab as salvage therapy for recurrent monoclonal gammopathy-induced C3 glomerulopathy in a kidney allograft. BMC Nephrol. **19**: 106.

Morton MR, Bannister K. (1993). Renal failure due to mesangiocapillary glomerulonephritis in pregnancy: Use of plasma exchange therapy. Clin Nephrol. **40**: 74–8.

Nargund P, Kambham N, Mehta K, et al. (2015). Clinicopathological features of membranoproliferative glomerulonephritis under a new classification. Clin Nephrol. **84**: 323–30.

Nasr SH, Valeri AM, Appel GB, et al. (2009). Dense deposit disease: Clinicopathologic study of 32 pediatric and adult patients. Clin J Am Soc Nephrol. **4**: 22–32.

Nester CM, Smith RJ. (2013). Treatment options for C3 glomerulopathy. Curr Opin Nephrol Hypertens. **22**: 231–7.

Nester CM, Smith RJ. (2016). Complement inhibition in C3 glomerulopathy. Semin Immunol. **28**: 241–9.

Nicolas C, Vuiblet V, Baudouin V, et al. (2014). C3 nephritic factor associated with C3 glomerulopathy in children. Pediatr Nephrol. **29**: 85–94.

Oosterveld MJ, Garrelfs MR, Hoppe B, et al. (2015). Eculizumab in pediatric dense deposit disease. Clin J Am Soc Nephrol. **10**: 1773–82.

Owen KR, Donohoe M, Ellard S, et al. (2004). Mesangiocapillary glomerulonephritis type 2 associated with familial partial lipodystrophy (Dunnigan-Köbberling syndrome). Nephron Clin Pract. **96**: c35–8.

Pickering MC, D'Agati VD, Nester CM, et al. (2013). C3 glomerulopathy: Consensus report. Kidney Int. **84**: 1079–89.

Ponticelli C, Glassock RJ. (2009). *Treatment of Primary Glomerulonephritis*. 2nd Edition. OUP, Oxford.

Ponticelli C, Glassock RJ. (2010). Posttransplant recurrence of primary glomerulonephritis. Clin J Am Soc Nephrol. **5**: 2363–72.

Prasto J, Kaplan BS, Russo P, et al. (2014). Streptococcal infection as possible trigger for dense deposit disease (C3 glomerulopathy). Eur J Pediatr. **173**: 767–72.

Rabasco C, Cavero T, Román E, et al. (2015). Effectiveness of mycophenolate mofetil in C3 glomerulonephritis. Kidney Int. **88**: 1153–60.

Radhakrishnan J, Halevy D. (2000). Cyclosporin treatment of glomerular diseases. Expert Opin Invest Drugs. **9**: 1053–63.

Ravindran A, Fervenza FC, Smith RJH, et al. (2018a). C3 glomerulopathy: Ten years' experience at Mayo Clinic. Mayo Clin Proc. **93**: 991–1008.

Ravindran A, Fervenza FC, Smith RJH, et al. (2018b). C3 glomerulopathy associated with monoclonal Ig is a distinct subtype. Kidney Int. **94**: 178–86.

Rennke H, Renounce H. (1995). Secondary membranoproliferative glomerulonephritis (nephrology forum). Kidney Int. **47**: 643–56.

Rousset-Rouvière C, Cailliez M, Garaix F, et al. (2014). Rituximab fails where eculizumab restores renal function in C3Nef-related DDD. Pediatr Nephrol. **29**: 1107–11.

Ruseva MM, Peng T, Lasaro MA, et al. (2016). Efficacy of targeted complement inhibition in experimental C3 glomerulopathy. J Am Soc Nephrol. **27**: 405–16.

Sahin H, Gok Oguz E, Akoglu H, et al. (2018). Successful treatment of posttransplant recurrent complement C3 glomerulopathy with eculizumab. Iran J Kidney Dis. **12**: 315–18.

Sanchez-Moreno A, de la Cerda F, Cabrera R, et al. (2014). Eculizumab in dense-deposit disease after renal transplantation. Pediatr Nephrol. **29**: 2055–9.

Savige J, Amos L, Ierino F, et al. (2016). Retinal disease in the C3 glomerulopathies and the risk of impaired vision. Ophthalmic Genet. **37**: 369–76.

Schena FP. (1999). Primary glomerulonephritides with nephrotic syndrome. Limitations of therapy in adult patients. J Nephrol. **12**: s125–30.

Servais A, Frémeaux-Bacchi V, Lequintrec M, et al. (2007). Primary glomerulonephritis with isolated C3 deposits: A new entity which shares common genetic risk factors with haemolytic uraemic syndrome. J Med Genet. **44**: 193–9.

Servais A, Noël LH, Dragon-Durey MA, et al. (2011). Heterogeneous pattern of renal disease associated with homozygous factor H deficiency. Hum Pathol. **42**: 1305–11.

Servais A, Noël LH, Frémeaux-Bacchi V, et al. (2013). C3 glomerulopathy. Contrib Nephrol. **181**: 185–93.

Servais A, Noël LH, Roumenina LT, et al. (2012). Acquired and genetic complement abnormalities play a critical role in dense deposit disease and other C3 glomerulopathies. Kidney Int. **82**: 454–64.

Sethi S, Fervenza FC. (2011). Membranoproliferative glomerulonephritis: Pathogenetic heterogeneity and proposal for a new classification. Semin Nephrol. **31**: 341–8.

Sethi S, Fervenza FC. (2012). Membranoproliferative glomerulonephritis: A new look at an old entity. N Engl J Med. **366**: 1119–31.

Sethi S, Fervenza FC. (2014). Pathology of renal diseases associated with dysfunction of the alternative pathway of complement: C3 glomerulopathy and atypical hemolytic uremic syndrome (aHUS). Semin Thromb Hemost. **40**: 416–21.

Sethi S, Fervenza FC, Smith RJ, Haas M. (2015). Overlap of ultrastructural findings in C3 glomerulonephritis and dense deposit disease. Kidney Int. **88**: 1449–50.

Sethi S, Fervenza FC, Zhang Y, et al. (2012). C3 glomerulonephritis: Clinicopathological findings, complement abnormalities, glomerular proteomic profile, treatment, and follow-up. Kidney Int. **82**: 465–73.

Sethi S, Fervenza FC, Zhang Y, et al. (2013). Atypical postinfectious glomerulonephritis is associated with abnormalities in the alternative pathway of complement. Kidney Int. **83**: 293–9.

Sethi S, Nasr SH, De Vriese AS, et al. (2015). C4d as a diagnostic tool in proliferative GN. J Am Soc Nephrol. **26**: 2852–9.

Sethi S, Quint PS, O'Seaghdha CM, et al. (2016). C4 glomerulopathy: A disease entity associated with C4d deposition. Am J Kidney Dis. **67**: 949–53.

Sethi S, Sullivan A, Smith RJ. (2014). C4 dense-deposit disease. N Engl J Med. **370**: 784–6.

Sethi S, Vrana JA, Fervenza FC, et al. (2016). Characterization of C3 in C3 glomerulopathy. Nephrol Dial Transplant. **32**: 459–65.

Simon P, Ramee MP, Boulahrouz R, et al. (2004). Epidemiologic data of primary glomerular diseases in Western France. Kidney Int. **66**: 905–8.

Singh L, Singh G, Bhardwaj S, et al. (2016). Dense deposit disease mimicking a renal small vessel vasculitis. J Am Soc Nephrol. **27**: 59–62.

Smith RJH, Alexander J, Barlow PN, et al. (2007). New approaches to the treatment of dense deposit disease. J Am Soc Nephrol. **18**: 2447–56.

Strife CF, McEnery P, McAdams J, et al. (1975). A third ultrastructural variant of membranoproliferative glomerulonephritis. Kidney Int. **8**: 454–9.

Strife CF, McEnery PT, McAdams AJ, et al. (1977). Membranoproliferative glomerulonephritis with disruption of the glomerular basement membrane. Clin Nephrol. **7**: 65–72.

Tarshish P, Bernstein J, Tobin T, et al. (1992). Treatment of mesangiocapillary glomerulonephritis with alternate-day prednisone. A report of the International study of kidney disease in children. Pediatr Nephrol. **6**: 123–30.

Tiller D, Clarkson A, Mathew T. (1981). A prospective randomized trial of the use of cyclophosphamide, dipyridamole and warfarin in membranous and membranoproliferative glomerulonephritis. In W Zurukzoglu, M Papadimitriou, M Sion, et al. (eds), *Proceedings of the 8th International Congress on Nephrology*, pp. 345–51. S Karger, Basel.

Varade W, Forrestal J, West C. (1990). Patterns of complement activation in idiopathic membranoproliferative glomerulonephritis: Types I, II, III. Am J Kidney Dis. **16**: 196–206.

Vernon KA, Gale DP, de Jorge EG, et al. (2011). Recurrence of complement factor H-related protein 5 nephropathy in a renal transplant. Am J Transplant. **11**: 152–5.

Walker PD, Ferrario F, Joh K, et al. (2007). Dense deposit disease is not a membranoproliferative glomerulonephritis. Mod Pathol. **20**: 605–16.

Warady B, Guggenheim S, Sedman A, et al. (1985). Prednisone therapy of membranoproliferative glomerulonephritis in children. J Pediatr. **107**: 702–7.

Welte T, Arnold F, Kappes J, et al. (2018). Treating C3 glomerulopathy with eculizumab. BMC Nephrol. **19**:7.

West CD, McAdams J, McConville J, et al. (1965). Hypocomplementemic and normocomplementemic persistent (chronic) glomerulonephritis: Clinical and pathological characteristics. J Pediatr. **23**: 459–67.

Wu J, Jaar BG, Briggs WA, et al. (2004). High-dose mycophenolate mofetil in the treatment of post-transplant glomerular disease in the allograft: A case series. Nephron Clin Pract. **98**: c61–6.

Xiao X, Pickering MC, Smith RJ. (2014). C3 glomerulopathy: The genetic and clinical findings in dense deposit disease and C3 glomerulonephritis. Semin Thromb Hemost. **40**: 465–71.

Xu X, Ning Y, Shang W, et al. (2016). Analysis of 4931 renal biopsy data in central China from 1994 to 2014. Ren Fail. **38**: 1021–3.

Yanagihara T, Hayakawa M, Yoshida J, et al. (2005). Long-term follow-up of diffuse membranoproliferative glomerulonephritis type I. Pediatr Nephrol. **20**: 585–90.

Yang Y, Denton H, Davies OR, et al. (2018). An engineered complement Factor H construct for treatment of C3 glomerulopathy. J Am Soc Nephrol. **29**: 1649–61.

Zand L, Kattah A, Fervenza FC, et al. (2013). C3 glomerulonephritis associated with monoclonal gammopathy: A case series. Am J Kidney Dis. **62**: 506–14.

Zand L, Lorenz EC, Cosio FG, et al. (2014). Clinical findings, pathology, and outcomes of C3GN after kidney transplantation. J Am Soc Nephrol. **25**: 1110–17.

Zhang Y, Nester CM, Holanda DG, et al. (2013). Soluble CR1 therapy improves complement regulation in C3 glomerulopathy. J Am Soc Nephrol. **24**: 1820–9.

Zhang Y, Nester CM, Martin B, et al. (2014). Defining the complement biomarker profile of C3 glomerulopathy. Clin J Am Soc Nephrol. **9**: 1876–82.

Zipfel PF, Skerka C, Chen Q, et al. (2015). The role of complement in C3 glomerulopathy. Mol Immunol. **67**: 21–30.

Zuber J, Fakhouri F, Roumenina LT, et al. (2012). Use of eculizumab for atypical haemolytic uraemic syndrome and C3 glomerulopathies. Nat Rev Nephrol. **8**: 643–57.

Chapter 9

Infection-related and renal-limited glomerulonephritis

Richard J Glassock, Lee Hebert,
Gabriella Moroni, and Claudio Ponticelli

Introduction and overview

The infection-related glomerulonephritides encompass a wide swath of epidemic and endemic diseases (Glassock et al., 2015). Bacteria, fungi, protozoa, nematodes, helminths, and viruses all contribute to the glomerular disease burden. Most of these have numerous and varied extrarenal manifestations and are commonly classified as secondary glomerular diseases. However, a few have mainly or exclusively renal involvement and can be classified within the rubric of primary glomerular disease, even though they are not truly idiopathic in nature. Acute post-infectious glomerulonephritis (APIGN) is a prototype of this form of infection-related glomerulonephritis. This group of glomerular diseases is characterized by intraglomerular inflammation and cellular proliferation resulting from immunological events triggered by a variety of organisms, mostly bacterial. In this condition the extrarenal manifestations are generally the consequence of disturbed kidney function, rather than any direct effect of the offending organism. The principal cause of APIGN is post-streptococcal glomerulonephritis (PSGN), which most often occurs in children following a pharyngeal infection with a particular strain of streptococci and has a favourable outcome. Alternatively, infection-related glomerulonephritis can be caused by an ongoing infection, which, at times, can be remarkably occult and difficult to detect. This is *not* a post-infectious nephritic process as the kidney injury occurs in parallel with the infection itself, not after the organism has been eradicated. This is an important nosologic distinction that has important treatment consequences (Glassock et al., 2015).

The ecology of infection-related glomerulonephritis is constantly changing as a result of alterations in hygienic conditions, improvement in vaccines, better antimicrobial therapy, and emergence of new or mutated microbial pathogens. For example, the spectrum of infection-related glomerulonephritis has changed significantly in the last few decades. The incidence of PSGN, particularly in its epidemic form, has progressively declined in many industrialized countries. In many countries, infection-related glomerular diseases are now caused by other Gram-positive bacteria (e.g. staphylococci), viruses (HIV, hepatitis B, hepatitis C), or protozoa (e.g. malaria). Also, while spontaneous recovery from APSGN within few weeks is still the rule in children, the prognosis is less certain in older adults, perhaps because of delay in diagnosis or underlying comorbidities. Other primary glomerular disease entities, e.g. IgA nephropathy and C3 glomerulopathy (see Chapter 7 and Chapter 8), can sometimes resemble APSGN in onset and clinical characteristics but have a much different longer-term prognosis. This chapter discusses the prototypical renal-limited forms of infection-related glomerulonephritis.

Post-streptococcal glomerulonephritis (PSGN)

Post-streptococcal glomerulonephritis (PSGN) usually develops after upper respiratory tract or skin infections and is caused by β-haemolytic streptococci of group A. PSGN predominantly affects children in epidemic or sporadic forms while it is much less common (<10 per cent of cases) in adults. The clinical manifestations may vary from subclinical forms with mild, easily missed urinary abnormalities to the acute forms characterized by the abrupt onset of macroscopic haematuria, decrease in glomerular filtration rate (GFR), fluid retention with consequent oedema, and hypertension (Table 9.1).

Pathology

In the acute phase, light microscopy shows a pattern of exudative glomerulonephritis, characterized by a diffuse and global involvement of the glomeruli. Hypercellularity, due both to cellular infiltration and endogenous cellular proliferation with consequent enlargement of the glomerular tuft, is the main characteristic. The cellular composition depends on the stage of the disease. In the acute phase, the prevailing proliferating cells are endothelial cells, while polymorphonuclear granulocytes are the predominant infiltrating cells (see Plate 15). Proliferation of mesangial cells, infiltrating macrophages, and lymphocytes are also present and have an appearance resembling membranoproliferative glomerulonephritis (with subendothelial electron dense deposits and C3 glomerulonephritis (C3GN; Nasr et al., 2013; Iseri et al., 2016; see also Chapter 8). Helper T-cells are in higher proportion in early stages of the disease while the amount of suppressor T-cells remains constant throughout the course of the disease. As a consequence of the hypercellularity, occlusion of the capillary lumens with reduced filtration surface area can be observed. Necrosis of the glomerular

Table 9.1 Main features of acute post-streptococcal glomerulonephritis (PSGN).

Pathology:	Hypercellularity of the glomeruli secondary to proliferation of resident cells and infiltration of inflammatory cells (polymorphonuclear leucocytes). By immunofluorescence C3 deposits are uniformly found in the mesangial cells and along the glomerular capillary walls and much less IgG deposition. Deposits of C1q tend to be scanty. C4d and MBL-associated serine protease (MASP) deposits are found in about 40% of cases deposits. On electron microscopy there are small sub-endothelial electron dense deposits and subepithelial 'humps' depending on the timing of renal biopsy.
Pathogenesis:	It is believed to be an immune complex disease. Antibodies directed against streptococcal antigens either may cross-react with some component of the GBM or may attack the antigens planted on the glomerular basement membrane (GBM), eliciting an inflammatory response. Some streptococcal antigens, once deposited in glomeruli, can activate the alternative complement pathway, in the absence of IgG, and thus lead to a lesion resembling C3 glomerulonephritis (see Chapter 8).
Aetiology:	The disease is triggered by infections caused by nephritogenic strains of β-haemolytic group A streptococci.
Clinical presentation:	The disease may be asymptomatic (only microscopic haematuria) or may present with an acute nephritic syndrome with microscopic or macroscopic haematuria, proteinuria, hypertension, and, rarely, rapidly progressive renal failure (see Table 8.2).
Epidemiology:	The disease is more frequent in children and in males. May occur in an epidemic or sporadic form. It tends to be less and less frequent in developed countries.
Prognosis:	The prognosis is generally favourable, particularly in children, as glomerulonephritis spontaneously recovers in a few weeks. Some adults presenting with nephritic syndrome or renal insufficiency may show persisting urinary abnormalities in the long term or may even develop renal failure. Whether these cases are bona-fide instances of PSGN or other diseases masquerading as PSGN (e.g. IgA nephropathy or C3 glomerulopathy) is controversial.
Treatment:	Salt, potassium, and water restriction is recommended in the first days after onset, particularly in oliguric patients. Diuretics, antihypertensive drugs, and antistreptococcal antibiotics may be required in the early phases. Antimicrobial therapy does little to alter the natural history of the disease, but does influence its spread among close contacts.

tufts is usually not seen, and if present should raise a suspicion of a systemic vasculitis (see Chapter 10). Few glomeruli may show extracapillary proliferation (crescents), often in a segmental distribution. The glomerular basement membrane (GBM) is generally normal. In some cases, with the trichrome stain, using oil immersion lens, it is possible to recognize tiny subepithelial deposits, the so-called *humps* (see Plate 12). Macrophages and lymphocytes are also present in the tubulo-interstitial areas. In few cases, an arteriolar fibrinoid necrosis may be seen.

In the resolving phases of the disease, proliferation of mesangial cells and matrix are predominant, neutrophils diminish progressively, while a few mononuclear cells may still be present in the capillary lumens. During this phase the capillary lumens are patent. The residual mesangial hypercellularity usually slowly resolves within months.

By immunofluorescence microscopy, granular immune deposits of C3 and, to a lesser extent, IgG are uniformly present in mesangial areas and along the glomerular capillary walls. IgG is present only transiently in the acute phase of the disease while C3 is present both in the early and in the late phases of the disease. IgM may be present in small amount and at lower intensity as well as IgA. Sorger and colleagues (1982) described three distinct immunofluorescent patterns. *The starry sky pattern*, which may be seen in the first weeks of the disease, is characterized by finely granular immune deposits in the capillary walls and to a lesser degree in the mesangium (see Plate 11). In the *garland pattern*, there are heavy confluent deposits of IgG and C3 along the capillary walls, which correlate with a large number of subepithelial 'humps' at electron microscopy. This pattern is usually associated with persistence of heavy proteinuria and worse long-term prognosis (Sorger et al., 1987). The *mesangial pattern* is defined by the presence of granular deposition of C3 in the stalk region of the glomerulus; immunoglobulins are not always present. This pattern is associated with mesangial hypercellularity and is most often found in the resolving phases of the disease (see also 'Mesangial proliferative glomerulonephritis' in Chapter 11). Deposits of C5b-9, Factor B, and CD59 are also found in most cases (Hisano et al., 2007). Typically, C1q deposition is absent or scanty, but C4d, MASP, MBL, and C4bp, indicating prominent activation of the lectin pathway, are found in about 40 per cent of patients (Hisano et al., 2007). Those without lectin pathway activation have characteristics indicating activation of the alternative pathway (resembling that of C3 glomerulopathy; see also Chapter 8).

On electron microscopy, the most characteristic feature in the acute phase of the disease is the presence of sub-epithelial electron dense deposits called *humps* as they resemble camel humps (see Plate 16). Humps usually resolve within four to six weeks leaving translucent or electron-lucent areas. These 'humps' can also be seen in other diseases (such as IgA vasculitis and C3 glomerulopathy) so they are not pathognomonic of PSGN. Small subendothelial and mesangial deposits are also observed, particularly in early disease, so C3GN must be in the differential diagnosis (see also Chapter 8).

Pathogenesis

On the basis of the clinical course of the disease together with evidence of the deposition of immunoglobulins and complement within the glomeruli, acute PSGN is often classified as an *immune-complex disease*. However, in spite of decades of investigations, the sequence leading to immune-complex formation and activation of complement and inflammation has not been completely clarified.

A first hypothesis suggested that some antibodies produced against streptococci antigens may cross-react with GBM antigens or with antigens planted on the glomerular cells surface. This hypothesis was supported by experimental studies showing that soluble glycoproteins of streptococcal nephritogenic strains were able to induce nephritis, that the injection of the antiserum of the affected animals induced nephritis in normal animals, and that antibodies against streptococcal cell membranes were able to cross-react with glomeruli in tissue section or isolated glomeruli (reviewed in Lange, 1980). In addition, in serum of patients with PSGN, antibodies to type-IV collagen, heparan sulphate, and laminin have been detected (Kefalides et al., 1993).

Alternatively, it has been hypothesized that nephritogenic streptococci can produce and release in the circulation proteins that have a particular affinity for normal glomerular sites. After lodging into the sites of the glomerulus, for which they have intrinsic affinity, the nephritogenic proteins would attract properdin or other molecules and activate the alternative (and lectin) pathway of complement. On the other hand, the nephritogenic proteins deposited in the glomerulus could act as planted antigens and bind to circulating antistreptococcal antibodies with subsequent immune complex formation in situ, activation of complement, and recruitment of inflammatory cells and of inflammatory mediators, including chemoattractants, proteases, cytokines, oxidants, and growth factors that, together with proliferating resident cells, can damage the glomerulus (Couser and Johnson, 2014). The involvement of other factors, such as local generation of terminal complement components, cell-mediated immunity, and apoptosis (Oda et al., 2007), has also been suggested, but their role in the pathogenesis of PSGN has not been completely clarified.

During the last several decades several streptococcal proteins have been investigated as possible nephritogenic antigens. A first candidate was a complex of intracellular anionic proteins called *endostreptosins*. Antibodies against endostreptosins were present in high titres in patients with PSGN and were able to react with glomeruli of affected patients. However, elevated titres of these antibodies have been documented also in patients with streptococcal infection but without glomerulonephritis. Further studies led to the isolation of the endostreptosins complex of proteins an antigen termed *pre-absorbing antigen* (Yoshizawa et al., 1992). Antibodies to pre-absorbing antigen were present in 30 out of 31 patients with PSGN and only in one out of 36 patients with streptococcal infection but without nephritis. This protein was the only one detected in the glomeruli of affected patients and was able to activate the alternative pathway of complement. *Nephritis strain-associated protein* (NSAP) is another potential antigen isolated from strains of streptococci derived from patients with PSGN. Anti-NSAP antibodies were found both in sera and in biopsy specimens from patients with PSGN.

An extracellular plasmin-binding protein secreted by nephritis-associated Group A streptococci identical to *streptococcal pyrogenic exotoxin B* (SPEB) and to a streptococcal proteinase has also been identified (Poon-King et al., 1993). This antigen is colocalized in the glomeruli with complement and immunoglobulins deposits, and is the only streptococcal antigen that has been demonstrated within the electron dense sub-epithelial deposits (humps) of PSGN (Batsford et al., 2005). The titres of anti-SPEB antibodies were found to be significantly higher in children with PSGN than in normal children, or in those with acute rheumatic fever or scarlet fever. In kidney biopsy specimens stained for SPEB, 67 per cent of PSGN were positive versus only 16 per cent of non-PSGN subjects. Anti-SPEB titres tended to rise rapidly after the onset of the disease reaching a peak after two weeks and decreasing slowly without returning to baseline after one year (Cu et al., 1998). Thus, a single attack can confer a long-term immunity, so explaining why recurrence of PSGN is extremely rare. Another nephritogenic antigen isolated from Group A streptococcus is the *nephritis-associated plasmin receptor* (NAPlr), a glyceraldeide-3-phosphate-dehydrogenase (GAPHD) whose nucleotide sequence shows high homology as well as similar functions to that of the plasmin receptor (Plr) of group A streptococcus. Significant glomerular deposition of NAPlr was documented in the early phases of PSGN, suggesting that the deposited NAPlr can entrap and maintain plasmin in the active form inducing glomerular damage (Yoshizawa et al., 2004). Further studies showed that glomerular plasmin activity was absent or weak in normal controls and in patients with rapidly progressive glomerulonephritis, while it was prominent in patients with PSGN and positive glomerular NAPlr, suggesting that NAPlr upregulates the glomerular plasmin activity (Oda et al., 2012). Cationic NAPlr and SPEB can facilitate immune-complex deposition and inflammation, as both antigens have been identified in the mesangium of biopsies of PSGN (Oda et al., 2010).

The immune-complex deposition in the glomeruli activates the complement cascade.

A prominent role of the alternative complement pathway has been suggested by numerous observations, but as mentioned earlier, in some patients the lectin pathway is activated as well (Hisano et al., 2007). Sethi and colleagues (2013) have advanced the notion that patients with pathologic features strongly suggesting PIGN who pursue a course of persisting haematuria and progress to advanced CKD (even in the absence of a symptomatic preceding streptococcal or other infection) designated as '*atypical PIGN*' frequently have disordered regulation of the alternative complement pathway. They studied 11 patients meeting their definition of atypical PIGN and ten had auto-antibodies to complement proteins or mutations in complement genes, including *C3Nef, CfH,* or *CfHR5* mutations. These abnormalities may have contributed to the persistence of disease and its progression in these cases. They resemble closely the cases described as C3GN; see also Chapter 8), indicating that the line drawn between PIGN and C3GN is a blurry one.

Aetiology

Based on a bulk of clinical and laboratory evidence accumulated during the last decades it has been ascertained that both specific nephritogenic strains of streptococci and a specific immune response by the host are required for the development of acute PSGN. Group A streptococci nephritogenic strains M types 1, 2, 4, and 12 are involved in upper respiratory tract infections, while M type 25, 45, 47, 49, 55, and 57 are involved in the skin infections (Rodriguez-Iturbe and Parra, 2001). The high diversity of group A streptococcus strains during outbreaks of PSGN can be seen not only in different countries, but also in the same country (Williamson et al., 2016). Rarely, also non-group A streptococci may be involved in the pathogenesis of glomerulonephritis. However, only a minority of patients infected with a nephritogenic streptococcal strains develop overt disease. The possibility of a genetic predisposition may be suggested by a higher incidence of HLA-DRB1*03011 in patients with PSGN (Ahn and Ingulli, 2008) and by prospective family studies showing the development of PSGN in 38 per cent of the siblings in cases of sporadic disease (Rodriguez-Iturbe et al., 1981). Due to the limited numbers of nephritogenic subtypes of streptococci, and long-lasting acquired immunity to these organisms, the development of repeated episodes of typical PSGN is uncommon. Patients with repeated bouts of 'nephritis' almost certainly have underlying IgA N or C3GN, rather than typical PSGN. The co-existence of PSGN and post-streptococcal acute rheumatic fever is also quite uncommon as the nephritogenic and rheumatogenic stains of β-haemolytic streptococci do not overlap.

Clinical presentation and features

The typical PSGN is generally preceded by infection of nephritogenic group A β- haemolytic streptococci in throat or skin. Exceptionally, the disease may occur following circumcision or spider bites. Throat streptococcal infection may be characterized either by pharyngitis alone or by a more severe disease with fever, cervical lymphadenopathy, and tonsillar exudate. Scarlet fever may be recognized by the rash due to an erythrogenic toxin which blanches on pressure which is more intense along antecubital fossae and axillae and is accompanied by enanthema consisting of punctuate erythema and petechiae on the soft palate. Streptococcal impetigo is characterized by grouped small vesicles, localized in exposed areas generally associated with regional lymphadenopathy. Vesicles cause intense itching, rapidly break, and become covered with thick crusts and heal without scarring.

After a latent period of one to two weeks for upper respiratory tract infection and three to six weeks for skin infection, the symptoms and signs of glomerulonephritis develop. During the latent period, one-third of patients develop microscopic haematuria.

Glomerulonephritis may present in a subclinical form or in an acute form. The subclinical forms are more frequent, exceeding the symptomatic cases four- or fivefold. Subclinical disease manifests solely with microscopic (non-visible) haematuria and a reduction of serum complement (C3, but not C4), sometimes associated with an increase in blood pressure. If a renal biopsy is performed endocapillary proliferation is present by light microscopy as a 'pattern of injury' but this is not a diagnostic feature as it can also occur in C3 glomerulopathy (see Chapter 8).

The typical clinical presentation of the acute forms is a nephritic syndrome without significant differences in the mode of presentation between sporadic and epidemic forms. Acute nephritic syndrome is characterized by the abrupt onset of transient oliguria, proteinuria (sometimes in a nephrotic range), haematuria (visible or non-visible), peripheral oedema, and hypertension. The typology of clinical presentation may vary with the age of the patient. Oedema of the face is sudden and very frequent, being present in >50 per cent of patients; in some cases, oedema involves the legs and sacrum. Anasarca, including ascites, is more common among young children. Transient oliguria of one to two weeks duration is described in about 50 per cent of patients, but anuria is rare. Hypertension occurs in 80 per cent of children (Dagan et al., 2016) and is also frequent in adults and elderly (Rodriguez-Iturbe and Haas, 2016). It is more severe in adults and in the elderly but not all patients require drug treatment. Hypertensive encephalopathy is a rare complication which may be associated with grand mal seizures. Congestive heart failure due to fluid volume expansion is the presenting symptoms in some patients, being much more frequent in older patients. Rare cases of posterior leukoencephalopathy (Ahn and Ingulli, 2008; Gupta et al., 2010) and autoimmune haemolytic anaemia (Cachat et al., 2003) have also been reported in patients with PSGN. Oliguria and fluid retention are partly due to decreased GFR resulting from the inflammatory glomerular reaction that progressively reduces the area of the glomerular capillaries. Renal blood flow is normal or reduced less than GFR and as a consequence the filtration fraction is depressed. The reduced GFR is not the only factor responsible for the sodium retention observed in these patients, as severe sodium retention can occur even in presence of mild reduction of GFR, probably as a consequence of an increased salt and water distal tubular reabsorption. In the acute phase of PSGN, sodium retention persists in spite of increased plasma levels of atrial natriuretic peptide, suggesting an impaired response of the kidney to this peptide (Ozdemir et al., 1992). Salt and water retention often results in dilutional anaemia, hypertension, and congestive heart failure (Glassock, 1988). The increased plasma levels of endothelin may also contribute to arterial hypertension and to the lack of response to atrial natriuretic peptide (Ozdemir et al., 1992). Plasma renin activity is severely depressed during acute episodes. Significant hyperkalaemia and mild metabolic acidosis is common early in the clinical presentation.

Haematuria is a constant finding in acute GN being macroscopic (visible) in one-third of the patients and microscopic (non-visible) in the remaining patients. Macroscopic haematuria rapidly disappears with the increase in the urine output, while dysmorphic microscopic haematuria usually persists longer. In addition to red blood cells, the urinary sediment is characterized by the presence of leukocytes (polymorphonuclear in the acute phases, mononuclear in the resolving phases), tubular cells, and granular, erythrocyte, and leukocyte casts.

Mild proteinuria is frequent but nephrotic syndrome (NS) is rare in children, being present only in around 4 per cent of cases, while NS is found in around 20 per cent of cases in adults and the elderly. Constitutional symptoms, including anorexia, malaise, nausea, vomiting, and bilateral loin pain, are common at presentation.

Overall, compared to children, the clinical presentation is more severe in adults, especially in in the elderly adult (Table 9.2). Dyspnoea, congestive heart failure, oliguria, marked proteinuria, and renal insufficiency are more frequent in adults and in older patients than in children. Rarely, the dominant picture

Table 9.2 Clinical presentation of acute post-streptococcal glomerulonephritis (PSGN).

	Children (Potter et al., 1982; Clark et al., 1988)	Adults (Baldwin., 1977)	Elderly (Melby et al., 1987; Washio et al., 1995)
Haematuria	97–100%	86%	100%
Macroscopic haematuria	30%	NA	NA
Proteinuria	47–80%	56–99%	92%
NS	4%	20–32%	20%
Renal failure	25–40%	38–51%	72–83%
Hypertension	50–60%	63–89%	81–86%
Cardiac failure	<5%	46%	43%

is that of rapidly progressive renal insufficiency. These cases are generally associated with diffuse crescents. Rapid progression to end-stage renal disease (ESRD) occurs in <0.5 per cent of the sporadic forms and is even rarer in the epidemic forms of PSGN.

During the first two weeks of active disease, C3 and total haemolytic complement levels are significantly depressed in >90 per cent of patients; C4 and C2 levels are usually normal or only mildly depressed. Marked reduction of C4 suggests an alternative diagnosis, e.g. systemic lupus erythematosus (SLE) or cryoglobulinaemic vasculitis. A role for the membrane attack complex (C5b–C9) in the pathogenesis of the disease has also been suggested (Matsell et al., 1994). In these patients, serum complement levels normalize within four weeks; however, occasionally it may take several months for this to occur. Failure of the C3 level to return to normal by eight weeks suggests atypical PSGN, C3GN, or dense deposit disease (DDD). In these cases, renal biopsy should be undertaken because of the therapeutic and prognostic implications.

The initial level of serum complement has no prognostic value. Rheumatoid factor is demonstrated in about one-third of patients and most patients show a low level of polyclonal cryoglobulinemia (Type III, composed of polyclonal IgG and IgM) in the acute phases of the disease. Hypergammaglobulinemia is present in about 90 per cent of patients. Anaemia is frequent in the early phases of the disease, due to dilutional phenomenon. Rarely, a haemolytic anaemia is present, suggesting atypical haemolytic-uraemia syndrome (aHUS; Izumi et al., 2005; Kakajiwala et al., 2016), but some (or even all) of these cases may represent the co-existence of aHUS and C3GN, rather than PSGN (see also Chapter 8).

Cultures for streptococcus in patients with PSGN are frequently positive in epidemic forms (around 70 per cent), while in sporadic forms they are positive only in 25 per cent of patients. Increasing titre of one or more antistreptococcal serum antibodies suggest recent infection. Antistreptolysin O titres are more frequently elevated in throat infection than in skin infection. Parra and colleagues (1998) found elevated antistreptolysin O titres only in one-third of patients with skin infections, while anti-DNAase titres were elevated in around 70 per cent. Antibody titres increase during the first week of infection and reach the peak at one month, then progressively decline over many months. Patients who are treated with antibiotics early in the course of infections or elderly patients may not have significant rise in antibodies titres, but the course of disease is not greatly modified.

Epidemiology

Acute PSGN most commonly affects children and young adults. The peak incidence is in the first decade of life; however, the disease may also occur in adults, including the elderly. Males are affected more commonly than females, the ratio often being 2:1. Pharyngitis and tonsillitis are more frequent in spring and in winter in temperate climates, while impetigo is more frequent in summer and in tropical areas.

As already described, the disease may present in epidemic or in sporadic forms. Many decades ago, a number of epidemic cases of acute PSGN were documented worldwide. During the recent decades epidemic PSGN is becoming rare in developed countries but continues to be reported from underdeveloped countries and cases tend to occur in closed communities with poor hygienic conditions (Rodriguez-Iturbe and Haas, 2016). The epidemics tend to be cyclic in certain areas with low socio-economic status or crowded living conditions, e.g. the Red Lake, Minnesota, Port of Spain, Trinidad, India, and Venezuela epidemics. The most recent epidemics have been described in Nova Serrana in Brazil, following the ingestion of unpasteurized cheese infected with *Streptococcus zooepidemicus* from bovine mastitis (Balter et al., 2000) and in the Northern territory of Australia (Marshall et al., 2011).

The incidence of the sporadic forms of PSGN is also decreasing in developed countries (Simon et al., 1994; Roy et al., 1990; Ilyas and Tolymat, 2008). Today, the global burden of severe group A streptococcal disease is concentrated largely in developing tropical countries and indigenous populations, e.g. Aboriginal Australians (Steer et al., 2007; Hoy et al., 2012; Chaturvedi et al., 2018).

Natural history and prognosis

The short- and long-term prognosis is excellent for patients with subclinical forms of PSGN. For patients presenting with an acute nephritic syndrome, the short-term prognosis is generally favourable in children. Less than 1 per cent of children die of complications of renal failure. The risk of death has also decreased in recent years in developed countries. However, the prognosis may be less favourable in underdeveloped areas, where death can occur mostly in children, adolescents, and young adults, particularly pregnant women (Hoy et al., 2012; Gunasekaran et al., 2015; Ramnathan et al., 2017). This makes urgent the realization of a group A streptococcus vaccine in epidemic regions (Ecxler and Kim, 2016).

More uncertain are the long-term outcomes. Excellent prognosis was reported in the earliest studies, but the patient follow-up was too short to draw firm conclusions. Specifically, most studies with long-term follow-up showed that the majority of children and adults with the *epidemic* form of PSGN had an excellent prognosis, with the development of ESRD in far less than 0.5 per cent (Nissenson et al., 1979; Pinto et al., 2015; VanDeVoorde, 2015). Persisting hypertension can occur uncommonly, especially in adults, and renal abnormalities can persist for many months, or even years, in 2 to 5 per cent of patients (Potter et al., 1982). Ten years after an acute episode of *epidemic* glomerulonephritis, hypertension was diagnosed in 45 per cent of 60 patients vs. 21 per cent of 48 community controls (Pinto et al., 2015).

More controversial are the results in the *sporadic* forms (Baldwin, 1977; Kasahara et al., 2001). The early literature on this subject (pre-1968) is confounded by the fact that some case of 'clinically apparent' PSGN may have actually been examples of an acute exacerbation of an unrecognized IgA nephropathy or C3 glomerulopathy (see also Chapter 7 and Chapter 8). Persistence of reduced GFR, abnormal proteinuria, and/or haematuria is more common in the sporadic forms. Thus, these cases may not have been PSGN but rather a disease that can closely mimic PSGN, such as IgA nephropathy or C3GN (see Chapter 7_and Chapter 8). There is agreement that patients with NS at presentation (Sorger et al., 1987), those with crescentic glomerulonephritis, and those with acute renal failure at presentation have a worse prognosis (Nissenson et al., 1979; Askenazi et al., 2006; Gunasekaran et al., 2015).

In addition, the prognosis is less favourable for adults than children, both for epidemic and sporadic forms. As discussed, the percentage of patients with persisting urinary abnormalities was higher for adults than for children in the Venezuelan epidemic outbreak (Garcia et al., 1981). Vogl and colleagues (1986) reported a complete recovery only in 59 per cent of adults with PSGN after a mean follow-up of 4.8 years. Whether these cases were true PSGN and not some other disease cannot be determined. The prognosis also may be less favourable in indigenous populations, such as Australian Aborigines (Hoy et al., 2012). Studies that depend solely on clinical diagnosis of PSGN not confirmed by renal biopsy can be misleading, as other diseases (such as IgAN or C3 glomerulopathy) can closely initially resemble PSGN (see Chapter 7 and Chapter 8).

Specific treatment

In patients with subclinical PSGN, no specific or symptomatic treatment is required, but patients should be advised to follow a moderate salt restriction and their blood pressure and body weight should be checked regularly.

In patients with symptomatic acute nephritic syndrome, bed rest is usually prescribed, although there is no evidence that it is necessary, with the exception of patients with congestive heart failure or severe hypertension with encephalopathy. Restriction of water and salt intake is recommended to prevent oedema, hypertension, and congestive heart failure. Even more efficacious are loop diuretics that may easily reverse oliguria in the early phases of the disease. Although hypertension is generally attributed to sodium and water retention, diuretics alone may be insufficient to control hypertension and it is advisable to administer antihypertensive agents. Good results have been reported with ACE inhibitors, which should be used with caution in patients with hyperkalaemia. In case of an emergency, oral nifedipine (0.25–0.5 mg/kg) or intravenous (IV) labetalol (0.2–1 mg/kg) may be administered and repeated if necessary to control hypertensive spikes.

Antibiotics are usually prescribed to eliminate the infecting organism, if present. In 2016, van Driel and colleagues reported that there were no clinically relevant differences in symptom resolution when comparing cephalosporins and macrolides with penicillin in the treatment of group A β-haemolytic streptococcal tonsillopharyngitis. Limited evidence in adults suggests cephalosporins are more effective than penicillin for relapse. Limited evidence in children suggests carbapenem is more effective than penicillin for symptom resolution. Based on these results, and considering the low cost and absence of resistance, penicillin can still be regarded as a first-choice treatment for both adults and children. These measures can resolve the streptococcal infection, but are of little help for reversing the glomerulonephritis, as the glomerular lesions are already established. Antimicrobial therapy is indicated primarily to prevent the spread of the nephritogenic streptococcus among close contacts. Prophylactic antimicrobials are not indicated in long-term management of PSGN.

Glucocorticoids and/or immunosuppressive agents are not indicated in the typical cases of acute PSGN. These drugs have been used with apparent success in a few rare cases with extensive glomerular crescents and rapidly progressive glomerulonephritis which may have a more severe prognosis. However, the evidence for their efficacy is very weak. While a few anecdotal reports (Vijayakumar, 2002; Raff et al., 2005; Baikunje et al., 2016) supported a potential benefit of glucocorticoids in crescentic PSGN, in a small randomized trial conducted in children with crescentic PSGN, treatment with prednisone, azathioprine, cyclophosphamide, dipyridamole, and anticoagulants did not offer advantages over supportive therapy (Roy et al., 1981).

Other infection-related glomerulonephritis

The frequency of typical PSGN in children and adults is progressively declining, at least in developed countries. However, other sporadic infection-related (often Staphyloccocal infections) glomerulonephritides are increasing, particularly in adults and in the elderly (Moroni et al., 2002; Nasr et al., 2011; Stratta et al., 2014).

Pathology

Renal biopsy shows a wide variety of findings including endocapillary proliferative, necrotizing crescentic and membranoproliferative glomerular lesions, and interstitial inflammations. By immunofluorescence microscopy, IgG and C3 are deposited and IgA is dominant or co-dominant with the IgG deposits in a number of cases (Satoskar et al., 2017). This infection-related nephritis is most common in diabetic subjects (Satoskar et al., 2017). On electron microscopy, mesangial, subendothelial, and subepithelial dense deposits with a hump-shaped appearance are present in almost all patients with IgA-dominant or co-dominant infection-related GN (Haas et al., 2008).

Pathogenesis

The pathogenetic mechanisms underlying non-PSGN infection-related glomerulonephritides have not been thoroughly investigated, but an immune-complex mechanism seems most likely. In infection-related GN with dominant or co-dominant deposition of IgA in glomeruli, a staphylococcal organism is commonly implicated (Satoskar et al., 2006; Satoskar et al., 2017; Worawichawong et al., 2011). Arakawa and colleagues (2006) found elevated titres of serum IgA against *S. aureus* cell membrane antigen and hypothesized that staphylococcal enterotoxin could act as a super-antigen triggering glomerulonephritis. A super-antigen can bind on antigen-presenting cells and then may interact with T-cells causing massive T-cell activation and production of large amounts of cytokines, including those with IgA class-switching functions (Koyama et al., 1995). In diabetic patients, the pathogenesis may be also related to increased serum levels of IgA and circulating immune complexes containing IgA as a consequence of subclinical mucosal infections (Eguchi et al., 1995).

Aetiology

Non-streptococcal bacterial infections, such as deep-seated staphylococcal and Gram-negative infections (cutaneous and visceral), and viral or protozoal infections (e.g. HIV, HCV, HBV, cytomegalovirus, malaria) and atypical sites of bacterial infections (pneumonia, endocarditis, osteomyelitis, urinary tract infections, phlebitis, deep-seated abscess) characterize these forms of infection-related glomerulonephritis. Commonly, these cases are secondary to an ongoing methicillin-resistant or sensitive staphylococcal skin or visceral infection (Satoskar et al., 2006; Nasr et al., 2007) and the nephritis is superimposed upon diabetic glomerulosclerosis. Hypocomplementaemia is also common (30–50 per cent) and simultaneous anti-neutrophil cytoplasmic antibody (ANCA) can be found (Satoskar et al., 2017).

Clinical presentation

Many patients with these disorders are immunocompromised with a background of alcoholism and drug addiction, or with underlying diseases such as malignancies, diabetes, or liver cirrhosis. Often the clinical presentation is not confined to the kidneys (multi-organ disease is common); thus, they are not renal limited, and the infection is ongoing. In addition, the clinical features are often more severe than in PSGN, with a high frequency of acute kidney injury (AKI), progressive CKD, and NS (Moroni et al., 2002; El-Husseini et al., 2005; Nasr et al., 2013; Natarajan et al., 2014).

Because a variety of infections can trigger an exacerbation an underlying unrecognized primary IgA nephropathy, it is often difficult to conclude if the disease is *de novo* or merely a manifestation of a latent (subclinical or lanthanic) form of IgA nephropathy triggered to display a clinically expressed disease. Features that favour IgA-dominant or co-dominant infection related over primary IgA nephropathy include presentation in older age or in a diabetic patient, AKI, documented staphylococcal infection, hypocomplementaemia, diffuse glomerular endocapillary hypercellularity with prominent neutrophil infiltration on light microscopy, stronger immunofluorescence staining for C3 than IgA, and the presence of subepithelial humps on electron microscopy (Nasr and D'Agati, 2011).

Natural history and outcome

The outcomes of IgA-dominant infection-related GN are much poorer than seen in typical PSGN. For example, the outcome reported by Nasr and colleagues (2008) in 52 patients (with IgA-dominant or co-dominant lesions) after a mean follow-up of 25 months was very poor, with 56 per cent of patients having various degrees of CKD at the last follow-up. Of the eleven patients with diabetes included in that study, all had impaired renal function at presentation. None of them recovered renal function and nine progressed to ESRD. Eighteen out of 41 patients (44 per cent) without diabetes had persistent renal dysfunction, and seven of them progressed to ESRD. The other eighteen patients were not included in the analysis because they had a follow-up <3 months; eight of them had persistent renal dysfunction, the other six were dialysis dependent, and 12 per cent died. The only significant predictor of ESRD on multivariate testing was an elevated serum creatinine at diagnosis. These data suggest that IgA-dominant or co-dominant infection-related GN should be considered a serious disease in adults, particularly in those with an immunocompromised background (such as diabetes). Cases of fatal pulmonary-renal syndrome can also occur in IgA dominant or co-dominant infection related glomerulonephritis (Saad et al., 2015). In cases not associated with IgA deposition, the prognosis depends on the age and comorbidity. In older patients with diabetes or malignancy, the prognosis is obviously poor. In a series, only 25 per cent of these patients recovered full renal function (Nasr et al., 2010).

Specific treatment

The supportive therapy in all forms of infection-related GN is similar to that described for PSGN and should be started early, particularly in immunocompromised patients. Detection and control of infection is vital and should be initiated as soon as possible.

The results reported with glucocorticoid therapy of non-PSGN infection-related GN are difficult to evaluate. Anecdotal cases of good response to IV high-dose steroids in patients with a high percentage of crescents have been reported. In a series, no significant differences in the remissions were seen between patients treated with glucocorticoids (44 per cent) and those given only symptomatic treatment (70 per cent); however, only patients with more severe disease received steroid therapy (Moroni et al., 2002). Nasr and colleagues (2008) treated 17 patients with IgA-dominant infection-related GN with glucocorticoids. The main indication for steroid therapy was impaired renal function with or without concomitant crescentic disease. Among treated patients, twelve of seventeen (70 per cent) had complete remission, 18 per cent persistent renal dysfunction, and 12 per cent progressed to ESRD. Among the other 23 patients who did not receive glucocorticoids, ten (43 per cent) entered complete remission. In another series of nine adults with acute glomerulonephritis and crescents, five patients received glucocorticoid treatment and had excellent responses; among the four patients not treated with steroids, two had significant kidney function impairment (Baikunje et al., 2016). Whether this marginal benefit is worth the risk, especially in the presence of diabetes, is very uncertain. No controlled trials of treatment have ever been reported. In the exceptional cases of acute crescentic glomerulonephritis associated with life-endangering pulmonary haemorrhage, the use of methylprednisolone (MP) pulses associated with plasmapheresis might be indicated (Koizumi et al., 2015). Parikh and colleagues (2017) have recently summarized the available data on treatment of both PSGN and non-PSGN infection-related nephritis. In their view, immunosuppression of any kind should be avoided in both conditions. Treatment of staphylococcal-associated glomerulonephritis (SAGN) with concomitant immunosuppression can be lethal (see Table 9.3).

Practical recommendations

Whether a patient with a suspected PSGN or another infection-related GN should be hospitalized or followed as an outpatient depends on the severity of the disease. Asymptomatic patients do not need hospitalization. Renal biopsy may be needed in case of persistence of microscopic haematuria, progressive renal failure, or development of heavy (nephrotic-range) proteinuria or uncertainties regarding the correct diagnosis, including the possibility of a drug-associated hypersensitivity interstitial nephritis. In the case of children with oedema, proteinuria, and hypertension, hospitalization is needed when there is a poor response to diuretics and/or antihypertensive agents, the risk of hypertensive encephalopathy being higher in these patients. Adults with acute nephritic syndrome should be hospitalized, particularly if NS and/or renal failure are present, due to the high risk of congestive heart failure.

The diagnostic evaluation includes tests needed to determine the cause of the acute nephritic syndrome (Box 9.1). The diagnosis of acute PSGN is usually easy. However, if the aetiological micro-organism is not identified it may be difficult to recognize at the beginning whether it is a typical PSGN or an atypical form of a non-PSGN infection-related GN. Moreover, a large number of other primary or secondary glomerular diseases may present with similar signs and symptoms. Acute GN and hypocomplementaemia may be seen in many systemic diseases, such a SLE and cryoglobulinemia or bacterial endocarditis. The more frequent diseases that may be included in the differential diagnosis

Table 9.3 Outcomes for staphylococcus-associated glomerulonephritis (SAGN) treated with immunosuppression.

Study	N	Pathogenic organisms	Immunosuppression regimen	Renal recovery rate (%)	CKD rate (%)	ESRD (%)	Mortality (%)
Nasr et al., 2011	22	Staph species only (46%; 50/109 patients had SAGN).	Corticosteroids only variable duration.	13.6	54.5	31.8	18.2
Montseny et al., 1995	17	17% of cases due to staphylococcal species.	Corticosteroids ± cyclophosphamide.	29	47	12	12
Nasr et al., 2008	17	24.4% of cases due to staphylococcal species.	Corticosteroids.	70	18	12	0
Boils et al., 2015	14	53% of cases due to staph species.	Corticosteroids ± cyclophosphamide.	28.6	42.9	7.1	23.5
Nagaba et al., 2012	2	MRSA* infection only; 8 patients followed and 2 received immunosuppression.	Corticosteroids.	N/A	N/A	N/A	100**
Satoskar et al., 2013	4	Staph species only; 8 patients followed and 4 received immunosuppression.	Corticosteroids.	0	100	25	0

*MRSA = methicillin resistant staphylococcus aureus

**Both patients died from sepsis.

Source: Data from Parikh SV, Alvarado AS, Hebert LA. (2017). The management of bacterial infection-associated glomerulonephritis. In AA Satoskar, T Nadasdy (eds), *Bacterial Infections of the Kidney*, pp 117–32. Springer International Publishing, New York.

Box 9.1 Diagnostic laboratory work-up for patients with acute nephritic syndrome

- Serum creatinine.
- Complete blood count with differential and platelet count.
- Urinalysis with urine sediment examination.
- Measurement of daily proteinuria (urine protein/creatinine ratio [UPCR] employing an intended 24-hour urine specimen (not a 'spot' UPCR).
- Anti-streptolysin O titre; anti-DNAase antibody.
- Culture of throat and skin lesions.
- Blood culture (if endocarditis or sepsis is suspected).
- Serum complement (C3 and C4) levels.
- Antinuclear antibodies.
- ANCA (anti-MPO and anti-PR3) and anti-GBM
- Plasma D-dimer assay (to screen for a hypercoagulable state).
- Serum rheumatoid factor.
- Serum free kappa and lambda light chain (in older adults).

are IgA nephropathy, lupus nephritis, C3GN, and cryoglobulinaemic vasculitis (with or without hepatitis C viral infection). IgA nephropathy is clinically characterized by haematuria, sometimes associated with arterial hypertension and some degree of renal dysfunction, but the C3 levels are most often normal. Some patients may have episodes of macroscopic haematuria often associated with throat or respiratory infection. The differential diagnosis may be difficult if haematuria occurs for the first time in a patient who is not known to be a carrier of IgA nephropathy.

Laboratory findings may orientate the diagnosis, as hypocomplementaemia suggests PSGN or IgA-dominant or co-dominant infection-related GN. However, these parameters may be normal in either disease, particularly in patients with PSGN presenting late in the course of the disease, after C3 levels have returned to normal. Lupus nephritis, C3 glomerulonephritis, DDD, and cryoglobulinaemic vasculitis and infective endocarditis or 'shunt' nephritis can also present with an acute nephritic syndrome associated with hypocomplementaemia. However, patients with SLE may have a constellation of extrarenal symptoms and biological markers that make the diagnosis easier in typical cases. More difficult may be the clinical diagnosis for patients with C3GN and DDD. NS is more frequent in these patients but some of them may have only moderate proteinuria. On the other hand, NS may occur also in in non-PSGN due to infection-related GN, particularly in adults. Cryoglobulinaemic patients are often carriers of hepatitis C virus. Although some patients with PSGN may also show circulating cryoglobulins, the amount of cryoglobulins and the levels of 'cryocrit' are usually more elevated in patients with cryoglobulinaemic GN and the cryoglobulins are typically of the mixed IgG/IgM variety (Type II cryoimmunoglobulins). Finally, the differential diagnosis with a rapidly progressive GN can be difficult on clinical grounds alone, particularly for those patients with PSGN or infection-related GN showing renal function deterioration. The determination of ANCA may help the differential diagnosis in a number of cases (see also Chapter 10). Viral forms of infection-related GN, such as parvovirus, may resemble lupus nephritis, including hypocomplementaemia.

Since most of the diseases producing the acute nephritic syndrome, infection-related or not, may be difficult to recognize at the beginning, the nephrologist has to choose between two options:

i. to perform a renal biopsy with light, immunofluorescence, and electron microscopy, to identify the underlying kidney disease; or

ii. to wait and see what is the short-term outcome (spontaneous remission or persisting disease).

The first option includes a minimal risk of biopsy-related complications, but offers the advantage of a prompt diagnosis and of prompt specific therapeutic intervention. Moreover, the result of renal biopsy may also give prognostic information. The second option is less expensive and avoids the possible complication caused by the biopsy. However, in case of wrong diagnosis it exposes the patient to the risks of a delayed diagnosis and specific treatment (if any). Although any single decision should be taken on the basis of a patient's history, clinical characteristics, and pertinent laboratory investigations (such as serology and complement levels), we are in favour of renal biopsy in case of a suspected symptomatic non-PSGN form of infection-related GN in adults, while in young children we prefer to wait for a few days before taking a decision, unless the patient presents with nephrotic proteinuria or renal dysfunction. Renal biopsy is not needed in typical PSGN, unless atypical features supervene during follow-up, such as persisting hypocomplementaemia.

Treatment remains mostly conservative (Table 9.4). An early and aggressive symptomatic treatment is of paramount importance in severe cases to prevent life-threatening complications such as congestive heart failure, hypertensive

Table 9.4 Practical recommendations for non-PSGN infection-related GN.

Hospitalization:	In children it is recommended only for cases with loop-diuretic-resistant oliguria or NS. Hospitalization is always recommended for adult and elderly patients.
Renal biopsy:	It is usually avoided in children with epidemic forms of typical PSGN and in those with sporadic forms without NS or signs of acute renal failure. It is recommended in children with persisting NS and/or renal dysfunction. Renal biopsy is recommended in many adult and elderly patients with PSGN. It is mandatory in adults with non-PSGN infection-related GN.
Conservative treatment:	An adequate course of appropriate antimicrobial agents is recommended, particularly in cases of non-PSGN Infection related GN, which are often caused by strains of *S. aureus* or by visceral infections. Water, sodium, and potassium restriction, and loop-diuretics should be administered if oedema or congestive heart failure is present, and antihypertensive agents should be added to manage arterial hypertension (caution with ACEi/ARB in case of hyperkalaemia). Hypertensive emergencies should be treated with IV nifedipine, labetalol, diazoxide, or nitroprusside.
Glucocorticoids:	Immunosuppression is not indicated. Evidence of benefit is very equivocal and the potential for harm (death form sepsis) is unequivocal. See text.

encephalopathy, and hyperkalaemia. Apart from the restriction of water, sodium, and potassium, the generous use of loop diuretics should be encouraged. In treating hypertension, the choice of the antihypertensive agent depends on the clinical conditions of the patient. ACE inhibitors and angiotensin-receptor blockers (ARBs) may be contraindicated in case of hyperkalaemia, while in the presence of congestive heart failure the use of the old non-selective β-blockers should be replaced by selective β-blockers or mixed α1–β adrenergic antagonists, possibly in association with ACE inhibitors or ARBs if there is not concomitant hyperkalaemia. Calcium-channel antagonists are particularly effective in case of severe hypertension. It is recommended to strictly monitor the blood pressure, particularly in oedematous children who are more susceptible to hypertensive encephalopathy. Calcium-channel blockers, IV labetalol, diazoxide, or nitroprusside should be immediately administered if this complication develops. Potassium binding resins or polymers should be given in oliguric patients with serum potassium levels ≥6 mEq/l.

There is no substantial body of evidence that glucocorticoids are useful in non-PSGN infection-related GN. Theoretically, these agents may reduce inflammation and accelerate the recovery of the acute NS, but we do not recommend their use in children with typical PSGN, as the syndrome spontaneously recovers in a few days. In adults with extensive extracapillary proliferation (crescents), high-dose glucocorticoids might be considered (see also Chapter 10); if an active infection is still present, such treatment would be an *unacceptable* risk. Finally, we recommend that all patients, particularly adults, are monitored regularly in the long-term to evaluate whether the disease may result in progressive impairment of kidney function. This is particularly true in those cases with initial hypocomplementaemia that does not resolve within eight weeks from the clinical onset of disease.

Infection-related glomerulonephritis and transplantation

To the best of our knowledge, only 11 cases of *de novo* infection-related acute GN have been reported in renal transplant recipients (Moroni et al., 2004; Plumb et al., 2006). In contrast with the typical PSGN, the location of the infection was variable, ranging from skin abscess to mycotic aortic aneurysm. The aetiological infections identified were mainly *staphylococcus*, but *E. coli* and *streptococci* were also identified in a few patients. The clinical presentation was an acute decline of graft function in all but one patient. The acute renal dysfunction resolved in most patients, but in the long term, three patients lost graft function and one died. It is difficult to ascertain whether progression was due to chronic allograft nephropathy, to glomerulonephritis, or both. Five patients were treated with MP pulse therapy and two of them eventually progressed to ESRD. Six patients did not receive glucocorticoids, and of these, one died and another one developed ESRD.

It may be concluded that infection-related glomerulonephritis is a possible, although uncommon, complication in renal transplant recipients. It has an unusual presentation and may have a poor outcome in the long term. The role of therapy is still undefined.

References

Ahn SY, Ingulli E. (2008). Acute poststreptococcal glomerulonephritis: An update. Curr Opin Pediatr. **20**: 157–62.

Arakawa Y, Shumizu Y, Sakurai H, et al. (2006). Polyclonal activation of IgA against *Staphylococcus aureus* cell membrane antigen in post-methicillin-resistant *S. aureus* infection glomerulonephritis. Nephrol Dial Transplant. **21**: 1448–9.

Askenazi DJ, Feig DI, Graham NM, et al. (2006). 3–5-year longitudinal follow-up of pediatric patients after acute renal failure. Kidney Int. **69**: 184–9.

Baikunje S, Vankalakunti M, Nikith A, et al. (2016). Post-infectious glomerulonephritis with crescents in adults: A retrospective study. Clin Kidney J. **9**: 222–6.

Baldwin DS. (1977). Poststreptococcal glomerulonephritis. A progressive disease? Am J Med. **62**: 1–11.

Balter S, Benin A, Pinto SWL, et al. (2000). Epidemic nephritis in Nova Serrana Brazil. Lancet. **355**: 1776–80.

Batsford SR, Mezzano S, Mihatsch M, et al. (2005). Is nephritogenic antigen in post-streptococcal glomerulonephritis pyrogen exotoxin B (SPE B) or GAPDH? Kidney Int. **68**: 1120–9.

Boils CL, Nasr SH, Walker PD, et al. (2015). Update on endocarditis-associated glomerulonephritis. Kidney Int. **87**: 1241–9.

Cachat F, Dunsmore K, Tufro A. (2003). Concomitant anuric post-streptococcal glomerulonephritis and autoimmune hemolytic anemia. Eur J Pediatr. **162**: 552–3.

Chaturvedi S, Boyd R, Kraus V. (2018). Acute post-streptococcal glomerulonephritis in the Northern territory of Australia: A review of data from 2009 to 2016 and comparison to literature. Am J Trop Med Hyg. **99**: 1643–8.

Clark G, White RHR, Glasgow EF, et al. (1988). Poststreptococcal glomerulonephritis in children: Clinicopathological correlation and long-term prognosis. Pediatr Nephrol. **2**: 381–8.

Couser WG, Johnson RJ. (2014). The etiology of glomerulonephritis. Role of infection and autoimmunity. Kidney Int. **86**: 905–14.

Cu GA, Mezzano S, Bannan JD, et al. (1998). Immunohistochemical and serological evidence for the role of streptococcal proteinase in acute post-streptococcal glomerulonephritis. Kidney Int. **54**: 819–26.

Dagan R, Cleper R, Davidovits M, et al. (2016). Post-infectious glomerulonephritis in pediatric patients over two decades: Severity-associated features. Isr Med Assoc J. **18**: 336–40.

El-Husseini AA, Sheashaa HA, Sabry AA, et al. (2005). Acute postinfectious crescentic glomerulonephritis: clinicopathologic presentation and risk factors. Int Urol Nephrol. **37**: 603–9.

Eguchi EK, Kagame M, Suzuki D, et al. (1995). Significance of high levels of serum IgA and IgA circulating immune complexes (IgA-CIC) in patients with non-insulin-dependent diabetes mellitus. J Diabetes Complications. **9**: 42–8.

Excler JM, Kim JH. (2016). Accelerating the development of a group A streptococcus vaccine: An urgent public health need. Clin Exp Vaccine Res. **5**: 101–7.

Garcia R, Rubio L, Rodriguez-Iturbe B. (1981). Long-term prognosis of epidemic post-streptococcal glomerulonephritis in Maracaibo: Follow-up studies 11–12 years after the acute episode. Clin Nephrol. **15**: 291–8.

Glassock RJ. (1988). Pathophysiology of acute glomerulonephritis. Hosp Pract **23**: 163–8.

Glassock RJ, Alvarado A, Prosek J, et al. (2015). Staphylococcus-related glomerulonephritis and post-streptococcal glomerulonephritis: Why defining 'post' is important in understanding and treating infection-related glomerulonephritis. Am J Kidney Dis. **65**: 826–32.

Gopalakrishnan N, Jeyachandran D, Abeesh P, et al. (2017). Infection-related glomerulonephritis in arenal allograft. Saudi J Kidney Transpl. **28**: 1421–6.

Gunasekaran K, Krishnamurthy S, Mahadevan S, et al. (2015). Clinical characteristics and outcome of post-infectious glomerulonephritis in children in southern India: A prospective study. Indian Pediatr. **82**: 896–903.

Gupta S, Goyal VK, Talukdar B. (2010). Reversible posterior leucoencephalopathy syndrome in post-streptococcal glomerulonephritis. Indian Pediatr. **47**: 274–6.

Haas M, Racusen LC, Bagnasco SM. (2008). IgA-dominant postinfectious glomerulonephritis: A report of 13 cases with common ultrastructural features. Hum Pathol. **39**: 1309–16.

Hisano S, Matsushita M, Fujita T, et al. (2007). Activation of the lectin complement pathway in post-streptococcal acute glomerulonephritis. Pathol Int. **567**: 351–7.

Hoy WE, White AV, Dowling A, et al. (2012). Post-streptococcal glomerulonephritis is a strong risk factor for chronic kidney disease in later life. Kidney Int. **81**: 1026–32.

Ilyas M, Tolaymat A. (2008). Changing epidemiology of acute post-streptococcal glomerulonephritis in Northeast Florida: A comparative study. Pediatr Nephrol. **23**: 101–6.

Iseri K, Iyoda M, Yamamoto Y, et al. (2016). Streptococcal infection-related nephritis (SIRN) manifesting membranoproliferative glomerulonephritis type I. Intern Med. **55**: 647–50.

Izumi T, Hyodo T, Kikuchi T, et al. (2005). An adult with acute post-streptococcal glomerulonephritis complicated by hemolytic uremic syndrome and nephrotic syndrome. Am J Kidney Dis. **46**: e59–63.

Kakajiwala A, Bhatti T, Kaplan BS, et al. (2016). Post-streptococcal glomerulonephritis associated with atypical hemolytic uremic syndrome: To treat or not to treat with eculizumab? Clin Kidney J. **9**: 90–6.

Kasahara T, Hayakawa H, Okabo S, et al. (2001). Prognosis of acute poststreptococcal glomerulonephritis (APSGN) is excellent in children when adequately diagnosed. Pediatr Int. **43**: 364–7.

Kefalides NA, Ohno N, Wilson CB, et al. (1993). Identification of antigenic epitopes in type IV collagen by use of synthetic peptides. Kidney Int. **43**: 94–100.

Koizumi M, Yahata K, Kaneko K, et al. (2015). Post-infectious acute glomerulonephritis with vasculitis and pulmonary hemorrhage. CEN Case Rep. **4**: 65–9.

Koyama A, Kobayashi M, Yamaguchi N, et al. (1995). Glomerulonephritis associated with MRSA infection: A possible role of bacterial superantigen. Kidney Int. **47**: 207–16.

Lange C. (1980). Antigenicity of kidney glomeruli. Evaluation by antistreptococcal cell membrane antisera. Transplant Proc. **12**: 82–7.

Marshall CS, Cheng AC, Markey PG, et al. (2011). Acute post-streptococcal glomerulonephritis in the Northern Territory of Australia: A review of 16 years data and comparison with the literature. Am J Trop Med Hyg. **85**: 703–10.

Matsell DG, Wyatt RJ, Gaber LW. (1994). Terminal complement complexes in acute poststreptococcal glomerulonephritis. Pediatr Nephrol. **8**: 671–6.

Melby PC, Musick WD, Luger AM, et al. (1987). Poststreptococcal glomerulonephritis in the elderly. Report of a case and review of the literature. Am J Nephrol. **7**: 235–40.

Montseny JJ, Meyrier A, Kleinknecht D, et al. (1995). The current spectrum of infectious glomerulonephritis: Experience with 76 patients and review of the literature. Medicine (Baltimore). **74**: 63–73.

Moroni G, Papaccioli D, Banfi G, et al. (2004). Acute post-bacterial glomerulonephritis in renal transplant patients: Description of three cases and review of the literature. Am J Transplant. **4**: 132–6.

Moroni G, Pozzi C, **Quaglini S**, et al. (2002). Long-term prognosis of diffuse proliferative glomerulonephritis associated with infection in adults. Nephrol Dial Transplant. **17**: 1204–11.

Nagaba Y, Hiki Y, Aoyama T, et al. (2012). Effective antibiotic treatment of methicillin-resistant *Staphylococcus aureus*-associated glomerulonephritis. Nephron. **92**: 297–303.

Nasr SH, D'Agati VD. (2011). IgA-dominant postinfectious glomerulonephritis: A new twist on an old disease. Nephron Clin Pract. **119**: c18–25.

Nasr SH, Fidler ME, Valeri AM, et al. (2011). Postinfectious glomerulonephritis in the elderly. J Am Soc Nephrol. **22**: 187–95.

Nasr SH, Markowitz GS, Stokes MB, et al. (2008). Acute postinfectious glomerulonephritis in the modern era. Medicine (Baltimore). **87**: 21–32.

Nasr SH, Radakrishnan J, D'Acati VD. (2013). Bacterial infection-related glomerulonephritis in adults. Kidney Int. **83**: 792–803.

Nasr SH, Share DS, Vargas MT, et al. (2007). Acute post-staphylococcal glomerulonephritis superimposed on diabetic glomerulosclerosis. Kidney Int. **71**: 1317–21.

Natarajan G, Ramanathan S, Jeyachandran D, et al. (2014). Follow-up study of post-infectious glomerulonephritis in adults: Analysis of predictors of poor outcome. Saudi J Kidney Dis Transpl. **25**: 1210–16.

Nissenson AR, Baraff LJ, Fine RN, et al. (1979). Poststreptococcal acute glomerulonephritis: Fact and controversy. Ann Intern Med. **91**: 76–80.

Oda T, Yoshizawa N, Yamakami K, et al. (2007). Significance of glomerular cell apoptosis in the resolution of acute post-streptococcal glomerulonephritis. Nephrol Dial Transplant. **22**: 740–8.

Oda T, Yoshizawa N, Yamakami K, et al. (2010). Localization of nephritis-associated plasmin receptor in acute poststreptococcal glomerulonephritis. Hum Pathol. **41**: 1276–85.

Oda T, Yoshizawa N, Yamakami K, et al. (2012). The role of nephritis-associated plasmin receptor (NAPlr) in glomerulonephritis associated with streptococcal infection. J Biomed Biotechnol. doi: 10.1155/2012/417675

Ozdemir S, Saatci U, Besbas N, et al. (1992). Plasma atrial natriuretic peptide and endothelin levels in acute post-streptococcal glomerulonephritis. Pediatr Nephrol. **6**: 519–22.

Parikh SV, Alvarado AS, Hebert LA. (2017). The management of bacterial infection-associated glomerulonephritis. In **AA Satoskar, T Nadasdy** (eds), *Bacterial Infections of the Kidney*, pp. 117–32. Springer International Publishing, New York.

Parra G, Rodríguez-Iturbe B, Batsford S, et al. (1998). Antibodies to streptococcal zymogen in the serum of patients with acute glomerulonephritis: A multicenter study. Kidney Int. **54**: 509–17.

Pinto SW, Mastroianni-Kirsztajn G, Sesso R. (2015). Ten-year follow-up of patients with epidemic post-infectious glomerulonephritis. PLoS One. **10**: e0125313.

Plumb TJ, Greenberg A, Smith SR, et al. (2006). Postinfectious glomerulonephritis in renal allograft recipients. Transplantation. **82**: 1224–8.

Poon-King R, Bannan J, Viteri A, et al. (1993). Identification of an extracellular plasmin binding protein from nephritogenic streptococci. J Exp Med. **178**: 759–63.

Potter EV, Lipschulz SA, Abidh S, et al. (1982). Twelve to seventeen-year follow-up of patients with poststreptococcal acute glomerulonephritis in Trinidad. N Engl J Med. **307**: 725–9.

Raff A, Hebert T, Pullman J, et al. (2005). Crescentic post-streptococcal glomerulonephritis with nephrotic syndrome in the adult: Is aggressive therapy warranted? Clin Nephrol. **63**: 375–80.

Ramanathan G, Abeyaratne A, Sundaram M, et al. (2017). Analysis of clinical presentation, pathological spectra, treatment and outcomes of biopsy-proven acute postinfectious glomerulonephritis in adult indigenous people of the Northern Territory of Australia. Nephrology (Carlton). **22**: 403–11.

Rodriguez-Iturbe B, Haas M. (2016). Post-streptococcal glomerulonephritis. In JJ Ferretti, DL Stevens, VA Fischetti (eds), *Streptococcus pyogenes: From Clinical Manifestations to Biology* [online]. University of Oklahoma Health Sciences Center, Oklahoma City, OK.

Rodriguez-Iturbe B, Parra G. (2001). Poststreptococcal glomerulonephritis. In S Massry, RJ Glassock (eds), *Textbook of Nephrology*. 4th Edition. pp. 667–72. Lippincott Williams & Wilkins, Philadelphia.

Rodriguez-Iturbe B, Rubio L, Garcia R. (1981). Attack rare of poststreptococcal glomerulonephritis in families. A prospective study. Lancet. **1**: 401–3.

Roy S 3rd, Murphy WM, Arant BS (1981). Post-streptococcal crescentic glomerulonephritis in children: Comparison of quintuple therapy versus supportive care. J Pediatr. **98**: 403–10.

Roy S 3rd, Stapleton FB. (1990). Changing perspectives in children with poststreptococcal acute glomerulonephritis. Pediatr Nephrol. **4**: 585–88.

Saad M, Daoud M, Nasr P, et al. (2015). IgA-dominant post-infectious glomerulonephritis presenting as a fatal pulmonary-renal syndrome. Int J Nephrol Renovasc Dis. **8**: 77–81.

Satoskar AA, Molenda M, Scipio P, et al. (2013). Henoch-Schönlein purpura-like presentation in IgA-dominant Staphylococcus infection-associated glomerulonephritis: A diagnostic pitfall. Clin Nephrol. **79**: 302–12.

Satoskar AA, Nadasdy G, Plaza JA, et al. (2006). Staphylococcus infection-associated glomerulonephritis mimicking IgA nephropathy. Clin J Am Soc Nephrol. **1**: 1179–86.

Satoskar AA, Suleiman S, Ayoub I, et al. (2017). Staphylococcal infection-associated GN: Spectrum of IgA staining and prevalence of ANCA in a single-center cohort. Clin J Am Soc Nephrol. **12**: 39–49.

Sethi S, Fervensza F, Zhang Y, et al. (2013). Atypical post-infectious glomerulonephritis is associated with abnormalities in the alternative pathway of complement. Kidney Int. **83**: 293–9.

Simon P, Ramée MP, Autuly V, et al. (1994). Epidemiology of primary glomerular disease in a French region. Variation according to period and age. Kidney Int. **46**: 1192–8.

Sorger K, Gessler U, Hubner FK, et al. (1982). Subtypes of acute postinfectious glomerulonephritis. Synopsis of clinical and pathological features. Clin Nephrol. **17**: 114–28.

Sorger K, Gessler U, Hubner FK, et al. (1987). Follow-up studies of three subtypes of acute postinfectious glomerulonephritis ascertained by renal biopsy. Clin Nephrol. **27**: 111–24.

Steer AC, Danchin MH, Carapetis JR. (2007). Group A streptococcal infections in children. J Paediatr Child Health. **43**: 203–13.

Stratta P, Musetti C, Barreca A, et al. (2014). New trends of an old disease: The acute postinfectious glomerulonephritis at the beginning of the new millennium. J Nephrol. **27**: 229–39.

VanDeVoorde RG, 3rd. (2015). Acute poststreptococcal glomerulonephritis: The most common acute glomerulonephritis. Pediatr Rev. **36**: 3–12.

van Driel ML, De Sutter AI, Habraken H, et al. (2016). Different antibiotic treatments for group A streptococcal pharyngitis. Cochrane Database Syst Rev. **9**: CD004406.

Vijayakumar M. (2002). Acute and crescentic glomerulonephritis. Indian J Pediatr. **69**: 1071–5.

Vogl W, Renke M, Mayer-Eichberger D, et al. (1986). Long-term prognosis of endocapillary glomerulonephritis of poststreptococcal type in children and adults. Nephron. **44**: 58–65.

Washio M, Katafuchi R, Oh T, et al. (1995). Poststreptococcal glomerulonephritis with the nephrotic range of proteinuria. Int J Nephrol Urol. **27**: 457–64.

Washio M, Oh Y, Okuda S, et al. (1994). Clinicopathological study of poststreptococcal glomerulonephritis in the elderly. Clin Nephrol. **41**: 265–70.

Williamson DA, Smeesters PR, Steer AC, et al. (2016). Comparative M protein analysis of *Streptococcus pyogenes* from pharyngitis and skin infection in New Zealand: Implications for vaccine development. BMC Infect Dis. **16**: 561.

Worawichawong S, Girard L, Trpkov K, et al. (2011). Immunoglobulin A-dominant postinfectious glomerulonephritis: Frequent occurrence in nondiabetic patients with *Staphylococcus aureus* infection. Hum Pathol. **42**: 279–84.

Yoshizawa N, Oshima S, Sagel I, et al. (1992). Role of a streptococcal antigen in the pathogenesis of acute poststreptococcal glomerulonephritis. J Immunol. **148**: 3110–16.

Yoshizawa N, Yamakami K, Fujino M, et al. (2004). Nephritis associate plasmin receptor and acute poststreptococcal glomerulonephritis: Characterization of the antigen and associated immune response. J Am Soc Nephrol. **15**: 1785–93.

Chapter 10

Renal-limited vasculitis (RLV)

Richard J Glassock and Patrick H Nachman

Introduction and overview

Definition

This chapter uses the term renal-limited vasculitis (RLV) to refer to a collection of disorders of widely different aetiology and pathogenesis having in common the development of destructive lesions of the glomerular capillaries, often leading to segmental necrosis of the capillary wall and proliferation of cells within Bowman's space (crescents) in the absence of any multi-system manifestations (Couser, 1988; Glassock et al., 1995; Falk et al., 1998; Pusey and Rees, 1998; Morgan et al., 2006; Lionaki et al., 2007). The resulting accumulation of cells gives rise to a 'crescent' (see ATLAS, PLATE 17) enveloping the glomerular tuft itself. Polymerization of fibrinogen in Bowman's space due to passage of fibrinogen through gaps in the damaged capillary wall, the elaboration of procoagulant factors by infiltrating monocytes, and impaired fibrinolysis all contribute to the pathogenesis of the crescent. Quite often the crescentic lesions are extensive involving a majority of glomeruli. Such patients also frequently manifest rapid and progressive deterioration of renal function leading to the clinical syndrome of *rapidly progressive glomerulonephritis*. Early and aggressive treatment can often delay or prevent the development of end-stage renal disease (ESRD).

Very often such lesions are also the consequence of disorders with multi-system manifestations, such as microscopic polyangiitis (MPA), granulomatosis with polyangiitis (GPA), or anti-GBM disease with alveolar haemorrhage (Goodpasture's Disease), but these clinic-pathologic-entities will be discussed only in passing here as this chapter focuses on the forms of vasculitis that are largely confined to the kidney. Serology is an extremely important tool for classifying RLV and other forms of crescentic and rapidly progressive glomerulonephritis (GN; Cornec et al., 2016). Table 10.1 provides aetiologic and pathogenetic classification of all forms of vasculitis that lead to crescentic GN.

Table 10.1 A classification of crescentic glomerulonephritis [GN]* according to serology (anti-glomerular basement membrane [GBM] antibody and anti-neutrophil cytoplasmic antibody [ANCA]) and immunofluorescence findings in renal biopsies.

Anti-glomerular basement membrane antibody mediated disease (Anti-GBM antibody positive, ANCA negative):	Primary (renal-limited) crescentic glomerulonephritis without pulmonary haemorrhage*
	Goodpastures's disease (with pulmonary haemorrhage)
	Secondary to another systemic disease (e.g. SLE)
	Superimposed on another primary glomerular disease (e.g. membranous nephropathy)
	Secondary to drugs, neoplasia, viruses, renal trauma, environmental exposure (hydrocarbons?)
	De novo in the transplant renal allograft in a patient with X-linked Alport syndrome
Immune complex-mediated disease (anti-GBM antibody negative, ANCA negative or positive):	Primary (renal-limited) glomerular disease with crescents*
	Superimposed on another primary glomerular disease (e.g. IgA nephropathy or membranous nephropathy)
	Multisystem disease (Lupus nephritis, HCV-related cryoglobulinaemia, IgA vasculitis)
	Secondary to infections, neoplasia, drugs, or other
Pauci-immune necrotizing and crescentic glomerulonephritis (ANCA-positive, anti-GBM antibody negative); also known as ANCA-associated crescentic glomerulonephritis:	Primary (renal-limited) glomerular disease with crescents (RLV)*
	Multisystem disease (systemic microscopic polyangiitis [MPA]; granulomatous polyangiitis [GPA; formerly Wegener's granulomatosis])
	Drug-induced (penicillamine, propylthiouracil, allopurinol, hydralazine, minocycline, levamisole, rifampicin)
	Viral- or environmental exposure-related (Parvovirus B19?; silica?)
Dual-antibody disease (anti-GBM antibody positive and ANCA positive):	Primary (renal-limited) disease*
	Multisystem disease, often with alveolar haemorrhage
Idiopathic pauci-immune necrotizing and crescentic glomerulonephritis (Anti-GBM antibody negative and ANCA-negative):	Primary (renal-limited) disease*
	Multisystem disease, sometimes with alveolar haemorrhage

* Forms of crescentic glomerulonephritis that are discussed in this chapter.

Pathology

The fundamental morphologic lesion of RLV is the destruction of the integrity of the glomerular capillary walls accompanied by accumulation of cells in Bowman's space—called crescents (see ATLAS, Plate 17)—believed to be derived from both proliferating and de-differentiated visceral and parietal epithelial cells (Ferrario and Rastaldi, 1998; Ng et al., 1999; Bariety et al., 2003, 2005; Thorner et al., 2008). Ruptures in the integrity of the capillary wall (gaps or focal discontinuities) are common if not universal (Bonsib, 1985). Similar gaps may appear in Bowman's capsule leading to the invasion of Bowman's space by T-cells, macrophages, and myofibroblasts from the adjacent interstitium (Ng et al., 1999). Proliferating podocytes and parietal cells of Bowman's capsule as well as macrophages and infiltration by lymphocytes contribute to the cellularity of the crescent (Lan et al., 1997; Ng et al., 1999; Bariety et al., 2003; Thorner et al., 2008). The accompanying glomerular capillary lesions are most often segmental, necrotizing GN or exudative and proliferative GN. The former is likely a manifestation of a microscopic form of polyangiitis. In the lesions resulting from angiitis (most often ANCA-associated, see below) the glomerular lesions are commonly of differing stage; acute lesions admixed with chronic lesions. Whereas, the glomerular lesions accompanying anti-GBM disease are almost always at the same stage of evolution. Early in the course of RLV the cellular proliferation in the crescent dominates, but later fibrosis ensues leading to glomerular scarring, obliteration and obsolescence. Crescents evolve from cellular, to fibrocellular, to fibrous lesions (Wiggins, 1998). This process may often develop quite rapidly, in a matter of weeks or months, or can develop over a more prolonged period. Various degrees of interstitial inflammation, particularly in a periglomerular location (associated with focal discontinuities of Bowman's capsule) may be seen. Extraglomerular vasculitis is relatively un-common, but can be observed. Granulomatous vasculitis is seldom seen in renal biopsies in RLV.

The underlying pathogenetic mechanisms responsible for RLV are a major determinant of the features observed by light, immunofluorescence (see ATLAS Plate 18), and electron microscopy. For example, in antiglomerular basement membrane (anti-GBM) antibody-mediated RLV, the glomerular tufts are often compressed by a proliferating crescent, capillary wall discontinuities (gaps) are common, the lesions are all at the same stage of evolution, IgG (IgG1 and/or IgG3, rarely IgG4) is deposited in a linear and continuous fashion along the inner aspect of the capillary wall, and no electron-dense deposits are seen (Turner and Rees, 1998). In immune complex-mediated RLV, there is often cellular proliferation within the glomerular tufts, gaps are less common, the lesions are of differing stages of evolution, granular deposits of IgG/IgM or IgA decorate the capillary loops and/or mesangium, and electron-dense deposits are seen in the subendothelial, intramembranous and/or subepithelial and mesangial distribution. In the ANCA-associated RLV, a fibrinoid and necrotizing lesion is often seen in the glomerular tufts, crescents are exuberant and cellular, gaps are common, the lesions are at various stages of evolution, only scant deposits of IgG/IgM ('pauci-immune') are seen, and no electron-dense deposits are observed (Falk et al., 1998). In the latter case, an extraglomerular 'angiitis' may be observed, but granulomatous angiitis is very uncommon. When crescentic GN is observed in ANCA and anti-GBM negative RLV scant deposits of C3 may occasionally be observed by immunofluorescence microscopy as well as small electron-dense deposits by electron microscopy (Sethi et al., 2017)

Regardless of the underlying pathogenetic mechanism, extensive deposits of partially or fully polymerized fibrin are interspersed between the proliferating cells in Bowman's space. Bridges between the basement membrane and Bowman's capsule appear early and the entry of Bowman's space to the proximal tubule is often occluded with cells and a fibrin clot (Le Hir et al., 2001), producing a form of intrarenal obstructive nephropathy. When extensive, these lesions may in part account for the rapid decline in glomerular filtration rate (GFR) observed in RLV. Co-existing acute tubular necrosis and/or interstitial nephritis can also contribute to the decline in renal function.

The extent of glomerular involvement may vary considerably from case to case, in part due to 'sampling error.' Most cases exhibiting a progressive decline in GFR will have >50 per cent of the glomeruli involved with crescents, and patients with oliguro-anuric acute kidney injury (AKI) may have 100 per cent of the glomeruli in the biopsy sample involved with crescents (Alchi et al., 2015). At the individual glomerular level, crescents can be segmental or circumferential, the latter having more ominous prognostic implications. Segmental crescents can resolve, leaving a focal scar or adhesion, but circumferential crescents frequently lead to total glomerular obsolescence, which may be followed by complete glomerular 'reabsorption,' leaving behind 'aglomerular' atrophic tubules (Kriz and Le Hir, 2005).

Pathogenesis

The pathogenetic mechanisms found to underlie RLV are quite heterogeneous (Pusey and Rees, 1998; see also Table 10.1).

About 10–15 per cent of cases will be due to anti-GBM disease consequent to the binding of auto-antibodies predominantly targeting epitopes on the alpha-3 chain of type IV collagen located in the globular NC-1 domain (the Goodpasture antigen) expressed uniformly along the inner aspect of the GBM (Kalluri et al., 1975; Turner and Rees, 1998; Borza et al., 2003; McAdoo and

Pusey, 2017)). Recently autoantibodies targeting epitopes on the NC-1 domain of the alpha-5 chain have also been described in a minority of patients with anti-GBM disease (Cui et al., 2016). The glomerular injury is due to local (not systemic) complement activation and polymorphonuclear leukocyte activation. These patients frequently have high levels of circulating anti-GBM antibody but normal serum complement levels. Although direct injury of the glomerular capillary wall, involving complement activation and polymorphonuclear leukocytes, is believed to be the main mechanism for the glomerular disease, it is very likely that T-cells may also be independently operative in the pathogenesis of the disease (Huang et al., 1994; Kitching et al., 1999; Salama et al., 2003). Both the alternative and classical pathways of complement activation are likely involved in tissue injury as C1q deposition is seen in about 25 per cent of cases of anti-GBM disease (Hu et al., 2013).

In another 10–15 per cent of cases of RLV, immune complexes are involved. This mechanism is either due to the formation of immune complexes in the circulation and their subsequent deposition in glomerular capillary tufts or to the in-situ formation of immune complex within the glomerular capillaries (Cameron, 1998; Holdsworth et al., 1998). The antigens involved in the immune complex-mediated form of RLV disease are quite diverse but are commonly not readily identifiable. Theoretically, they can range from replicating exogenous antigens (bacteria, viruses) to autologous antigen (nuclear antigens, tumour antigens). The immunoglobulin component of the immune complex may be IgG and or IgM, but when IgA is dominant then IgA nephropathy or IgA vasculitis is diagnosed (see Chapter 7).

Immune complex-mediated crescentic GN is most often due to a multisystem disease (such as lupus nephritis). Circulating ANCA may be concomitantly present in some cases of immune complex-mediated RLV (Scaglione et al., 2017). Immune complex-mediated RLV can also arise as a complication of another primary glomerular disease (e.g. membranous nephropathy, or C3 glomerulopathy; see Chapter 6 and Chapter 8)

In about 50–80 per cent of cases of RLV, an ANCA mechanism is involved (Morgan et al., 2006). ANCA are directed to either myeloperoxidase (MPO) or to proteinase-3 (PR-3) or rarely both (as measured by ELISA and purified antigens). Dual anti-MPO and anti-PR3 antibodies are uncommon and when present strongly suggests drug-induced disease (Pendergraft et al., 2014; Pendergraft and Niles, 2014); especially when combined with auto-antibodies to other leucocyte enzymes such as anti-lactoferrin or anti-elastase antibodies (Choi et al., 1999, 2000) or a very high titre of anti-MPO antibodies. Levamisole-induced ANCA vasculitis is particularly frequently accompanied by many auto-antibodies, including both anti-MPO and anti-PR3 ANCA.

Conversion from one ANCA serotype to another during the course of disease evolution also suggests a drug-induced aetiology (Choi et al., 2000) Anti-MPO auto-antibodies predominate in RLV; about 80 per cent of cases involve this immune mechanism. Anti-MPO auto-antibodies are also quite frequently observed in drug-associated ANCA vasculitis, mostly due to hydralazine or propylthiouracil (Choi et al., 2000). Thus, *all* patients with anti-MPO RLV, especially those with very high titres of MPO-ANCA or multiple co-existing auto-antibodies (e.g. anti-nuclear, anti-IgG, anti-histone, etc.) should be carefully interviewed regarding the recent use of agents thought to cause ANCA vasculitis (Choi et al., 2000)

The MPO-ANCA commonly gives a perinuclear or p-ANCA pattern on indirect immunofluorescence (IIF) using alcohol-fixed, buffy-coat human leukocytes, whereas the PR-3 ANCA most commonly give a cytoplasmic or c-ANCA pattern on similarly prepared leukocyte substrates. The precise mechanism by which ANCA arise is still debated, but it is clear that these auto-antibodies activate neutrophils and cause them to injure capillary walls in the glomeruli and in blood vessels elsewhere (Jennette and Falk, 2008). Local as well as systemic complement activation (especially via the alternative pathway) may be a prominent feature of the disorder depending on the nature of the antigen–antibody systems involved (Xiao et al., 2007; Jennette et al., 2013; Gou et al., 2013; Fukui et al., 2016; Chen et al., 2017), although serum complement levels are rarely below the normal range. Cytokines most likely also participate in the pathogenesis of the glomerular injury seen in ANCA vasculitis (Feldman and Pusey, 2006), including tumour necrosis factor-α. Concomitant production of anti-plasminogen and plasminogen activator auto-antibodies can inhibit fibrinolysis and predispose to fibrinoid necrosis and thrombophilia in ANCA vasculitis (Berden et al., 2010; In a moderate number (about 10–30 per cent) of cases of RLV, both anti-GBM and ANCA mechanisms co-exist and, in a small number of cases (<10 per cent), no anti-GBM, immune complexes or ANCA mechanism can be identified (Rutgers et al., 2005; Lionaki et al., 2007). It is entirely possible, even likely, that antibody-independent, T-cell-mediated processes are involved in some or even most forms of RLV (Tipping and Holdsworth, 2006), and such mechanism may explain in part the uncommon finding of negative anti-GBM and ANCA in cases of non-immune complex-mediated RLV. In addition, it is important to note that fragments of ceruloplasmin in the serum may obscure the detection of MPO-ANCA by interfering with the binding of anti-MPO directed at certain MPO. Removal of this ceruloplasmin fragment by isolation of purified IgG converts an anti-MPO negative serum to a positive one (Roth et al., 2013). Complement activation via the alternative pathway may participate in the pathogenesis of glomerular injury in some of these cases of ANCA- and anti-GBM negative forms of RLV (Sethi et al., 2017). Mounting data points to the role of complement activation via the alternative pathway in ANCA GN and vasculitis (Xiao et al., 2007; Jennette et al., 2013; Gou et al., 2013).

Regardless of the fundamental immunopathological mechanisms, the glomerular crescent forms and evolves by proliferation of visceral and parietal epithelial cells, polymerization of fibrin (from fibrinogen escaping into Bowman's space through the 'gaps'), infiltration with monocytes, macrophages, and T-cells, and invasion by myofibroblastic cells from the interstitium. These processes are driven by local accumulation of chemical mediators such as interleukin-1 (IL-1), tumour necrosis factor (TNF-α), macrophage chemotactic protein-1 (MCP-1), macrophage inflammatory factor (MIF), membrane prothrombinase, and transforming growth factor (TGF)-β production (Khan et al., 2005). An important role may be played by transcription factors T-bet and Jun D. T-bet is a transcription factor that is essential for T helper (Th)1 lineage commitment and optimal IFN-gamma production by CD4(+) T cells. Phoon and colleagues (2008) showed that T-bet directs Th1 responses that induce renal injury in experimental CrGN. Behmoaras and colleagues (2008) demonstrated that the activator protein-1 (AP-1) transcription factor JunD, a major determinant of macrophage activity, is strongly associated with susceptibility to crescent formation. Eventually the TGFβ-stimulated myofibroblasts from the interstitium differentiate into fibroblasts secreting collagens I, III, and IV, leading to the organization and fibrosis of the crescent (Wiggins, 1998).

Aetiology

Not surprisingly, the aetiology of RLV is very diverse and in many cases entirely unknown, even though its pathogenesis can be accurately described in most instances (>90 per cent; de Lind van Wijngaarden et al., 2008). Secondary forms of RLV undoubtedly occur in infectious disease such as hepatitis B or C, malignant neoplasia (e.g. lung cancer), drug exposure (e.g. hydralazine, propylthiouracil, levamisole), autoimmune disease (e.g. systemic lupus erythematosus, SLE), or in association with multisystem diseases such as Goodpasture's disease (anti-GBM disease with nephritis and pulmonary haemorrhage), systemic granulomatosis with polyangiitis (GPA; formerly Wegener's granulomatosis), microscopic polyangiitis (MPA), IgA vasculitis, and eosinophilic granulomatosis with polyangiitis (EGPA; formerly Churg-Strauss allergic granulomatosis). These secondary forms of RLV or systemic vasculitis are not the primary focus of this chapter. Thus, from an aetiological standpoint this chapter will deal with anti-GBM-mediated disease, without pulmonary involvement (no alveolar haemorrhage), immune complex disease arising *de novo* without systemic features, and the renal-limited form of ANCA-associated vasculitis (also called pauci-immune necrotizing and crescentic GN, or combinations thereof, and ANCA/anti-GBM negative RLV). A background of heavy exposure to silica may be ascertained in patients with ANCA-associated RLV (Hogan et al., 2007). Several hypotheses have been put forward to possibly explain the cause of ANCA-associated RLV (de Lind van Wijngaarden et al., 2008; Yang et al., 2008). A mechanistic connection between complementary peptides on organisms and ANCA formation has been postulated (Preston and Falk, 2011). Lysosomal membrane protein-2 (LAMP-2) having similarity to epitopes on fimbriated bacteria provoking anti-LAMP-2O auto-antibodies have been suggested to be involved in some case of vasculitis; however, such antibodies appear to be quite uncommon in the US (Roth et al., 2012). It seems quite clear that not all anti-MPO antibodies are pathogenic in ANCA RLV or systemic disease. The pathogenicity of anti-MPO antibodies is largely determined by the epitope with which they react (Roth et al., 2013). Aberrant glycosylation of MPO (and exposure of neo-epitopes) might explain the propensity for developing anti-MPO auto-antibodies in patients with anti-GBM disease (Yu et al., 2017). Antibodies to MPO can also aggravate anti-GBM disease in experimental animals (Heeringa et al, 1996)

Viral infections (influenza, hantavirus), occult neoplasia (lymphoma, lung carcinoma), exposure to volatile hydrocarbons, obstructive uropathy, or renal trauma (extra-corporeal shock wave lithotripsy) might be aetiological factors in some cases of anti-GBM antibody RLV (Ma et al., 1978; Stevenson et al., 1995; Billheden et al., 1997; Maes et al., 1999; Xenocostas et al., 1999; Borza et al., 2005; Weschler et al., 2008; Glassock, 2016). Drug exposure is an important cause of ANCA-associated RLV, especially due to anti-MPO (See Box 10.1 for listing; Pendergraft and Niles, 2014). Recently, anti-TNF-α therapy in rheumatologic conditions and use of sofosbuvir for treatment of hepatitis C infection has been associated with development of ANCA vasculitis (Ginsberg et al., 2016; Ahmad et al., 2017).

Clinical presentation and features

In addition to a rapid progressive decline in renal function, other clinical features of GN are usually present, including dysmorphic haematuria, erythrocyte casts, and modest glomerular proteinuria, usually < 2.0 g/day (Glassock et al., 1995). Nephrotic syndrome (NS) is relatively uncommon, seen in less than 15 per cent of cases at presentation, and more frequently in immune complex-mediated RLV. Hypertension is quite variable and may be entirely absent (Glassock et al., 1995). The onset of RLV is usually rather abrupt with overt symptoms and signs suggesting GN such as gross

Box 10.1 Drug-associated forms of ANCA vasculitis (renal-limited and systemic)

- Hydralazine
- Allopurinol
- Sulfasalazine*
- Minocyline*
- Propylthiouracil and methimazole
- Penicillamine*
- Levamisole-contaminated cocaine
- Rifampicin
- Aminoguanidine (an experimental drug, not clinically available)
- Sofosbuvir (and perhaps other direct acting antiviral) therapy for hepatitis C viral infection
- Anti-TNF alpha therapy for rheumatoid arthritis/ankylosing spondylitis

* these agents are not commonly associated with ANCA conversion; see Choi et al., 2000.

haematuria (Glassock et al., 1995). In the absence of specific treatment, the disorder rapidly culminates in features of renal failure (weakness, nausea, vomiting, and easy fatigability). Nevertheless, insidious development of renal failure over several months may also occur. It can be suspected in patients who present with relatively advanced renal failure associated with interstitial fibrosis and tubular atrophy, but no preceding symptoms or signs and typically no history of extrarenal manifestations of active vasculitis. An antecedent 'viral-like' illness is not uncommon and mild arthralgias, myalgias, and low-grade fever may occasionally be seen, especially in immune complex and ANCA-associated CrGN.

By definition (see 'Aetiology'), evidence of multisystem, extrarenal involvement (other than that explained by 'uraemia') is lacking in *primary RLV*, but vascular congestion resulting from greatly impaired GFR and fluid retention may cause pulmonary oedema and even mild haemoptysis. Frank pulmonary haemorrhage should not occur in primary RLV disease and, if present, suggests a multisystem disorder such as Goodpasture's syndrome due to anti-GBM disease or pulmonary angiitis (MPA or GPA), SLE, IgA vasculitis, or cryoimmunoglobulinaemia. Concomitant cutaneous leukocytoclastic vasculitis ('palpable purpura') suggests IgA vasculitis, lupus nephritis, or MPA/

GPA (Jennette et al., 1994) or drug-associated vasculitis (especially levamisole) (Pendergraft WF 3rd, 2014). Upper and lower airway involvement (otitis, sinusitis, tracheitis, bronchitis) suggests GPA. Mononeuritis multiplex suggests polyangiitis, especially that associated with chronic viral hepatitis (hepatitis B viral infection). Purpura, splenomegaly, and liver abnormalities suggest chronic hepatitis C virus-associated cryoimmunoglobulinaemia (Johnson et al., 1994). Patients with anti-PR3 ANCA-associated RLV, GPA, or MPA may be at increased risk for venous thrombo-embolism due to concomitant antibody to plasminogen (preventing normal fibrinolysis; Bautz et al., 2008; see also Chapter 1).

Overall, both males and females are affected in nearly equal proportions (Glassock et al., 1995). Anti-GBM antibody-mediated RLV is seen most frequently in older females compared to anti-GBM-associated pulmonary-renal syndrome (Goodpasture's disease), which tends more common in younger men. (Turner and Rees, 1998) Immune complex and ANCA-associated RLV are seen in all ages but are much more common in older individuals, especially ANCA-associated RLV (Jennette and Falk, 1990). The combination of ANCA and anti-GBM-mediated RLV is seen more commonly in older females.

Renal function, as assessed by serum creatinine or estimated GFR, is often impaired at discovery or shortly thereafter in RLV. It then rapidly worsens over several weeks or months. Uncommonly, a slowly evolving course can be observed, typically in anti-GBM disease with low-titre of antibodies (Segelmark et al., 2012) Oligo-anuric acute renal failure may be the presenting feature in patients with severe, fulminating disease with extensive crescentic involvement of glomerular and a very unfavourable prognosis. Urinalyses are almost always abnormal with dysmorphic hematuria (often with numerous acanthocytes and erythrocyte casts) and modest proteinuria (<2.0 g/day). Very heavy proteinuria and early development of hypoalbuminaemia is distinctly uncommon, except in immune complex-mediated RLV. Blood pressure is normal or only modestly elevated in the majority of patients; elevated blood pressure is more likely to occur in immune complex-mediated RLV, especially with glomerular infiltration with monocytes, as might be associated with cryoglobulinaemia C3 glomerulopathy (see Chapter 8). Very severe or malignant hypertension should make one suspicious of polyarteritis nodosa, renal arterial occlusive disease, athero-embolic renal disease, scleroderma renal crisis, thrombotic microangiopathy, or malignant nephrosclerosis with fibrinoid necrosis of renal arterioles (Glassock et al., 1995).

A new entity, unfortunately called 'atypical anti-GBM disease' has recently emerged (Nasr et al., 2016). These cases are characterized by non-crescentic, non-vasculitic renal disease showing 'ultra-linear' deposition of IgG along the capillary wall without any detectable classical anti-GBM antibody in the circulation. The renal lesions are endocapillary proliferative GN, MesPGN, MPGN, or FSGS. Thrombotic microangiopathy (TMA) is common and the Ig deposits are monoclonal in about 50 per cent of cases. NS, often with haematuria, is common but pulmonary haemorrhage is rare. The course is usually an indolent one to ESRD rather than a rapidly progressive course. Treatment is unknown. Some of these cases may have been diagnosed as 'antibody-negative anti-GBM disease'. Classical anti-GBM disease (as discussed herein), with circulating anti-GBM antibodies may uncommonly also behave in an 'atypical fashion', with relapses and intermittent periods of anti-GBM negative serological tests (see McAdoo and Pusey, 2017; Glassock, 2016). Fibrillary GN with non-congophillic, fibrillary deposits of IgG can occasionally mimic true anti-GBM disease by IF, but EM and staiunig for DNAJb9 will always disclose the true nature of the disease (Glassock, 2016) (see also Chapter 11)

Laboratory features, especially serology, are *crucial* for the identification of the underlying pathogenic mechanism of RLV (Cornec et al., 2017), which will then guide therapy and assist in prognostication (see Table 10.2). Anti-GBM-mediated RLV is characterized by circulating anti-GBM antibodies (best measured by a commercially available ELISA assay using recombinant human COLIVA3NCI antigen; Turner and Rees, 1998; Borza et al., 2003). About 95 per cent of patients will be positive if specimens are taken early in the course of disease before treatment is begun. False-positive assays are very uncommon. A 'false negative' anti-GBM assay can be seen in IgG4 mediated disease (Segelmark et al., 1990; Glassock, 2016). The titre of the anti-GBM antibody is only weakly correlated with the severity of the renal disease. Most of the anti-GBM antibody is IgG (usually IgG1 or IgG3, rarely IgG4 subclass) but rarely it may be IgA (Border et al., 1979; Segelmark et al., 1990). About 30 per cent of patients with anti-GBM disease may also present with concomitant ANCA (usually MPO-ANCA) and about five per cent of those with ANCA vasculitis have

Table 10.2 Factors affecting the prognosis of crescentic glomerulonephritis.

Clinical	Pathology
◆ Age at onset of disease	◆ Extent of crescentic involvement (% normal glomeruli)
◆ Infectious/drug aetiology	
◆ Renal function at discovery (oliguria, dialysis dependency)	◆ Nature of the crescent (cellular, fibrocellular, fibrous)
◆ Serology (ANCA, anti-GBM, dual antibody)	◆ Extent of glomerulosclerosis
	◆ Extent of chronic tubulo-interstitial fibrosis lesions
◆ Timeliness of institution of treatment	
◆ Genetics (HLA)	◆ Disruption of Bowman's capsule

concomitant anti-GBM antibodies (Levy et al., 2004), so *all* patients with RLV must be assessed for both anti-GBM and ANCA, regardless of their clinical presentation (see 'Induction therapy for RLV'; Rutgers et al., 2005). C3 and C4 levels are most often normal or increased and cryoimmunoglobulins are absent in anti-GBM-mediated disease. However, hypocomplementaemia can be seen in some patients with ANCA vasculitis (Manenti et al., 2015) and this may have prognostic significance (see 'Prognostic factors'). In anti-GBM disease a lower titre of antibody to the immunodominant GBM epitope is associated with a better renal outcome (Segelmark et al., 2003)

In immune complex-mediated RLV the serological findings are quite varied according to the underlying disease. Antistreptolysin O titre may be increased and C3 decreased in post-streptococcal disease (see also Chapter 9). Serum C3 and or C4 may also be abnormally low (e.g. in SLE or in cryoglobulinaemia with chronic hepatitis C viral infection, in monoclonal immunoglobulin deposition diseases, or in C3 glomerulopathy; see Chapter 8 and 9).

In ANCA-associated RLV, the ANCA levels measured by IIF and antigen-specific ELISA assays are increased, most often (about 70–75 per cent) MPO-ANCA in RLV. The sensitivity and specificity for these assays are best when they are used together (Hagen et al., 1998). In ANCA-associated RLV the sensitivity and specificity are around 85–90 per cent and 95 per cent, respectively, but since these assays are not standardized, one must know the characteristics of the individual laboratory performing the test in order to interpret its diagnostic value.

Up to one-third of patients with anti-GBM disease also have circulating ANCA (Savage and Lockwood, 1990; Hellmark et al., 1997; Kalluri et al., 1997; Rutgers et al., 2005; Cui et al., 2011; McAdoo et al., 2017, McAdoo et al., Pusey, 2017a). Both anti-MPO specific P-ANCA and anti-PR3 specific C-ANCA can occur in patients with anti-GBM disease, but anti-MPO is most common (about 80 per cent). Interestingly, no differences in the antigenic specificity of anti-GBM antibodies were detected between sera with or without concurrent expression of ANCA (Hellmark et al., 1997). Co-existence of ANCA in patients with anti-GBM antibodies is commonly associated with small vessel vasculitis in organs in addition to lung and kidney (Levy et al., 2004), but RLV can also occur (McAdoo et al., 2017).

Epidemiology

Renal-limited vasculitides are relatively uncommon disorders. The multisystem forms are seen much more frequently. Anti-GBM antibody nephritis is seen worldwide but is rather rare (Turner and Rees, 1998), with an incidence rate of 0.5–1.0 new cases diagnosed per million population per year. It is more common in Caucasians and Asians of Chinese ancestry in black populations.

It may be more common in the spring and summer months. It may even occur in mini-epidemics or clusters of cases, suggesting an environmental (viral?) aetiology (Canney et al., 2016; McAdoo and Pusey, 2016). The occurrence of anti-GBM disease as a form of RLV are seen more commonly in older women. Younger males have a tendency to have a multisystem presentation, with alveolar haemorrhage and rapidly progressive GN. The disease is very rare in children younger than ten years of age and is very seldom seen over the age of 75 years. Susceptibility to anti-GBM disease is largely controlled by the HLA-DRB1 genes on chromosome 6. DRB1*15 and *04 increase susceptibility and DRB1*07 is protective (Fisher et al., 1997) Immune complex-mediated RLV not secondary to a systemic disease is rather uncommon, probably similar to anti-GBM disease.

ANCA-associated RLV is much more common, with an annual incidence rate of around 5–20 newly diagnosed cases per million population, depending on the region. According to the extensive experience of the Mayo Clinic from 1996 to 2015, the incidence and prevalence of ANCA vasculitis (both systemic and renal limited forms) in Olmstead County residents was 20 per million per year and 350 per million, respectively (Berti et al., 2018). There is a marked predilection to affect older individuals (over age 50 years), both males and females (Gaskin and Pusey, 1998). Caucasians, Hispanics, and Asians (Chinese) are most commonly affected (Li et al, 2016) and the disorder is less common in black populations. There may be differences in frequency between regions, such as Southern and Northern Europe. MPO-ANCA vasculitis is the preponderant serotype in China where PR3-ANCA is rare. (Li et al., 2016) No seasonal differences in occurrence of ANCA-associated RLV have been consistently noted.

Natural history of RLV

Data concerning the natural history of RLV in the pre-treatment eras are quite limited and do not separate the various pathogenctic subcategories discussed. It is generally believed that GN with extensive circumferential crescents (>50 per cent glomerular involvement) seldom undergoes spontaneous remission and that survival with endogenous renal function for more than 6–12 months in the absence of specific treatment is uncommon (Cameron, 1977). Lesser degrees of crescentic involvement (e.g. <20 per cent glomerular involvement), especially when superimposed on another glomerular disease (e.g. post-streptococcal GN; see also Chapter 9), may spontaneously Patients with moderate crescentic involvement (30–50 per cent of glomeruli) may have a more indolent course, but if untreated, will still probably progress to ESRD. When biopsy samples contain relatively few glomeruli (<10 per core), it may be difficult to estimate the true extent of glomerular involvement with crescents (Glassock et al., 1995) due to sampling error considerations. Prognostication based on the degree of crescentic involvement should be made with great caution if the numbers of glomeruli in the biopsy specimen are limited.

Thus, nearly every patient with RLV and extensive glomerular involvement (as defined here with >50 per cent glomerular crescents) and probably also those with a much lower percentage of crescents should be considered as candidates for aggressive therapy (see 'Specific treatment'), especially if the biopsy sample is limited, unless treatment is contraindicated by excessive risks or unless clinical and morphologic parameters strongly suggest an unfavourable outcome even with aggressive treatment (see 'Specific treatment'). Assessing futility of treatment based on clinical and morphological findings at discovery of RLV is possible, but there is always some residual uncertainty. With early and aggressive treatment with immunosuppression, patient survival and renal survival at five and ten years can be dramatically improved (Chen et al., 2016) but relapses and complications of treatment can contribute to morbidity and to mortality (Flossman et al., 2011). The factors that can be used to assess the prognosis for outcome (freedom from ESRD, death, relapse of disease after initial induction therapy) are outlined as follows (see also Box 10.1).

Prognostic factors

Treatment timeliness

As will be discussed later, the *single* most important factor affecting prognosis is the speed with which treatment is instituted following recognition and categorization of disease. A delay in treatment can allow the disease-related damage to glomeruli to become irreversible (Little and Pusey, 2004). An adverse effect on prognosis is engendered by delay in diagnosis and initiating treatment especially if this allows the development of dialysis dependence and/or oligo-anuria in anti-GBM disease (with or without concomitant ANCA), but when ANCA alone is found, or the RLV lesions are more suggestive of a pauci-immune vasculitis (see 'Pathology') then recovery may be possible even in dialysis-dependent patients with aggressive therapy (Lee et al., 2014).

Age and gender

Overall, the age and gender of patients may influence prognosis, largely because of the age-associated difference and the prevalence of the underlying subtypes of RLV, the predilection for subtypes to affect certain genders, and the rising risk of complications in older patients (Cameron, 1977; Glassock et al., 1995; Flossman et al., 2011). Modified treatment regimens (reduced steroids, reduced CYC) may be helpful in reducing risks of serious adverse events in older and elderly adults (Pagnoux et al., 2015). The prognosis for older patients with combined ANCA-associated RLV and anti-GBM disease appears particularly grim (Bonsib et al., 1993). However, in a large retrospective review, McAdoo and colleagues (2017) found that dialysis-dependent dual antibody disease (anti-GBM + ANCA) had a better prognosis than anti-GBM antibody alone. Children with RLV secondary to a well-recognized streptococcal illness or exposure to drugs (such as anti-thyroid medications) may have a favourable prognosis, particularly with mild crescentic involvement (Cameron, 1977). Nevertheless, age alone is not a powerful determinant of prognosis. Even in children, the outcome of the disease is mainly related to timely diagnosis and treatment (Dewan et al., 2008).

Proteinuria

The magnitude of proteinuria at discovery has no particular short-term prognostic significance in RLV. Following treatment, however, persistent proteinuria or the emergence of nephrotic-range proteinuria may indicate a poor long-term outcome. This may be a manifestation of 'oligonephronia' resulting from irreversible damage to a large population of nephrons with maladaptive functional and morphologic changes (e.g. focal and segmental glomerulosclerosis) in the residual hyperfunctioning nephrons (see also Chapter 5).

Renal function

Severe acute onset of oligo-anuric renal failure is usually a reflection of very extensive crescentic involvement or an associated tubulo-interstitial lesion (e.g. acute tubular necrosis or acute tubulo-interstitial nephritis) and the former usually confers a worse prognosis. Patients with anti-GBM antibody-mediated RLV treated *before* the onset of dialysis dependency (e.g. a serum creatinine ≤ 6.8 mg/dl or 600 μm/l) have an improved prognosis ; Levy et al., 2001). Patients with ANCA-associated RLV may sustain and maintain substantial short-term improvement in renal function even if treatment is delayed to dialysis dependency, depending on the treatment regimen used () (Falk et al., 1990; Hauer et al., 2002; Hogan et al., 2005; Mukhtyar et al., 2008; Pagnoux et al., 2008); however, this conclusion is still a subject of debate and inquiry. Although serum creatinine levels at the time of presentation and the initiation of therapy are important predictors of renal outcome (survival free of dialysis), there is no absolute level of serum creatinine above which treatment is deemed universally futile and other parameters, e.g. oligo-anuria and renal biopsy findings, may be helpful in estimating the likelihood of renal recovery with treatment (Hogan et al., 2005; Alchi et al., 2015; Lee et al., 2014). A low eGFR (<15 ml/min/1.73 m^2) at presentation was an independent negative prognostic factor for patient survival in ANCA vasculitis in a large retrospective study (n = 535) conducted by the European Vasculitis Study Group (Flossman et al., 2011).Oligo--anuria at presentation is an indication of a low likelihood of recovery, even with aggressive treatment in anti-GBM disease (Alchi et al, 2015)

Renal morphology and pathogenetic subtype

In general, the extent of crescentic involvement of the glomeruli (usually assessed by counting the percentage of normal glomeruli in the biopsy specimen) relates to prognosis (and response to treatment)). In the ANCA-associated subtype, Berden and colleagues (2010) proposed a morphological classification that aids in prognosis determination (see Table 10.3). The utility of this system has been validated independently in ANCA-associated RLV and systemic vasculitis (Nohr et al., 2014; Unlu et al., 2013).

A focal lesion characterized by ≥50 per cent of normal glomeruli generally has a more favourable prognosis with a 90 per cent or greater renal survival (with therapy) after five years of follow-up. When ≥50 per cent of the glomeruli display cellular crescents the prognosis (with therapy) is less favourable, with a renal survival of about 75 per cent at five years or more. When ≥50 per cent of the glomeruli are globally sclerotic the prognosis (even with therapy) is very poor, with a renal survival of about 25 per cent or less after five to seven years of follow up. The mixed class with <50 per cent normal glomeruli, < 50 per cent cellular crescents, and <50 per cent globally sclerotic glomeruli has an intermediate prognosis with a renal survival of about 60 per cent at five years or more of follow-up. Circumferential ('full moon') crescents seem to have an adverse

Table 10.3 Classification for prognosis determination in ANCA-associated glomerulonephritis.

Q1	Are there ≥50% globally sclerotic glomeruli?	*If yes, it is Sclerotic Class*
		If no, move to question 2
Q2	Are there ≥50% normal glomeruli?	*If yes, it is Focal Class*
		If no, move to question 3
Q3	Are there ≥50% cellular crescents?	*If yes, it is Crescentic Class*
		If no, it is Mixed Class

Biopsies should be scored for glomerular lesions in the following order:
Globally sclerotic glomeruli → normal glomeruli→ cellular crescentic glomeruli.
Any biopsies that do not have a majority of one of the above phenotypes will
  automatically be in the Mixed Class.

Source: data from Berden AE, Ferrario F, Hagen EC, et al. (2010). Histopathologic classification of ANCA-associated glomerulonephritis. J Am Soc Nephrol. 21: 1628–36.

impact on prognosis, compared to segmental crescents (Unlu et al., 2013). The combination of circumferential fibrocellular glomerular crescents involving 100 per cent of the glomeruli and oligo-anuria is particularly ominous.

Renal functional impairment in patients with RLV may also be the consequence of associated tubulo-interstitial lesions (e.g. acute tubule necrosis, tubulo-interstitial nephritis). Tubule atrophy, interstitial inflammation, and fibrosis can adversely impact prognosis and response to treatment (Berden et al., 2012).

Disruption of Bowman's capsule, which allows for invasion of the crescent with interstitium-derived myofibroblasts, also indicates a poor outcome (Ferrario et al., 1994). An associated renal thrombotic microangiopathy is not uncommon (10–15 per cent) among RLV or systemic disease due to ANCA (Chen et al., 2015), and is accompanied by more serve disease and a much worse prognosis.

The pathogenic subtype of the lesion is an important determinant of prognosis (see 'Serology'), especially if treatment is instituted late in the course of disease. Very extensive crescentic involvement in anti-GBM antibody-mediated disease (few or no normal glomeruli) indicates a very poor outcome (Cameron, 1977; Glassock et al., 1995). For example, a very high titre of circulating anti-GBM antibodies, 100 per cent crescentic involvement, and oligo-anuria with dialysis-dependence in RLV indicates a very poor prognosis, even with aggressive therapy (see 'Specific treatment') in anti-GBM antibody-mediated disease (Levy et al., 2001; van Daalen et al., 2017). But dialysis-dependent patients with combined anti-GBM and ANCA disease may have a better outcome with aggressive therapy than with anti-GBM disease only (Van Daalen et al., 2017;. Patients with ANCA-associated RLV unassociated with anti-GBM may also have a poor prognosis when extensive glomerular involvement (<2 per cent normal glomeruli) is accompanied by severe interstitial fibrosis, but with aggressive therapy a small fraction (ten per cent) may recover useful renal function even if they have required dialysis therapy for treatment of rapidly progressive renal failure (See 'Specific treatment'; de Lind van Wijngaarden et al., 2006, 2007).

Patients with combined ANCA and anti-GBM-associated RLV behave more like severe anti-GBM antibody-only disease than severe ANCA-only-associated disease (Levy et al., 2004; McAdoo et al., 2017), except that relapse is much more frequent in dual antibody-positive RLV than in anti-GBM-mediated RLV (McAdoo et al., 2017) and some patients may recover renal function even if dialysis dependent at discovery (Van Daalen et al., 2017). Extensive endocapillary proliferation with subepithelial 'humps' unaccompanied by glomerulosclerosis or tubulo-interstitial atrophy and fibrosis may be associated with a more favourable outcome, especially with a background of an acute infectious disease

(Cameron, 1977; Neild et al., 1983). Extensive necrotizing lesions of the glomerular capillary tuft, frequently of varying age, cellularity, and fibrosis, as is seen commonly in ANCA-associated RLV, may also be associated with the persistence of proteinuria and impaired renal function even with initially successful treatment. The late emergence of heavy proteinuria, hypertension, and progressive renal failure is a common sequela of very severe initial disease (Leaker and Neild, 1991). As mentioned, this latter process may be non-immunologically mediated and related to haemodynamic maladaptations occurring in surviving nephrons (see also Chapter 2). Therapy designed to modify these adaptations (e.g. RAS inhibition) may have a salutary effect on long-term prognosis (Leaker and Neild, 1991; see also Chapter 2). Patients with combined ANCA and anti-GBM who are dialysis dependent seem to respond better to therapy, including plasmapheresis, and may recover renal function with aggressive therapy (McAdoo et al., 2017).

Serology

The pre-therapy titre of auto-antibodies (e.g. anti-GBM, ANCA) correlates rather poorly with disease severity and renal outcome, at least in those patients with RLV. The relationship of ANCA levels to clinical disease activity is very complex and involves epitope specificity of the antibodies, subclass of IgG, type of assay, and treatment regimens (Fussner and Specks, 2015). Overall, high initial levels of anti-GBM antibodies are more associated with a poor outcome than high levels of ANCA (Jennette and Falk, 1991; Herody et al., 1993; Lionaki et al., 2007; Segelmark et al., 2003). In a large series, however, the titre of anti-GBM antibodies neither correlated with the fraction of crescentic glomeruli nor with serum creatinine (Fischer and Lager, 2007). Patients with non-dialysis-dependent anti-GBM RLV may have better outcomes when the titre of anti-GBM antibody is low at presentation (Segelmark et al., 2003). Thus, initial serologic studies in anti-GBM antibody-mediated disease are primarily useful for diagnosis but may have some utility in prognosis. A possible exception may be represented by patients with both anti-GBM antibodies and anti-MPO ANCA who may have worse renal survival than patients with anti-MPO ANCA only, at least in some series (Levy et al., 2004; Rutgers et al., 2005).

Whether serial serologic monitoring of ANCA (anti-MPO and/or anti-PR-3) or anti-GBM antibody titres following successful induction therapy may have value in predicting subsequent relapses is also disputed (Specks et al, 2015a). Relapses of anti-GBM antibody disease after successful therapy are quite uncommon (<5 per cent) (Glassock, 2016) and monitoring of antibody levels after successful initial therapy is not needed, unless a clinical recurrence is evident (see 'Relapsing disease'). The available data relating relapse to serology in

ANCA-associated RLV is more extensive for C-ANCA/PR3-ANCA than for P-ANCA/MPO-ANCA. The literature on the subject also lacks homogeneity on the testing methodology and the definition of significant changes in titres. However, a substantial (fourfold or greater) rise in ANCA titre after reaching a nadir post-therapy or conversion from negative to positive ANCA serology may herald a clinical relapse (Han et al., 2003), but the positive predictive value of such a change in titre for a relapse is only about 60–80 per cent (Cohen Tervaert et al., 1990; Davenport et al., 1995; de'Oliviera et al., 1995) and the timing of a relapse may be delayed by many months. Relapse is well known to be far more common in anti-PR3-positive patients (>50 per cent) compared to anti-MPO-positive patients with ANCA-associated RLV or systemic disease about 10–15 per cent), so monitoring is likely to be of greater value in the patient with anti-PR-3-positive disease. Some studies have suggested that patients with PR3-ANCA may benefit from a prophylactic approach of reinstituting therapy when ANCA reappears or titre increases (Cohen Tervaert et al., 1990). However, in an analysis of serially obtained PR3-ANCA titres as part of the large randomized and controlled trial of etanercept in GPA, increases in ANCA titres were not associated with relapse (Finkelman et al., 2007). At this point in time, there is little evidence to support the notion that serial ANCA testing (especially in anti-MPO-positive patients) can be used effectively and safely to predict future relapses and guide 'pre-emptive' increases in the intensity of (or re-institution of) immunosuppression. In a large retrospective study, only 50 per cent of patients had experienced a relapse within 18 months of the rise in ANCA titre, and it was recommended that immunosuppressive therapy *not* be determined by changes in ANCA titre alone (Kemma et al., 2015). Nevertheless, some patients may exhibit a consistent and recurring pattern of a rising ANCA titres preceding each clinical relapse of disease (this is mostly found in patients with PR3-ANCA). Such patients might become candidates for a prophylactic approach to therapy with immunosuppressive agents (including rituximab (RTX), azathioprine (AZA), or mycophenolate mofetil (MMF) (see 'Specific treatment'). A negative ANCA test at the time of renission is associated with a lowser risk of subsequent relapse (Morgan et al, 2017). ANCA sub-type can influence prognosis. For example, patients with anti-PR3 ANCA vasculitis (less common in ANCA-associated RLV) may respond better to RTX than to cyclophosphamide (CYC) plus AZA (see 'Plasmapheresis for induction'), especially with relapsing disease (Unizony et al., 2016).

Serum complement levels (C3/C4) are typically normal in anti-GBM or ANCA-associated RLV, but C3 levels (but not C4 levels) below the median (<120mg/dL) at diagnosis the long-term prognosis for patient survival is adversely affected (Augusto et al., 2016). Thus, hypocomplementaemia at presentation is an indication of serious organ damage and confers an unfavourable prognosis (Fukui et al., 2016)

There is both a genetically determined predisposition to anti-GBM and ANCA-associated RLV and systemic vasculitis as well as an influence of underlying genetic makeup on prognosis (Rhamattulla et al., 2016). Certain alleles at the HLA chromosome (chromosome 6), e.g. HLA DR-2 and/or B-7 may determine the severity of disease and its outcome (Rees et al., 1984;; Borgmann and Haubnitz, 2004; Tsuchiya et al., 2006; Heckmann et al., 2008). The DRB1*15 allele is an established risk factor for anti-PR3 ANCA vasculitis (Cao et al., 2011) and similar alleles also increase susceptibility to anti-GBM disease Gene-specific hypomethylation of the proteinase 3 promoter gene (*PRTN3*) and myeloperoxidase gene (*MPO*) is associated with an increase in active disease and relapses in ANCA vasculitis (Jones et al., 2017). However, at the present time these genetic influences on susceptibility, severity, and prognosis are mainly of research interest and they do not have any role in therapeutic decision making. An alpha-1-antitrypsin deficiency may rarely be encountered. Interestingly, in a large genome-wide association study, GPA or PR3-ANCA-associated disease were significantly associated with single nucleotide polymorphisms of the SERPINA1 gene, which encodes for alpha-1-antitrypsin, the enzymatic targets of which includes PR3 (Lyons et al., 2012).

Other

The incidence of malignancies influencing long-term survival is increased in ANCA- vasculitis (Rahmatulla et al., 2015). This is almost entirely accounted for by non-melanoma skin cancers and is likely an effect of immunosuppression. The risk of bladder and haematological malignancies has been decreasing due to lower cumulative doses of alkylating agents used to control the disease (Rahmatulla et al., 2015)

Specific treatment of ANCA-positive, anti-GBM negative RLV (ANCA-associated small vessel vasculitis—ANCA-SVV)

Overview

Data on the treatment of renal-limited ANCA positive, pauci-immune necrotizing and crescentic GN is derived from the literature of ANCA-associated small vessel vasculitis, including GPA and MPA (Little and Pusey, 2004). There is much less data directly derived specifically from patients with RLV.

Treatment of RLV is generally divided into an *induction* phase (three to six months) where the goal is to achieve a complete or partial remission of the renal manifestations and a *maintenance* phase (often lasting for several years), when necessary, where the goal is to prevent relapses at the lowest risk of side-effects. The *induction* treatment of severe ANCA-associated RLV rests primarily on the use of intravenous (IV) methylprednisolone (MP), high-dose oral glucocorticoids, and oral or IV CYC or RTX. In patients with mild-to moderate RLV associated with anti-MPO antibodies, oral MMF plus high-dose prednisolone may also be both effective and safe, but RTX may be the preferred option, unless patients are intolerant or allergic to RTX or the agent is not available). (Reviewed in Cornec et al., 2017).

Induction therapy for RLV

Corticosteroids for induction

Steroids alone are not satisfactory treatment for ANCA vasculitis or RLV, and they are always combined with some form of immunosuppression (Nachman et al., 1996). Initiation of therapy with *pulse MP* (usually 7–15 mg/kg/day for three days) is used to curb the active inflammation as soon as possible (Bolton and Couser,1979, , Little and Pusey, 2004). This is followed by oral prednisone or prednisolone at a daily dosage of 1 mg/kg/day (not to exceed 80 mg/day for the first month of therapy). Prednisone or prednisolone is then tapered over the second month to alternate-day dosing and subsequently decreased by 10 mg/day every week until they are eventually discontinued by the end of the third to fifth month. In the large randomized-controlled PEXIVAS trial, patients treated with a more rapid taper and a cumulatively reduced dose of oral prednisone (resulting in half the cumulative dose) had non-inferior outcomes to those who received full dose (Walsh M et al., 2013; Merkel P et al.) The rate of decrease in glucocorticoid dosing should be tailored based on an assessment of each patient's disease activity and risks. Prophylactic trimethoprim-sulfamethoxazole should be administered during the high-dose steroid therapy to minimize the risk of a pneumocystis infection. Prolongation of steroid therapy (>5 mg/day) in ANCA vasculitis beyond six months is associated with a greater risk of infection but not a decreased risk of relapse (McGregor et al., 2012).

Cyclophosphamide for induction

Cyclophosphamide (CYC) was introduced for treatment of GPA by Wolff and Fauci in 1968. Due to the pronounced beneficial effect on natural history of this disease, CYC has never been examined in a controlled trial compared to a placebo or steroids alone. The beneficial role of CYC in the treatment of acute, severe ANCA-associated RLV is evidenced by the substantial improvement in the rate of remission (from 56 per cent to 85 per cent) and a threefold decrease in the risk of relapse that is associated with the use of this drug compared to steroids alone (Nachman et al., 1996). CYC may be administered as a daily oral regimen or as monthly IV pulses. When the IV route is used, it is usually started at a dose of 0.5 g/m^2 of body surface area, which is subsequently increased to a maximum dose of 1 g/m^2. This dose is adjusted to maintain the two-week leukocyte nadir at more than 3000/mm^3. When the daily oral regimen is used, CYC is given at 1.5–2 mg/kg/day, adjusting the dose to maintain the leukocyte count above 3000/mm^3 throughout therapy. CYC is traditionally continued for a total of three to six months, depending on the patient's response to treatment. The optimal route of CYC therapy (daily oral vs. IV pulse) was examined in a randomized controlled trial (de Groot et al., 2010; Harper et al., 2012) which demonstrated that the IV regimen allows for a ~twofold smaller cumulative dose of CYC than the oral regimen and is associated with a decrease in the rate of clinically significant neutropenia. However, it does not lead to any difference in time to remission, likelihood of a remission, or long-term outcomes, compared to daily oral CYC, and the risk of relapse may be higher. The regimen of daily oral CYC is associated with a decreased risk of relapse (Guillevin et al., 1997; Harper et al., 2012). Overall relapse rate was 40 per cent in the pulse IV CYC and 21 per cent in the oral CYC group after four years of follow-up (Harper et al., 2012). However, despite the increase in relapse rate with the IV CYC regimen, the final outcomes of patients (death or ESRD) are no different between the two-dose regimen after a follow-up of about four years (Harper et al., 2012); thus, either approach to a CYC dosing regimen for induction is reasonable. IV CYC used with steroids and plasmapheresis can be quite effective in dialysis-dependent patients with ANCA RLV (Pepper et al., 2013), but dosage needs to be adjusted appropriately. Secondary analyses of randomized trials have suggested that anti-PR3 positive patients with ANCA vasculitis respond better to RTX than to CYC for induction of remission, especially in relapsing disease (see 'Relapsing disease'; Unizony et al., 2016). No such relationship between serology and treatment response was observed in MPO-ANCA vasculitis.

Rituximab for induction
Rituximab has a long history of use in ANCA vasculitis (Eriksson, 2005). As a result of two pivotal randomized controlled trials (RCTs; RAVE and RITUXIVAS) (Stone et al., 2010; Jones et al., 2010) RTX, a chimeric anti-CD20 monoclonal antibody (see Chapter 2) has been added to the therapeutic armamentarium for ANCA vasculitis, including RLV. In the RAVE trial, 197 patients with either GPA or MPA as *de novo* or relapsing disease, the majority of whom had renal manifestations, were randomized in a double-blind, double-dummy

fashion to receive either daily oral CYC (2 mg/kg/day) or RTX (375 mg/m^2 per week for four weeks) and followed for up to 18 months. Both groups received similar initial high steroid dosing followed by gradual tapering regimen. After attaining remission (usually within three months but up to six months), patients in the RTX group were followed without further therapy for relapses for an additional 12–15 months (Specks et al., 2013), while those in the CYC group were maintained on oral azathioprine (AZA; 2 mg/kg/day) and followed for a comparable period of time. The primary end-point was complete remission of all disease active without the use of any prednisone at six months. All patients were ANCA positive (2/3 anti-PR3 and 1/3 anti-MPO) at baseline. A serum creatinine of >4.0 mg/dl and/or life-threatening pulmonary haemorrhage were exclusion factors in the trial.

After six months, 64 per cent of patients in the RTX group and 53 per cent in the CYC group met the primary outcome criteria. These results met the pre-specified criterion of non-inferiority. The results in the CYC group for patients who were relapsing at entry were inferior to those in the RTX group. No difference in effectiveness of CYC or RTX was seen in those with moderately severe renal disease (serum creatinine levels of 1.5–4.0 mg/dl or mild-to-moderate non-life threatening pulmonary haemorrhage). Adverse events were similar, except for leukopenia in the CYC group, as expected. B-cell depletion was more rapid in the RTX group, but both groups attained marked peripheral B-cell (CD-19 counts) depletion. After 18 months of the study, 39 per cent of RTX-only treated patients and 33 per cent of the CYC-AZA patients maintained a remission (Specks et al., 2013). Reconstitution of B-cells occurred at about six to nine months in the RTX group (see 'Prevention of relapses'). ANCA levels fell during the initial six months of treatment in both groups, but up to 50 per cent remained positive at the end of the six-month induction period. This study lead to the approval of RTX by the US Food and Drug Administration for induction of remission in GPA and MPA (and by inference, ANCA-associated RLV as well).

Combinations of RTX and lower doses of CYC were also effective in the RITUXIVAS study (Jones et al., 2010). Such combinations have also been used successfully for induction of remissions in observational trials (Niles et al., 2011). As mentioned, RTX may be preferred for induction of remission in patients with anti-PR3 ANCA vasculitis, specifically in relapsing disease (Unizony et al., 2016). Additionally, a protocol involving additional doses of RTX after the conventional initial course has shown more prolonged remissions, but this protocol has not yet been tested in a randomized clinical trial (Rocatello et al., 2017). The benefits of RTX or CYC therapy for patients with ANCA vasculitis and severe renal disease appears comparable (Geetha et al., 2015, 2016). In a cohort study using a combined regimen of RTX, low-dose CYC, and shortened course of corticosteroids, followed by maintenance with AZA or MMF was associated with significantly improved patient and renal survival and relapse rate compared to a propensity-matched retrospective control group treated with CYC and corticosteroids (McAdoo, et al., 2018).

Ofatumumab, a second-generation anti-CD20 monoclonal antibody, may also be effective for induction of remissions in ANCA vasculitis, and may also be useful in RTX-resistant cases (McAdoo et al., 2018). RTX therapy has also been reported to fail to manage the extra-reanl granulomatous manifestations of GPA, at least in some cases (Aries et al , 2005). Long term studies have generally supported a beneficial effect of RTX in ANCA Vasculitis (Stasi, et al, 2006)

Mycophenolate mofetil (MMF) for induction
The effectiveness of MMF for induction of a remission in ANCA vasculitis has been less rigorously tested than for CYC or RTX. Small uncontrolled, open label studies have demonstrated encouraging results (Joy et al., 2005; Stassen et al., 2007; Silva et al., 2011; Han et al., 2011; Chaigne et al., 2013). In a small open-label, randomized controlled study from China, patients with ANCA-associated vasculitis (predominantly anti-MPO) were assigned to MMF or monthly IV CYC. At six months, the complete remission rate was 78 per cent in the MMF group and 47 per cent in the CYC group. Side-effects were approximately equal in the two groups (Hu et al., 2008). Adverse events increase when GFR was reduced.

In a pilot study using MMF plus steroids in anti-MPO positive mild-to-moderate vasculitis (some of the subjects had renal limited disease) achieved a remission rate of 76 per cent by 60 months (Silva et al., 2010). In a retrospective review of 51 cases, 57 per cent had relapsing disease, 89 per cent responded by about four months (Koukoulaki and Jayne, 2006). In most of these studies MMF was used in doses of 1–3 g/day (average 2 g/day) and ANCA titres fell with therapy. Relapses were common when treatment was withdrawn, or dosage reduced) (Koukoulaki and Jayne, 2006). Severe adverse events were uncommon, and mainly gastrointestinal or infectious in nature. Similar results have been reported by Han and colleagues (2011) in a prospective trial of MMF versus IV CYC in MPA. Due to interindividual variability in the pharmacokinetics of MMF, better results may be obtained if drug levels (MPA) and area under the curve (AUC) kinetics are monitored during therapy with MMF (Chainge et al., 2013). It is possible that enteric-coated mycophenolate sodium may be superior to MMF, but this is not well established (Jones et al., 2014). Long-term outcomes are quite favourable in Chinese patients (Chen al., 2016), most of whom have anti-MPO ANCA vasculitis.

On balance, it appears that MMF combined with steroids can be a useful and effective approach to ANCA vasculitis with renal involvement (including ANCA RLV) mainly in anti-MPO-associated disease of a non-life-threatening nature (Silva et al., 2010). However, relapses are common (see 'Relapsing disease'). MMF may be especially useful in those patients who are unable to take or tolerate CYC or RTX (Stassen et al., 2007).

Plasmapheresis for induction

The addition of *plasmapheresis* (also called apheresis or plasma exchange; PLEX) to induction therapy with glucocorticoids and CYC, RTX, or MMF for ANCA-associated vasculitis has been considered of potential benefit for patients presenting with advanced renal failure (creatinine >500 micromol/l or dialysis-requiring renal failure or with life-endangering diffuse alveolar haemorrhage.

In a large, multicentre controlled trial (MEPEX Trial; Jayne et al., 2007), 137 patients with a new diagnosis of ANCA vasculitis confirmed by renal biopsy and severe renal failure (Serum creatinine >5.8 mg/dl; >510 μm/l) were randomly assigned to either treatment with plasmapheresis (n = 70), or 3000 mg of IV MP (n = 67). Both groups received standard-of-care therapy with oral CYC and oral prednisone followed by AZA for maintenance. Plasmapheresis consisted of seven treatment sessions within 14 days of study entry with a volume of 60 ml/kg on each occasion; the replacement was with five per cent albumin. Fresh frozen plasma at the end of the procedure was used in patients who were at risk of haemorrhage (or in subjects who have recently [<72 hours] undergone a percutaneous renal biopsy). Compared to pulse MP, plasmapheresis was associated with a significant increase in renal recovery at three months (69 per cent of patients who received plasmapheresis vs. 49 per cent of patients in the IV MP group), and of dialysis-free survival at 12 months. The hazard ratio for ESRD over 12 months for the plasmapheresis versus MP groups was 0.47 (95 per cent; CI: 0.24–0.91, P = 0.03). Long-term follow-up of the MEPEX trial patients did not clearly demonstrate any lasting beneficial effect of plasmapheresis in patients with dialysis-dependent ANCA vasculitis (Walsh et al., 2013). The uncertainty around the role of plasmapheresis led to the conduct of the much larger PEXIVAS trial (reported only in abstract form at the time of writing). In this randomized controlled trial of 704 patients with ANCA vasculitis and eGFR < 50 ml/min/1.73 m^2 (including 204 with baseline Cr > 5.8 mg/dl), the addition of plasmapheresis to background immunosuppression with corticosteroids plus CYC or RTX was not associated with a reduction in death or end stage kidney disease (NCT#00987389; Walsh M. 2013; Merkel P 2018).

Full publication of this landmark trial is eagerly awaited and it may transform clinical practice concerning use of plasmapheresis in treatment of ANCA vasculitis (without concomitant anti-GBM antibody). Importantly, a sub-group analysis of the 69 patients from the MEPEX trial who presented with dialysis-dependent acute renal failure at the beginning of this trial (de Lind van Wijngaarden et al., 2007) revealed that the point at which the chance of dying from therapy with plasmapheresis exceeds that of the chance of re-covery was reached only in patients with severe tubular atrophy and <2 per cent of glomeruli remaining normal. This analysis suggests that there is essen-tially no histological determinant that would render a trial of therapy futile in the management of patients with ANCA vasculitis presenting with ad-vanced renal failure. Among patients who require haemodialysis, those who do recover sufficient renal function nearly always do so within the first three months of treatment (Nachman et al., 1996; de Lind van Wijngaarden et al., 2007). In a retrospective analysis of outcomes of 46 patients receiving main-tenance immunosuppression while requiring chronic dialysis, no patient died of active vasculitis (Weidanz et al., 2007). Rather, the major cause of death was infection, and the vast majority of non-fatal infections occurred in patients receiving immunosuppression. Importantly, the relapse rate post-dialysis was significantly less than pre-dialysis (RR 0.4, 95 per cent; CI: 0.15–0.98, P = 0.044). This study suggests that the risk of fatal and non-fatal infection is higher than the risk of relapse or death from active disease (Lionaki et al., 2009). Considering that most patients who will recover renal function after suffering acute renal failure from RLV do so in the first three months after initiation of dialysis (Nachman et al., 1996; de Lind van Wijngaarden et al., 2007), a rational approach would be to discontinue immunosuppressive therapy in all patients who do not have clinical evidence for active disease and who have not recovered renal function by that point. Plasmapheresis continues to be recommended in patients with anti-GBM disease, and, as mentioned, patients with combined ANCA and anti-GBM disease who are dialysis dependent may respond better to immunosuppression plus intensive plasmapheresis (McAdoo et al., 2017).

Other agents
Although the use of CYC and/or RTX has emerged as preferred therapy for ANCA RLV (and systemic ANCA vasculitis), novel agents continue to attract attention, particularly for refractory or mild cases (Tervaert et al., 2001). The use of *methotrexate* in lieu of CYC, RTX, or MMF has been advocated for patients suffering from mild ANCA vasculitis without significant renal impairment (Sneller et al., 1995). In an RCT of induction therapy among patients with 'early'

ANCA vasculitis comparing weekly methotrexate to daily oral CYC, the rate of remission at six months was comparable among the two treatment groups (De et al., 2005). However, the onset of remission in methotrexate-treated patients with relatively extensive disease was delayed. Methotrexate was also associated with a significantly higher rate of relapse than CYC (69.5 per cent vs. 46.5 per cent), and 45 per cent of relapses occurred while patients were receiving methotrexate (De Groot et al., 2005). Importantly, methotrexate is relatively contraindicated for patients with renal impairment. The dose of methotrexate must be reduced in patients with a creatinine clearance <80 ml/min, and its use is contraindicated when creatinine clearances are <10 ml/min. Overall, the role of methotrexate in ANCA vasculitis appears to be limited to a very select group of patients with mild renal and extrarenal disease. It is not appropriate for patients with RLV and decreased renal function.

Calcineurin inhibitors (CNI; cyclosporine or tacrolimus) have been used sparingly for induction of a remission in ANCA vasculitis because of the demonstrated efficacy of CYC-, RTX-, or MMF-based regimens (Allen, 1993). Also, these agents may have value in preventing relapses or, rarely, in patients who are intolerant of other disease-remitting agents (Haubitz et al., 1998; Ramachandran et al., 2015), but there are no randomized trials.

Deoxyspergualin (gusperimus) and leflunomide might have potential utility for induction therapy in ANCA vasculitis, but the information available is too limited to make any recommendation (Tervaert et al., 2001; Furuta and Jayne, 2014). These agents might find a niche in treatment of relapses or in those patients refractory to standard induction therapy (Birck et al., 2003).

Complement (C) inhibition is an emerging new therapy for ANCA vasculitis. The rationale for this approach is provided by evidence for involvement of the alternative and lectin pathways of C activation in pathogenesis of the disease (Chen et al., 2017). A recently completed phase 2 RCT of a C5a receptor inhibitor (Avacopan; CCX168) has shown efficacy as a steroid-sparing alternative when added to standard immunosuppressive therapy with CYC or RTX in treatment of ANCA-associated vasculitis (CLEAR trial; Jayne et al., 2017). Further studies exploring the value of complement inhibition in ANCA vasculitis are in progress (e.g.; NCT# 02994927; and NCT03712345).

Management of induction therapy-resistant disease

Unresponsiveness to initial induction therapy for ANCA vasculitis (including RLV) is uncommon in the absence of severe renal disease (Lee et al., 2014). In a retrospective analysis of 155 patients with ANCA vasculitis and severe renal disease at presentation (median eGFR = 7.1 ml/min/1.73 m^2; 87 per cent requiring haemodialysis), Lee and colleagues (2014) found that non-response at four months after induction therapy (primarily with CYC and steroids) was approximately 50 per cent. Only five per cent of patients remaining on dialysis at four months eventually regained renal function. Importantly, no futility threshold at presentation could be identified, but prolonged immunosuppressive therapy beyond four months was very unlikely to have any benefit for patients who remained dialysis dependent.

Several agents have been evaluated as adjunctive therapy for patients with disease resistant to induction of a remission by conventional therapy with glucocorticoids and CYC. Before the introduction of RTX to the armamentarium, adjunctive therapy with IVIg (single course of a total of 2 gm/kg) was evaluated in a RCT in patients with persistently active ANCA vasculitis despite conventional therapy. Patients treated with IVIg experienced a more rapid decline in disease activity (as measured by a 50 per cent reduction in systemic vasculitis activity scores) and C-reactive protein at months one and three, but there was no significant difference between the two groups after three months with respect to disease activity or frequency of relapse (Jayne et al., 2000). IVIg has significant anti-inflammatory and immunomodulating properties (see Chapter 3).

Since the introduction of RTX, the combined use of CYC and RTX appears to have supplanted other combination therapies (including concomitant use of IVIg) for patients with severe ANCA vasculitis who fail to respond, or continue to progress, despite initial therapy with CYC and plasmapheresis.

Alemtuzumab (Campath-1H[*]) is a humanized monoclonal IgG1 antibody directed against the CD52 antigen expressed on the surface of peripheral blood lymphocytes, monocytes, and macrophages (Kirk et al., 2003). Treatment with alemtuzumab leads to complement-mediated lysis, antibody-dependent cellular cytotoxicity, and induction of apoptosis of target cells and results in depletion of T-cells and B-cells (Isaacs et al., 1996). Alemtuzumab has been used to treat a select group of 71 patients with refractory or multiply relapsing ANCA vasculitis, often with severe extrarenal vasculitis (Jayne, 2002). These patients received at least one course of 134mg IV alemtuzumab over five days. Clinical remission on no immunosuppression was achieved in 65 per cent of patients. Unfortunately, this treatment regimen was associated with high rates of serious infection and death (mortality rate of 0.09 per patient year), and 60 per cent experienced a relapse with a median relapse-free survival of 9.2 months. Alemtuzumab has also been associated (paradoxically) with the development of anti-GBM antibody nephritis (Clatworthy et al., 2008). The use of alemtuzumab should best be restricted to very severe, resistant cases, and in settings with experience using this medication. It would not ordinarily be used in treatment of RLV.

Tumour necrosis factor (TNF)-α is thought to play an important role in the pathogenesis of ANCA vasculitis based on in vitro and in vivo data (Lamprecht et al., 2007). The chimeric monoclonal antibody directed against TNF-α, *infliximab*, was evaluated in a small, open-label, uncontrolled case series of patients where infliximab was used in conjunction with corticosteroids, and either CYC or other immunosuppressive agents. In the largest of these studies, which included 32 patients with acute or resistant disease, infliximab was associated with a remission rate of 88 per cent and a relapse rate of 20 per cent (Booth et al., 2004). These promising results are seriously mitigated, however, by an elevated rate of serious infectious complications. In addition, the use of TNF inhibitors has paradoxically been associated with an increased risk of developing an auto-immune disease resembling systemic lupus erythematosus. TNF inhibitors play a very limited, if any, role in management of ANCA RLV, except perhaps in treatment refractory cases (McAdoo and Pusey, 2017b)Deoxyspergualin, an immunosuppressant agent (15-deoxyspergualin) is thought to be effective in some auto-immune diseases. Experience is limited in RLV, but preliminary observations suggest efficacy in refractory cases of systemic ANCA vasculitis. No randomized controlled trials have been conducted. Leukopenia is common (Birck et al., 2003).

Relapsing disease

Overview

All forms of ANCA-associated vasculitis have a tendency to relapse after induction of a remission, less so after a complete compared to partial remission. Relapsing ANCA-associated vasculitis responds to immunosuppression with glucocorticoids and other agents with a similar response rate as the initial disease (Nachman et al., 1996), however relapsing ANCA positive RLV without anti-GBM antibodies seems to respond better to RTX than to CYC (See RAVE trial above (Stone et al, 2010, Specks, 2015) . Relapses in ANCA vasculitis and RLV are difficult to predict and reliable, verified biomarkers suitable for this purpose are largely lacking but continue to be sought (Specks, 2015).

Patients with a history of relapsing disease pose a particular challenge because they are subject to the cumulative toxic effects of glucocorticoids and other agents. Due to the serious consequences of high cumulative dosage of CYC (oncogenesis, myelotoxicity, gonadal toxicity and aspermatogenesis, cystitis, and bladder cancer and infections), there has been a strong the impetus to find alternatives to CYC for maintenance of remission, especially for patients with mild-to-moderate disease

Several agents have been evaluated for maintenance immunosuppressive therapy with a goal to prevent future relapses. These *prophylactic* studies must be clearly differentiated from *treatment of* an established relapse. In evaluating studies of prevention of relapse, important considerations should be kept in mind:

- The *risk* of relapse is not uniform among all patients with ANCA vasculitis. Depending on the number of risk factors, the incidence of relapse may vary from 26 per cent over a median of 62 months, to 47 per cent over a median of 39 months (Hogan et al., 2005).

- Serial ANCA titres may have utility in predicting relapse (especially anti-PR3 antibodies) (Han et al., 2003), as disease relapses are particularly likely to occur in anti-PR3 ANCA vasculitis.

- Anti-PR3 antibodies are less frequently identified in RLV compared to anti-MPO antibodies.

- Relapse tends to be less common in RLV mediated by anti-MPO antibodies, and even persistence of anti-MPO antibodies may be accompanied by stable or inactive disease (auto-antibodies directed to 'non-pathogenic' MPO epitopes).

A reduced level of circulating CD5 + CD24^{hi} + CD38^{hi} + B-cells at the time of peripheral B cell reconstitution after RTX induction therapy may portend a higher risk of relapse in ANCA vasculitis treated with CYC and steroids (Bunch et al., 2013; Aybar et al., 2015; Bunch et al., 2015), perhaps by impairing immunomodulatory endogenous production of Il-10. However, this result has not been confirmed in an analysis of CD5 + B-cells in patients treated with CYC or RTX (Unizony et al., 2015). High levels of urinary soluble CD163 (sCD163) which is a glycosylated membrane protein exclusively expressed on monocytes and macrophages and is presumed to be shed by glomerular crescent macrophages have also been reported to be a sensitive and specific marker of active (crescentic) renal vasculitis but not with non-renal exacerbations of vasculitis (O'Reilly et al., 2016; Free and Falk, 2016). Prospective studies are needed to validate the utility of these findings compared to other common and inexpensive biomarkers of renal vasculitis, such as serial urinalyses (Free and Falk, 2016). Box 10.2 shows factors contributing to a higher risk of relapse (adapted from Morgan et al., 2017; Goceroglu et al., 2016).

- The efficacy of a drug regimen in *preventing* relapse can only be assessed if compared to a placebo or active comparator.

- Therefore, in order to convincingly demonstrate efficacy in preventing relapse, a study should target a population at high and predictable risk for relapse, followed for a sufficiently long period of time, and include a control group treated with placebo or an active comparator.

Box 10.2 Factors that have been associated with a higher risk of relapse in ANCA-associated vasculitis (including RLV)

- Younger age.
- Better renal function at discovery.
- Clinical diagnosis of GPA and anti-PR3 antibody positive at discovery (this does not pertain to RLV).
- Pulmonary vasculitis (alveolar haemorrhage or pulmonary nodules or cavities) (this does not pertain to RLV).
- Upper respiratory tract involvement (this does not pertain to RLV).
- Use of IV pulse CYC therapy for induction.
- Too rapid steroid withdrawal (?—controversial).
- Persisting ANCA + at time of conversion from induction to maintenance regimens, especially with anti-PR3 positive ANCA (not consistently observed).
- Conversion from negative to positive ANCA after remission (the effect upon relapses of a rise in ANCA titre is less convincing unless the titre rise is fourfold or greater).
- MMF or methotrexate for induction and/or maintenance compared to AZA (controversial).

- Unfortunately, many published reports on the subject have been open-label, uncontrolled cohort studies with a small number of patients followed over a relatively short period of time. Recent controlled trials have partially remedied this deficiency.

Prevention of relapses

It is important the note that the studies and trials of relapse prevention reviewed here have all been conducted in patients with systemic ANCA-vasculitis. Although these trials included a minority of patients with RLV (or intentionally excluded them from the study), the necessity for and benefit of these interventions in preventing relapse of renal vasculitis have not been formally evaluated and cannot be directly deduced from these studies. There is currently little direct evidence that patients with RLV and MPO-ANCA require maintenance immunosuppression for the prevention of relapse.

Trimethoprim-sulfamethoxazole (co-trimoxazole)

The only placebo-controlled study evaluated benefit of co-trimoxazole in the prevention of relapses in patients with GPA: no studies of prevention of relapses in RLV using co-trimoxazole have been conducted. In this study, co-trimoxazole was effective in preventing systemic relapses involving the nose and upper respiratory tract, but no benefit was seen in disease affecting the kidneys or other organ systems (Guillevin et al., 1999).

Azathioprine (AZA)

If the patient has reached a complete remission after three months of treatment with CYC, switching from CYC to oral AZA is effective and useful in decreasing exposure to the cumulative toxic effects of CYC. Oral AZA (1–3 mg/kg/day) is then continued for 12–18 months or longer, depending on the response and side-effects. This regimen offers the advantage of limiting the use of CYC and results in similar rates of remission and relapse as the CYC-only-based therapy in a large randomized and controlled study (CYCAZAREM; Jayne et al., 2003). Patients whose PR3-ANCA titres remain positive at the time of the switch to AZA may have about a twofold increased risk of subsequent relapse when compared to patients whose ANCA titres have reverted to negative (Sanders et al., 2006). This finding has not been confirmed in a more recent prospective randomized trial of extended vs. standard duration maintenance therapy with AZA (Sanders et al., 2016)

Although not specifically designed to demonstrate the ability of AZA to *prevent* relapses (compared to a placebo for example), the CYCAZAREM study established that substituting AZA for CYC after three to six months of induction therapy versus 12 months resulted in similar rates of relapse (Jayne et al., 2003) over the short term (Jayne et al., 2003). Whether converting to AZA at 12 months versus three to six months is best, remains uncertain as long-term follow-up has shown poor outcomes in both strategies (Walsh et al., 2014). Relapses of ANCA vasculitis can occur during AZA maintenance or after its discontinuation, at about the same rate (one relapse per 113–117 patient months of AZA therapy regardless of the duration of maintenance therapy (> or < 18 months; de Joode et al., 2017). Lower relapse-free survival was associate with IV CYC induction and anti-PR3 ANCA.

MMF

The efficacy of MMF compared to AZA in preventing relapses was examined in a randomized trial (IMPROVE) by the European Vasculitis Study Group. The results of this trial strongly suggest that MMF appears inferior to AZA for maintenance of remission in patients who are induced with a CYC–steroid regimen (Hiemstra et al., 2010). After a three-year observation period, relapses occurred in 55 per cent of the MMF-treated patients and in 38 per cent of the AZA-treated groups. MMF is not suggested for maintenance therapy of ANCA vasculitis, unless patients are intolerant of AZA or cannot receive RTX (see 'Rituximab'). Variability in the efficacy of MMF might be attributed to heterogeneity of pharmacokinetics. Therapeutic blood level monitoring of MPA might improve results (Schaier et al., 2015).

Rituximab

Observational studies have strongly suggested that periodic (every four to six months) RTX (500–1000 mg) administration, for continuous B-cell depletion, after induction of a remission, is effective prophylaxis for relapses (Pendergraft et al., 2014; Rhee et al., 2010). Such an approach can allow for a substantial decline in other immunosuppressive and steroid therapy without exacerbating the risk of relapse. Prolonged RTX therapy (Median 2.1 years, maximum seven years) has so far been free of major side-effects, except for a 10 per cent prevalence of late-onset neutropenia (Rhee et al., 2010) and a ten per cent prevalence of hypogammaglobulinaemia (Pendergraft et al., 2014). In the largest study to date, Pendergraft and colleagues at Boston's Massachusetts General Hospital found major relapse in six per cent of patients with anti-MPO ANCA and four per cent in patients with anti-PR3 ANCA using the continuous B-cell depletion regimen. Patient survival was excellent, but advanced age (>80 years) was a mortality risk. It is of some interest that despite continuous B-cell depletion in the peripheral blood, over 50 per cent of the patients with anti-MPO ANCA and 25 per cent of the patients with anti-PR3 ANCA had positive titres throughout the study period. Despite its limitations as an uncontrolled study where confounding variables (e.g. intense observation and clinical care) might have influenced the outcomes, these studies suggest that continual prophylactic use of RTX in ANCA vasculitis (probably including RLV) can substantially reduce the relapse rate and the burden of immunosuppression at very acceptable level of adverse event rates, but the very long-term complications of RTX in this setting are unknown, and the optimal duration of treatment is also uncertain (de Joode et al., 2015)

The French Vasculitis Study Group conducted a randomized trial comparing the efficacy of AZA (in gradually diminishing dosage) to periodic RTX (500 mg RTX on day 0 and 14, and repeated at six, 12, and 18 months without steroids) after induction of a complete remission using a CYC-prednisone regimen (Guillevin et al., 2014). At month 28, major relapse had occurred in 29 per cent of the AZA group and in five per cent of the RTX group. The frequency of severe adverse events was similar in both groups. Tapering doses of

AZA might have contributed to the higher risk of relapse in the AZA group, but the effects of RTX on relapse rates found in the observational trials mentioned earlier were confirmed. Other ongoing trials (RITAZAREM, NCT# 01697267 [Gopaluni et al., 2017]) are examining the relative benefits of RTX (1000 mg every four months for five doses) or AZA 2 mg/kg/day in relapsing forms of ANCA vasculitis in which a remission has been induced with RTX + steroids. The primary end-point is time to disease relapse. Follow up is anticipated to be 36 months.

The optimal dose and frequency of RTX therapy for the maintenance of remission was evaluated in a randomized controlled trial comparing an 'as needed' dosing regimen based on ANCA and CD19 + B-cells compared to regular systematic infusions of 500 mg IV every six months (MAINRITSAN-II; Charles et al., 2018). The relapse rate did not differ significantly when RTX dosing was directed either by a reappearance of CD19+ B lymphocytes or of ANCA, or by a marked increase in ANCA titer as compared to a fixed schedule RTX therapy (500 mg IV every 6 months) after a 28-month follow-up. Fewer RTX infusions were given to the tailored dosing regimen group.In October, 2018 the US FDA approved the use of RTX (according to the protocol used in the MAINRITSAN-I trial) for use in follow-up treatment of GPA, MPA and RLV.

TNF inhibition

The efficacy and safety of the TNF receptor–Fc fusion protein *etanercept* in the maintenance of remission among patients with Wegener's granulomatosis was evaluated in a randomized controlled trial. In that study, etanercept or placebo were added to a regimen of daily oral CYC or methotrexate and corticosteroids. The use of etanercept failed to affect the rate or the severity of relapses, and was associated with a higher rate of solid tumours (Stone, 2003).

Methotrexate or leflunomide

Methotrexate is similarly effective and safe compared to AZA for prevention of relapses in systemic ANCA-associated vasculitis (Pagnoux et al., 2008). Whether this is also true for RLV is unknown. One prospective, multicentre RCT compared the use of *methotrexate* to *leflunomide* in 54 patients with the diagnosis of GPA (Metzler et al., 2007). All patients received induction therapy with prednisone and oral CYC (2 mg/kg/day) for six months. In the methotrexate group, patients were then started on 7.5 mg/week orally, and then titrated upward to 15 mg/week by week five, and 20 mg/week after week eight. Leflunomide was started with a loading dose of 100 mg/day orally for the first three days, followed by 20 mg/day for up to four weeks and continued at 30 mg/day thereafter. This study was terminated early because of a significantly higher rate of major and minor relapse in the methotrexate group compared with the leflunomide group. Significant adverse events occurred in the leflunomide group, including hypertension, persistent leukopenia, and peripheral neuropathy in one patient. It appears from this study that methotrexate is inferior to leflunomide in preventing relapse of GPA. Its effect on RLV is uncertain. Whether a lower dose of leflunomide would be equally as effective but associated with fewer side-effects remains to be determined.

Treatment of relapses

Mild relapses can often be satisfactorily treated with a temporary increase in steroid dosage (Miloslavsky et al., 2015), but repetitive relapses will require a more aggressive approach. Retreatment of relapses with RTX and steroids seems to be both safe and very effective (Miroslavsky et al., 2014). In the absence of controlled trials use of other agents, e.g. AZA, MMF, CNI, or MTX, cannot be recommended. The RAVE trial (Stone et al., 2010; see also 'Rituximab for induction') showed superiority of RTX plus steroids over oral CYC plus steroids for re-induction of a remission in relapsing ANCA vasculitis. Therefore, at this time, RTX plus steroids (with steroid dosage lower than used for induction of remission unless the relapse is very severe) seems to be the preferred regimen for treatment of relapsing ANCA vasculitis, probably including RLV.

The use of six-monthly pulses of IVIg (0.5 g/kg/day × four days) was evaluated for the treatment of relapse occurring while on glucocorticoids and/or immunosuppressants (CYC, AZA, methotrexate, or MMF; Martinez et al., 2008) in a small open label, uncontrolled study of 22 patients. IVIg was added to the immunosuppressant regime the patient was receiving with good initial response. Patients with renal dysfunction should receive a sucrose-free formulation of IVIg in order to minimize the risk of osmotic agent-induced acute renal failure (Dickenmann et al., 2008). The use of IVIg has been largely supplanted by that of RTX and is seldom used in contemporary management of RLV.

ANCA negative and anti-GBM negative renal-limited pauci-immune necrotizing/crescentic GN vasculitis

About 5–10 per cent of patients with pauci-immune necrotizing and crescentic GN without systemic manifestations (RLV) may present with persistently negative ANCA and anti-GBM antibody tests. These patients are typically treated according to the same guidelines as for patients who are ANCA positive. The number of these patients is small, and no specific therapeutic studies or outcome measures have been published specifically for this group of patients. A therapeutic dilemma occurs when such patients present with advanced renal failure or diffuse pulmonary haemorrhage (i.e. with indication for plasmapheresis). Here again, there is unfortunately no data to support or refute the use of plasmapheresis in this situation. Because of the severity of these presentations and the narrow window of opportunity to intervene successfully, we have erred on the side of providing plasmapheresis in these circumstances. It is conceivable that these patients have auto-antibodies to either other antigens or to epitopes of PR3 or MPO that are not readily detected by the currently available tests (Hellmich et al., 2007; Roth et al., 2012). It is noteworthy that such patients were indeed included in the MEPEX controlled trial of plasmapheresis vs. MP (Jayne et al., 2007).

ANCA-negative and anti-GBM negative immune complex-mediated RLV

As already described, ANCA and anti-GBM negative immune complex-mediated crescentic GN are quite often secondary to infections, malignancy, or auto-immune diseases such as SLE, or superimposed on another primary glomerular disease (such as IgA nephropathy or membranous nephropathy (see Chapter 6 and Chapter 7). Truly 'idiopathic' primary immune complex GN (immune complex-mediated RLV) is very uncommon. Therefore, prior to commencing immunomodulating and anti-inflammatory therapy, patients with apparently 'idiopathic' immune complex-mediated RLV should undergo a thorough screen for occult malignancy, other auto-immune disease (e.g. SLE), or infection. As noted previously, drug-associated RLV is usually anti-MPO ANCA positive and the lesions are typically pauci-immune necrotizing and crescentic GN. There is no direct information on the treatment of primary ('idiopathic') immune complex RLV. The separation of 'pauci-immune' from 'immune complex' RLV can be difficult. The treatment of such patients is therefore mirrored on that of ANCA-positive patients or patients with lupus nephritis using pulse *IV MP* followed by *oral glucocorticoids* and RTX or IV or oral CYC for patients with moderate or severe renal impairment and glomerular crescents involving >20 per cent of glomeruli. Patients with milder form of disease, lesser crescentic involvement, and relatively well-preserved renal function may conceivably receive therapy with oral glucocorticoids and MMF (1–1.5 g twice daily).

ANCA-negative, and anti-GBM-positive RLV (anti-GBM disease)

This section discusses the management of anti-GBM disease unaccompanied by pulmonary haemorrhage or associated with co-existing ANCA.

The standard treatment for anti-GBM disease consists of oral *glucocorticoids*, oral CYC, and intensive *plasmapheresis* (Turner and Rees, 1998; Levy et al., 2001). Plasmapheresis consists of removal of 50 ml/kg (for a maximum of 4l) of plasma with replacement with a five per cent albumin solution, performed daily for at least 14 days or until circulating antibody levels become undetectable (Levy et al., 2001; McAdoo and Pusey, 2017). Typically, in anti-GBM disease the titres of anti-GBM antibody decline rapidly with adequate therapy and frequency of plasmapheresis sessions. With adequate plasmapheresis dosage anti-GBM antibody levels typically become negative by eight weeks, with rare exceptions. (Savage et al., 1986). About 50 per cent of patients should clear circulating anti-GBM antibody within four weeks. Anti-GBM antibody levels will decay slowly even without treatment but this may take many months and, rarely, more than a year. In those patients with pulmonary haemorrhage, clotting factors should be replaced by administering fresh-frozen plasma at the end of each plasmapheresis treatment. Similarly to the regimen described for ANCA-associated vasculitis, prednisone is started at 1 mg/kg/day (for a maximum dose of 60 mg/day) and tapered after the first month over a period of four to five months. The role of high-dose IV MP pulses (7mg/kg/day × three days for a maximum dose of 500 mg/day) remains unproven in the treatment of anti-GBM disease. Nonetheless, the urgent nature of the clinical process prompts some nephrologists to administer MP as part of induction therapy. No data is available as to the optimal modality or duration of CYC therapy, but the IV administration of CYC is generally not recommended. At London's Hammersmith Hospital, CYC is given orally (2–3 mg/kg/day) for up to three months. A reduced dosage of CYC should be used if severe renal failure is present or in patients who are dialysis dependent, and in the absence of pulmonary haemorrhage, treatment should be discontinued after 8–12 weeks if there is no recovery of renal function (Levy et al., 2001).

Using this regimen, patient survival is approximately 85 per cent with 40 per cent progression to ESRD (Lockwood et al., 1976; Madore et al., 1996; Pusey et al., 1983; Pusey, 1990; McAdoo and Pusey, 2017). These results are better than those before the introduction of plasmapheresis, when patient survival was <50 per cent with a near 90 per cent rate of ESRD. In a retrospective analysis of 71 patients treated with plasmapheresis, prednisolone, and CYC, patient and renal survival were excellent among patients presenting with a serum creatinine <500 μmol/l (5.7 mg/dl) (100 per cent and 95 per cent respectively at one year and 94 per cent at a median follow up of 90 months). Among patients presenting with a serum creatinine >500 μmol/l but not needing dialysis, patient and renal survival were 83 per cent and 82 per cent, respectively at one year and 80 per cent and 50 per cent respectively, long term. In contrast, the outcome at one year of patients on dialysis was significantly worse, with 65 per cent patient survival and only eight per cent renal survival (Levy et al., 2001). Therefore, if plasmapheresis is to be effective, it must be initiated as early as possible in the course of the disease. Although no absolute degree of crescent formation alone predicted irreversible renal failure, no patient who required immediate dialysis and had 100 per cent crescents on renal biopsy recovered renal function (Levy et al., 2001). Oligo-anuria at presentation is also an ominous finding, indicating a high likelihood of progression to ESRD, despite aggressive therapy (Alchi et al., 2015). These findings underscore the importance of early recognition of the anti-GBM positive forms of RLV. Combination therapy with corticosteroids, CYC, and PLEX has a pronounced beneficial effect on both renal and patient survival (Cui et al., 2011), providing it is begun before dialysis dependency ensues.

Once remission of anti-GBM disease is achieved with immunosuppressive and plasmapheresis therapy, recurrent (relapsing) disease occurs only rarely (<3 per cent) (Levy et al., 2001; McAdoo and Pusey, 2017 Glassock, 2017). Similarly, the recurrence of anti-GBM disease after renal transplantation is also rare, especially when transplantation is delayed until after disappearance of anti-GBM antibody in the circulation (Almkuist et al., 1981; see 'Transplantation'). Because of the rarity of relapses, the course of immunosuppression can be brief (three to six months) and maintenance immunosuppression is not required. Rarely, repeated plasmapheresis and continued immunosuppression, sometimes using RTX, can be required for relapsing disease. (Touzot et al., 2015; Glassock, 2017; McAdoo and Pusey, 2017). Following titres of anti-GBM antibody may be of value to assess the success of treatment but this is not well established. Re-biopsy is seldom if ever indicated

While combinations of CYC, steroids, and plasmapheresis remain the 'gold-standard' of therapy for anti-GBM-mediated RLV, regimens employing RTX + steroids and plasmapheresis have been used for induction of remission with some success in anecdotal cases or small series (Touzot et al., 2015), particularly in the rare cases of relapsing disease (Glassock, 2017). In patients intolerant of CYC or at high risk of CYC-related complications (e.g. the elderly patient), and those unable to receive or intolerant of RTX, AZA, or MMF can be substituted for the CYC. The use of RTX and steroids alone, without plasmapheresis, for induction of remission has not been evaluated and its use should be discouraged until data showing efficacy and safety has been made available. Very rarely, anti-GBM disease may be complicated with a thrombotic microangiopathy due to the simultaneous presence of ADAMT3-13 inhibiting auto-antibodies. RTX may be a valuable adjunctive agent, along with plasmapheresis, in such cases (Vega-Cabrera et al., 2013).

It is tempting to speculate on a clinical role for IgG endopeptidase therapy in anti-GBM disease. Rapid inactivation of antibody (in a matter of minutes to hours) would be expected, and this approach might be useful in situations where plasmapheresis is not immediately available (Jordan et al., 2017).

ANCA positive, anti-GBM-positive disease (dual antibody disease) with RLV

The treatment of patients with both anti-GBM auto-antibodies and ANCA in the absence of multi-system involvement (RLV) follows the same treatment regimen as described for ANCA vasculitis and anti-GBM RLV individually. If recognized early, plasmapheresis in addition to anti-inflammatory (steroids) and immunomodulating (CYC, MMF, or RTX) therapy is indicated. In a retrospective analysis comparing patients with anti-GBM (n = 13), MPO-ANCA (n = 46) and both (n = 10), 'double positive' patients and those with anti-GBM autoantibodies presented with significantly higher serum creatinine (10.3 ± 5.6 mg/dl and 9.6 ± 8.1 mg/dl, respectively) than patients with MPO-ANCA alone (5.0 ± 2.9 mg/dl). Thus, one-year renal survival was best among patients with MPO-ANCA alone (63 per cent) as compared to the double positive group (10.0 per cent p = 0.01) and the anti-GBM group (15.4 per cent; p = 0.17; Rutgers et al., 2005). Patient survival at one year was best among patients with anti-GBM alone, although the differences did not reach statistical significance. RTX may be a useful agent for therapy of dual-positive anti-MPO vasculitis and anti-GBM antibody disease, but this is mainly based on anecdotes rather than clinical trials (Huang et al., 2016).

In patients who have both circulating anti-GBM and ANCA, the chance of recovery of renal function may be better than that of patients with anti-GBM alone. In these patients, immunosuppressive therapy should not be withheld, even in those presenting with advanced renal failure requiring dialysis (Jayne et al., 1990; Levy et al., 2004; Rutgers et al., 2005).

Practical recommendations

The general principles that should guide therapy of RLV are given in Table 10.4. These treatment paradigms are driven by a combination of clinical features, serologic findings and immunohistological characteristics.

ANCA-positive RLV with pauci-immune necrotizing and crescentic GN

Patients with severe ANCA-positive RLV and pauci-immune necrotizing and crescentic GN presenting with *de novo* (non-relapsing) disease should receive induction therapy with pulse MP (7–14 mg/kg; 500–1000 mg) for three days,

Table 10.4 Initial therapy of renal-limited vasculitis (with crescentic glomerulonephritis) based on pathogenetic category and dialysis-dependency*

Category	Dialysis-independent	Dialysis-dependent
Anti-GBM (only)	Oral or IV glucocorticoids, oral cyclophosphamide, plasmapheresis	Conservative,[a] especially if oliguro- anuric and 100% crescents
Immune complex (with or without concomitant ANCA)	Oral or IV glucocorticoids, oral or IV cyclophosphamide	Oral or IV glucocorticoids, oral or IV cyclophosphamide[b] (possibly with plasmapheresis)
ANCA-associated (without anti-GBM)	Oral or IV glucocorticoids, oral or IV cyclophosphamide or RTX or MMF	Oral or IV glucocorticoids, oral or IV cyclophosphamide[b] or RTX + Plasmapheresis[c]
Dual antibody (ANCA plus anti-GBN)	Same as for anti-GBM alone	Same as for anti-GBM alone (depending on level of anti-GBM antibody and underlying pathology) (?)
Non-anti-GBM or ANCA (idiopathic)	Same as for ANCA alone	Same as for ANCA alone

See also Table 10.1

*Dialysis-dependency defined as requiring for treatment of renal failure for >1 week.

[a]Some patients may receive therapy as for dialysis-independent patients if acute onset of renal failure and very cellular (non-fibrotic) crescents present.

[b]Reduced dosage of cyclophosphamide may be required.

[c]Plasmapheresis is currently recommended in patient with severe renal failure, but this recommendation may not withstand based on the results of the PEXIVAS trial.

RTX = Rituximab

followed by prednisone (1 mg/kg/day, not to exceed 60 mg/day) for the first two to four weeks, followed by a taper over the subsequent four months. The rapidity with which prednisone dosage is tapered can be individualized based on the severity of disease activity and the appearance of adverse effects of corticosteroids. The preliminary results of the PEXIVAS trial indicate that prednisone taper may be performed faster than has traditionally been done without a significant impact on treatment effectiveness. It is reasonable to start induction therapy with pulse IV CYC (0.5–0.75 g/m^2 body surface area every four weeks for up to twelve to twenty-four weeks, oral CYC (2 mg/kg/day) for three to six months, or RTX (375 mg/m^2 weekly $\times$ 4). Dosage reduction for CYC are needed for those patients with severe renal failure. Regimens that combine RTX with low-dose CYC for induction of a remission can also be considered. Patients with less severe ANCA positive RLV can be started on MMF (2 g/day) instead of CYC. In ANCA-positive RLV that has been previously treated with CYC but is now relapsing, the use of an RTX-based regimen is preferred.

Patients who are in clinical remission, complete or partial, can be switched after three to four months to a maintenance regimen with AZA, 2 mg/kg/day titrated to keep the WBC count >3000 cells/mm^3) or to RTX maintenance with infusions of 500–1000 mg every four to six months. MMF monotherapy is not advised for remission maintenance unless patients are intolerant of AZA or unable to receive RTX. CYC should not be used for maintenance therapy. Methotrexate is seldom, if ever, used for maintenance of remission therapy in this group of patients

The optimal duration of maintenance therapy is unclear. Only one study to date has formally evaluated whether long (four years) maintenance therapy with AZA was superior to a shorter course (two years). In this study, the longer duration of maintenance therapy was not associated with a demonstrable benefit, although these results are mitigated by the small size of the trial (Sanders et al., 2016). Patients who are at high risk of relapse with a history of at least one risk factor (PR3-ANCA at presentation, younger age, IV CYC induction, rapid steroid withdrawal, partial remission, see Box 10.2), should receive maintenance therapy for 12–18 months after complete remission is attained. On the other hand, maintenance therapy with AZA, MMF, or RTX might be unnecessary after a successful induction of a complete remission in patients with no risk factors for relapse (e.g. MPO-ANCA at presentation), in complete remission after induction, and sero-negative for ANCA.

Patients with advanced renal failure requiring or nearing the need for dialysis from rapidly progressive GN, should receive a course of plasmapheresis in addition to glucocorticoids and CYC or RTX. This recommendation may however change with the full release of the PEXIVAS trial (NCT#00987389; Walsh M. 2013; Merkel P 2018). When RTX is used along with plasmapheresis the dose of RTX should be given at the end of the plasmapheresis session and not repeated for 48 hours. Patients with persistent or progressive disease despite glucocorticoids, CYC, or RTX might benefit from the addition of plasmapheresis or the other main therapy (i.e. adding RTX to patients initially treated with CYC and vice versa). IV gamma globulin (IVIg) or perhaps TNF receptor inhibitors (e.g. infliximab; Feldman and Pusey, 2006) can be considered, but both of these approaches need further investigation for efficacy and safety.

The treatment of disease relapse should be tailored to the severity of the disease. Patients with a severe relapse and loss of GFR, should receive therapy with glucocorticoids and RTX as discussed earlier. Patients with mild-to-moderate relapse (with mild upper respiratory tract disease) may receive therapy with daily glucocorticoids alone or combined with and AZA or MMF. Patients who suffer a relapse while on maintenance therapy with AZA or MMF should be treated with RTX. Cyclosporin has been used successfully to treat ANCA-positive RLV, but a high relapse rate is to be expected (Allen et al., 1993). Cyclosporin has also been used successfully to prevent reactivation of disease, but this has not been subjected to a randomized trial (especially in comparison to MMF, AZA, or RTX maintenance regimens; Haubitz et al., 1998) and this approach is not widely used or recommended for routine use in ANCA positive or negative RLV.

ANCA and anti-GBM-negative renal limited pauci-immune necrotizing and crescentic GN

Treatment of patients with RLV who are persistently ANCA and anti-GBM antibody negative follows the same recommendations as for those with a positive ANCA test.

Immune complex-mediated RLV GN (ANCA-negative or -positive and anti-GBM antibody negative)

In the absence of evidence for underlying systemic auto-immune disease, infection, or occult malignancy, or an underlying alternate primary glomerular disease, the treatment of 'idiopathic' immune complex-mediated RLV GN, with or without ANCA consists of daily glucocorticoids, with consideration for induction therapy with pulse MP and CYC, RTX for patients with more advanced renal impairment or extensive crescent formation seen on biopsy; or MMF for patients with well-preserved renal function. Plasmapheresis may also be used, but without any clear evidence of benefit if the patient is nearing dialysis requirement and has extensive crescents on renal biopsy

Anti-GBM-mediated RLV

These patients should receive induction with oral glucocorticoids, CYC, and plasmapheresis as mentioned. Patients with severe renal disease should probably also receive pulse MP for induction (7 mg/kg/day ×3 [≤ 500 mg/day]). The risk–benefit ratio of such therapy should be carefully assessed for an individual patient presenting at or near dialysis, as the likelihood of dialysis-free survival at 12 months is only in the order of ten per cent. Long-term (beyond six months) maintenance immunosuppression is usually not needed due to the rarity of relapses. RTX therapy combined with high-dose steroids is not gener-ally recommended for induction therapy, unless the patient is intolerant of CYC or is suffering from a rare relapse (McAdoo and Pusey, 2017). In older patients, AZA or MMF can be substituted for CYC. Reduced dosage of CYC is needed when severe renal failure is present. Combinations of RTX and low-dose CYC might be considered in patients at higher risk of potential CYC-related compli-cations (Jones et al., 2010; Niles, 2011)

Anti-GBM and ANCA (dual positive) RLV

These patients should receive induction therapy with pulse glucocorticoids, CYC, or RTX, *and* plasmapheresis as described for anti-GBM antibody-positive patients. Such patients with severe renal impairment may have a better prog-nosis than those with anti-GBM alone, but this is not consistently found, and in general the outcome of the disease in these patients with therapy is similar to those with anti-GBM disease only, at comparable degrees of renal function at presentation.

Transplantation

ANCA-positive RLV with pauci-immune necrotizing and crescentic GN

Renal transplantation is well-recognized as an option of renal replacement therapy in patients with ANCA-associated RLV without systemic small vessel vasculitis (GPA or MPA). Successful renal transplantation in patients with ANCA-associated RLV has been reported in patients who were in full remis-sion and with negative ANCA titres, in patients with positive ANCA titres (Morin et al., 1993; Frasca et al., 1996; Rostaing et al., 1997; Gera et al., 2007; Ponticelli, Moroni and Glassock., 2011; Geetha et al., 2011; Goceroglu et al., 2015), and even in patients with evidence of active vasculitis at the time of transplantation (Schmitt et al., 1993). Geetha and colleagues (2011) described extensive experience in 85 patients with ANCA vasculitis (most of whom had MPA or GPA). Living donors were used in 69 or 85 cases (81 per cent). At the time of grafting, 29 of 85 (34 per cent) subjects were ANCA-positive, and the vasculitis relapse rate was 0.02 per patient years. Graft and patient survival at five years were 98 per cent and 93 per cent, respectively. In a large retrospective study from six Dutch Hospitals, the post-transplantation recurrence rate was only 2.8 per cent per patient year and non-renal relapses were easily manage-able. However, four of 11 patients with recurrent disease within the first five years ultimately lost their grafts, so clinical vigilance and early detection and treatment of recurrences are vital to optimize results of renal transplantation in this group of patients (Goceroglu et al., 2015). Although uncommon, recurrent systemic vasculitis after transplantation has been described as occurring from a few days (Reaich et al., 1994) to several years post-transplantation (Fogazzi et al., 1993). Reported recurrences after transplantation involve a spectrum of various organs and are not limited to the transplanted kidney.

Based on a pooled analysis (Nachman et al., 1999), the presence of ANCA at transplantation does not appear to increase the rate of relapse post-transplantation. Patients with a clinical diagnosis of GPA had a relative risk of relapse of 2.75 when compared with patients with MPA or RLV alone. Conversely, ANCA pattern (c-ANCA or p-ANCA) or antigen specificity (PR3 or MPO) was not associated with differences in recurrence rate post-transplantation. In the reported series the most common post-transplant immunosuppressive therapies were antibody induction, glucocorticoids, MMF, and tacrolimus. The overall and death censored graft survivals were 94 per cent and 100 per cent, respectively, at five years post-transplantation. Non-renal recurrence is uncommon. There is no consistent body of information indicating that a negative ANCA test is necessary prior to transplantation in order to avoid recurrence of disease in the graft. The prognosis for ANCA-positive renal transplant recipients is good also in the long-term. In a retrospective study the ten-year patient survival was 87 per cent in ANCA vasculitis patients vs. 90 per cent well matched controls and the ten-year death-censored graft survivals were 84 and 100 per cent, respectively (Moroni et al., 2007).

A review of the reports of recurrent ANCA vasculitis post-transplantation reveals a good response to steroids and CYC in the treatment of relapsing disease. RTX therapy of post-transplant relapses of ANCA vasculitis is highly successful (Geetha et al., 2007). Use of RTX for post-transplant relapse of ANCA vasculitis should now replace the use of CYC.

In summary, renal transplantation is a beneficial option in the management of patients with ANCA-positive RLV and ESRD. Although the presence of circulating ANCA is not a sufficient contraindication to transplantation, it is current practice not to perform transplantation in patients with clinically active vasculitis, but to delay surgery until the disease is in remission. Whether there is a need to wait a certain period of time after remission is attained before proceeding to transplantation is not well established. It is not advised to delay transplantation for a patient in remission for that reason alone.

Anti-GBM disease

The risk of recurrent disease in renal allografts is low (<5 per cent) for patients with anti-GBM disease. Although recurrence of anti-GBM disease after transplantation has been reported (Khandelwal et al., 2004), its frequency is very low, especially in patients who have negative anti-GBM titres at the time of transplantation. Traditionally, renal transplantation has been delayed for six to 12 months after the anti-GBM titres become negative, although there is no direct evidence to substantiate this recommendation. Nevertheless, it seems reasonable to delay transplantation until negative (or very low and stable) anti-GBM titres are attained. In cases of recurrent disease post-transplantation, patients should be treated with pulse MP, oral CYC, and/or RTX and plasma-pheresis (Khandelwal et al., 2004).

References

Ahmad YK, Tawfeek S, Sharaf-Eldin M, et al. (2017). Anti-nuclear cytoplasmic antibody-associated vasculitis: A probable adverse effect of sofosbuvir treatment in chronic hepatitis C patients. Hosp Pharm. **52**: 294–301.

Alchi B, Griffiths M, Sivalingam M, et al. (2015). Predictors of renal and patient outcomes in anti-GBM disease: Clinicopathologic analysis of a two-centre cohort. Nephrol Dial Transplant. **30**: 814–21.

Allen N, Caldwell D, Rice J, et al. (1993). Cyclosporin A therapy for Wegener's granulomatosis. In WL Gross (ed), *ANCA Associated Vasculitides: Immunological and Clinical Aspects*, pp. 473–6. Plenum Press, New York.

Almkuist RD, Buckalew VM Jr, Hirszel P, et al. (1981). Recurrence of anti-glomerular basement membrane antibody mediated glomerulonephritis in an isograft. Clin Immunol Immunopathol. **18**: 54–60.

Aries PM, Hellmich B, Both M, et al. (2005). Lack of efficacy of rituximab in Wegener's granulomatosis with refractory granulomatous manifestations. Ann Rheum Dis. **65**: 853–8.

Augusto JF, Langs V, Demiselle J, et al. (2016). Low serum complement C3 levels at diagnosis of renal ANCA-associated vasculitis is associated with poor prognosis. PLoS One. **11**: e0158871.

Aybar LT, McGregor JG, Hogan SL, et al. (2015). Reduced CD5(+) CD24(hi) CD38(hi) and interleukin-10(+) regulatory B-cells in active anti-neutrophil cytoplasmic autoantibody-associated vasculitis permit increased circulating autoantibodies. Clin Exp Immunol. **180**: 178–88.

Bariety J, Hill GS, Mandet C, et al. (2003). Glomerular epithelial-mesenchymal transdifferetiation in pauci-immune crescentic glomerulonephritis. Nephrol Dial Transplant. **18**: 1777–84.

Bariety J, Bruneval P, Mayrier A, et al. (2005). Podocyte involvement in human crescentic glomerulonephritis. Kidney Int. **68**: 1109–19.

Bautz DJ, Preston GA, Lionaki S, et al. (2008). Antibodies with dual reactivity to plasminogen and complementary PR3 in PR3-ANCA vasculitis. J Am Soc Nephrol. **19**: 2421–9.

Behmoaras J, Bhangal G, Smith J, et al. (2008). Jund is a determinant of macrophage activation and is associated with glomerulonephritis susceptibility. Nat Genet. **40**: 553–9.

Berden AE, Nolan SL, Morris HL, et al. (2010). Anti-plasminogen antibodies compromise fibrinolysis and associate with renal histology in ANCA-associated vasculitis. J Am Soc Nephrol. **21**: 2169–79.

Berden AE, Ferrario F, Hagen EC, et al. (2010). Histopathologic classification of ANCA-associated glomerulonephritis. J Am Soc Nephrol. **21**: 1628–36.

Berden AE, Jones RB, Erasmus DD, et al. (2012). Tubular lesions predict renal outcome in antineutrophil cytoplasmic antibody-associated glomerulonephritis after rituximab therapy. J Am Soc Nephrol. **23**: 313–21.

Berti A, Cornec-Le Gall E, Cornec D, et al. (2018). Incidence, prevalence and chronic renal damage of anti-neutrophil: Cytoplasmic antibody associated glomerulonephritis in a 20-year population-based cohort. Nephrol Dial Transplant. doi: 10.1093/ndt/gfy250

Billheden J, Boman J, Stegmayr B, et al. (1997). Glomerular basement membrane antibodies in hantavirus disease (hemorrhagic fever with renal syndrome). Clin Nephrol. **48**: 137–40.

Bolton WK, Couser WG (1979). Intravenous pulse methylprednisolone therapy of acute crescentic rapidly progressive glomerulonephritis. Am J Med. 66:495-502**Bonsib SM.** (1985). Glomerular basement membrane discontinuities: Scanning electron microcopic study of acellular glomeruli. Am J Pathol. **19**:357–60.

Bonsib SM, Goeken JA, Kemp JD, et al. (1993). Coexistent anti-neutrophil cytoplasmic antibody and antiglomerular basement membrane antibody associated disease: Report of six cases. Mod Pathol. **6**: 526–30.

Border WA, Baehler RW, Bhathena D, et al. (1979). IgA antibasement membrane nephritis with pulmonary hemorrhage. Ann Intern Med. **91**: 21–5.

Borgmann S, Haubnitz M. (2004). Genetic impact of pathogenesis and prognosis of ANCA-associated vasculitides. Clin Exp Rheumatol. **6**: s79–s86.

Borza DB, Chedid MF, Colon S, et al. (2005). Recurrent Goodpastures disease in a monoclonal IgA1-kappa antibody autoreactive with the alpha1/alpha2 chains of type IV collagen. Am J Kidney Dis. **45**: 397–406.

Borza DB, Neilson EG, Hudson BG, et al. (2003). Pathogenesis of Goodpasture's syndrome: A molecular perspective. Semin Nephrol. **23**: 522–31.

Booth A, Harper L, Hammad T, et al. (2004). Prospective study of TNF-alpha blockade with infliximab in anti-neutrophil cytoplasmic antibody-associated systemic vasculitis. J Am Soc Nephrol. **15**: 717–21.

Birck R, Warnatz K, Lorenz HM, et al. (2003). 15-Deoxyspergualin in patients with refractory ANCA-associated systemic vasculitis: a six-month open-label trial to evaluate safety and efficacy. J Am Soc Nephrol. **14**: 440–7.

Bunch DO, McGregor JG, Khandoobhai NB, et al (2013). Decreased CD5+ B cells in active ANCA vasculitis and relapse after rituximab. Clin J Am Soc Nephrol. **8**: 382–91.

Bunch DO, Mendoza CE, Aybar LT, et al (2015). Gleaning relapse risk from B cell phenotype: Decreased CD5 + B cells portend a shorter time to relapse after B cell depletion in patients with ANCA-associated vasculitis. Ann Rheum Dis. **74**: 1784–6.

Cameron JS. (1977). The long-term outcome of glomerular disease. In RW Schrier, Gottschalk AR (eds). *Diseases of the Kidney*, pp. 1929–35. Little Brown, Boston.

Cameron JS. (1998). Crescentic nephritis secondary to infection, systemic disease and other glomerulopathies. In C Pusey, A. Rees (eds), *Rapidly Progressive Glomerulonephritis*, pp. 207–35. Oxford University Press, Oxford.

Canney M, O'Hara PV, McEvoy CM, et al. (2016). Spatial and temporal clustering of anti-glomerular basement membrane disease. Clin J Am Soc Nephrol. **11**: 1392–9.

Cao Y, Schmitz JL, Yang J, et al. (2011). DRB1*15 allele is a risk factor for PR3-ANCA disease in African Americans. J Am Soc Nephrol. **22**: 1161–7.

Chaigne B, Gatault P, Darrouzain F, et al. (2013). Mycophenolate mofetil in patients with anti-neutrophil cytoplamic antibody-associated vasculitis: A prospective pharmacokinetics and clinical study. Clin Exp Immunol. **176**: 172–9.

Charles P, Terrier B, Perrodeau É, et al. (2018). Comparison of individually tailored versus fixed-schedule rituximab regimen to maintain ANCA-associated vasculitis remission: Results of a multicentre, randomised controlled, phase III trial (MAINRITSAN2). Ann Rheum Dis. **77**: 1143–9.

Chen M, Jayne DRW, Zhao MH. (2017). Complement in ANCA-associated vasculitis: Mechanisms and implications for management. Nat Rev Nephrol. **13**: 359–67.

Chen SF, Wang H, Huang YM, et al. (2015). Clinicopathologic characteristics and outcomes of renal thrombotic microangiopathy in anti-neutrophil cytoplasmic autoantibody-associated glomerulonephritis. Clin J Am Soc Nephrol. **10**: 750–8.

Chen Y, Gao E, Yang L, et al. (2016) Long-term outcome of mycophenolate mofetil treatment for patients with microscopic polyangiitis: An observational study in Chinese patients. Rheumatol Int. **36**: 967–74.

Choi HK, Merkel PA, Tervaert JW, et al. (1999). Alternating antineutrophil cytoplasmic antibody specificity: Drug-induced vasculitis in a patient with Wegener's granulomatosis. Arthritis Rheumatol. **42**: 384–8.

Choi HK, Slot MC, Pan G, et al. (2000). Evaluation of antineutrophil cytoplasmic antibody seroconversion induced by minocycline, sulfasalazine, or penicillamine. Arthritis Rheumatol. **43**: 2488–92.

Choi HK, Merkel PA, Walker AM, Niles JL. (2000). Drug-associated antineutrophil cytoplasmic antibody-positive vasculitis: Prevalence among patients with high titers of antimyeloperoxidase antibodies. Arthritis Rheumatol. **43**: 405–13.

Clatworthy MR, Wallin EF, Jayne DR. (2008). Anti-glomerular basement membrane disease after alemtuzumab. N Engl J Med. **359**: 768–9.

Cohen Tervaert JW, Huitema MG, Hene RJ, et al. (1990). Prevention of relapses in Wegener's granulomatosis by treatment based on antineutrophil cytoplasmic antibody titre. Lancet. **336**: 709–11.

Cornec D, Cornec-Le Gall E, et al. (2016). ANCA-associated vasculitis—clinical utility of using ANCA specificity to classify patients. Nat Rev Rheumatol. **12**: 570–9.

Cornec D, Cornec-Le Gall E, Specks U. (2017). Clinical trials in antineutrophil cytoplasmic antibody-associated vasculitis: What we have learnt so far, and what we still have to learn. Nephrol Dial Transplant. **32**: i37–i47.

Couser WG. (1988). Rapidly progressive glomerulonephritis: classification, pathogenetic mechanisms, and therapy. Am J Kidney Dis. **11**: 449–64.

Cui Z, Zhao MH, Jia XY, Wang M, et al. (2016). Antibodies to α5 chain of collagen IV are pathogenic in Goodpasture's disease. J Autoimmun. **70**: 1–11.

Cui Z, Zhao J, Jia XY, et al. (2011). Anti-glomerular basement membrane disease: Outcomes of different therapeutic regimens in a large single-center Chinese cohort study. Medicine (Baltimore). **90**: 303–11.

Davenport A, Lock RJ, Wallington T. (1995). Clinical significance of the serial measurement of autoantibodies to neutrophil cytoplasm using a standard indirect immunofluorescence test. Am J Nephrol. **15**: 201–7.

de Groot K, Adu D, Savage CO. (2001). The value of pulse cyclophosphamide in ANCA-associated vasculitis: Meta-analysis and critical review. Nephrol Dial Transplant. **16**: 2018–27.

de Groot K, Rasmussen N, Bacon PA, et al. (2005). Randomized trial of cyclophosphamide versus methotrexate for induction of remission in early systemic antineutrophil cytoplasmic antibody-associated vasculitis. Arthritis Rheumatol. **52**: 2461–9.

de Groot K, Harper L, Jayne DR, et al. (2009). Pulse versus daily oral cyclophosphamide for induction of remission in antineutrophil cytoplasmic antibody-associated vasculitis: A randomized trial. Ann Intern Med. **150**: 670–80.

de Joode AAE, Sanders JSF, Puéchal X, et al. (2017). Long-term azathioprine maintenance therapy in ANCA-associated vasculitis: Combined results of long-term follow-up data. Rheumatology (Oxford). **56**: 1894–901

de Joode AA, Sanders JS, Rutgers A, et al. (2015). Maintenance therapy in antineutrophil cytoplasmic antibody-associated vasculitis: Who needs what and for how long? Nephrol Dial Transplant. **30**: i150–8.

de Lind van Wijngaarden RA, et al. (2006). Clinical and histologic determinants of renal outcome in ANCA-associated vasculitis. A prospective analysis of 100 patients with severe renal involvement. J Am Soc Nephrol. **17**:2264–74

de Lind van Wijngaarden RA, Hauer HA, et al. (2007). Chances of renal recovery for dialysis-dependent ANCA-associated glomerulonephritis. J Am Soc Nephrol. **18**: 2189–97.

de Lind van Wijngaarden RA. (2008). Hypotheses on the etiology of antineutrophil cytoplasmic autoantibody associated vasculitis. The cause is hidden, but the result is known. Clin J Am Soc Nephrol. **3**: 237–52.

De Groot K, Rasmussen N, Bacon PA, et al. (2005). Randomized trial of cyclophosphamide versus methotrexate for induction of remission in early systemic antineutrophil cytoplasmic antibody-associated vasculitis. Arthritis Rheumatol. **52**: 2461–69.

De'Oliviera J, Gaskin G, Dash A, et al. (1995). Relationship between disease activity and anti-neutrophil cytoplasmic antibody concentration in long-term management of systemic vasculitis. Am J Kidney Dis. **25**: 380–9.

Dewan D, Gulati S, Sharma RK, et al. (2008). Clinical spectrum and outcome of crescentic glomerulonephritis in children in developing countries. Pediatr Nephrol. **23**: 389–94.

Dickenmann M, Oettl T, Mihatsch MJ. (2008). Osmotic nephrosis: Acute kidney injury with accumulation of proximal tubular lysosomes due to administration of exogenous solutes. Am J Kidney Dis. **51**: 491–503.

Eriksson P. (2005). Nine patients with anti-neutrophil cytoplasmic antibody-positive vasculitis successfully treated with rituximab. J Intern Med. **257**: 540–8.

Falk RJ, Hogan S, Carey TS, et al. (1990). Clinical course of anti-neutrophil; cytoplasmic auto-antibody associated glomerulonephritis and systemic vasculitis. The Glomerular Disease Collaborative Network. Ann Intern Med. **113**: 656–63.

Falk R, Jenette C, Nachman P, et al. (1998). Pathogenesis of systemic vasculitis. In C Pusey, A Rees (eds), *Rapidly Progressive Glomerulonephritis*, pp. 148–85. Oxford University Press, Oxford.

Feldmann M, Pusey CD. (2006). Is there a role for TNF-alpha in anti-neutrophil cytoplasmic antibody-associated vasculitis? Lessons from other chronic inflammatory diseases. J Am Soc Nephrol. **17**: 1243–52.

Ferrario F, Tadros MT, Napodano P, et al. (1994). Critical re-evaluation of 41 cases of 'idiopathic' crescentic glomerulonephritis. Clin Nephrol. **41**: 1–9.

Ferrario F, Rastaldi MP (1998). Pathology of rapidly progressive glomerulonephritis. In C Pusey, A. Rees (eds), *Rapidly Progressive Glomerulonephritis*, pp. 207–35. Oxford University Press, Oxford.

Finkelman JD, Lee AS, Hummel AM, et al. (2007). ANCA are detectable in nearly all patients with active severe Wegener's granulomatosis. Am J Med. **120**: 643.e9–14.

Fischer EG, Lager DJ. (2007). Anti-glomerular basement membrane glomerulonephritis: A morphologic study of 80 cases. Am J Clin Pathol. **125**: 445–50.

Fisher M, Pusey CD, Vaughn RW, et al. (1997). Susceptibility to anti-glomerular basement membrane disease is strongly associated with HLA-DRB1 genes. Kidney Int. **51**: 222–9.

Flossmann O, Berden A, de Groot K, et al. (2011). Long-term patient survival in ANCA-associated vasculitis. Ann Rheum Dis. **70**: 488–94.

Fogazzi GB, Banfi G, Allegri L, et al. (1993). Late recurrence of systemic vasculitis after kidney transplantation involving the kidney allograft. Advances in Experimental Medicine and Biology. **336**: 503–6.

Frasca GM, Neri L, Martello M, et al. (1996). Renal transplantation in patients with microscopic polyarteritis and anti-myeloperoxidase antibodies: Report of three cases. Nephron. **72**: 82–5.

Free ME, Falk RJ. (2016). The search for a biomarker of relapse in ANCA-associated vasculitis. J Am Soc Nephrol. **27**: 2551–3.

Fukui S, Iwamoto N, Umeda M, et al. (2016). Antineutrophilic cytoplasmic antibody-associated vasculitis with hypocomplementemia has a higher incidence of serious organ damage and a poor prognosis. Medicine (Baltimore). **95**: e4871.

Furuta S, Jayne D. (2014). Emerging therapies in antineutrophil cytoplasm antibody-associated vasculitis. Curr Opin Rheumatol. **26**: 1–6.

Fussner LA, Specks U. (2015). Can antineutrophil cytoplasmic antibody levels be used to inform treatment of pauci-immune vasculitis? Curr Opin Rheumatol. **27**: 231–40.

Gaskin G and Pusey C. (1998). Clinical aspects of systemic vasculitis. In C Pusey, A Rees (eds), *Rapidly Progressive Glomerulonephritis*, pp. 207–35. Oxford University Press, Oxford.

Geetha D, Eirin A, True K, et al. (2011). Renal transplantation in antineutrophil cytoplasmic antibody-associated vasculitis: A multicenter experience. Transplantation. **91**: 1370–5.

Geetha D, Seo P, Specks U, et al. (2007). Successful induction of remission with rituximab for relapse of ANCA-associated vasculitis post-kidney transplant: Report of two cases. Am J Transplant. **7**: 2821–5.

Geetha D, Hruskova Z, Segelmark M, et al. (2016). Rituximab for treatment of severe renal disease in ANCA associated vasculitis. J Nephrol. **29**: 195–201.

Geetha D, Specks U, Stone JH, et al. (2015). Rituximab versus cyclophosphamide for ANCA-associated vasculitis with renal involvement. J Am Soc Nephrol. **26**: 976–85.

Gera M, Griffin MD, Specks U, et al. (2007). Recurrence of ANCA-associated vasculitis following renal transplantation in the modern era of immunosupression. Kidney Int. **71**: 1296–1301.

Ginsberg S, Rosner I, Slobodin G, et al. (2016). Etanercept treatment-related c-ANCA-associated large vessel vasculitis. Clin Rheumatol. **35**: 271–3.

Glassock R, Cohen A, Adler S. (1995). Primary glomerular disease. In **BM Brenner** (ed), *The Kidney*, pp. 1402–10. Saunders, Philadelphia.

Glassock RJ. (2016). Atypical anti-glomerular basement membrane disease: Lessons learned. Clin Kidney J. **9**: 653–6.

Göçeroğlu A, Berden AE, Fiocco M, et al. (2016). ANCA-Associated glomerulonephritis: Risk factors for renal relapse. PLoS One. **11**: e0165402.

Göçeroğlu A, Rahmattulla C, Berden AE, et al. (2016). Outcome of renal transplantation in antineutrophil cytoplasmic antibody-associated glomerulonephritis. Transplantation. **100**: 916–24.

Gou SJ, Yuan J, Wang C, et al. (2013). Alternative complement pathway activation products in urine and kidneys of patients with ANCA-associated GN. Clin J Am Soc Nephrol. **8**: 1884–91.

Gopaluni S, Smith RM, Lewin M, et al. (2017). Rituximab versus azathioprine as therapy for maintenance of remission for anti-neutrophil cytoplasm antibody-associated vasculitis (RITAZAREM): Study protocol for a randomized controlled trial. Trials. **18**: 112.

Gou SJ, Yuan J, Chen M, et al. (2013). Circulating complement activation in patients with anti-neutrophil cytoplasmic antibody-associated vasculitis. Kidney Int. **83**: 129–37.

Guillevin L, Cohen P, Gayraud M, et al. (1999). Churg–Strauss syndrome. Clinical study and long-term follow-up of 96 patients. Medicine (Baltimore). **78**: 26–37.

Guillevin L, Cordier JF, Lhote F, et al. (1997). A prospective, multicenter, randomized trial comparing steroids and pulse cyclophosphamide versus steroids and oral cyclophosphamide in the treatment of generalized Wegener's granulomatosis. Rheumatol. **40**: 2187–98.

Guillevin L, Pagnoux C, Karras A, et al. (2014). Rituximab versus azathioprine for maintenance in ANCA-associated vasculitis. N Engl J Med. **371**: 1771–80.

Hagen EC, Daha MR, Hermans J, et al. (1998). Diagnostic value of standardized assays for anti-neutrophil cytoplasmic antibodies in idiopathic systemic vasculitis: EC/BCR project for ANCA Assay Standardization. Kidney Int. **53**: 743–53.

Han WK, Choi HK, Roth RM, et al. (2003). Serial ANCA titers: Useful tool for prevention of relapses in ANCA-associated vasculitis. Kidney Int. **63**: 1079–85.

Han F, Liu G, Zhang X, et al. (2011). Effects of mycophenolate mofetil combined with corticosteroids for induction therapy of microscopic polyangiitis. Am J Nephrol. **33**: 185–92.

Harper L, Morgan MD, Walsh M, et al. (2012). Pulse versus daily oral cyclophosphamide for induction of remission in ANCA-associated vasculitis: Long-term follow-up. Ann Rheum Dis. **71**: 955–60.

Haubitz M, Koch KM, Brunkhorst R. (1998). Cyclosporin for the prevention of disease re-activation in relapsing ANCA-associated vasculitis. Nephrol Dial Transplant. **13**: 2074–6.

Hauer HA, Bajema IM, Van Houwelingen HC, et al. (2002). Determinants of outcome in ANCA-associated glomerulonephritis: A prospective clinico-histopatholgical analysis of 96 patients. Kidney Int. **62**: 1732–43.

Heckmann M, et al. (2008). The Wegener's granulomatosis trait lcous on Chromosome 6p21.3 as characterized by taqSNP genotyping. Ann Rheum Dis. **67**: 972–9.

Heeringa P, Brouwer E, Klok PA, et al. (1996). Autoantibodies to myeloperoxidase aggravate mild anti-glomerular-basement-membrane-mediated glomerular injury in the rat. Am J Pathol. **149**: 1695–706.

Hellmark T, Niles JL, Collins AB, et al. (1997). Comparison of anti-GBM antibodies in sera with or without ANCA. J Am Soc Nephrol. **8**: 376–85.

Hellmich B, Csernok E, Fredenhagen G, et al. (2007). A novel high sensitivity ELISA for detection of antineutrophil cytoplasm antibodies against proteinase-3. Clin Exp Rheumatol. **25**: S1–S5.

Herody M, Bobrie G, Gouarin C, et al. (1993). Anti-GBM disease: Predictive value of clinical, histological and serological data. Clin Nephrol. **40**: 249–55.

Hiemstra TF, Walsh M, Mahr A, et al. (2010). Mycophenolate mofetil vs azathioprine for remission maintenance in antineutrophil cytoplasmic antibody-associated vasculitis: A randomized controlled trial. JAMA. **304**: 2381–8.

Hogan SL, Falk RJ, Chin H, et al. (2005). Predictors of relapse and treatment resistance in antineutrophil cytoplasmic antibody-associated small-vessel vasculitis. Ann Intern Med. **143**: 621–31.

Hogan SL, et al. (2007). Association of silica exposure with anti-neutrophil cytoplasmic autoantibody small-vessel vasculitis: A population-based, case-control study. Clin J Am Soc Nephrol. **2**: 290–9.

Holdsworth SR, Erlich JH, Tipping PG. (1998). Immunopathogenesis of crescentic glomerulonephritis. In C Pusey, A Rees (eds), *Rapidly Progressive Glomerulonephritis*, pp. 12–42. Oxford University Press, Oxford.

Hu SY, Jia XY, Yang XW, et al. (2013). Glomerular C1q deposition and serum anti-C1q antibodies in anti-glomerular basement membrane disease. BMC Immunol. **14**: 42.

Hu W, Liu C, Xie H, et al. (2008). Mycophenolate mofetil versus cyclophosphamide for inducing remission of ANCA vasculitis with moderate renal involvement. Nephrol Dial Transplant. **23**: 1307–12.

Huang XR, Holdsworth SR, Tipping PG (1994). Evidence for delayed type hypersensitivity mechanisms in glomerular crescent formation. Kidney Int. **46**: 69–78.

Huang J, Wu L, Huang X, et al. (2016). Successful treatment of dual-positive anti-myeloperoxidase and anti-glomerular basement membrane antibody vasculitis with pulmonary-renal syndrome. Case Rep Nephrol Dial. **6**: 1–7.

Isaacs JD, Manna VK, Rapson N, et al. (1996). CAMPATH-1H in rheumatoid arthritis: An intravenous dose-ranging study. B J Rheum. **35**: 231–40.

Jayne D, Rasmussen N, Andrassy K, et al. (2003). A randomized trial of maintenance therapy for vasculitis associated with antineutrophil cytoplasmic autoantibodies. N Engl J Med. **349**: 36–44.

Jayne DR. (2002). Campath-1H (anti-CD52) for refractory vasculitis: Retrospective Cambridge experience 1989–1999. Cleve Clin J Med. **69**: SII–129.

Jayne DR, Chapel H, Adu D, et al. (2000). Intravenous immunoglobulin for ANCA-associated systemic vasculitis with persistent disease activity. Q J Med. **93**: 433–9.

Jayne DR, Gaskin G, Rasmussen N, et al. (2007). Randomized trial of plasma exchange or high-dosage methylprednisolone as adjunctive therapy for severe renal vasculitis. J Am Soc Nephrol. **18**: 2180–8.

Jayne DR, Marshall PD, Jones SJ, et al. (1990). Autoantibodies to GBM and neutrophil cytoplasm in rapidly progressive glomerulonephritis. Kidney Int. **37**: 965–70.

Jayne DRW, Bruchfeld AN, Harper L, et al. (2017) Randomized trial of C5a receptor inhibitor avacopan in ANCA-associated vasculitis. J Am Soc Nephrol. **28**: 2756–67.

Jennette JC, Falk RJ. (1990). Antineutrophil cytoplasmic autoantibodies and associated diseases: a review. Am J Kidney Dis. **15**: 517–29.

Jennette JC, Falk RJ. (1991). Diagnostic classification of antineutrophil cytoplasmic autoantibody-associated vasculitides. Am J Kidney Dis. **18**: 184–7.

Jennette JC, Falk RJ. (2008). New insights into the pathogenesis of vasculitis-associated with anti-neutrophil cytoplasmic autoantibodies. Curr Opin Rheumatol. **20**: 55–60.

Jennette JC, Milling DM, Falk RJ. (1994). Vasculitis affecting the skin: A review. Arch Dermatol. **130**: 899–906.

Jennette JC, Xiao H, Hu P. (2013). Complement in ANCA-associated vasculitis. Semin Nephrol. **33**: 557–64.

Johnson RJ, Willson R, Yamabe H, et al. (1994). Renal manifestations of hepatitis C virus infection. Kidney Int. **46**: 1255–63.

Jones BE, Yang J, Muthigi A, et al. (2017). Gene-specific DNA methylation changes predict remission in patients with ANCA-associated vasculitis. J Am Soc Nephrol. **28**: 1175–87.

Jones RB, Tervaert JW, Hauser T, et al. (2010). Rituximab versus cyclophosphamide in ANCA-associated renal vasculitis. N Engl J Med. **363**: 211–20.

Jones RB, Walsh M, Chaudhry AN, et al. (2014). Randomized trial of enteric-coated mycophenolate sodium versus mycophenolate mofetil in multi-system autoimmune disease. Clin Kidney J. **7**: 562–8.

Jordan SC, Lorant T, Choi J, et al. (2017) IgG endopeptidase in highly sensitized patients undergoing transplantation. N Engl J Med. **377**: 442–53.

Joy MS, Hogan SL, Jennette JC, et al. (2005). A pilot study using mycophenolate mofetil in relapsing or resistant ANCA small vessel vasculitis. Nephrol Dial Transplant. **20**: 2725–32.

Kalluri R, Danoff T, Neilson EG. (1995). Murine anti-alpha3(IV) collagen disease: A model of human Goodpasture syndrome and anti-GBM nephritis. J Am Soc Nephrol. **6**: 833.

Kalluri R, Meyers K, Mogyorosi A, et al. (1997). Goodpasture syndrome involving overlap with Wegener's granulomatosis and anti-glomerular basement membrane disease. J Am Soc Nephrol. **8**: 1795–800.

Kemna MJ, Damoiseaux J, Austen J, et al. (2015). ANCA as a predictor of relapse: Useful in patients with renal involvement but not in patients with nonrenal disease. J Am Soc Nephrol. **26**: 537–42.

Keogh KA, Wylam ME, Stone JH, et al. (2005). Induction of remission by B lymphocyte depletion in eleven patients with refractory antineutrophil cytoplasmic antibody-associated vasculitis. Arthritis Rheumatol. **52**: 262–8.

Khan SB, Cook HT, Bhangal G, et al. (2005). Antibody blockade of the TNF-alpha receptor reduces inflammation and scarring in experimental crescentic glomerulonephritis. Kidney Int. **67**: 1812–20.

Khandelwal M, McCormick BB, Lajoie G, et al. (2004). Recurrence of anti-GBM disease 8 years after renal transplantation. Nephrol Dial Transplant. **19**: 491–4.

Kirk AD, Hale DA, Mannon RB, et al. (2003). Results from a human renal allograft tolerance trial evaluating the humanized CD52-specific monoclonal antibody alemtuzumab (CAMPATH-1H). Transplantation. **76**: 120–9.

Kitching AR, Tipping PG, Holdsworth SR. (1999). Il-12 directs severe renal injury, crescent formation and the Th1 responses in murine glomerulonephritis. Eur J Immunol. **29**: 1–10.

Klemmer PJ, Chalermskulrat W, Reif MS, et al. (2003). Plasmapheresis therapy for diffuse alveolar hemorrhage in patients with small-vessel vasculitis. Am J Kidney Dis. **42**: 1149–53.

Koukoulaki M, Jayne DR. (2006). Mycophenolate mofetil in anti-neutrophil cytoplasm antibodies-associated systemic vasculitis. Nephron Clin Pract. **102**: c100–7.

Kriz W, Le Hir M. (2005). Pathways to nephron loss starting from glomerular disease-insights form animal models. Kidney Int. **67**: 404–19.

Lamprecht P, Till A, Steinmann J, et al. (2007). Current state of biologicals in the management of systemic vasculitis. Ann N Y Acad Sci. **1110**: 261–70.

Lan HY, Nikolic-Paterson DJ, Mu W, et al. (1997). Local macrophage proliferation in the pathogenesis of glomerular crescent formation in rat glomerular basement membrane (GBM) glomerulonephritis. Clin Exp Immunol. **110**: 233–40.

Le Hir M, Keller C, Eschmann V, et al. (2001). Podocyte bridges between the tuft and Bowman's capsule: An early event in experimental crescentic glomerulonephritis. J Am Soc Nephrol. **12**: 2060–171.

Leaker B, Neild GH. (1991). Effect of enalapril on proteinuria and renal function in patients with healed severe crescentic glomerulonephritis. Nephrol Dial Transplant. **6**: 936–8.

Lee T, Gasim A, Derebail VK, et al. (2014). Predictors of treatment outcomes in ANCA-associated vasculitis with severe kidney failure. Clin J Am Soc Nephrol. **9**: 905–13.

Levy JB, Turner AN, Rees AJ, et al. (2001). Long-term outcome of anti-glomerular basement membrane antibody disease treated with plasma exchange and immunosuppression. Ann Int Med. **134**: 1033–42.

Levy JB, Hammad T, Coulthart A, et al. (2004). Clinical features and outcome of patients with both ANCA and anti-GBM antibodies. Kidney Int. **66**: 1535–40.

Li ZY, Ma TT, Chen M, et al. (2016). The prevalence and management of anti-neutrophil cytoplasmic antibody-associated vasculitis in China. Kidney Dis (Basel). **1**: 216–23.

Lionaki S, Jennette JC, Falk RJ. (2007). Anti-neutrophil cytoplasmic (ANCA) and anti-glomerular basement membrane (GBM) autoantibodies in necrotizing and crescentic glomerulonephritis. Semin Immunopathol. **29**: 459–74.

Lionaki S, Hogan SL, Jennette CE, et al. (2009). The clinical course of ANCA small-vessel vasculitis on chronic dialysis. Kidney Int. **76**: 644–51.

Little MA, Pusey CD. (2004). Rapidly progressive glomerulonephritis: Current and evolving treatment strategies. J Nephrol. **8**: 510–19.

Lockwood CM, Rees AJ, Pearson TA, et al. (1976). Immunosuppression and plasma-exchange in the treatment of Goodpasture's syndrome. Lancet. **1**: 711–15.

Lyons PA, Rayner TF, Trivedi S, et al. (2012). Genetically distinct subsets within ANCA-associated vasculitis. N Engl J Med. **367**: 214–23.

McAdoo SP, Tanna A, Hrušková Z, et al. (2017). Patients double-seropositive for ANCA and anti-GBM antibodies have varied renal survival, frequency of relapse, and outcomes compared to single-seropositive patients. Kidney Int. **92**: 693–702.

McAdoo SP, Pusey CD. (2016). Clustering of Anti-GBM Disease: Clues to an Environmental Trigger? Clin J Am Soc Nephrol. **11**: 1324–6.

McAdoo SP, Pusey CD. (2017a). Anti-glomerular basement membrane disease. Clin J Am Soc Nephrol. **12**: 1162–72.

McAdoo SP, Pusey CD. (2017b) Is there a role for TNFα blockade in ANCA-associated vasculitis and glomerulonephritis? Nephrol Dial Transplant. **32**: i80–8.

McAdoo SP, Bedi R, Tarzi R, et al. (2016). Ofatumumab for B-cell depletion therapy in ANCA-associated vasculitis: A single-centre case series. Rheumatology (Oxford). **55**: 1437–42.

McAdoo SP, Medjeral-Thomas N, Gopaluni S, et al. (2018). Long-term follow-up of a combined rituximab and cyclophosphamide regimen in renal anti-neutrophil cytoplasm antibody-associated vasculitis. Nephrol Dial Transplant. **33**. doi: 10.1093/ndt/gfx378

McGregor JG, Hogan SL, Hu Y, et al. (2012). Glucocorticoids and relapse and infection rates in anti-neutrophil cytoplasmic antibody disease. Clin J Am Soc Nephrol. **7**: 240–7.

Ma KW, Golbus SM, Kaufman R, et al. (1978). Glomerulonephritis with Hodgkin's disease and herpes zoster. Arch Pathol Lab Med. **102**: 527–9.

Madore F, Lazarus JM, Brady HR. (1996). Therapeutic plasma exchange in renal diseases. J Am Soc Nephrol. **7**: 367–86.

Maes B, Vanwalleghem J, Kuypers D, et al. (1999). IgA anti-glomerular basement membrane disease associated with bronchial carcinoma and monoclonal gammopathy. Am J Kidney Dis. **33**: E3.

Manenti L, Vaglio A, Gnappi E, et al. (2015). Association of serum C3 concentration and histologic signs of thrombotic microangiopathy with outcomes among patients with ANCA-associated renal vasculitis. Clin J Am Soc Nephrol. **10**: 2143–51.

Martinez V, Cohen P, Pagnoux C, et al. (2008). Intravenous immunoglobulins for relapses of systemic vasculitides associated with antineutrophil cytoplasmic autoantibodies: Results of a multicenter, prospective, open-label study of twenty-two patients. Arthritis Rheumatol. **58**: 308–17.

Metzler C, Miehle N, Manger K, et al. (2007). Elevated relapse rate under oral methotrexate versus leflunomide for maintenance of remission in Wegener's granulomatosis. Rheumatology (Oxford). **46**: 1087–91.

Miloslavsky EM, Specks U, Merkel PA, et al. (2014). Rituximab for the treatment of relapses in antineutrophil cytoplasmic antibody-associated vasculitis. Arthritis Rheumatol. **66**: 3151–9.

Miloslavsky EM, Specks U, Merkel PA, et al. (2015). Outcomes of nonsevere relapses in antineutrophil cytoplasmic antibody-associated vasculitis treated with glucocorticoids. Arthritis Rheumatol. **67**: 1629–36.

Morgan MD, Harper L, Williams J, et al. (2006). Anti-neutrophil cytoplasm-associated glomerulonephritis. J Am Soc Nephrol. **17**: 1224–34.

Morgan MD, Szeto M, Walsh M, et al. (2017). Negative anti-neutrophil cytoplasm antibody at switch to maintenance therapy is associated with a reduced risk of relapse. Arthritis Res Ther.**19**: 129–36.

Morin MP, Thervet E, Legendre C, et al. (1993). Successful kidney transplantation in a patient with microscopic polyarteritis and positive ANCA [letter]. Nephrol Dial Transplant. **8**: 287–88.

Moroni G, Torri A, Gallelli B, et al. (2007). The long-term prognosis of renal transplant in patients with systemic vasculitis. Am J Transplant. **7**: 2133–9.

Mukhtyar C, et al. (2008). Outcomes from studies of anti-neutrophil cytoplasmic antibody associated vasculitis: A systematic review by the European League Against Rheumatism systemic vasculitis task force. Ann Rheum Dis. **67**: 1004–10.

Nachman PH, Hogan SL, Jennette JC, et al. (1996). Treatment response and relapse in antineutrophil cytoplasmic autoantibody-associated microscopic polyangiitis and glomerulonephritis. J Am Soc Nephrol. **7**: 33–9.

Nachman PH, Segelmark M, Westman K, et al. (1999). Recurrent ANCA-associated small vessel vasculitis after transplantation: A pooled analysis. Kidney Int. **56**: 1544–50.

Nasr SH, Collins AB, Alexander MP, et al. (2016 The clinicopathologic characteristics and outcome of atypical anti-glomerular basement membrane nephritis. Kidney Int. **89**: 897–908.

Neild GH, Cameron JS, Ogg CS, et al. (1983). Rapidly progressive glomerulonephritis with extensive glomerular crescent formation. Q J Med. **52**: 395–416.

Ng YY, Fan JM, Mu W, et al. (1999) Glomerular-epithelial-myofibroblast transdifferentiation in the evolution of glomerular crescent formation. Nephrol Dial Transplant. **14**:2860–72.

Niles J. (2011). Rituximab in induction therapy for anti-neutrophil cytoplasmic antibody (ANCA) vasculitis. Clin Exp Immunol. **164**: 27–30.

Nohr E, Girard L, James M, et al. (2014) Validation of a histopathologic classification scheme for antineutrophil cytoplasmic antibody-associated glomerulonephritis. Hum Pathol. **45**: 1423–9.

O'Reilly VP, Wong L, Kennedy C, et al. (2016). Urinary soluble CD163 in active renal vasculitis. J Am Soc Nephrol. **27**: 2906–16.

Pagnoux C, Hogan SL, Chin H, et al. (2008) Predictors of treatment resistance and relapse in antineutrophil cytoplasmic antibody-associated small-vessel vasculitis: Comparison of two independent cohorts. Arthritis Rheumatol. **58**: 2908–18.

Pagnoux C, Quéméneur T, Ninet J, et al (2015). Treatment of systemic necrotizing vasculitides in patients aged sixty-five years or older: Tesults of a multicenter, open-label, randomized controlled trial of corticosteroid and cyclophosphamide-based induction therapy. Arthritis Rheumatol. **67**: 1117–27.

Pagnoux C, Mahr A, Hamidou MA, et al. (2008). Azathioprine or methotrexate maintenance for ANCA-associated vasculitis. N Engl J Med. **359**: 2790–803.

Pendergraft WF 3rd, Niles JL. (2014). Trojan horses: Drug culprits associated with antineutrophil cytoplasmic autoantibody (ANCA) vasculitis. Curr Opin Rheumatol. **26**: 42–9.

Pendergraft WF 3rd, Herlitz LC, Thornley-Brown D, et al. (2014). Nephrotoxic effects of common and emerging drugs of abuse. Clin J Am Soc Nephrol. **9**: 1996–2005.

Pendergraft WF 3rd, Cortazar FB, Wenger J, et al. (2014). Long-term maintenance therapy using rituximab-induced continuous B-cell depletion in patients with ANCA vasculitis. Clin J Am Soc Nephrol. **9**: 736–44.

Pepper RJ, Chanouzas D, Tarzi R, et al. (2013). Intravenous cyclophosphamide and plasmapheresis in dialysis-dependent ANCA-associated vasculitis. Clin J Am Soc Nephrol. **8**: 219–24.

Phoon RK, Kitching AR, Odobasic D, et al. (2008). T-bet deficiency attenuates renal injury in experimental crescentic glomerulonephritis. J Am Soc Nephrol. **1**: 477–85.

Ponticelli C, Moroni G, Glassock RJ.(2011) Recurrence of secondary glomerular disease after renal transplantation. Clin J Am Soc Nephrol.;6:1214-21

Preston G, Falk R. (2011). Autoimmunity: Does autoantigen complementarity underlie PR3-ANCA AAV? Nat Rev Rheumatol. **7**: 439–40.

Pusey CD. (1990). Plasma exchange in immunological disease. Prog Clin Biol Res. **337**: 419–24.

Pusey CD, Lockwood CM, Peters DK. (1983). Plasma exchange and immunosuppressive drugs in the treatment of glomerulonephritis due to antibodies to the glomerular basement membrane. Int J Artif Organs. **6**: 15–18.

Pusey C, Rees A. (eds). (1998). *Rapidly Progressive Glomerulonephritis.* Oxford University Press, Oxford.

Reaich D, Cooper N, Main J. (1994). Rapid catastrophic onset of Wegener's granulomatosis in a renal transplant. Nephron. **67**: 354–7.

Rees A, Peters DK, Amos N, et al. (1984). The influence of HLA-linked genes on the severity of anti-GBM antibody mediated nephritis. Kidney Int. **26**: 445–50.

Rahmattulla C, Berden AE, Wakker SC. (2015). Incidence of malignancies in patients with antineutrophil cytoplasmic antibody-associated vasculitis diagnosed between 1991 and 2013. Arthritis Rheumatol. **67**: 3270–8.

Rahmattulla C, Mooyaart AL, van Hooven D, et al. (2016). Genetic variants in ANCA-associated vasculitis: A meta-analysis. Ann Rheum Dis. **75**: 1687–92.

Ramachandran R, Tiwana S, Prabhakar D, et al. (2015). Successful induction of granulomatosis with polyangiitis with tacrolimus. Indian J Nephrol. **25**: 46–9.

Rhee EP, Laliberte KA, Niles JL. (2010). Rituximab as maintenance therapy for anti-neutrophil cytoplasmic antibody-associated vasculitis. Clin J Am Soc Nephrol. **5**: 1394–400.

Roccatello D, Sciascia S, Rossi D, et al. (2017). The '4 plus 2' rituximab protocol makes maintenance treatment unneeded in patients with refractory ANCA-associated vasculitis: A 10-year observation study. Oncotarget. **8**: 52072–7

Rostaing L, Modesto A, Oksman F, et al. (1997). Outcome of patients with antineutrophil cytoplasmic autoantibody-associated vasculitis following cadaveric kidney transplantation. Am J Kidney Dis. **29**: 96–102.

Roth AJ1, Ooi JD, Hess JJ. (2013). Epitope specificity determines pathogenicity and detectability in ANCA-associated vasculitis. J Clin Invest. **123**: 1773–83.

Roth AJ, Brown MC, Smith RN, et al. (2012). Anti-LAMP-2 antibodies are not prevalent in patients with antineutrophil cytoplasmic autoantibody glomerulonephritis. J Am Soc Nephrol. **23**: 545–55.

Rutgers A, Slot M, van Passen P, et al. (2005). Coexistence of anti-glomerular basement membrane antibodies and myeloperoxidase-ANCAs in crescentic glomerulonephritis. Am J Kidney Dis. **46**: 253–62.

Salama AD, Chaudhry AN, Holthaus KA, et al. (2003). Regulation by CD28 + lymphocytes of auto-antigen specific T-cell responses in Goodpasture's (anti-GBM) disease. Kidney Int. **64**: 1685–94.

Sanders JS, Huitma MG, Kallenberg CG, et al. (2006). Prediction of relapses in PR3-ANCA-associated vasculitis by assessing responses of ANCA titres to treatment. Rheumatology (Oxford). **45**: 724–9.

Sanders JS, de Joode AA, DeSevaux RG, et al (2016) Extended versus standard azathioprine maintenance therapy in newly diagnosed proteinase-3 anti-neutrophil cytoplasmic antibody-associated vasculitis patients who remain cytoplasmic anti-neutrophil cytoplasmic antibody-positive after induction of remission: A randomized clinical trial. Nephrol Dial Transplant. **31**: 1453–9.

Savage CO, Pusey CD, Bowman C, et al. (1986). Antiglomerular basement membrane antibody mediated disease in the British Isles 1980-4. Br Med J (Clin Res Ed). **292**: 301–4.

Savage CO, Lockwood CM. (1990). Antineutrophil antibodies in vasculitis. Adv Nephrol. **19**: 225–36.

Scaglioni V, Scolnik M, Catoggio LJ, et al. (2017). ANCA-associated pauci-immune glomerulonephritis: Always pauci-immune? Clin Exp Rheumatol. **35**: 55–8.

Schaier M, Scholl C, Scharpf D, et al. (2015). High interpatient variability in response to mycophenolic acid maintenance therapy in patients with ANCA-associated vasculitis. Nephrol Dial Transplant. **30**: i138–45.

Schmitt WH, Haubitz M, Mistry N, et al. (1993). Renal transplantation in Wegener's granulomatosis [letter]. Lancet. **342**: 860.

Segelmark M, Butkowski R, Wieslander J. (1990). Antigen restriction and IgG subclasses among anti-GBM autoantibodies. Nephrol Dial Transplant. **5**: 991–6.

Segelmark M, Dahlberg P, Wieslander J. (2012). Anti-GBM disease with a mild relapsing course and low levels of anti-GBM autoantibodies. Clin Kidney J. **5**: 549–51.

Segelmark M, Hellmark T, Wieslander J. (2003). The prognostic significance in Goodpasture's disease of specificity, titre and affinity of anti-glomerular-basement-membrane antibodies. Nephron Clin Pract. **94**: c59–68.

Sethi S, Zand L, De Vriese AS, et al. (2017). Complement activation in pauci-immune necrotizing and crescentic glomerulonephritis: Results of a proteomic analysis. Nephrol Dial Transplant. **32**: i139–45.

Silva F, Specks U, Kalra S, et al. (2011). Mycophenolate mofetil for induction and maintenance of remission in microscopic polyangiitis with mild to moderate renal involvement: A prospective, open-label pilot trial. Clin J Am Soc Nephrol. **5**: 445–53.

Sneller MC, Hoffman GS, Talar-Williams C, et al. (1995). An analysis of forty-two Wegener's granulomatosis patients treated with methotrexate and prednisone. Arthritis Rheumatol. **38**: 608–13.

Specks U, Merkel PA, Seo P, et al. (2013). Efficacy of remission-induction regimens for ANCA-associated vasculitis. N Engl J Med. **369**: 417–27.

Specks U. (2015). Accurate relapse prediction in ANCA-associated vasculitis: The search for the Holy Grail. J Am Soc Nephrol. **26**: 505–7.

Specks U.(2015) Pro: Should all patients with anti-neutrophil cytoplasmic antibody-associated vasculitis be primarily treated with rituximab? Nephrol Dial Transplant. ;**30**:1083-7.

Stasi R, Stipa E, Poeta GD, et al. (2006). Long-term observation of patients with anti-neutrophil cytoplasmic antibody-associated vasculitis treated with rituximab. Rheumatology (Oxford). **45**: 1342–6.

Stassen PM, Cohen Tervaert JW, et al. (2007). Induction of remission in active anti-neutrophil cytoplasmic antibody-associated vasculitis with mycophenolate mofetil in patients who cannot be treated with cyclophosphamide. Ann Rheum Dis. **66**: 798–802.

Stevenson A, Yaqoob M, Mason H, et al. (1995). Biochemical markers of basement membrane disturbances and occupational exposure to hydrocarbons and mixed solvents. Q J Med. **88**: 23–8.

Stone JH. (2003). Limited versus severe Wegener's granulomatosis: baseline data on patients in the Wegener's granulomatosis etanercept trial. Arthritis Rheumatol. **48**: 2299–309.

Stone JH, Merkel PA, Spiera R, et al. (2010). Rituximab versus cyclophosphamide for ANCA-associated vasculitis. N Engl J Med. **363**: 221–32.

Tervaert JW, Stegeman CA, Kallenberg CG. (2001). Novel therapies for anti-neutrophil cytoplasmic antibody-associated vasculitis. Curr Opin Nephrol Hypertens. **10**: 211–7.

Thorner PS, Ho M, Eremina V, et al. (2008). Podocytes contribute to the formation of glomerular crescents. J Am Soc Nephrol. **19**: 495–502.

Tipping PG, Holdwworth SR. (2006). T-cells in crescentic glomerulonephritis. J Am Soc Nephrol. **17**: 1253–63.

Touzot M, Poisson J, Faguer S, et al. (2015). Rituximab in anti-GBM disease: A retrospective study of 8 patients. J Autoimmun. **60**: 74–9.

Tsuchiya N, Kobayashi S, Hashimoto H, et al. (2006). Association of HLA-DRB*0901-DQB1*0303 haplotype with microscopic piolyangiitis in Japanese. Genes Immun. **7**: 81–4.

Turner AN, Rees AJ. (1998). Anti-glomerular basement membrane disease. In C Pusey, A Rees (eds), *Rapidly Progressive Glomerulonephritis*, pp. 108–24. Oxford University Press, Oxford.

Unlu M, Kiremitci S, Ensari A, et al. (2013) Pauci-immune necrotizing crescentic glomerulonephritis with crescentic and full moon extracapillary proliferation: Clinico-pathologic correlation and follow-up study. Pathol Res Pract. **209**: 75–82.

Unizony S, Villarreal M, Miloslavsky EM, et al. (2016). Clinical outcomes of treatment of anti-neutrophil cytoplasmic antibody (ANCA)-associated vasculitis based on ANCA type. Ann Rheum Dis. **75**: 1166–9.

Unizony S, Lim N, Phippard DJ, et al. (2015). Peripheral CD5 + B cells in antineutrophil cytoplasmic antibody-associated vasculitis. Arthritis Rheumatol. **67**: 535–44.

van Daalen EE, Jennette JC, McAdoo SP, et al. (2017) Predicting outcome in patients with anti-GBM glomerulonephritis. Clin J Am Soc Nephrol. **13**: 63–72.

Vega-Cabrera C, Del Peso G, Bajo A, et al (2013). Goodpasture's syndrome associated with thrombotic thrombocytopenic purpura secondary to an ADAMTS-13 deficit. Int Urol Nephrol. **45**: 1785–9.

Walsh M, Casian A, Flossmann O, et al. (2013). Long-term follow-up of patients with severe ANCA-associated vasculitis comparing plasma exchange to intravenous methylprednisolone treatment is unclear. Kidney Int. **84**: 397–402.

Walsh M, Merkel PA, Peh CA, et al (2013). Plasma exchange and glucocorticoid dosing in the treatment of anti-neutrophil cytoplasm antibody associated vasculitis (PEXIVAS): Protocol for a randomized controlled trial. Trials. **14**: 73.

Walsh M, Faurschou M, Berden A, et al. (2014). Long-term follow-up of cyclophosphamide compared with azathioprine for initial maintenance therapy in ANCA-associated vasculitis. Clin J Am Soc Nephrol. **9**: 1571–6.

Weschsler E, Yang T, Jordan SC, et al. (2008). Anti-glomerular basement membrane disease in an HIV-infected patient. Nat Clin Pract Nephrol. **4**: 167–71.

Weidanz F, Day CJ, Hewins P, et al. (2007). Recurrences and infections during continuous immunosuppressive therapy after beginning dialysis in ANCA-associated vasculitis. Am J Kidney Dis. **50**: 36–46.

Wiggins RC. (1998). Rapidly progressive glomerulonephritis: resolution and scarring. In C Pusey, A Rees. (eds), *Rapidly Progressive Glomerulonephritis*, pp. 43–58. Oxford University Press, Oxford.

Xenocostas A, Jothy S, Collins B, et al. (1999). Anti-glomerular basement membrane glomerulonephritis after extra-corporeal shock wave lithotripsy. Am J Kidney Dis. **13**: 128–32.

Xiao H, Schreiber A, Heeringa P, et al. (2007). Alternative complement pathway in the pathogenesis of disease mediated by anti-neutrophil cytoplasmic antibodies. Am J Pathol. **170**: 52–64.

Yang J, Bautz DJ, Lionaki S, et al. (2008). ANCA patients have T-cells responsive to complementary PR-3 antigen. Kidney Int. **74**: 1159–69.

Yu JT, Li JN, Wang J, et al. (2017). Deglycosylation of myeloperoxidase uncovers its novel antigenicity. Kidney Int. **91**: 1410–19.

Chapter 11

Other primary glomerular diseases

Claudio Ponticelli and Gabriella Moroni

Fibrillary glomerulonephritis

Fibrillary glomerulonephritis (FGN) is a glomerular disease characterized histologically by a diffuse increase in mesangial matrix due to deposits having an ultrastructural fibrillary structure, which are usually negative for Congo-Red stained but positive for immunoglobulin deposition. Most patients present with proteinuria, often in a nephrotic range, microhaematuria, and hypertension. Most patients with FGN present with significant renal insufficiency and have a poor outcome despite immunosuppressive therapy (Table 11.1). Although FGN and immunotactoid glomerulopathy (ITG) have quite similar light microscopical and clinical features, the current opinion is that they represent two separate diseases. FGN is an idiopathic (primary) condition characterized by polyclonal immune deposits with restricted gamma isotypes. By contrast, ITG is more properly classified as a monoclonal immunoglobulin deposition disease as it contains monoclonal IgG deposits and has a significant association with underlying monoclonal paraproteinaemia and hypocomplementaemia (Fogo et al., 1993; Bridoux et al., 2002; Rosenstock et al., 2003). The recent discovery that most cases of primary or FGN, but no case of ITG, showed immunohistochemistry glomerular deposits of the DNAJ Homolog Subfamily B Member 9 (DNAJB9) confirms that FGN and ITG are two different diseases (Nasr et al., 2017).

Pathology

Light microscopy: FGN may show different histological patterns. According to Rosenstock and colleagues (2003), the most common pattern (44 per cent of patients) was MPGN, with mesangial expansion, foci of mesangial interposition, and replication of glomerular basement membrane (GBM). Isolated mesangial proliferation or sclerosis was seen in 21 per cent of cases. A pattern of diffuse endocapillary proliferation was observed in 15 per cent of cases. About 7 per cent of patients had a membranous-like pattern with subepithelial fibrillar deposits.

Table 11.1 Main characteristics of fibrillary glomerulonephritis (FGN).

Pathology	The most common histologic pattern is membranoproliferative glomerulonephritis with fibrillar deposits located in the sub-epithelium and in the mesangium. By immunohistochemistry glomerular deposits of DNAJB9 are seen. On electron microscopy fibrils are randomly arranged and intermingled with the mesangial matrix.
Pathogenesis	DNAJB9 could potentially be the precursor fibril protein and the autoantigen triggering an autoimmune response. The predominant IgG1 could lead to the formation of the fibrillary deposits and classical complement pathway activation would participate in the final glomerular injury.
Aetiology	The aetiology is unknown. FGN is frequently associated with other diseases, including diabetes mellitus, malignancy, hepatitis C, etc.
Clinical presentation	Patients present with proteinuria, which is in a nephrotic range in about 50% of cases. Haematuria is frequent. Most patients have renal insufficiency at presentation and about 60% are hypertensive. Rarely FGN presents as a rapidly progressive glomerulonephritis.
Prognosis	Most untreated patients progress to ESRD. However, rare cases of spontaneous remission have been also reported.
Treatment	No specific treatment is available. The disease only rarely responds to glucocorticoids or other immunosuppressive drugs. RTX seems to be more effective, but no more than 30% may obtain remission or a halted progression.

In the remaining 13 per cent there was advanced glomerular sclerosis. Cellular or fibrocellular crescents were seen in 31 per cent of all biopsies (Plate 19).

Immunofluorescence: This displays diffuse, glomerular positivity for IgG (almost 100 per cent of cases), IgM (about 50 per cent), C3 (86–100 per cent), and less frequently for IgA and C1q. Although IgG4 is the most frequent IgG, all the subclasses of IgG may be found. The deposits are usually polyclonal. Glomerular deposits are diffuse, in some cases irregular, predominantly located in the subepithelium and more rarely in the mesangium. These immunofluorescence findings can overlap with other forms of immune-mediated glomerulonephritis, with ITG, and with renal amyloidoses. FGN deposits frequently do not react with histochemical dyes Congo Red and Thioflavin T, although exceptions to this rule can occur (Alexander et al., 2018).

Immunochemistry: By immunohistochemistry, strong, homogeneous, smudgy DNAJB9 staining of glomerular deposits can be seen. This represents a highly sensitive and specific biomarker for FGN. Such deposits are not seen in ITG (Nasr et al., 2017; Andeen et al., 2018).

Electron microscopy: The distinctive features are infiltration of glomerular structures by fibrils, which are more frequently detected in the mesangium (98 per cent) or within the GBM (92 per cent). Fibrils are randomly arranged and intermingled with the mesangial matrix or GBM. They usually have a diameter comprised between 12 nm and 24 nm, larger than amyloid fibrils but smaller than the fibrils seen in ITG (Alpers and Kowalewska, 2008). Unfortunately, size alone is not sufficient for a differential diagnosis between FGN and ITG, as microtubules with a diameter between 16 nm and 22 nm have been reported. Moreover, the distinction between fibrils and microtubules requires meticulous morphologic analysis on high-quality, ultra-thin sections. Immunoelectron microscopy can help in determining whether DNAJB9 is localized to FGN fibrils. The fibrils must be distinguished from diabetic fibrillosis in patients with concomitant diabetes (Gonul et al., 2006). The discovery of DNAJB9 as a pathognomic marker of FGN obviates the requirement of electron microscopy to make a diagnosis and clearly identifies FGN as a primary renal disease in most cases.

Pathogenesis

The pathogenesis of FGN is largely unknown. Considering the high abundance of DNAJB9 in FGN deposits and its localization to individual FGN fibrils, DNAJB9 could potentially be the precursor fibril protein and the auto-antigen in FGN. It is possible that during endoplasmic reticulum stress, a misfolded DNAJB9 molecule is formed (possibly facilitated by protein post-translational modification) and deposited in glomeruli through entrapment and/or interaction with glomerular constituents, which then triggers an auto-immune response (Nasr et al., 2017). The predominant IgG1 could lead to the formation of the typical Congo-Red-negative fibrillary deposits and classical complement pathway activation would participate in the final glomerular injury (Andeen et al., 2018). However, FGN can exist in Congo-Red positive as well as Congo-Red negative forms (Alexander et al., 2018). Mass spectrometry and DNAJB9 immunohistochemistry can be useful in making this distinction (Alexander et al., 2018). Identification of circulating anti-DNAJB9 auto-antibodies or altered circulating forms of DNAJb9 as a diagnostic tool is anticipated.

Aetiology

The aetiology of FGN is unknown and the disease is considered as a primary glomerular disease. In about one-third of cases FGN may be associated with diabetes mellitus, malignancy, hepatitis C, or autoimmune diseases (Nasr et al., 2011).

Clinical presentation

FGN may occur at any age, but often presents at an age between 55 and 60 years. The disease occurs more frequently in women (Fogo et al., 1993; Rosenstock et al., 2003). Patients typically present with proteinuria, which is in a nephrotic range in about 50 per cent of cases. Haematuria is frequent. Most patients have renal insufficiency of various degrees at presentation and about 60 per cent are hypertensive. Rarely, FGN can masquerade as crescentic GN with 'pseudo-linear' IgG deposits and resemble anti-GBM disease (Thomas et al., 2016; Payan-Schober et al., 2017; see also Chapter 10). These cases may account for a small fraction of so-called 'atypical' anti-GBM disease with linear IgG deposits with no detectable circulating anti-GBM antibody.

Epidemiology

FGN is very rare, occurring in approximately 1 per cent of native kidney biopsies in several large biopsy series obtained from Western countries (Alpers and Kowalewska, 2016). In a retrospective French review, only nine cases of FGN were found by reviewing the biopsies of 15 nephrology departments between 1980 and 1997 (Bridoux et al., 2002). At New York's Columbia University Renal Pathology Laboratory, the diagnosis of FGN was made in 0.6 per cent of 10,108 renal biopsies, and 90 per cent of patients were Caucasian (Rosenstock et al., 2003). However, a higher prevalence of FGN in the Black population was observed in a report from North Carolina (Payan Schober et al., 2017). This may represent a selection bias.

Natural history

The outcome for patients with FGN is frequently poor, especially if superimposed crescentic disease is present. Progression to end-stage renal disease (ESRD) occurs in approximately half of the patients within two years from presentation (Fogo et al., 1993). Serum creatinine at presentation and severity of interstitial fibrosis at initial renal biopsy are independent predictors of progression (Rosenstock et al., 2003). In a single-centre series of 61 patients followed in mean for 52 months, three patients had complete remission, five patients had partial remission, 26 patients had chronic kidney disease, and 27 patients progressed to ESRD. Most of these patients were given immunosuppressive therapy (Nasr et al., 2011). In a French series, among 14 patients who were not given immunosuppressive therapy, 12 progressed to renal failure (Javaugue et al., 2013). A documented case of spontaneous clinical and histologic regression of FGN has been reported (Sekulic et al., 2017).

Specific treatment

The apparent role of Ig in the pathogenesis of FGN has led to a variety of immunotherapies. However, only transient response to glucocorticoids and immunosuppressive drugs has been reported in some patients with FGN. Single cases of response to fludarabine (Rosenstock et al., 2003) or Acthar gel (Madan et al., 2016) have been reported. In a review of 27 patients with FGN, chronic kidney disease progressed in 12 of 14 patients who were not given immunosuppressive therapy, ten of whom reached ESRD; renal response occurred in six of 13 patients who received immunosuppressive therapy, with rituximab (RTX) in five patients or cyclophosphamide in one patient (Javaugue et al., 2013). In another study, RTX therapy was associated with non-progression of renal disease in four of 12 patients with FGN. At the time of treatment, these non-progressors had better renal function and shorter time from diagnosis to treatment than progressors (Hogan et al., 2014). Other anecdotal reports showed good response to RTX (Collins et al., 2008; Chaudary et al., 2014; Lebler et al., 2018). However, rare cases of fatality after RTX in FGN have also been reported (Sainz-Prestel et al., 2013).

Practical recommendations

Although FGN is a rare disease, its prevalence is probably under-appreciated. As a matter of fact, electron microscopy is not performed routinely, and without ultramicroscopic examination or immunohistochemistry, the diagnosis of glomerular deposition diseases is often overlooked. It is possible that some cases diagnosed as membranoproliferative or membranous glomerulonephritis actually mask an underlying FGN. Once a diagnosis of fibrillary deposits is made or suspected, staining with DNAJB9 allows a rapid and accurate diagnosis of FGN. The differential diagnosis with cryoglobulinaemia, monoclonal gammopathy, or lupus nephritis is usually easy on the basis of clinical and laboratory features. Until the discovery of the role of DNAJB9, the differential diagnosis between FGN and ITG was difficult, mainly based on the diameter, the morphology, and the array of fibrils evaluated with a properly calibrated electron microscope. Today, studies using detection of DNAJB9 should resolve this conundrum.

The therapeutic approach in FGN remains challenging. The disease is rare and the reports on therapeutic attempts are scanty. Symptomatic treatment should be maximized (see Chapter 2). Treatment with glucocorticoids or cyclophosphamide may be tried but very few patients will respond. RTX may halt or slow the progression in about 30–40 per cent of cases. Theoretically, agents that interfere with Ig production, i.e. fludarabine or alemtuzumab, might be of benefit, but information about their efficacy in FGN is lacking. Open label trials of ACTH gel are underway and publication of the results are eagerly anticipated (Tumlin J, personal communication, 2018).

Transplantation

By reviewing the literature, Samaniego and colleagues (2001) reported 14 cases of FGN patients who received renal transplantation. Histological recurrence was diagnosed in six patients (44 per cent); four of them lost their allograft respectively four, five, 11, and 13 years after transplantation. Another patient died with stable graft function seven years after transplantation. Rosenstock and colleagues (2003) reported two further cases. One patient had no clinical evidence of recurrence eight years after transplantation with normal creatinine and no proteinuria. The other patient died four years after transplantation due to colon cancer with a stable creatinine of 2.2 mg/dl. In a large single-centre series, 14 patients with FGN received kidney transplant. After a mean follow-up of 51 months, five patients (36 per cent) had biopsy-proven recurrence of FGN. Two of these patients lost their allograft because of recurrent disease and subsequently received a second transplant that was lost again because of recurrent disease in one, whereas the second patient had no recurrence (Nasr et al., 2011). In Australia and New Zealand data, 13 FGN patients experienced comparable outcomes to other ESRD patients for both ten-year patient survival and renal-allograft survival (Mallett et al., 2015). Thus, renal transplantation may be considered as a viable option for patients with FGN, but with the expectation of a frequent recurrence of the same disease in the renal allograft, which may impair long-term graft survival. A case of *de novo* FGN has also been reported after renal transplantation (Gough et al., 2005).

Collagenofibrotic glomerulopathy

Collagenofibrotic glomerulopathy is an extremely rare primary glomerular disease in which accumulation of collagen III fibrils progressively accumulates within the mesangial matrix and subendothelial space. The disease has been included in the classification of primary glomerular diseases by the World Health Organization (Churg et al., 1995). Pathological features include lobulation and enlargement of glomeruli due to massive accumulation of fibrillar material as seen at ultramicroscopic examination. Clinically the disease is characterized by

Table 11.2 Main characteristics of collagenofibrotic glomerulopathy.

Pathology	Glomeruli appear expanded with a lobular aspect caused by eosinophilic subendothelial and mesangial deposits. Immunochemistry shows abundant staining for type-III collagen in mesangium and GBM. On electron microscopy there is a wide accumulation of fibrillar material in the mesangium and subendothelial space.
Pathogenesis	The disease is probably related to an increase in serum type III procollagen peptide leading to abnormal subendothelial and mesangial deposits of collagen III.
Aetiology	Unknown, no good evidence for a genetic transmission.
Clinical presentation	Most patients present with proteinuria in a nephrotic range, hypertension, and anaemia.
Prognosis	The disease may follow an unremitting course leading about half of patients to ESRD within ten years from presentation.
Treatment	No specific treatment is available.

proteinuria, often in a nephrotic range, hypertension, and slow progression to renal failure. There is a typical increase in serum type-III procollagen peptide (PIIINP) levels. Most of the few reported cases have been observed in Japan (Alchi et al., 2007) or in India (Reddy et al., 2017), suggesting a geographic or ancestral influence (Table 11.2).

Pathology

Light microscopy: Glomeruli appear expanded by eosinophilic, mesangial, and subendothelial deposits that confer a clear lobular aspect to glomeruli. Congo-Red and thioflavin T stains are negative. There is neither mesangial cell proliferation nor cell infiltration (Plate 20). Peripheral capillary walls are thick and often show double-contour appearance, similar to that seen in membranoproliferative glomerulonephritis (MPGN) type 1 (see Chapter 8). In advanced stages, tubular atrophy and interstitial fibrosis are present, capillary lumens are narrowed by the expanded mesangium and thickened capillary walls, and glomeruli show a nodular appearance suggestive of Kimmelstiel-Wilson lesions in patients with diabetic nephropathy (Alchi et al., 2007).

Immunofluorescence: In some patients, no staining can be seen (Kurien et al., 2015). In other cases, focal and segmental staining for IgM, IgG, and C3 may be found in subendothelial deposits. However, in a well-documented case of collagenofibrotic glomerulopathy, all IgA, IgG, and IgM immunoglobulins, complement, and light chains were detected in the subendothelial space and capillary walls of the glomeruli (Fukami et al., 2014). Immunohistochemistry shows abundant staining for type-III collagen in the expanded mesangium and thickened glomerular capillary walls.

Electron microscopy: It is necessary for a definite diagnosis. The lamina densa of glomerular basement membrane (GBM) is unremarkable (Patel and Cimbaluk, 2016). The extracellular space of the mesangium and subendothelial space of the GBM are markedly expanded, giving a lucent or lytic appearance to these structures (Nimmagadda et al., 2017). In both spaces, there is a marked accumulation of fibrillar material. The fibres have a transverse band structure, with a distinctive periodicity of approximately 60 nm—exactly the same as that of type-III collagen. The fibres tend to be curved or frayed, forming irregularly arranged bundles on longitudinal section and a flower-like or ragged, moth-eaten appearance on cross-section (Alchi et al., 2007; see also Plate 21).

Pathogenesis

The disease is clearly related to abnormal glomerular deposits of type-III collagen, a ubiquitous structural protein of the extracellular matrix that is particularly abundant in tissues showing elastic properties, such as skin, blood vessels, and various internal organs. In normal human kidney, type-III collagen is present only in the interstitium and blood vessels, but not in glomeruli. It may be found in the glomerular mesangium in patients with various types of glomerulonephritis and in the vascular pole in patients with progressive renal disease.

It is still unknown whether in collagenofibrotic glomerulopathy abnormal collagen originates from within the glomeruli or derives from an extrarenal source (Iskandar and Herrera, 2015; Kurien et al., 2015). Glomerular epithelial cells potentially can synthesize type-III collagen. However, it is unclear whether epithelial cells or even endothelial cells are responsible for the production and/or deposition of type-III collagen fibres in this disease. Alternatively, type-III collagen glomerulopathy might be a systemic disorder with abnormal metabolism of type-III collagen (Iskandar and Herrera, 2015). The finding of abnormally high serum PIIINP levels suggests the systemic nature of this condition, a hypothesis also supported by the rising of PIIINP after transplantation (Suzuki et al., 2004), and by the association of collagenofibrotic glomerulopathy with systemic Hodgkin's lymphoma (Soni et al., 2011). On the other hand, increases in serum and urine procollagen type-III peptide can be seen in advanced renal fibrosis and are not specific to collagenofibrotic glomerulopathy (Kurien et al., 2015).

Aetiology

The causes are entirely elusive. Although the disease is mostly sporadic, a few cases occurred in siblings whose parents had no renal disease (Aoki et al., 2015; Chen et al., 2017). This led to the assumption that collagenofibrotic glomerulopathy is a genetic disease transmitted as an autosomal recessive trait (Gubler et al., 1993), but numbers of patients and families analysed to date have not allowed an inheritance pattern to be definitely established (Alchi et al., 2007).

Clinical presentation

The disease usually presents as an isolated, sporadic form in adults (Kurien et al., 2015; Anhita et al., 2016; Nimmagadda et al., 2017; Reddy et al., 2017). Rarely, a familial form with autosomal recessive inheritance may present in children (Gubler et al., 1993). The most common presenting feature is proteinuria, which may reach the nephrotic range in approximately 60 per cent of patients. About two-thirds of patients have hypertension at the time of presentation. Anaemia is frequent even before renal failure develops (Patro et al., 2011). The main specific laboratory finding is represented by elevated serum PIIINP levels. Elevated serum levels of hyaluronan, a glycosaminoglycan found in the extracellular spaces of most tissues, were found in three of four patients with collagenofibrotic glomerulopathy (Goto et al., 2014). However, the reasons for these elevated levels of hyaluronan are unknown as serum levels of the enzyme hyaluronidase were normal, and hyaluronan was not deposited in the mesangial or subendothelial spaces.

Epidemiology

Most cases reported in the literature occurred in Asian patients, particularly in Japanese and Indian populations. However, rare cases have also been observed in Caucasian patients (Imbasciati et al., 1991; Gubler et al., 1993; Ferreira et al., 2009). Most cases occurred sporadically, but familial cases transmitted according to an apparently autosomal recessive trait have also been described (Gubler et al., 1993).

Natural history

The disease is usually progressive both in children and adults, although the renal functional deterioration may be slow (Duggal et al., 2012). However, it is difficult to establish the long-term prognosis as in many reported cases the follow-up was relatively short. A Japanese retrospective investigation on patients followed by different hospitals reported a ten-year renal survival rate of 49 per cent (Suzuki et al., 2004).

Specific treatment

Specific treatment is not available. Theoretically, glucocorticoids might be of some help as these agents may suppress type-III collagen synthesis in the dermis. Hisakawa and colleagues (1998) treated a 68-year- old Japanese man with prednisolone (40 mg/d) and reported some improvement of renal function, anaemia, and proteinuria, which paralleled decreases in serum PIIINP levels.

Symptomatic treatment should be directed to control hypertension, correct anaemia, and reduce proteinuria with ACE inhibitors and angiotensin receptor blockers (see also Chapter 2).

Practical recommendations

The diagnosis of this disease is quite difficult and it is easy to miss. Although there is markedly elevated serum precursor type-III collagen protein in circulation, the diagnosis is usually made by kidney biopsy (Cohen, 2012). The histological pattern may resemble that of a MPGN, but in collagenofibrotic disease there is no glomerular hypercellularity and at immunofluorescence IgG and C3 deposits, when present, are scanty and focal. With light microscopy, a differential diagnosis with thrombotic micro-angiopathy may be difficult, but the clinical features and ultrastructural investigation may orientate towards a correct diagnosis. Amyloidosis may be ruled out as the type-III collagen deposits do not stain with Congo-Red or thioflavin T. The electron microscopy is needed for a correct differential diagnosis with other fibrillary diseases. In type-III collagen glomerulopathy, electron-dense immune complex-type deposits usually are not present; however, subendothelial dense deposits can be seen infrequently. Unique microtubular structures as seen in immunotactoid glomerulopathy, fibrin, and amyloid fibrils are not observed. In contrast to nail-patella syndrome, the lamina densa of the GBM in patients with collagenofibrotic glomerulopathy is of normal thickness and lacks the lucent areas, or the so-called 'moth-eaten appearance'. Various degrees of effacement of epithelial foot processes usually are seen. The differential diagnosis with nail-patella syndrome, another type-III collagen glomerulopathy owing to mutations in the gene *LMX1B*, is easy as nail-patella syndrome is a multisystem disorder with orthopaedic and cutaneous manifestations.

Unfortunately, however, when the diagnosis is made there is not an available specific treatment. A trial with glucocorticoids may be attempted, following proteinuria and serum PIIINP levels to evaluate the response. Otherwise, patients should be given symptomatic therapy.

Transplantation

At the best of our knowledge, only one young Japanese woman received a kidney transplantation. Her post-operative course was uneventful with good renal function three years after transplantation. The immunosuppression consisted of methylprednisolone, tacrolimus, and basiliximab. Although urinary protein was negative, the serum level of PIIIP gradually increased, suggesting new collagen production in the graft and the presence of a systemic factor that stimulated collagen-III production (Suzuki et al., 2004).

Thin basement membrane nephropathy (TBMN)

Thin basement membrane nephropathy (TBMN) is a primary glomerular disorder characterized clinically by isolated microscopic haematuria and pathologically by diffuse uniform thinning of GBM on electron microscopy examination (Table 11.3). Numerous names have been used for the disease, but TBMN is the preferred term as it refers to a renal disorder that is associated with observable structural changes in the GBM. In the majority of cases, TBMN is caused by a disorder of type-IV collagen (COL4), a fundamental component of GBM. This disorder depends on mutations of *COL4A3/COL4A4* genes responsible for the synthesis of the alpha 3/4 chains of type-IV collagen. TBMN is often discovered incidentally and usually has a good long-term prognosis. However, some adults with TBMN have proteinuria >0.5 g/day or renal impairment and may progress to ESRD in an advanced age. About 50 per cent of cases of TBMN show a familial aggregation most often in an autosomal dominant pattern. Unlike X-linked Alport syndrome, affected-father-to-affected-son transmission may be seen.

Pathology

Light microscopy: The glomeruli appear normal or show mild mesangial cellular proliferation and matrix expansion. Slight attenuation of the GBM sometimes can be observed by Jones methenamine silver or periodic acid-Schiff stains, suggesting GBM thinning.

Immunofluorescence: It is usually negative but there is sometimes positivity for IgM or C3 and rarely IgG or IgA.

Electron microscopy: It reveals the typical feature of TBMN, i.e. uniform thinning of the GBM. However, the diagnosis may be difficult as the GBM thickness varies with age, sex, and the different methods of tissue preparation and

Table 11.3 Main characteristics of thin basement membrane nephropathy (TBMN).

Pathology	At optic microscopy the glomeruli appear normal. Immunofluorescence is negative. On electron microscopy there is a uniform thinning of GBM.
Pathogenesis	In TBMN there are defects of type IV collagen, a fundamental component of GBM. These defects are caused by heterozygous mutations of *COL4A3* or *COL4A4* genes which are responsible for the synthesis of collagen IV.
Aetiology	In many cases, TBMN is an inherited disorder of type-IV collagen. At least 50% of patients with TBMN have an autosomal dominant transmission.
Clinical presentation	The disease is usually asymptomatic in children and young adults. In these cases, TBMN can be diagnosed by the discovery of dysmorphic microscopic haematuria or by an occasional macroscopic haematuria. With advancing age, a consistent number of patients may develop proteinuria or chronic kidney disease. The differential diagnosis with Alport syndrome may be difficult. Extrarenal signs and symptoms are absent in TBMN. Genetic heterozygous mutations in either *COL4A3* or *COL4A4* can be detected in TBMN whereas homozygosity or combined heterozygosity of *COL4A3* or *COL4A4*, or hemizygosity for a single defective *COL4A5* allele in males characterize autosomal recessive Alport syndrome.
Prognosis	Most patients do not show any progression of the disease but proteinuria and progressive renal failure may develop in older patients.
Treatment	If proteinuria or hypertension develop, ACE-inhibitors or angiotensin receptor blockers are recommended.

measurement (Foster et al., 2005). The GBM thinning in TBMN is uniform; it appears as a trilaminar structure with a central lamina densa and an inner lamina rara interna and an outer lamina rara externa. The mean thickness in adults ranges from 321 nm to 370 nm ± 50 nm (Tryggvason and Patrakka, 2006). In children, the GBM thickness is 150 nm at birth, 200 nm at age one year, and approaches thickness in adults at age 11 years (Vogler et al., 1987). The criteria for TBMN in adolescents and in adults vary from 200 nm (Cosio et al., 1996) to 264 nm (Gauthier et al., 1989). The difference may be partly explained by the technical differences in tissue processing. The World Health Organization has proposed a threshold of 250 nm for adults and 180 nm for children between 2 and 11 years of age (Churg et al., 1995).

Sometimes, rare regions are observed with laminations, microgranular formation, or regional thickening, features which are typically seen in Alport syndrome, a genetic disorder characterized by renal, cochlear, and ocular involvement, and caused by an inherited defect in type-IV collagen due to mutations in genes encoding the α3, α4, or α5 chains of type-IV collagen. To render differential diagnosis more difficult, electron microscopic analysis at early stages of Alport syndrome can reveal uniform thinning of the GBM similar to that seen in TBMN (Craver et al., 2014). Three-dimensional morphological evaluation by low vacuum scanning electron microscopy may be useful for a differential diagnosis in these difficult cases. The GBMs show characteristic coarse meshwork appearances in Alport syndrome, and thin and sheet-like appearances in TBMN. At the cut side view of the capillary wall, the GBMs in Alport syndrome appear as fibrous inclusions between a podocyte and an endothelial cell, while the GBMs in TBMN show thin linear appearances (Okada et al., 2014). Immunohistochemical evaluation of the type-IV collagen α3 to α5 chains in renal biopsy can also differentiate between TBMN and early stages of Alport syndrome with thin GBM, as these chains usually are either absent or abnormally distributed in Alport syndrome (Haas, 2009). Normal children and some patients with minimal change nephropathy or other glomerulonephritis may also show thin GBM, but thinning is usually focal and not uniform as in TBMN.

Pathogenesis

In the majority of cases, TBMN is a genetic disorder of type-IV collagen mainly related to mutations in locus *COL4A3/COL4A4*. Type-IV collagen is a specific triple-helical structural component of basement membranes. There are six distinct collagen IV α chains, α1 to α6. The most common form of type-IV collagen molecules contains α1 and α2 chains in a 2:1 ratio. In GBM, this form of collagen IV is replaced after birth by molecules with the chain composition α3:α4:α5 encoded respectively by genes *COL4A3* and *COL4A4* (situated on chromosome 2) and *COL4A5* (on the X chromosome). Collagen IV is essential for the integrity of GBM, as well as for some other specialized basement membranes in the inner ear and lens capsule. The development of autosomal dominant TBMN usually involves heterozygous mutations in either *COL4A3* or *COL4A4*. A large number of mutations in *COL4A3* and *COL4A4* have been identified in TBMN, and most of these are single nucleotide substitutions that are different in each family (Weber et al., 2016; Xu et al., 2016).

While males or females who are heterozygous for *COL4A3* or *COL4A4* mutations usually manifest as TBMN, those who are homozygous or combined heterozygotes develop autosomal-recessive Alport syndrome, a disorder caused by mutations in *COL4A3*, *COL4A4*, and *COL4A5*. *COL4A5* mutations are associated with X-linked Alport syndrome, which represents 80–85 per cent of cases and is more severe in boys than in girls. Mutations in *COL4A3* or *COL4A4* are associated with autosomal Alport syndrome (Thorner, 2007). *COL4A3* and *COL4A4* genes can also be involved in hereditary focal segmental glomerulosclerosis (FSGS). In 13 Cypriot families clinically affected with TBMN microscopic haematuria, mild proteinuria, and variable degrees of renal impairment, a dual diagnosis of FSGS and TBMN was made in 20 biopsied cases. Out of 236 family members genetically studied, 127 (53.8 per cent) carried a heterozygous mutation of *COL4A3* or *COL4A4*. None of the heterozygous patients had any extrarenal manifestation, supporting the diagnosis of TBMN. During follow-up of up to three decades, 31 of 82 patients (37.8 per cent) developed chronic renal failure and 16 (19.5 per cent) reached ESRD. Next-generation sequencing of these patients failed to reveal a second mutation in any of the *COL4A3/A4/A5* genes, supporting that true heterozygosity for *COL4A3/A4* mutations predisposes to FSGS and chronic renal failure (Voskarides et al., 2007; Pierides et al., 2009). Functional studies in these patients supported a potential role of the unfolded protein response cascade in modulating the final phenotype in patients with collagen IV nephropathies (Papazachariou et al., 2014). By performing next-generation sequencing on 70 families with hereditary FSGS, Malone and colleagues (2014) discovered that seven of these families had rare or novel variants in *COL4A3* or *COL4A4*. The predominant clinical finding in these families was proteinuria associated with haematuria. In all seven families, there were individuals with nephrotic-range proteinuria and histologic features of FSGS by light microscopy. In another study, pathogenic mutations of *COL4A3-5* were found in 22 per cent of patients with FSGS and a familial history of renal disease (Gast et al., 2016). It is also possible that membranes in other tissues may be affected in TBMN (Gale et al., 2016; Savige, 2016; Chen et al., 2018).

In summary, many different mutations of collagen IV genes *COL4A3*, *COL4A4*, and *COL4A5* may cause TBMN, autosomal recessive Alport syndrome, and even a lesion of FSGS. However, testing for *COL4A3* and *COL4A4* mutations to diagnose TBMN is difficult because of the frequent polymorphism of these genes and the likelihood of a further gene locus. From a clinical point of view, simultaneous next-generation sequencing of all three *COL4A3/COL4A4/COL4A5* genes may be recommended as the most expedient approach to diagnosing collagen IV-related GBM nephropathies (Nabais-Sa et al., 2015).

Aetiology

In most cases, TBMN is an inherited disorder of type IV collagen. At least 50 per cent of patients with TBMN have an autosomal dominant transmission. Patients with TBMN are heterozygous for mutations in either *COL4A3* or

COL4A4 similarly to female individuals with mutations in one *COL4A5* allele, which are carriers for X-linked Alport syndrome in male individuals. Recently, a mis-sense variant in the fibronectin1 gene was identified in members of a Chinese family with haematuria or TBMN. A male patient in this family progressed to ESRD (Yuan et al., 2016).

Clinical presentation

TBMN is often diagnosed in children and young adults when there is persistent dysmorphic haematuria, with no or mild proteinuria, without other renal or extrarenal abnormalities. Many patients have relatives with isolated microhaematuria. At least a single episode of macroscopic haematuria is observed in 5–22 per cent of patients, typically manifesting after exercise or during infection. Exceptionally, in patients with macroscopic haematuria, erythrocyte casts may cause tubular obstruction and acute kidney injury (Lim et al., 2015). Occasionally, the haematuria disappears with time, but with advancing age a consistent number of patients may develop proteinuria and even progressive chronic kidney disease associated with hypertension.

Such a clinical picture can also be seen in Alport syndrome. A detailed family history and genetic testing can allow a differential diagnosis. Alport syndrome is usually inherited as an X-linked or autosomal recessive trait, while TBMN is usually autosomal dominant (Chan and Gale, 2015). In other instances, a differential diagnosis with initial phases of IgA nephropathy may be difficult. Renal biopsy with ultramicroscopy and immunohistochemical evaluation can allow a differential diagnosis. However, in a number of cases it may be difficult to establish whether patients are affected by a form of TBMN caused by heterozygous *COL4A3* or *COL4A4* mutations, by a disease caused by mutations of other genes, or by a co-existent renal disease. Indeed, in about two-thirds of cases, TBMN is associated with other glomerular diseases, more frequently IgA nephropathy and FSGS (Qazi and Bastani, 2015; Zurawski et al., 2016).

Epidemiology

TBMN is the most common cause of persistent glomerular haematuria in children and adults. However, the exact prevalence of the disease is difficult to assess, as the diagnosis is made mostly on the basis of persistent haematuria combined with minimal proteinuria, whereas the number of electron microscopic analyses of renal biopsies showing thinned GBM are by far less common. Moreover, TBMN may be detected in various types of glomerulonephritis. This may explain a large disparity in the prevalence of TBMN in the general population that has been estimated to range between 1 and 10 per cent (Tryggvason and Patrakka, 2006). TBMN has been reported in all geographic regions of the world and in all ancestries, but most cases have been reported in developed countries. Haematuria has been diagnosed at all ages. It is still uncertain whether the disease is or not more frequent in females. Exact prevalence of the disease is difficult to appreciate as not all the patients have persistent isolated microscopic haematuria, many of them are not submitted to renal biopsy, and electron microscopic analyses is performed only in a limited number of cases.

Natural history

TBMN is often considered to be a benign disease. In the great majority of patients TBMN does not show any impairment of renal function over time. Some patients followed for up to 30 years maintained a persistent microhaematuria, sometimes with intervals of episodes of macroscopic haematuria. However, a number of patients may develop proteinuria and chronic kidney disease. The prevalence of these abnormalities depends on the age of patients and the concomitant mutation of other genes or the concomitant presence of other glomerular disorders (e.g. IgA N). A prospective regional study in the Netherlands showed that the vast majority of patients with TBMN had chronic asymptomatic microscopic haematuria frequently associated with hypertension in late middle age; about 15 per cent of patients with TBMN had, in addition, substantial proteinuria associated in the majority of cases with the lesions of FSGS. In 5 per cent of cases a nephrotic syndrome was observed, occasionally associated with FSGS tip variety lesions (Van Paassen et al., 2004). In an Italian multicentre study, eight out of 38 adults with TBMN (21 per cent) followed up for 12–240 months showed signs of disease progression or hypertension (Frascà et al., 2005). In a Spanish study, 16 of 32 patients with TBMN showed proteinuria >0.5 g/day. At the end of a long-term follow-up (198 months in proteinuric patients and 210 months in patients without proteinuria) the prevalence of hypertension was 68 per cent in proteinuric patients, compared with 12 per cent in non-proteinuric patients. A slow decline of renal function was observed in proteinuric patients, although no patient developed ESRD. Multiple bilateral kidney cysts were found in 56 per cent of proteinuric patients, suggesting that development of cysts may influence the outcome of the disease (Sevillano et al., 2014). In a large study on Cypriot families with 127 mutation carriers (MCs), microscopic haematuria was the only urinary finding in patients under age 30. The prevalence of haematuria alone fell to 66 per cent between 31 and 50 years, to 30 per cent between 51 and 70 years, and to 23 per cent over age 71. Proteinuria with chronic renal failure developed in 8 per cent of MCs between 31 and 50 years, in 25 per cent between 51 and 70 years, and in 50 per cent over 71 years. Altogether, 18 of these 127 MCs (14 per cent) developed ESRD at a mean age of 60 years (Pierides et al., 2009). The risk of renal failure would be particularly strong in subjects carrying the variant NEPH3 gene (Voskarides et al., 2017). On the basis of these results, TBMN cannot be considered a benign renal condition in a substantial number of patients, particularly those in late age. This conclusion has obvious implications for potential living donors who are found to have a TBMN lesion in pre-transplant evaluations (see 'Transplantation').

Specific treatment

Most patients with TBMN do not require any treatment. Patients showing signs of progressive renal disease may benefit from treatments that may reduce proteinuria, i.e. ACE-inhibitors, angiotensin-receptor blockers, spironolactone, and vitamin D (Garsen et al., 2015). In the exceptional cases of noncrescentic pulmonary-predominant anti-GBM disease with concurrent TBMN plasmapheresis, corticosteroids and cyclophosphamide are recommended (Singhal et al., 2018).

Practical recommendation

The first problem for the nephrologist confronted by a patient with persistent microscopic haematuria is to accurately and fully assess the diagnosis. A careful study of the urine sediment by phase contrast microscopy showing more than 75–80 per cent distorted (dysmorphic) red blood cells is very strongly suggestive of a glomerular disease. The finding of >4–5 per cent acanthocytes (ring-formed cells with one or more protrusions of different shape and size) is essentially equivalent to a diagnosis of glomerular disease. To ascertain the diagnosis of TBMN, a renal biopsy with ultrastructural examination is absolutely necessary and indispensable. As mentioned previously, the differential diagnosis with Alport syndrome may be difficult and the threshold for deciding whether GBM may be considered *thin* has been differently estimated and is variable with age. Moreover, while many investigators think in TBMN that there is a uniform thinning of GBM, some investigators pointed out that a considerable number of patients with TBMN display segmental GBM attenuation (Ivany et al., 2006). Immunohistochemical evaluation of the type IV collagen α3–α5 chains may help for the differential diagnosis as these chains are usually absent in Alport syndrome. Some clinical features may help in the differential diagnosis. Typical Alport syndrome findings, such as hearing loss, lenticonus, and retinopathy, develop usually first during adolescence. Approximately 95 per cent of the hemizygous female carriers of X-linked Alport syndrome have haematuria, but they cannot easily be distinguished from individuals with authentic TBMN without a study of the presence of the α3–α5 chains of type IV collagen in glomeruli, Bowman's capsule, tubular basement membrane, or skin basement membrane. However, knowledge about hearing loss, lenticonus, or retinopathy in other relatives can give a hint about X-linked Alport syndrome. Sequencing of the *COL4A3* and *COL4A4* genes is possible in specialized laboratories. It would be important to be able to provide DNA sequencing of the *COL4A3, COL4A4, and COL4A5* genes for making an accurate genetically-based diagnosis of TBMN and the various forms of Alport syndrome.

Despite the good outcome for many years, a considerable number of patients with TBMN may develop renal function impairment, most often in association with the appearance of proteinuria. It is therefore recommended that patients with a diagnosis of TBMN are regularly monitored, at least once a year, to check the absence of significant proteinuria, arterial hypertension, and/or renal function impairment.

Transplantation

In case of reappearance of microhaematuria after transplantation, one should investigate whether the donor was affected by Alport syndrome or IgA nephropathy before defining microhaematuria as a sign of recurrence.

Donation from individuals with TBMN remains controversial because the risk for the donor is largely unknown. Two small series collected information about 13 living kidney donors with TBMN. All the donors maintained normal renal function and were free of hypertension, and proteinuria over follow-ups ranging from 15 to 76 months (Koushik et al., 2005; Choi et al., 2018). The Expert Guidelines for the Management of Alport Syndrome and Thin Basement Membrane Nephropathy recommended that individuals with TBMN may be kidney donors if they have normal blood pressure, proteinuria, and renal function, and if a biopsy can exclude Alport syndrome (Savige et al., 2013).

By electron microscopy follow-up biopsy basement membrane thickness appeared normal in two allografts from donors with TBMN; the recipients did not show haematuria (Choi et al., 2012). In our experience, a young patient with Alport syndrome received the kidney from his father with TBMN. After 21 years the transplanted kidney is still functioning with an estimated GFR of 61 ml/min and mild proteinuria < 0.5 g/day. The father is still alive with normal kidney function.

Lipoprotein glomerulopathy (LPG)

Lipoprotein glomerulopathy (LPG) is a rare disorder in which lipoprotein thrombi are seen in glomerular capillaries. The disease may be familial or sporadic. It mainly affects Japanese or Chinese patients but cases have been reported also in Europe, the US, and Brazil. The disease usually presents with protein-uria and hypertension, and frequently progresses to renal failure (Table 11.4). Glomeruli on biopsy are large, their capillaries contain pale-staining amorphous thrombi staining positive for lipid (Oil Red-O stains) in non-ethanol fixed specimens. Although total cholesterol, low-density lipoprotein (LDL), cholesterol, or triglyceride levels are usually elevated, the only lipid abnormality seen in every patient with LPG has been increased serum apolipoprotein E (apoE) levels. These elevated apoE levels are determined in part by the binding activities of apoE to the LDL receptor, LDL receptor-related protein, and VLDL receptor.

Table 11.4 Main characteristics of lipoprotein glomerulopathy (LPG).

Pathology	Light microscopy shows marked dilatation of the capillary lumen of glomeruli by a pale stained substance. On electron microscopy the substance appears composed by granules and vacuoles of various sizes forming concentric lamellae. Immunochemical studies show deposits of apolipoproteins A, B, and E.
Pathogenesis	The disease probably results by interactions between genetic factors and kidney intrinsic factors, e.g. thermodynamic destabilization and enhanced aggregation of apoE3. In LPG there are mutations in apolipoprotein E causing arginine substitution with proline or cysteine. These variants produce structural changes in apolipoproteins E that may diminish their capacity to bind to LDL receptor and may decrease their uptake from endothelial and mesangial cells. Abnormal apolipoproteins E concentrate and aggregate in the glomerular flow and deposit in capillary walls or around the mesangium. Accumulation of abnormal lipoproteins may be facilitated by dysfunction of Fc receptors that dysregulate the uptake and clearance of lipoproteins.
Aetiology	LPG is an inherited disease caused by heterozygous mutations of apoE genes leading to a substitution of a single amino acid residue or amino acid deletion. The majority of patients with LPG have apoE Sendai or apoE Kyoto, suggesting that these apoE variants have a founder effect.
Clinical presentation	Proteinuria and hypertriglyceridaemia are constant features. Most patients present with a nephrotic syndrome.
Prognosis	About half of patients may develop ESRD but the rate of progression is extremely variable.
Treatment	Lipid-lowering agents including fibrates may obtain improvement of proteinuria and plasma levels of apoE and may halt the progression of the disease in a number of patients.

Epidemiology

According to Saito and Matsunaga (2014), about 150 cases of LPG have been reported in the literature. Of these, most cases were from the eastern area of Japan and some patients were Chinese. However, cases also have been described in Europe (Mourad et al., 1998; Magistroni et al., 2013) and in the US (Rovin et al., 2007; Boumendjel et al., 2010). Among the reported cases, about one-third of patients had a positive family history.

Pathology

Light microscopy: shows marked dilatation of the capillary lumen in glomeruli, which are filled by a pale stained lipoprotein rich material with typical layered structure.(Plate 22). Increased mesangial matrix, extracellular lipid accumulation, and focal mesangiolysis may be seen and focal segmental sclerosis also may occur in some cases (Tsimihodimos and Elisaf, 2011). Atypical histopathological features with a substantial amount of foamy macrophage infiltration in the glomeruli rarely can be seen (see Plate 22; Takasaki et al., 2015). It should be noted that foamy appearing glomeruli can also be seen in lecithin-cholesterol acyltransferase deficiency and in conditions that contain numerous histiocytes, including crystal-storing histiocytosis, macrophage-activating syndrome, and thrombotic microangiopathy (Kaur and Sethi, 2016).

Immunofluorescence: usually shows no deposits of immunoglobulins or complement. Immunohistochemical studies in snap-frozen renal sections show thrombus-like substances containing lipid droplets of apolipoproteins A, B, and E (Saito et al., 2006; Zhang et al., 2008).

Electron microscopy: shows thrombus-like substances in glomerular capillaries composed of granules and vacuoles of various sizes, forming concentric lamellae, like a fingerprint (Plate 23).

Pathogenesis

The current hypothesis is that LPG is an inherited disease in which apoE gene mutations lead to substitution of a single amino acid residue or amino acid deletion inducing the formation of abnormal apoE that deposit in the glomeruli (Saito and Matsunaga, 2014). These apoE polymorphisms, including three common phenotypes (E2, E3, E4) and a variety of rare mutations, can affect blood cholesterol and triglyceride levels (Matsunaga and Saito, 2014). Most mutations are located in or close to the LDL receptor-binding domain. They are heterozygous and among mis-sense mutations four are proline-for-arginine substitutions, and three are cysteine-for-arginine substitutions (Pasquariello et al., 2014). The substitution of the proline residue for arginine residue in apoE produces severe structural changes in the middle of the helix in apoE and may alter the three-dimensional conformation of the protein. These changes reduce the affinity of apoE for the LDL receptor and also decrease its uptake by endothelial cells. In three common apoE3 variants, it has been documented that hereditary mutations induce a generalized unfolding of the N-terminal domain of apoE3. The folding perturbations in apoE can lead to structural destabilization of abnormal lipoproteins containing apoE, which may concentrate and aggregate in the glomerular flow, forming lipoprotein thrombi that deposit in capillary walls or around the mesangium. These data suggest that apoE3 N-terminal domain unfolding due to mutation may constitute a common mechanism underlying the protein's association with the pathogenesis of LPG (Georgiadou et al., 2013). Cases of LPG in which arginine was substituted by proline are thermodynamically destabilized and aggregation-prone. It has been reported that a thermodynamic destabilization and enhanced aggregation of apoE3 also occurs in LPG associated with nonproline apoE3 mutations, suggesting a common mechanism behind the pathogenesis of LPG (Katsarou et al., 2018). Some apoE variants of LPG, such as apoE Kyoto (Arg25Cys) and apoE5 (Gln3Lys), may produce lipid peroxidation and a direct damage to glomerulus, suggesting a potential role of oxidative stress in LPG (Miyata et al., 1999). Recently, a case of LPG with apoE2 Chicago and apoE5 (Glu3Lys) mutations in the same allele has been reported (Kodera et al., 2017). Moreover, the negatively charged apoE variants can cause hypertriglyceridaemia, which in turn promotes the increase in apoE, apoC-III, and electronegative LDL. It should be also pointed out that apoE is synthesized in the human kidney and regulates mesangial cell proliferation and matrix overproduction in experimental models. Therefore, apoE seems to act as an autocrine regulator of mesangial and glomerular function, and intrarenal dysfunction induced by apoE abnormality may contribute to the induction of LPG (Saito et al., 2006).

A possible pathogenetic role may also be played by impairment of macrophage activity resulting from deficit of Fc receptors. A dysfunction of mesangial Fc receptors may dysregulate the uptake and clearance of LDL leading to the accumulation of lipoproteins in mesangial and endothelial cells, with formation of lipoprotein thrombi, lipid granules, and apoA and apoE deposits with a fingerprint pattern (Ito et al., 2012).

Aetiology

In 1997, Oikawa and colleagues detected high concentrations of apoE in three patients with LPG and identified an apoE2 variant in them. The patients' DNA sequences were analysed, and a nucleotide G to C point mutation in exon 4 of the apoE gene was confirmed in each patient. This mis-sense mutation denoted amino acid substitution of the proline residue for arginine residue at position 145 of apoE. This apoE2 variant (Arg145Pro) was termed apoE Sendai, representing the name of the city where the patients lived. Subsequently, an apoE3 variant called Kyoto (Arg25 Cys) was discovered (Matsunaga et al., 1999), followed by a number of other variants called apoE Tokyo, apoE Maebashi, apoE Guangzhou, apoE Tsukuba, etc (Chen, 2014). Even in Caucasian patients, an apoE Las Vegas (Ala152→Asp) and an apoE Modena (Arg150→Cys) were identified (Bomback et al., 2010; Magistroni et al., 2013). The discovery of novel mutants in apoE suggested that lipoproteins with these variants have an aetiological role in LPG. However, the majority of patients with LPG have apoE Sendai or apoE Kyoto, suggesting that these apoE variants have a founder effect. Rarely, two mis-sense mutations can occur in a patient (Li et al., 2014). The causative role of apoE mutations was confirmed by the demonstration that LPG may be induced by virus-mediated transduction of apoE Sendai in apoE-knockout mice (Saito et al., 2006).

Clinical presentation

Although the age at presentation may range from four to 69 years, most afflicted patients are in the third and fourth decades of life (Sam et al., 2006). Blood pressure in most patients is normal or moderately elevated. Protein excretion exceeds 1 g/day in almost all patients, and about 60 per cent of patients are nephrotic and present with oedemas. Microscopic haematuria is usually absent. One-third of patients have impaired renal function at presentation. Most patients have type-III hyperlipoproteinaemia, with predominance of triglycerides (Zhang et al., 2008; Saito and Matzunaga, 2014). In detailed assays for plasma lipoproteins isolated by means of ultracentrifugation, high cholesterol levels in very-low-density and intermediate density lipoprotein fractions were observed. In a review, all except one patient had elevated plasma apoE levels, ranging from 4.0 to 38 mg/dL (Sam et al., 2006).

Natural history

It is difficult to know the outcome for patients with LPG, as many of the described cases had a short-term follow-up. It is likely that most patients have a relentless course to ESRD.

Saito and colleagues (2006) reported that half of the patients developed renal failure 1–27 years after clinical onset. Rare cases of acute renal failure have also been reported. Among them, one patient with LPG and malignant hypertension developed a thrombotic microangiopathy that led to irreversible renal failure (Wu et al., 2013).

Specific treatment

Glucocorticoids, immunosuppressants, and anticoagulants are ineffective (Luo et al., 2008). Immunoadsorption onto protein A, lipopheresis, and double filtration plasmapheresis obtained significant but transient reduction of proteinuria and plasma apoE values (Xin et al., 2009; Magistroni et al., 2013; Li et al., 2014). Intensive therapy using lipid-lowering agents, including fibrates, was reported to halt the progression of renal dysfunction (Sam et al., 2006), and even to obtain regression of histological changes at renal biopsy (Ieri et al., 2003; Kodera et al., 2017). In a large study, 16 patients with apo Kyoto mutation were treated with fenofibrate for over 12 months at doses able to keep serum triglycerides and apoE levels <100 mg/dl. Six patients reached complete remission of proteinuria and eight reached partial remission (Hu et al., 2014). The effectiveness of fibrates was confirmed in Chinese patients (Chen et al., 2014). This data show that the progressive outcome of LPG may be improved by reducing the serum levels of triglyceride-lipoproteins containing apoE and also suggest that hyperlipidaemia mediated by the environment is an important factor in the development of LPG, although LPG essentially is based on the genetic abnormality of apoE. Recent data in mice reported that adipose triglyceride lipase deficiency can induce renal lipid accumulation, proteinuria, and glomerular filtration barrier dysfunction. These effects may be partially reversed by the antioxidant N-acetylcysteine (Chen et al., 2017).

Practical recommendations

LPG is an exceptionally rare disorder and its diagnosis can be easily missed. According to Saito and colleagues (2006) the diagnosis should be suspected in the presence of:

i. mild to severe proteinuria;

ii. dilatation of glomerular capillary lumina with pale-stained substances on light microscopy;

iii. stone or sand-like granules occupying the capillary lumina on electron microscopy (so-called lipoprotein thrombi); and or

iv. type-III hyperlipoproteinaemia with high apoE concentration, usually associated with a heterozygous apoE phenotype, E2/3 or E2/4, but sometimes with uncommon types, such as E1/3 or others.

Treatment of LPG should be based on symptomatic therapy, maximizing the doses of fibrates and statins, under strict surveillance of creatine-phosphokinase enzyme levels in the serum in order to detect and prevent rhabdomyolysis. Immunoadsorption with protein A, plasmapheresis, or lipopheresis may obtain a significant reduction of proteinuria and serum levels of apoE. An attempt with acetylcysteine might be tried in patients with LPG refractory to treatment.

Transplantation

Recurrence has been reported in the few patients who received a kidney allograft either from living or deceased donors, suggesting a pathogenic role of humoral component(s) resulting from abnormal lipoprotein metabolism, presumably linked to apoE and other genetic or acquired factors (Miyata et al., 1999). Although the majority of patients lost their allograft after recurrence, a few transplant recipients with LPG maintained stable graft function 10–14 years after histological recurrence was documented (Mourad et al., 1998; Cheung et al., 2014).

'Pure' mesangial proliferative glomerulonephritis (MesPGN)

This clinicopathological entity is an uncommon cause of primary glomerular disease (Churg et al., 1995). It is more often associated with a systemic illness, predominantly SLE and other auto-immune diseases, and infections (Table 11.5).

'Pure' mesangial proliferative glomerulonephritis (MesPGN) must also be separated from other primary glomerular diseases that can manifest pathologically as a diffuse mesangial proliferative lesion, including IgA nephropathy, IgM nephropathy, C3 glomerulonephritis, C1q nephropathy, 'atypical' anti-GBM disease, or resolving post-infectious glomerulonephritis, that may be distinguished by immunofluorescence microscopy and patterns of immunoglobulins and complement components deposition. The group of disorders included in the rubric of 'pure' MesPGN are undoubtedly very heterogeneous (Griveas et al., 2009). This section considers the collection of primary glomerular disorders having in common some degree of pathological mesangial cell hypercellularity unaccompanied by any disturbance in the architecture of the peripheral capillary wall, and in which IgA, IgM, and C1q nephropathy have been excluded by an appropriate immunofluorescence microscopy study of a renal biopsy. This novel form of glomerular injury should be separated from secondary MPGN and from the primary form of C3 glomerulopathy caused by dysregulation of the alternative pathway of complement. Most of the patients classified as pure MesPGN will have some combination of proteinuria and haematuria, and nephrotic syndrome may also develop (Alexopoulos et al., 2000; Nasr et al., 2009). *In summary*, patients with MesPGN and proteinuria represent a heterogeneous group with different clinical courses despite

Table 11.5 Main characteristics of 'pure' mesangial proliferative glomerulonephritis (MesPGN).

Pathology	Mesangial hypercellularity in all of the lobules, with at least three nucleated cells per glomerular lobule. Mesangial matrix may be increased. The peripheral capillary walls are thin and delicate. No necrosis or crescents. Scattered deposits of IgG and /or C3 in mesangium (but not IgA or IgM). Electron dense deposits in the mesangium may be observed.
Pathogenesis	Unknown. Mesangial cell proliferation might be caused by a number of factors. In turn, injured mesangial cells might cause foot process effacement and proteinuria. Some features might suggest that it is an 'immune complex' disease.
Aetiology	Unknown but some cases might be a resolving form of post-infectious disease.
Clinical presentation	Usually glomerular haematuria with variable degrees of proteinuria, including the nephrotic syndrome.
Prognosis	Variable. Persisting nephrotic syndrome may be feature of an evolution to FSGS and progressive renal failure.
Treatment	A trial with steroids or calcineurin inhibitors may be indicated for severe nephrotic syndrome and/or progressive course. Patients who respond with complete or partial remission may have a favourable outcome.

a similar morphological appearance in initial biopsies (Arias and Taborada Murillo, 2017). Some patients may respond to treatment and maintain stable renal function but others will progress to ESRD, often with the development of persistent, steroid-resistant nephrotic syndrome and superimposed focal and segmental glomerular sclerosis (FSGS) or, more rarely, crescentic glomerulonephritis.

Pathology

Light microscopy: Mesangial hypercellularity is usually defined by at least three nucleated (non-polymorphonuclear, non-monocytic) cells (presumptively mesangial cells) per mesangial zone or lobule. In MesPGN, the hypercellularity is rather uniformly expressed among all of the lobules, although it varies in degree. Mesangial matrix may be increased. The peripheral capillary walls are thin. Necrosis, exudation (presence of) circulating polymorph nuclear or monocytic leukocytes (see Plate 24), segmental sclerosis, adhesions, crescents, and thickening of the periphery of the capillary walls are absent. Milder degrees of mesangial hypercellularity are quite common in other primary glomerular diseases, including minimal change disease (MCD).

Immunofluorescence: According to the definition used here, deposits of IgA, IgM, C3, or C1q should be absent or inconspicuous. When polyclonal IgG deposits are present by immunofluorescence and electron-dense deposits are found by ultramicroscopy, an immune-complex mediated disorder may be suspected. However, a fraction of cases has no immune deposits or may present scattered mesangial deposits of IgG and C3. Cases with C3-only deposits may represent C3GN or stages of an acute, post-streptococcal glomerulonephritis (see Chapter 8 and Chapter 9). Isolated C3 deposits may also be seen in C3 glomerulopathy associated with abnormalities in the complement regulatory factors. Monoclonality of the IgG deposits strongly suggest an underlying monoclonal immunoglobulin deposition disease, with a phenotype mimicking an immune-complex glomerulonephritis (Nasr et al., 2004). Rarely, linear deposits of IgG are seen in cases of 'atypical' anti-GBM disease (See Chapter 10).

Electron microscopy: The hypercellularity of the mesangium can be easily demonstrated. Electron dense deposits are quite variable, but often present. There may be focal foot process effacement, but when this is very extensive, the diagnosis of MCD or FSGS should be considered, especially when the mesangial hypercellularity is mild or moderate and when diffuse foot process effacement is observed in electron microscopy.

Pathogenesis

The pathogenesis of MesPGN is largely unknown and most likely heterogeneous. Mesangial cells and their matrix form the central stalk of the glomerulus and are part of a functional unit interacting closely with endothelial cells and podocytes (Schlondorff and Banas, 2009). Mesangial cells are relatively quiescent cells, but a number of mitogenic signals can cause their activation and proliferation; in turn, proliferating mesangial cells may lead to mesangial sclerosis, podocyte injury, foot process effacement, and proteinuria. Research aimed to identify the factors involved in mesangial cell activation has been mainly made in Thy1 nephritis. In this model, several factors have been demonstrated to play a role in controlling mesangial cell proliferation, including platelet-derived growth factor-Beta, mitogen-activated protein kinase-1, cell cycle proteins, cyclin E and CDK2 (Chen et al., 2014), and T-type calcium channels (Cove-Smith et al., 2013). A role may also be played by nestin, a type VI intermediate filament protein which is expressed mostly in nerve cells but is also constitutively expressed in podocytes. A study in vitro demonstrated that nestin can promote proliferation of isolated mesangial cells, while blocking of nestin results in inhibition of cell proliferation (Daniel et al., 2008). Very rarely, linear deposits of IgG are found by immunofluorescence, possibly indicating a role for anti-GBM auto-antibodies.

Aetiology

The aetiology of MesPGN is unknown, but the clinical and pathological features often suggest that an infectious disease is involved. The late discovery of MesPGN with isolated deposits of C3 and persistent haematuria may suggest a resolving form of post-streptococcal glomerulonephritis or a C3 GN (see Chapter 8 and Chapter 9).

Clinical presentation

The typical presentation for MesPGN is a combination of glomerular haematuria and proteinuria. Nephrotic syndrome may be present. Renal function is typically normal, but progression of disease may be seen, especially if the lesion evolves to FSGS. A large series of patients with monoclonal IgG reported that 49 per cent had nephrotic syndrome, 68 per cent renal insufficiency, and 77 per cent haematuria at presentation. A monoclonal serum protein was detected in 30 per cent of patients (Nasr et al., 2009). Complement levels are normal and serological evaluation for SLE, vasculitis, and infection are negative.

Many patients have isolated recurrent gross or microscopic haematuria with minimally elevated levels of urinary protein excretion. Since renal biopsies are seldom carried out in these clinical situations, the overall occurrences of MesPGN may have been underestimated.

Epidemiology

The incidence and prevalence of MesPGN is not well known. Among patients presenting with nephrotic syndrome, MesPGN is quite uncommon, accounting for under 5 per cent of cases. Mild degrees of mesangial proliferation may accompany other lesions, such as MCD and FSGS, so it is possible that some cases may mistakenly be assigned to the category of MesPGN, at least initially. As discussed previously, IgA nephropathy, IgM nephropathy, C1q nephropathy, SLE and resolving post-infectious glomerulonephritis need to be excluded. Ascertainment bias (indications for renal biopsy) may contribute to the relative infrequency of MesPGN in descriptions of prevalence.

Natural history

The evolution of MesPGN is not well understood. It is very clear that some patients may evolve into a picture of typical FSGS. When the mesangial cell proliferation is mild, many cases cannot be clinically distinguished from the evolution of the MCD. Spontaneous remission may develop, but more often the disease persists and if nephrotic syndrome is present, progression to FSGS and renal failure is more common. Patients with isolated glomerular haematuria or those with minimal degrees of proteinuria tend to have a benign evolution.

Specific treatment

The efficacy and safety of various proposed treatment regimens are very uncertain. Due to their likely benign prognosis, patients with isolated microscopic haematuria or those with minimal degrees of proteinuria (<1.0 g/day) probably do not require any therapy, other than vigorous control of blood pressure. Those with nephrotic syndrome have usually been treated with oral glucocorticoids in a fashion similar to that described for FSGS. A response (partial or complete remission) is observed in about 50–70 per cent of patients so treated. Patients who respond to therapy (completely or partially) have a benign course similar to that of MCD. It has been reported that responders are usually older and have normal renal function at presentation, while non-responders tend to be younger and progress to ESRD, especially if they have impaired renal function at first assessment (Alexopoulos et al., 2000). However, in another small series, neither age nor plasma creatinine at presentation were predictive of response to steroids, cyclophosphamide, or cyclosporine (Griveas et al., 2009). A role for azathioprine or mycophenolate is unknown, but many patients resistant to the effects of glucocorticoids and with persistent nephrotic syndrome and worsening renal function are offered these options, with variable results. Cyclosporine or tacrolimus have been anecdotally effective, particularly when there is a high suspicion of an underlying FSGS.

Practical recommendations

Patients with MesPGN and isolated haematuria and/or minimal proteinuria do not require any specific therapy other than control of blood pressure. Those with more severe degrees of proteinuria, including nephrotic syndrome, should be given a trial of oral glucocorticoids similar to that recommended for FSGS. If the patient proves to be 'steroid-resistant' and still has relatively well-preserved renal function (serum creatinine of <2.0 mg/dl) a trial of either cyclophosphamide or a calcineurin inhibitor could be considered. A therapeutic role for mycophenolate or azathioprine is still uncertain. There is no information about the role of RTX.

Transplantation

In a study on 26 patients with allograft MesPGN, the disease recurred in 89 per cent patients. A detectable paraprotein was found in 20 per cent of cases. During a mean follow up of 87 months, 11 patients lost their allograft within a mean of 36 months from diagnosis. Median graft survival was 92 months. Independent predictors of graft loss were a higher degree of peak proteinuria and longer time from implantation to diagnosis (Said et al., 2018).

IgM nephropathy

The lesion of IgM nephropathy was first described by Cohen, Border, and Glassock (1978). This original description incited much controversy since deposits of IgM were often found 'non-specifically' in many disorders, including MCD and FSGS (Brugnano et al., 2016). Thus, some held that IgM nephropathy was not a 'clinicopathologic' entity. However, the diagnosis of IgM nephropathy is more properly restricted to a group of patients manifesting:

  i. haematuria and variable degrees of proteinuria, including the nephrotic syndrome;
 ii. diffuse and generalized mesangial deposits of IgM accompanied by discrete electron dense deposits in the mesangium at renal biopsy;
iii. variable but distinct degrees of mesangial proliferation without obvious segmental sclerosis; and
 iv. exclusion of systemic disease (see Table 11.6).

Widely scattered mesangial IgM deposits in a biopsy that reveals features quite compatible with the minimal change lesion are not sufficient to define IgM nephropathy. In addition, a renal biopsy which reveals the characteristic features of FSGS and also shows segmental deposits of IgM is *not* IgM nephropathy. Thus, in part, a diagnosis of IgM nephropathy is one of exclusion. Many, indeed most, patients with IgM nephropathy will also display features of MesPGN (see 'Pure' mesangial proliferative glomerulonephritis) and vice versa; thus, there is substantial overlap between mesangial proliferative and IgM nephropathy in the literature.

Pathology

Light microscopy: The spectrum of morphologic alterations ranges from minor changes, to variable degrees of mesangial proliferation, usually of mild to moderate degree (Kasap et al., 2008). The glomeruli appear hypercellular in the mesangial zones, but the peripheral capillary walls are thin, delicate and free of proteinaceous deposits. No FSGS should be observed, but there may be a variable increase in the mesangial matrix. Variable degrees of interstitial fibrosis and/or mononuclear cell infiltration can be seen.

Immunofluorescence: By definition, heavy diffuse and generalized deposits of IgM must be present in the mesangial zones. Lesser degrees of IgG and or IgA

Table 11.6 Main characteristics of IgM nephropathy.

Pathology	At light microscopy glomeruli may appear normal or may show mild to moderate mesangial proliferation. Immunofluorescence shows diffuse and generalized mesangial IgM deposition, often with C3 in the same distribution. Electron dense deposits may be present in the mesangium.
Pathogenesis	Glomerular IgM and complement activation might represent a common final pathway of injury to the glomerulus after toxic, haemodynamic, metabolic, or immunologic insults.
Aetiology	Unknown. No known infectious agent produces this lesion. The disease can be associated with FSGS.
Clinical presentation	Glomerular haematuria and/or nephrotic syndrome.
Prognosis	The natural course may be benign for patients with non-nephritic proteinuria. The disease may evolve to FSGS and renal failure if associated with persisting nephrotic syndrome.
Treatment	Some patients (50%) may respond to glucocorticoids, calcineurin inhibitors, and/or RTX. Treatment programs are similar to those used for primary FSGS.

may also be seen. C3 and C1q deposition are quite common and may be intense. The C3 deposits are in the same pattern as the IgM deposits.

Electron microscopy: Small discrete electron dense deposits are regularly found in the mesangium, but there are no deposits in or on the capillary walls. Increase in mesangial matrix and mesangial cell proliferation can also be observed. The podocyte foot process effacement is not uniformly distributed, unless severe proteinuria is present. Extensive and diffuse foot process effacement with a more focal distribution of IgM and no electron dense deposits should suggest a minimal change lesion with superimposed non-specific IgM deposition, instead of IgM nephropathy.

Pathogenesis

The pathogenesis of IgM nephropathy is unknown. Natural IgM autoantibodies are rapidly produced to inhibit pathogens and abrogate inflammation mediated by invading microorganisms and host neoantigen. Natural IgM has ten antigen combining sites. These multiple sites can enable even low-affinity IgM to activate complement via the classical pathway within the glomerulus (Strassheim et al., 2013; Lobo, 2017). These characteristics allow IgM to provide an initial defence against infection and to promote the healing of wounded cells. However, it remains to be proven whether IgM can deposit in the kidney on its own and initiate glomerular injury, or if it only does so after some other glomerular insult (Mubarak and Nasri, 2014). Recent studies showed that IgM binds to neo-epitopes exposed after insults to the glomerulus and contributes to the progression of glomerular damage in a mouse model of non-sclerotic glomerular disease (Panzer et al., 2015). These findings support a role for IgM in inducing glomerular injury and glomerulosclerosis (Platt and Cascalho, 2015). Thus, glomerular IgM and complement activation may represent a common final pathway of injury to the glomerulus after toxic, haemodynamic, metabolic, or immunologic insults.

Aetiology

The aetiology of IgM nephropathy is unknown. It is possible that certain antigens in the environment (or food) which preferentially elicit IgM responses may be responsible for the genesis of this disease (Vanikar, 2013). Some data suggest that genetic factors may be involved in the mechanism of the disease. In eight patients with biopsy-proven IgM nephropathy belonging to three unrelated families, immunogenetic studies showed the recurrence of an extended haplotype (Scolari et al., 1990).

Clinical presentation

The clinical presentation of IgM nephropathy is quite varied. In a series of 57 adults, 39 per cent of patients presented with the nephrotic syndrome, 49 per cent presented with non-nephrotic proteinuria, and 39 per cent had eGFR <60 ml/min (Connor et al., 2017). Exceptionally, IgM nephropathy may present as a crescentic glomerulonephritis (Kazy and Mubarak, 2014). Serum C3 levels are normal and there is no serological evidence of a systemic 'auto-immune', neoplastic or infectious disease. IgM levels may be elevated, while IgA levels are normal. Various ages may be affected and males are affected twice as commonly as females. Rarely, a familial aggregation may be observed. Cases associated with familial Mediterranean fever have been reported (Peru et al., 2008).

Epidemiology

The reported frequency of IgM nephropathy in literature has varied widely from 2 per cent to 18.5 per cent (Mubarak and Kasi, 2012). However, these data should be taken with caution since reports including patients with MCD or FSGS and 'non-specific' IgM deposition overestimated the frequency. Indeed, a large retrospective study reported a 1.8 per cent prevalence of IgM nephropathy (Connor et al., 2017). The disease apparently has a world-wide distribution. There is no evidence that it is increasing in frequency unlike FSGS.

Natural history

The natural history of the untreated disorder is not well understood as most reports included patients who were actively treated. It does seem clear that many, if not all, patients evolve over time into a picture more compatible with a lesion of FSGS. The outcome is much poorer for those with persistent nephrotic syndrome than those presenting with haematuria and/or low-grade proteinuria. In a large series of 110 patients with presumed IgM nephropathy, including both paediatric and adult patients with nephrotic syndrome or minor urinary abnormalities, during 15 years of follow-up, 36 per cent of patients developed renal insufficiency and 23 per cent reached ESRD (Myllymäki et al., 2003). Hypertension at the time of renal biopsy and high serum C3 can predict poor outcome (Myllymäki et al., 2006). In another series in adults, serum creatinine had doubled in 31 per cent of patients at five years (Connor et al., 2017). Spontaneous remissions may occur, but are rather infrequent. Interstitial fibrosis and global glomerulosclerosis indicate a less favourable outcome.

Specific treatment

In the absence of controlled trials, it is difficult to determine the efficacy of treatment. In retrospective uncontrolled observations, about 60 per cent of proteinuric patients responded to steroids, but frequent relapses and steroid dependence were frequent (Zeis et al., 2001; Myllimäki et al., 2003; Mokhtar, 2011). At any rate, complete or partial remission is associated with an improved prognosis. Cytotoxic drugs may be helpful in few steroid resistant cases, but cyclosporine proved to be superior to cyclophosphamide in an American paediatric series (Swartz et al., 2009). Tacrolimus and RTX with or without steroids have also been used. About 40 per cent of patients entered complete remission followed, however, by frequent relapses (Connor et al., 2017).

Practical recommendations

Patients with isolated haematuria and/or minimal proteinuria need not be treated other than to control blood pressure, if elevated. Patients with nephrotic syndrome should receive a trial of oral glucocorticoids using the regimen described for treatment of FSGS (Chapter 5). Relapsing diseases should be treated in the manner described for the MCD (Chapter 4). Steroid-resistant cases might be given a trial of oral cyclophosphamide (10–12 weeks) or a calcineurin inhibitor (six months), but the overall effectiveness and safety for this approach is not well understood and no controlled trials are available to guide the approach to treatment.

Transplantation

Recurrence of IgM nephropathy in the renal transplant can occur (Salmon et al., 2004). Good results with a combination of plasmapheresis, IV immuno-globulins, and RTX have been reported in a patient with early recurrence of nephrotic syndrome (Westphal et al., 2006).

C1q nephropathy

The clinicopathologic entity known as C1q nephropathy was first described by Jennette and Hipp (1985). Like IgA nephropathy and IgM nephropathy, it is defined by immunofluorescence examination of renal biopsy material. Such studies reveal the characteristic presence of heavy deposits of C1q in the glom-erular mesangium, usually accompanied by IgG and/or IgM and by C3 in a similar distribution. The disease is uncommon. A consensus definition on the diagnosis of C1q nephropathy is lacking and its existence as a distinct clinical disease entity remains controversial. C1q nephropathy has been thought to be a subgroup of primary FSGS, while other reports suggest that C1q nephropathy is not a single disease entity, but that it may be a combination of several disease groups (Mii et al., 2009). In cases defined as C1q nephropathy no features indi-cative of a systemic 'auto-immune' disease should be present (clinically or sero-logically), and nephrotic syndrome with progressive renal failure is common (Table 11.7).

C1q nephropathy is more frequently seen in children and young adults (Wenderfer et al., 2010; Mokhtar and Jalalah, 2015) but exceptionally the dis-ease may occur also in the elderly (Zhao et al., 2014). The disease is uncommon but cases have been reported everywhere in the world. The disorder seems to be more common in subjects of African ancestry but this may be due to a selection bias.

Pathology

Light microscopy: The features by light microscopy are quite varied and can include minimal change lesion or FSGS (Vizjak et al., 2008). The latter le-sion is the most common in most series. Some investigators believe that C1q nephropathy should be classified as a variant of 'idiopathic' FSGS (Markowitz et al., 2003). Collapsing lesions have been observed but necrosis and crescents are uncommon, seen in <5 per cent of cases. Other cases with a pattern of MesPGN have been described as an immune complex variant (Maleshappa and Vankalakunti, 2013).

Immunofluorescence microscopy: The characteristic feature is intense granular or amorphous deposition of C1q. Staining for C1q is evident in all cases of

Table 11.7 Main characteristics of C1q nephropathy.

Pathology	Light microscopy findings are highly variable but FSGS, mesangial proliferation and membranoproliferative patterns are common. The disease is characterized by marked mesangial deposition of C1q, often with immunoglobulins, resembling lupus nephritis (but without any serological features of SLE).
Pathogenesis	C1q deposition in mesangium might result from binding to Fc portion of IgM and IgG either via direct interactions with surface-bound Ig or via trapping of circulating immune complexes.
Aetiology	Unknown. Lesion has features suggesting SLE but serology and clinical findings are negative for an auto-immune disease.
Clinical presentation	Nephrotic syndrome with haematuria and progressive renal failure is common.
Prognosis	It is variable but it is often poor especially in the presence of persisting nephrotic syndrome and histological features of FSGS.
Treatment	Most patients are resistant to therapy.

C1q nephropathy (by definition), either in dominant or codominant fashion, mainly in the mesangium. Polyclonal IgG and IgM along with C3 deposits are also seen in 85–95 per cent of cases. IgA deposition is much less frequent. The staining with these immunoglobulins is less intense as C1q.

Electron microscopy: Mesangial electron-dense deposits are found quite frequently. They can also be seen in subendothelial and subepithelial area in cases of morphologic appearances of proliferative glomerulonephritis or FSGS (Vizjak et al., 2008). Tubuloreticular inclusions are seen rarely (in contradistinction to lupus nephritis).

Pathogenesis

The mechanisms of C1q deposition in the mesangium are unknown. However, the immunopathologic features of the disorder suggest that C1q deposition in the mesangium may result from binding to the Fc portion of IgM and IgG, either via direct interactions with surface-bound Ig or via trapping of circulating immune complexes. C1q might also recognize and bind neo-epitopes on apoptotic cells or might bind directly to ligands or receptors present on the surface of mesangial cells. Less likely mechanisms include a passive trapping of C1q due to the fluid phase formation of C1q-antiC1q antibody complex or cross reactivity with an antigen similar to C1q. The disease might be a part of the spectrum of minimal change lesion and FSGS. However, the presence of mesangial electron-dense deposits would argue against the disease being mediated by podocytes injury.

Aetiology

The aetiology of C1q nephropathy is unknown. The possibility that the disease may be triggered by viral infection cannot be ruled out.

Clinical presentation

The clinical features of C1q nephropathy are quite varied. Presentation ranges from asymptomatic proteinuria or haematuria to frank nephritic or nephrotic syndromes. Hypertension and renal insufficiency at the time of diagnosis are common findings. Hypertension is present in about 50 per cent of patients. Signs and laboratory features of a systemic auto-immune disease (such as SLE) are uniformly absent. Males outnumber females by about 1.8:1. Any age may be affected, but most cases are seen in children and in young adults. Renal insufficiency at the time of presentation is quite frequent. Exceptional cases of crescentic glomerulonephritis and rapidly progressive course have been reported (Gupta et al., 2015). The C3 levels are normal, and anti-C1q auto antibodies are absent (unlike Lupus nephritis). Very rarely, vasculitis or tubulo-interstitial nephritis and hypocomplementaemia may be observed.

Epidemiology

C1q nephropathy is an uncommon condition. It accounts for 0.2–2.5 per cent in biopsies from children and adults and from 2.1 to 9.2 per cent in paediatric biopsies. The prevalence is up to 16.5 per cent among renal biopsies in children with nephrotic syndrome and persistent proteinuria. There is a slight male preponderance at 68 per cent (Devasahayam et al., 2015). It apparently has a world-wide distribution.

Natural history

Persisting proteinuria and nephrotic syndrome is the rule. Spontaneous remissions are uncommon, but have been reported to occur (Nishida et al., 2000). Renal insufficiency is eventually seen in the majority of cases, but the final prognosis depends on the morphological pattern. A lesion of FSGS portends a poor outcome (Kanodia et al., 2015), while a pattern of minimal change disease and mesangial C1q deposition can show good response to steroids, although relapses are frequent (Gunasekara et al., 2014).

Specific treatment

The treatment of C1q nephropathy is uncertain, but poor response to gluco-corticoid therapy (10–20 per cent complete or partial remission) is to be expected (Kersnik-Levart et al., 2005; Tibor-Fulop et al., 2015). Patients with the minimal change lesion may respond better than those with the lesion of FSGS. Glucocorticoid therapy may be associated with a somewhat higher like-lihood of a partial remission (Hisano et al., 2008), but no controlled trials are available to validate this effect. In a study on eight steroid-resistant children with C1q nephropathy, cyclosporine obtained complete remission in seven children, while one child became steroid dependent (Kanemoto et al., 2013). Impaired renal function at presentation usually will indicate unresponsiveness to therapy. However, in a child and in an adult, both presenting with impaired renal function and massive proteinuria, RTX was effective in preserving renal function in one patient and eliminated the need for haemodialysis in the other (Sinha et al., 2011). Other sporadic cases of successful treatment with RTX have been reported (Ramachandran et al., 2017). LDL apheresis has also been used with success (Ito et al., 2016).

Practical recommendations

A trial of oral glucocorticoids similar to that described for treatment of FSGS could be tried. A better response would be expected in those with the MCD lesion than those with a lesion of FSGS. In steroid-dependent or steroid-resistant patients an attempt with calcineurin inhibitors or RTX may be justified. A complete or partial remission would likely be associated with an improved long-term outcome. Patients with persistent proteinuria should be treated with ACE inhibitors and/or angiotensin receptor blockers.

Transplantation

No reports of recurrence of C1q nephropathy in a renal allograft have yet appeared. However, it is possible that some of the recurrences reported in patients with 'primary' or 'idiopathic' FSGS may have been in patients with unrecognized C1q nephropathy in which immunofluorescence microscopy was not performed. Cases of *de novo* post-transplant C1q nephropathy have been reported. Said and colleagues (2010) observed intense mesangial staining for C1q on immunofluorescence in 24 renal transplant recipients with a mean age at transplant of 31 years. None of the patients were diagnosed with C1q nephropathy in the native kidney or had any features of SLE. The glomerular pattern on light microscopy was mesangial hypercellularity (46 per cent), FSGS

(21 per cent), or no lesions (33 per cent). Mesangial electron-dense deposits were seen in 82 per cent of cases. On follow-up (mean one year) of the ten patients without rejection, most had stable creatinine with no or stable proteinuria, and none lost their graft. The authors concluded that C1q-dominant mesangial deposition in the renal allograft is a morphological pattern with no apparent clinical significance in the majority of patients.

Idiopathic nodular glomerulosclerosis

This enigmatic clinicopathologic entity, also called diabetic nephropathy without diabetes (DNND), is characterized by glomerular lesions virtually indistinguishable from the diabetes-related Kimmelstiel–Wilson lesions, but developing in the absence of any abnormality in glucose homeostasis (Helzenberg et al., 1999; Tanaka et al., 2016). The nodular glomerulosclerosis pattern can rarely occur in MPGN, light or heavy chain deposition disease, amyloidosis, fibrillary and immunotactoid glomerulonephritis, and chronic hypoxic or ischemic conditions. Only when these entities can be excluded can a diagnosis of DNND be made (Balafa et al., 2016). It is a quite rare disorder, occurring in <0.5 per cent of native renal biopsy specimens (see Table 11.8).

Pathology

Light microscopy: The glomeruli reveal diffuse and nodular mesangial sclerosis (Plate 25), and thickening of the GBM. Severe, arteriolo-, and arterial-hyalinosis sclerosis is present in 100 per cent of the reported cases. Communication between peripheral capillary loops and peripheral vascular mesangial channels can be seen. By electron microscopy, mesangial channels show angulated, irregular borders with lining cells compatible with endothelium and surrounded by mesangial matrix. No basement membranes were identified surrounding the mesangial channels. These findings support the existence of vascular mesangial channels in nodular diabetic glomerulopathy and suggest neovascularization and altered blood flow within these glomeruli (Cossey et al., 2016).

Immunofluorescence: Linear albumin deposits on GBM may be present but glomerular deposits of immunoglobulin or complement are lacking. This facilitates a differential diagnosis with light chain deposition disease or C3 glomerulonephritis with lobular aspects.

Electron microscopy: Electron dense deposits are absent. No fibrillary deposits are seen. There are granular deposits on mesangium, and GBM. This lesion must be distinguished from diabetic fibrillosis on this basis (Gonul et al., 2006).

Table 11.8 Main characteristics of idiopathic nodular glomerulosclerosis (DNND).

Pathology	Intercapillary nodular and diffuse mesangial sclerosis, closely resembling the diabetes-related Kimmelstiel–Wilson lesion by light, immunofluorescent and electron microscopy. Diabetes, light chain deposition diseases, thrombotic microangiopathy and C3 glomerulonephritis with a membranoproliferative pattern must be excluded.
Pathogenesis	The presence of vascular mesangial channels suggests neovascularization and altered blood flow within glomeruli in DNND. Since the disease usually occurs in older subjects with hypertension, history of smoking, and obesity, it might represent a special form of atherosclerotic or metabolic glomerulopathy than can occur even without diabetes.
Aetiology	Unknown. DNND might be due to glomerular endothelial cell injury from cigarette smoking and/or intermittent hypoxia
Clinical presentation	Proteinuria, nephrotic syndrome and progressive renal failure are frequent. Hypertension is common but glucose intolerance and proliferative retinopathy are absent (by definition)
Treatment	Cessation of smoking. Control of blood pressure and proteinuria with renin-angiotensin-system inhibitors.

Pathogenesis

The pathogenesis of DNND is unclear. The disease is frequently associated with cardiovascular risk-factors, such as hypertension, obesity, and smoking. The strong association to excessive and prolonged cigarette smoking has suggested that a chronic injury to the endothelium induced by components of cigarette smoke combined with transient hypoxia, even in the absence of an abnormality in glucose homeostasis, can give rise to lesions resembling diabetic nodular glomerulosclerosis (Nasr and D'Agati, 2007). A possible role for insulin resistance has been hypothesized (Filippone et al., 2014). These data support the hypothesis that DNND could be a special form of atherosclerotic or metabolic glomerulopathy than can occur even without diabetes (Lopez-Revuelta et al., 2015). In a series of 17 patients with DNND, none of the patients fulfilled criteria for diabetes. However, intermittently elevated blood glucose or borderline-high HgbA1c levels were frequently reported (Hamrahian et al., 2018). In a smoker with DNND, overexpression and podocyte expression of glomerular advanced glycation end products (AGEs) and their receptor (RAGE) were seen. This data suggests that AGEs–RAGE system may be activated by smoke (Nakamura et al., 2018).

Aetiology

The aetiology of DNND is unknown. A possible role of genetic and environmental factors has been hypothesized, but not demonstrated.

Clinical presentation

The patients are typically over age 65 years, male or female, and have had long-standing hypertension. A history of heavy smoking can almost invariably be obtained (Nasr and D'Agati, 2007; Wu et al., 2014). Many patients are obese and may have intermittent increase of blood glucose, but a history of diabetes is typically absent. Renal insufficiency, heavy proteinuria (including the nephrotic syndrome) and hypertension are very common. However, patients neither obese nor hypertensive but with a severe form of the disease have been described (Chandragiri et al., 2016). Blood sugar and haemoglobin A1c are normal. Complement levels are normal. No monoclonal immunoglobulin paraproteins are present in serum or urine. Hypercholesterolaemia and extra-renal vascular disease are also very common. The absence of fibrillary deposits by electron microscopy excludes diabetic fibrillosis and fibrillary glomerulonephritis.

Epidemiology

The disorder is rather uncommon. By a complete review of the literature, Lopez-Revuelta and colleagues (2015) could find 95 cases of DNND described between 1994 and 2015. Males and females appear to be about equally affected, but most are older adults. The lesion has not yet been observed in children. Its geographic distribution is unknown.

Natural history

A progressive course to ESRD is seen in over 50 per cent of patients. The median time from biopsy to ESRD was one year (1–3.5) in the review of Lopez-Revuelta and colleagues (2015). Interstitial fibrosis and arteriosclerosis at biopsy, elevated serum creatinine at discovery, and persistent nephrotic range proteinuria are indicators of an adverse prognosis. Spontaneous remissions are very infrequent if they occur at all.

Specific treatment

There is no proven effective therapy for DNND. Patients should be encouraged to stop smoking, lose weight, and should have their blood pressure brought under strict control (<130/80 mmHg), preferably with renin-angiotensin inhibitors. There are no indications for the use glucocorticoids or cytotoxic agents.

Transplantation

No information is yet available regarding the recurrence of this disorder in the renal allograft.

C4 glomerulopathy

In 2014 Sethi, Sullivan and Smith reported a case of C4 Dense Deposit Disease (DDD). In 2016, a case of C4 DDD associated with thrombotic microangiopathy and acute renal failure was described (Ali et al., 2016). Additional cases of C4-positive proliferative glomerulonephritis were reported (Sethi et al., 2016). These few reported cases outline a novel type of complement glomerulopathy characterized by glomerular C4 staining (Sethi et al., 2014; see also Chapter 8).

Pathology

Light microscopy: shows a picture of MPGN, with mesangial and endocapillary hypercellularity. The glomerular capillary walls appear extremely thick. Staining with periodic acid–Schiff shows ribbon-like material lining the GBM. In two cases thrombotic microangiopathic lesions were seen (Ali et al., 2016; Parrott et al., 2017).

Immunofluorescence: microscopy shows bright C4d staining along the capillary walls and absent or minimal C1q, C3, and immunoglobulin.

Electron microscopy: shows mesangial and subendothelial large osmiophilic dense deposits. Lesions similar to C3GN or DDD have been observed (Sethi et al., 2016; see also Chapter 8). Laser microdissection and mass spectrometry of glomeruli shows large to moderate numbers of spectra matching C4 (Sethi et al., 2016).

Pathogenesis

Although the pathogenesis of C4 glomerulopathy has yet to be defined, overactivity of the lectin pathway of complement activation is likely involved. The lectin pathway, like the classical (immunoglobulin-dependent) pathway, activates C2 and C4 (and not C1q), but in contrast to the classical complement pathway, the lectin pathway does not recognize an antibody bound to its target. The lectin pathway starts with mannose-binding lectin (MBL) or ficolin binding to mannose, glucose or other sugars.

Clinical presentation

In the series of Sethi and colleagues (2016), all three patients presented with proteinuria, and two patients also had haematuria. Kidney function was preserved in two patients, whereas one patient presented with declining kidney function. Complement assays of the classical and alternative pathways were normal, but activity of the lectin pathway was markedly elevated. In another report, a young pregnant woman presented with new onset hypertension and proteinuria at 18 weeks gestational age (Parrott et al., 2017).

Natural history and treatment

Little information is available about the outcome and treatment of this novel glomerulopathy. Apart from the usual symptomatic treatment aimed to reduce proteinuria, arterial hypertension and possible consequences (see Chapter 2), an attempt with glucocorticoids, immunosuppressive drugs, or RTX might be suggested for progressing patients with a picture of MPGN. Due to the possible involvement of lectin pathway of complement, eculizumab might also be used in resistant cases.

References

Alchi B, Nishi S, Narita I, et al. (2007). Collagenofibrotic glomerulopathy: Clinicopathologic overview of a rare glomerular disease. Am J Kidney Dis. **49**: 499–506.

Alexander MP, Dasari S, Vrana JA, et al. (2018). Congophilic fibrillary glomerulonephritis: A case series. Am J Kidney Dis. **72**: 325–36.

Alexopoulos E, Papagianni A, Stangou M, et al. (2000). Adult-onset idiopathic nephrotic syndrome associated with pure diffuse mesangial hypercellularity. Nephrol Dial Transplant. **15**: 981–7.

Ali A, Schlanger L, Nasr SH, et al. (2016). Proliferative C4 dense deposit disease, acute thrombotic microangiopathy, a monoclonal gammopathy, and acute kidney failure. Am J Kidney Dis. **67**: 479–82.

Alpers CE, Kowalewska J. (2008). Fibrillary glomerulonephritis and immunotactoid glomerulopathy. J Am Soc Nephrol. **19**: 34–7.

Andeen NK, Yang HY, Dai DF, et al. (2018). DnaJ Homolog Subfamily B Member 9 Is a Putative Autoantigen in Fibrillary GN. J Am Soc Nephrol. **29**: 231 9.

Anitha A, Vankalakunti M, Siddini V, et al. (2016), Type III collagen disorders: A case report and review of literature. Indian J Pathol Microbiol. **59**: 75–7.

Aoki T, Hayashi K, Morinaga T, et al. (2015), Two brothers with collagenofibrotic glomerulopathy. CEN Case Rep. **4**: 85–9.

Arias LF, Taborada-Murillo A. (2017). Mesangial proliferative glomerulonephritis: A glomerular disease or a non-specific morphological change? Nephrology (Carlton). **22**: 575.

Balafa O, Liapis G, Pavlakou P. (2016). 'Diabetic nephropathy' in a non-diabetic patient. Pathol Res Pract. **212**: 1199–201.

Bomback AS, Song H, D'Agati VD, et al. (2010). A new apolipoprotein E mutation, apoE Las Vegas, in a European-American with lipoprotein glomerulopathy. Nephrol Dial Transplant. **25**: 3442–6.

Boumendjel R, Papari M, Gonzalez M. (2010). A rare case of lipoprotein glomerulopathy in a white man: An emerging entity in Asia, rare in the white population. Arch Pathol Lab Med. **134**: 279–82.

Bridoux F, Hugue V, Coldefy O, et al. (2002). Fibrillary glomerulonephritis and immunotactoid (microtubular) glomerulopathy are associated with distinct immunologic features. Kidney Int. **62**: 1764–75.

Brugnano R, Del Sordo R, Covarelli C, et al. (2016). IgM nephropathy: Is it closer to minimal change disease or to focal segmental glomerulosclerosis? J Nephrol. **29**: 479–86.

Chan MM, Gale DP. (2015). Isolated microscopic haematuria of glomerular origin: Clinical significance and diagnosis in the 21st century. Clin Med (Lond).**15**: 576–80.

Chandragiri S, Raju S, Mukku KK, et al. (2016). Idiopathic nodular glomerulosclerosis: Report of two cases and review of literature. Indian J Nephrol. **26**: 145–8.

Chaudhary A, Gyamlani G, Cossey NL, et al. (2014). Successful use of rituximab in fibrillary glomerulopathy. Ren Fail. **36**: 1151–4.

Chen D, Li Y, Mei Y, et al. (2014). miR-34a regulates mesangial cell proliferation via the PDGFR-β/Ras-MAPK signaling pathway. Cell Mol Life Sci. **71**: 4027–42.

Chen N, Pan X, Xu Y, et al. (2017). Two brothers in one Chinese family with collagen type III glomerulopathy. Am J Kidney Dis. **50**: 1037–42.

Chen W, Jiang Y, Han J, et al. (2017). Atgl deficiency induces podocyte apoptosis and leads to glomerular filtration barrier damage. FEBS J. **284**: 1070–81.

Chen Y. (2014). Lipoprotein glomerulopathy in China. Clin Exp Nephrol. **18**: 218–19.

Chen Y, Colville I, Ierino F, et al. (2018). Temporal retinal thinning and the diagnosis of Alport syndrome and thin basement membrane nephropathy. Ophthalmic Genet. **39**: 208–14.

Cheung CY, Chan AOK, Chan GPT, et al. (2014). Long-term outcome of kidney transplantation in a patient with coexisting lipoprotein glomerulopathy and fibrillary glomerulonephritis Clin Kidney J. **7**: 396–8.

Choi SR, Ahn S, Min SK, et al. (2018). Midterm outcome of kidney transplantation from donors with thin basement membrane nephropathy. Transplantation. **102**. e180–4.

Choi SR, Sun YO, Lim JH, et al. (2012). The role of kidney biopsy to determine donation from prospective kidney donors with asymptomatic urine abnormalities. Transplant Proc. **44**: 11–13.

Churg J, Bernstein J, Glassock R. (1995). *Renal Disease: Classification and Atlas of Glomerular Diseases*. 2nd Edition. Igaku-Shoin, New York.

Cohen AH. (2012). Collagen type III glomerulopathies. Adv Chronic Kidney Dis. **19**: 101–6.

Cohen AH, Border WA, Glassock RJ. (1978). Nephrotic syndrome with glomerular mesangial IgM deposits. Lab Invest. **38**: 610–19.

Collins M, Navaneethan SD, Chung M, et al. (2008). Rituximab treatment of fibrillary glomerulonephritis. Am J Kidney Dis. **52**: 9958–62.

Connor TM, Aiello V, Griffith M, et al. (2017). The natural history of immunoglobulin M nephropathy in adults. Nephrol Dial Transplant. **32**: 823–9.

Cosio FG, Falkenhain ME, Sedmark DD. (1996). Association of thin glomerular basement membrane with other glomerulopathies. Kidney Int. **46**: 471–74.

Cossey LN, Hennigar RA, Bonsib S, et al. (2016). Vascular mesangial channels in human nodular diabetic glomerulopathy. Hum Pathol. **48**: 148–53.

Cove-Smith A, Mulgrew CJ, Rudyk O, et al. (2013). Anti-proliferative actions of T-type calcium channel inhibition in Thy1 nephritis. Am J Pathol. **183**: 391–401.

Craver R, Crespo-Salgado J, Aviles D. (2014). Laminations and microgranule formation in pediatric glomerular basement membranes. Fetal Pediatr Pathol. **33**: 321–30.

Daniel C, Albrecht H, Lüdke A, et al. (2008). Nestin expression in repopulating mesangial cells promotes their proliferation. Lab Invest. **88**: 387–97.

Devasahayam J, Erode-Singaravelu G, Bhat Z, et al. (2015). C1q nephropathy: The unique underrecognized pathological entity. Anal Cell Pathol (Amst). 2015: 490413.

Duggal R, Nada R, Rayat CS, et al. (2012). Collagenofibrotic glomerulopathy-A review. Clin Kidney J. **5**: 7–12.

Ferreira RD, Custódio FB, Guimarães CS, et al. (2009). Collagenofibrotic glomerulopathy: Three case reports in Brazil. Diagn Pathol. **4**: 33.

Filippone EJ, Gupta A, Farber JL. (2014). Normoglycemic diabetic nephropathy. The Role of Insulin Resistance. Case Rep Nephrol Urol. **4**: 137–43.

Fogo A, Qureshi N, Horn RG. (1993). Morphologic and clinical features of fibrillary glomerulonephritis versus immunotactoid glomerulopathy. Am J Kidney Dis. **22**: 367–77.

Foster K, Markowitz GS, D'Agati VD. (2005). Pathology of thin basement membrane nephropathy. Semin Nephrol. **25**: 149–58.

Frascà GM, Onetti-Muda A, Mari F, et al. (2005). Thin glomerular basement membrane disease: clinical significance of a morphological diagnosis--A collaborative study of the Italian Renal Immunopathology Group. Nephrol Dial Transplant. **20**: 545–51.

Fukami K, Yamagishi SI, Minezaki T, et al. (2014). First reported case of collagenofibrotic glomerulopathy with a full-house pattern of immune deposits. Clin Nephrol. **81**: 290–5.

Gale DP, Oygar DD, Lin F, et al. (2016). A novel *COL4A1* frameshift mutation in familial kidney disease: The importance of the C-terminal NC1 domain of type IV collagen. Nephrol Dial Transplant. **31**: 1908–14.

Garsen M, Sonneveld R, Rops AL, et al. (2015). Vitamin D attenuates proteinuria by inhibition of heparanase expression in the podocyte. J Pathol. **237**: 472–81.

Gast C, Pengelly RJ, Lyon M, et al. (2016). Collagen (COL4A) mutations are the most frequent mutations underlying adult focal segmental glomerulosclerosis. Nephrol Dial Transplant. **31**: 961–70.

Gauthier B, Trachtman H, Frank R, et al. (1989). Familial thin basement membrane nephropathy in children with asymptomatic microhematuria. Nephron. **51**: 502–8.

Georgiadou D, Stamatakis K, Efthimiadou EK, et al. (2013). Thermodynamic and structural destabilization of apoE3 by hereditary mutations associated with the development of lipoprotein glomerulopathy. J Lipid Res. **54**: 164–76.

Gonul II, Gough J, Jim K, et al. (2006). Glomerular mesangial fibrillary deposits in a patient with diabetes mellitus. Int Urol Nephrol. **38**: 767–72.

Goto S, Nakai K, Ito J, et al. (2014). Marked elevation of serum hyaluronan levels in collagenofibrotic glomerulopathy. Intern Med. **53**: 1801–4.

Gough J, Yilmaz A, Yilmaz S, et al. (2005). Recurrent and *de novo* glomerular immune-complex deposits in renal transplant biopsies. Arch Pathol Lab Med. **129**: 231–3.

Griveas I, Stavianoudakis G, Karanikas E, et al. (2009). The role of pure diffuse mesangial hypercellularity in patients with proteinuria. Ren Fail. **31**: 192–5.

Gubler MC, Dommergues JP, Foulard M, et al. (1993). Collagen type III glomerulopathy: A new type of hereditary nephropathy. Pediatr Nephrol. **7**: 354–60.

Gunasekara VN, Sebire NJ, Tullus K (2014). C1q nephropathy in children: Clinical characteristics and outcome. Pediatr Nephrol. **29**: 407–13.

Gupta R, Sharma A, Agarwal SK, et al. (2015). C1q nephropathy and isolated CD59 deficiency manifesting as necrotizing crescentic glomerulonephritis: A rare association of two diseases. Saudi J Kidney Dis Transpl. **26**: 1274–8.

Haas M. (2009). Alport syndrome and thin glomerular basement membrane nephropathy: A practical approach to diagnosis. Arch Pathol Lab Med. **133**: 224–32.

Hamrahian M, Mollaee M, Anand M, et al. (2018). Impaired glucose metabolism-A potential risk factor for idiopathic nodular glomerulosclerosis: A single center study. Med Hypotheses. **121**: 95–8.

Herzenberg AM, Holden JK, Singh S, et al. (1999). Idiopathic nodular glomerulosclerosis. Am J Kidney Dis. **34**: 560–4.

Hisakawa N, Yasuoka N, Nishiya K, et al. (1998). Collagenofibrotic glomerulonephropathy associated with immune complexes. Am J Nephrol. **18**: 134–41.

Hisano S, Fukuma Y, Segawa Y, et al. (2008). Clinicopathologic correlation and outcome of C1q nephropathy. Clin J Am Soc Nephrol. **3**: 1637–43.

Hogan J, Restivo M, Canetta PA, et al. (2014). Rituximab treatment for fibrillary glomerulonephritis. Nephrol Dial Transplant. **29**: 1925–31.

Hu Z, Huang S, Wu Y, et al. (2014). Hereditary features, treatment, and prognosis of the lipoprotein glomerulopathy in patients with the APOE Kyoto mutation. Kidney Int. **85**: 416–24.

Ieiri N, Hotta O, Taguma Y. (2003). Resolution of typical lipoprotein glomerulopathy by intensive lipid-lowering therapy. Am J Kidney Dis. **41**: 244–9.

Imbasciati E, Gherardi G, Morozumi K, et al. (1991). Collagen type III glomerulopathy: A new idiopathic glomerular disease. Am J Nephrol. **11**: 422–9.

Iskandar SS, Herrera GA. (2015). Glomerular diseases with organized deposits. In JC Jennette, FG Silva, JL Olsan, et al. (eds), *Hiptenstall's Pathology of Kidney*. 7th edition, pp. 1029–31. Wolters Kluwer: Philadelphia.

Ito Y, Inoue T, Okada H. (2016). Successful treatment of C1q nephropathy by low-density lipoprotein apheresis. Ther Apher Dial. **20**: 530–1.

Ito K, Nakashima H, Watanabe M, et al. (2012). Macrophage impairment produced by Fc receptor gamma deficiency plays a principal role in the development of lipoprotein glomerulopathy in concert with apoE abnormalities. Nephrol Dial Transplant. **27**: 3899–907.

Ivany B, Pap R, Ondrik Z. (2006). Thin basement membrane nephropathy: Diffuse and segmental types. Arch Pathol Lab Med. **130**: 1533–7.

Javaugue V, Karras A, Glowacki F, et al. (2013). Long-term kidney disease outcomes in fibrillary glomerulonephritis: A case series of 27 patients. Am J Kidney Dis. **62**: 679–90.

Jennette JC, Hipp CG. (1985). Immunohistopathologic evaluation of C1q in 800 renal biopsy specimens. Am J Clin Pathol. **83**: 415–20.

Kanemoto K, Ito H, Anzai M, et al. (2013). Clinical significance of IgM and C1q deposition in the mesangium in pediatric idiopathic nephrotic syndrome. J Nephrol. **26**: 306–14.

Kanodia KV, Vanikar AV, Patel RD, et al. (2015). C1q nephropathy in India: A single-center study. Saudi J Kidney Dis Transpl. **26**: 398–403.

Kasap B, Türkmen M, Sarioğlu S, et al. (2008). The relation of IgM deposition to clinical parameters and histomorphometry in childhood mesangial proliferative glomerulonephritis. Pathol Res Pract. **204**: 149–53.

Katsarou M, Stratikos E, Chroni A, et al. (2018). Thermodynamic destabilization and aggregation propensity as the mechanism behind the association of apoE3 mutants and lipoprotein glomerulopathy. J Lipid Res. **59**: 2339–48.

Kaur A, Sethi S. (2016). Histiocytic and nonhistiocytic glomerular lesions: Foam cells and their mimickers. Am J Kidney Dis. **67**: 329–36.

Kazi J, Mubarak M. (2014). IgM nephropathy presenting as full-blown crescentic glomerulonephritis: First report in the literature. Nefrologia. **34**: 423–4.

Kersnik Levart T, Kenda RB, Avgustin Cavić M, et al. (2005). C1Q nephropathy in children. Pediatr Nephrol. **20**(12): 1756–61.

Kodera H, Mizutani Y, Sugiyama S, et al. (2017). A case of lipoprotein glomerulopathy with apoE Chicago and apoE (Glu3Lys) treated with fenofibrate. Case Rep Nephrol Dial. **7**: 112–20.

Koushik R, Garvey C, Manivel JC, et al. (2005). Persistent, asymptomatic, microscopic hematuria in prospective kidney donors. Transplantation. **80**: 1425–9.

Kurien AA, Larsen CP, Cossey LN. (2015). Collagenofibrotic glomerulopathy. Clin Kidney J. **8**: 543–7.

Leibler C, Moktefi A, Matignon M, et al. (2018). Rituximab and fibrillary glomerulonephritis: Interest of B-cell reconstitution monitoring. J Clin Med. 7(11): 430.

Li W, Wang Y, Han Z, et al. (2014). Apolipoprotein e mutation and double filtration plasmapheresis therapy on a new Chinese patient with lipoprotein glomerulopathy. Kidney Blood Press Res. **39**: 330–9.

Lim AK, Brown S, Simpson I, et al. (2015). Acute kidney injury due to glomerular haematuria and obstructive erythrocyte casts associated with thrombocytopaenia and thin basement membrane disease: A case report. BMC Nephrol. **16**: 180.

Lobo PI. (2017). Role of natural IgM autoantibodies (IgM-NAA) and IgM anti-leukocyte antibodies (IgM-ALA) in regulating inflammation. Curr Top Microbiol Immunol. **408**: 89–117.

López-Revuelta K, Abreu AA, Gerrero-Márquez C. (2015). Diabetic nephropathy without diabetes. J Clin Med. **4**: 1403–27.

Luo B, Huang F, Liu Q, et al. (2008). Identification of apolipoprotein E Guangzhou (arginine 150 proline), a new variant associated with lipoprotein glomerulopathy. Am J Nephrol. **28**: 347–53.

Madan A, Mijovic-Das S, Stankovic A, et al. (2016). Acthar gel in the treatment of nephrotic syndrome: A multicenter retrospective case series. BMC Nephrol. **17**: 37.

Magistroni R, Bertolotti M, Furci L, et al. (2013). Lipoprotein glomerulopathy associated with a mutation in apolipoprotein E. Clin Med Insights Case Rep. **6**: 189–96.

Malleshappa P, Vankalakunti M. (2013). Diverse clinical and histology presentation in C1q nephropathy. Nephrourol Mon. **5**: 787–91.

Mallett A, Tang W, Hart G, et al. (2015). End-Stage kidney disease due to fibrillary glomerulonephritis and immunotactoid glomerulopathy: Outcomes in 66 consecutive ANZDATA Registry cases. Am J Nephrol. **42**: 177–84.

Malone AF, Phelan PJ, Hall G, et al. (2014). Rare hereditary *COL4A3/COL4A4* variants may be mistaken for familial focal segmental glomerulosclerosis. Kidney Int. **86**: 1253–9.

Markowitz GS, Schwimmer JA, Stokes MB, et al. (2003). C1q nephropathy: A variant of focal segmental glomerulosclerosis. Kidney Int. **64**: 1232–40.

Matsunaga A, Saito T. (2014). Apolipoprotein E mutations: A comparison between lipoprotein glomerulopathy and type III hyperlipoproteinemia. Clin Exp Nephrol. **18**: 220–4.

Matsunaga A, Sasaki J, Komatsu T. (1999). A novel apolipoprotein E mutation, E2 (Arg25Cys), in lipoprotein glomerulopathy. Kidney Int. **56**: 421–7.

Mii A, Shimizu A, Masuda Y, et al. (2009). Current status and issues of C1q nephropathy. Clin Exp Nephrol. **13**: 263–74.

Miyata T, Sugiyama S, Nangaku M, et al. (1999). Apolipoprotein E2/E5 variants in lipoprotein glomerulopathy recurred in transplanted kidney. J Am Soc Nephrol. **10**: 1590–5.

Mokhtar GA. (2011). IgM nephropathy: Clinical picture and pathological findings in 36 patients. Saudi J Kidney Dis Transpl. **22**: 969–75.

Mokhtar GA, Jalalah SM. (2015). A clinicopathological study of C1q nephropathy at King Abdulaziz University. Iran J Kidney Dis. **9**: 279–85.

Mourad G, Djamali A, Turc-Baron C, et al. (1998). Lipoprotein glomerulopathy: A new cause of nephrotic syndrome after renal transplantation. Nephrol Dial Transplant. **13**: 1292–94.

Mubarak M, Kasi JI. (2012). IgM nephropathy revisited. Nephrourol Mon. **4**: 603–8.

Mubarak M, Nasri H. (2014). IgM nephropathy: Timely response to a call for action. J Renal Inj Prev. **3**: 5–6.

Myllymäki J, Saha H, Mustonen J, et al. (2003). IgM nephropathy: Clinical picture and long-term prognosis. Am J Kidney Dis. **41**: 343–50.

Myllymäki J, Saha H, Pasternack A, et al. (2006). High serum C3 predicts poor outcome in IgM nephropathy. Nephron Clin Pract. **102**: c122–7.

Nabais Sá MJ, Storey H, Flinter F, et al. (2015). Collagen type IV-related nephropathies in Portugal: Pathogenic *COL4A3* and *COL4A4* mutations and clinical characterization of 25 families. Clin Genet. **88**: 456–61.

Nakamura N, Taguchi K, Myazono Y, et al. (2018). AGEs–RAGE overexpression in a patient with smoking-related idiopathic nodular glomerulosclerosis. CEN Case Rep. **7**: 48–54.

Nasr SH, D'Agati VD. (2007). Nodular glomerulosclerosis in the nondiabetic smoker. J Am Soc Nephrol. **18**: 2032–6.

Nasr SH, Markovitz GS, Stokes MB, et al. (2004). Proliferative glomerulonephritis with monoclonal IgG deposits: A distinct entity mimicking immune-complex glomerulonephritis. Kidney Int. **65**: 85–96.

Nasr SH, Satoskar A, Markovitz GS, et al. (2009). Proliferative glomerulonephritis with IgG deposits. J Am Soc Nephrol **20**: 2055–64.

Nasr SH, Valeri AM, Cornell LD, et al. (2011). Fibrillary glomerulonephritis: A report of 66 cases from a single institution. Clin J Am Soc Nephrol. **6**: 775–84.

Nasr SH, Vrana JA, Dasari S, et al. (2017). DNAJB9 is a specific immunohistochemical marker for fibrillary glomerulonephritis. Kidney Int Rep. **3**: 56–64.

Nimmagadda S, Mukku K, Devaraju SR, et al. (2017). Unusual cause of glomerular deposition disease: Collagenofibrotic glomerulopathy. Indian J Nephrol. **27**: 62–5.

Nishida M, Kawakatsu H, Komatsu H, et al. (2000). Spontaneous improvement in a case of C1q nephropathy. Am J Kidney Dis. **35**(5): E22.

Oikawa S, Matsunaga A, Saito T, et al. (1997). Apolipoprotein E Sendai (arginine 145 proline): A new variant associated with lipoprotein glomerulopathy. J Am Soc Nephrol. **8**: 820–3.

Okada S, Inaga S, Kitamoto K, et al. (2014). Morphological diagnosis of Alport syndrome and thin basement membrane nephropathy by low vacuum scanning electron microscopy. Biomed Res. **35**: 345–50.

Panzer SE, Laskowski J, Renner B, et al. (2015). IgM exacerbates glomerular disease progression in complement-induced glomerulopathy. Kidney Int. **88**: 528–37.

Papazachariou L, Demosthenous P, Pieri M, et al. (2014). Frequency of *COL4A3/COL4A4* mutations amongst families segregating glomerular microscopic hematuria and evidence for activation of the unfolded protein response. Focal and segmental glomerulosclerosis is a frequent development during ageing. PLoS One. **9**: e115015.

Parrott J, Fields TA, Parrish M. (2017). Previable pre-eclampsia diagnosed by renal biopsy in setting of novel diagnosis of C4 glomerulopathy. Case Rep Obstet Gynecol. 2017: Art ID 8698670.

Pasquariello A, Pisciotta L, Sampietro T, et al. (2014). Lipoprotein glomerulopathy: Molecular characterization of three Italian patients and review of the literature. J Genet Disor Genet Reports **3**: 1–7.

Patel S, Cimbaluk D. (2016). Collagenofibrotic glomerulopathy. Kidney Int. **89**: 1221–30.

Patro KC, Jha R, Sahay M, Swarnalatha G. (2011). Collagenofibrotic glomerulopathy: Case report with review of literature. Indian J Nephrol. **21**: 52–5.

Payan Schober F, Jobson MA, Poulton CJ, et al. (2017). Clinical features and outcomes of a racially diverse population with fibrillary glomerulonephritis. Am J Nephrol. **45**: 248–56.

Peru H, Elmaci AM, Akin F, et al. (2008). An unusual association between familial Mediterranean fever and IgM nephropathy. Med Princ Pract. **17**: 255–7.

Pierides A, Voskarides K, Athanasiou Y, et al. (2009). Clinico-pathological correlations in 127 patients in 11 large pedigrees, segregating one of three heterozygous mutations in the *COL4A3/COL4A4* genes associated with familial haematuria and significant late progression to proteinuria and chronic kidney disease from focal segmental glomerulosclerosis. Nephrol Dial Transplant. **24**: 2721–9.

Platt JL, Cascalho M. (2015). IgM in the kidney: A multiple personality disorder. Kidney Int. **88**: 439–41.

Qazi RA, Bastani B. (2015). Co-existence of thin basement membrane nephropathy with other glomerular pathologies: A single center experience. J Nephropathol. **4**: 43–7.

Ramachandran R, Bharati J, Jha V. (2017). Successful treatment of C1q nephropathy with CD19 targeted rituximab therapy. Nephrology (Carlton). 22: 265.

Reddy MHK, Kumar ACV, Chandra VS, et al. (2017). Collagenofibrotic glomerulopathy. Indian J Nephrol. 27: 331–3.

Rosenstock JL, Markowitz GS, Valeri AM, et al. (2003). Fibrillary and immunotactoid glomerulonephritis: Distinct entities with different clinical and pathologic features. Kidney Int. 63: 1450–61.

Rovin BH, Roncone D, McKinley A, et al. (2007). FAPOE Kyoto mutations in European Americans with lipoprotein glomerulopathy. N Engl J Med. 357: 2522–4.

Said SM, Cornell LD, Valeri AM, et al. (2010). C1q deposition in the renal allograft: A report of 24 cases. Mod Pathol. 23: 1080–8.

Said SM, Cosio FG, Valeri AM, et al. (2018). Proliferative glomerulonephritis with monoclonal immunoglobulin G deposits is associated with high rate of early recurrence in the allograft. Kidney Int. 94: 159–69.

Sainz-Prestel V, Hernandez-Perez J, Rojas-Rivera J, et al. (2013). Rituximab-associated lung disease in fibrillary glomerulonephritis. Clin Kidney J. 6: 510–12.

Saito T, Matsunaga A. (2014). Lipoprotein glomerulopathy may provide a key to unlock the puzzles of renal lipidosis. Kidney Int. 85: 243–5.

Saito T, Matsunaga A, Oikawa S. (2006). Impact of lipoprotein glomerulopathy on the relationship between lipids and renal diseases. Am J Kidney Dis. 47: 199–211.

Saito T, Matsunaga A, Ito K, et al. (2014). Topics in lipoprotein glomerulopathy: An overview. Clin Exp Nephrol. 18: 214–17.

Salmon AH, Kamel D, Mathieson PW. (2004). Recurrence of IgM nephropathy in a renal allograft. Nephrol Dial Transplant. 19: 2650–2.

Sam R, Wu H, Yue L, et al. (2006). Lipoprotein glomerulopathy: A new lipoprotein E mutation with enhanced glomerular binding. Am J Kidney Dis. 47: 539–48.

Samaniego M, Nadasdy GM, Laszik Z, et al. (2001). Outcome of renal transplantation in fibrillary glomerulonephritis. Clin Neph. 55: 159–66.

Satoskar AA, Calomeni E, Nadasdy G, et al. (2008). Fibrillary glomerulonephritis with splenic involvement: A detailed autopsy study. Ultrastruct Pathol. 32: 113–21.

Savige J. (2016). A further genetic cause of thin basement membrane nephropathy. Nephrol Dial Transplant. 31: 1908–14.

Savige J, Gregory M, Gross O, et al. (2013). Expert guidelines for the management of Alport syndrome and thin basement membrane nephropathy. J Am Soc Nephrol. 24: 364–75.

Savige J, Rana K, Tonna S, et al. (2003). Thin basement membrane nephropathy. Kidney Int. 64: 1169–78.

Schlondorff D, Banas B. (2009). The mesangial cell revisited: No cell is an island. J Am Soc Nephrol. 20: 1179–87.

Scolari F, Scaini P, Savoldi S, et al. (1990). Familial IgM mesangial nephropathy: A morphologic and immunogenetic study of three pedigrees. Am J Nephrol. 10: 261–8.

Sekulic M, Nasr SH, Grande JP, et al. (2017). Histologic regression of fibrillary glomerulonephritis: The first report of biopsy-proven spontaneous resolution of disease. Clin Kidney J. 10: 738–74.

Sethi S, Quint PS, O'Seaghdha CM. (2016). C4 glomerulopathy: A disease entity associated with C4d deposition. Am J Kidney Dis. 67: 949–53.

Sethi S, Sullivan A, Smith RJ. (2014). C4 dense-deposit disease. N Engl J Med. **370**: 784–6.

Sevillano AM, Gutierrez E, Morales E, et al. (2014). Multiple kidney cysts in thin basement membrane disease with proteinuria and kidney function impairment. Clin Kidney J. **7**: 251–6.

Singhal P, Ren KYM, Curtis BM, et al. (2018). Atypical noncrescentic antiglomerular basement membrane disease with concurrent thin basement membrane nephropathy. Kidney Int Rep. **3**: 991–6.

Sinha A, Nast CC, Hristea I, et al. (2011). Resolution of clinical and pathologic features of C1q nephropathy after rituximab therapy. Clin Exp Nephrol. **15**: 164–70.

Soni SS, Gowrishankar S, Nagarik AP, et al. (2011). Collagenofibrotic glomerulopathy in association with Hodgkin's lymphoma. Saudi J Kidney Dis Transpl. **22**: 126–9.

Strassheim D, Renner B, Panzer S, et al. (2013). IgM contributes to glomerular injury in FSGS. J Am Soc Nephrol. **24**: 393–406.

Suzuki T, Okubo S, Ikezumi Y, et al. (2004). Favorable course of collagenofibrotic glomerulopathy after kidney transplantation and questionnaire survey about the prognosis of collagenofibrotic glomerulopathy. Nihon Jinzo Gakkai Shi. **46**: 360–4.

Swartz SJ, Eldin KW, Hicks MJ, et al. (2009). Minimal change disease with IgM + immunofluorescence: A subtype of nephrotic syndrome. Pediatr Nephrol. **24**: 1187–92.

Takasaki S, Maeda K, Joh K, et al. (2015). Macrophage infiltration into the glomeruli in lipoprotein glomerulopathy. Case Rep Nephrol Dial. **5**: 204–12.

Tanaka A, Nakamura T, Sato E, et al. (2016). Progressive idiopathic nodular glomerulosclerosis mimicking diabetic nephropathy without abnormal glycemic metabolism. Nephrology (Carlton). **21**(12): 1074–5.

Thomas JA, Vasin D, Lin M, et al. (2016). A case of mistaken identity: Fibrillary glomerulonephritis masquerading as crescentic anti-glomerular basement membrane disease. Clin Nephrol. **85**: 114–20.

Thorner S. (2007). Alport syndrome and thin basement membrane nephropathy. Nephron Clin Pract. **106**: c82–8.

Tibor Fülöp T, Csongrádi É, Lerant AA, et al. (2015). Resolution of C1q deposition but not of the clinical nephrotic syndrome after immunomodulating therapy in focal sclerosis. J Nephropathol. **4**: 54–8.

Tsimihodimos V, Elisaf M. (2011). Lipoprotein glomerulopathy. Curr Opin Lipidol. **22**: 262–9.

Tryggvason K, Patrakka J. (2006). Thin basement nephropathy. J Am Soc Nephrol. **17**: 813–22.

Vanikar A. (2013). IgM nephropathy: Can we still ignore it. J Nephropathol. **2**: 98–103.

Van Paassen P, Van Breda Vriesman PJC, Van Rie H, et al. (2004). Signs and symptoms of thin basement membrane nephropathy: A prospective regional study on primary glomerular disease. The Limburg Renal Registry. Kidney Int. **66**: 900–13.

Vizjak A, Ferluga D, Rozic M, et al. (2008). Pathology, clinical presentations, and outcomes of C1q nephropathy. J Am Soc Nephrol. **19**: 2237–44.

Vogler C, McAdams AJ, Homan SM, et al. (1987). Glomerular basement membrane and lamina densa in infants and children: An ultrastructural evaluation. Pediatr Pathol. **7**: 527–34.

Voskarides K, Damianou L, Neocleous V, et al. (2007). *COL4A3/COL4A4* mutations producing focal segmental glomerulosclerosis and renal failure in thin basement membrane nephropathy. J Am Soc Nephrol. **18**: 3004–16.

Voskarides K, Stefanou C, Pieri M, et al. (2017). A functional variant in NEPH3 gene confers high risk of renal failure in primary hematuric glomerulopathies. Evidence for predisposition to microalbuminuria in the general population. PLoS One. **12**(3): e0174274.

Weber S, Strasser K, Rath S, et al. (2016). Identification of 47 novel mutations in patients with Alport syndrome and thin basement membrane nephropathy. Pediatr Nephrol. **31**: 941–55.

Wenderfer SE, Swinford RD, Braun MC. (2010). C1q nephropathy in the pediatric population: pathology and pathogenesis. Pediatr Nephrol. **25**: 1385–96.

Westphal S, Hansson S, Mjörnstedt L, et al. (2006). Early recurrence of nephritic syndrome (immunoglobulin M nephropathy) after renal transplantation successfully treated with combinations of plasma exchanges, immunoglobulin, and rituximab. Transplant Proc. **38**: 2659–60.

Wu Y, Chen X, Yang Y, et al. (2013). A case of lipoprotein glomerulopathy with thrombotic microangiopathy due to malignant hypertension. BMC Nephrol. **14**: 53.

Wu J, Yu S, Tejwani V, Mao M, et al. (2014). Idiopathic nodular glomerulosclerosis in Chinese patients: A clinicopathologic study of 20 cases. Clin. Exp Nephrol. **18**: 865–75.

Xin Z, Zhihong L, Shijun L, et al. (2009). Successful treatment of patients with lipoprotein glomerulopathy by protein A immunoadsorption: A pilot study. Nephrol Dial Transplant. **24**: 864–9.

Xu Y, Guo M, Dong H, et al. (2016). A Novel *COL4A4* mutation identified in a Chinese family with thin basement membrane nephropathy. Sci Rep. **6**: 20244.

Yuan L, Xu H, Yuan J, et al. (2016), A novel FN1 variant associated with familial hematuria: TBMN? Clin Biochem. **49**: 816–20.

Zeis PM, Kavazarakis E, Nakopoulou L, et al. (2001). Glomerulopathy with mesangial IgM deposits: Long-term follow up of 64 children. Pediatr Int. **43**: 287–92.

Zhang B, Liu ZH, Zeng CH, et al. (2008). Clinicopathological and genetic characteristics in Chinese patients with lipoprotein glomerulopathy. J Nephrol. **21**: 110–17.

Zhao Y, Fan H, Bao BY, et al. (2014). C1q nephropathy in an old woman with acute renal failure: A case report and literature review. Ren Fail. **36**: 1136–8.

Żurawski J, Burchardt P, Moczko J, et al. (2016). The presence of thin glomerular basement membranes in various glomerulopathies. Ultrastruct Pathol. **40**: 77–82.

Index